Physicochemical Principles of Pharmacy

Physicochemical Principles of Pharmacy

FIFTH EDITION

Alexander T Florence CBE, DSc, FRSE, FRPharmS
The School of Pharmacy, University of London, UK

David Attwood PhD, DSc, CChem, FRSC
School of Pharmacy and Pharmaceutical Sciences
University of Manchester, UK

Pharmaceutical Press

Published by the Pharmaceutical Press

1 Lambeth High Street, London SE1 7JN, UK

© Royal Pharmaceutical Society of Great Britain 2011

(**PhP**) is a trade mark of Pharmaceutical Press

Pharmaceutical Press is the publishing division of the
Royal Pharmaceutical Society

First, second and third editions published by
Palgrave (formerly Macmillan Press Ltd) 1981, 1988, 1998
Third edition reprinted 2004, 2005
Fourth edition 2006
Fourth edition reprinted 2007, 2009
Fifth edition 2011

Typeset by Thomson Digital, Noida
Printed in Great Britain by TJ International, Padstow, Cornwall, UK

ISBN 978 0 85369 984 2

Contents

Preface

Physicochemical Principles of Pharmacy emerged first in 1981, partly as a result of the authors' frustration when teaching physical pharmacy to undergraduate pharmacy students that there was no European book that covered the subject using pharmaceutical examples to illustrate the topics. Having been brought up ourselves on a diet of physical chemistry of little obvious pharmaceutical relevance, we decided we should write a book that illustrated pharmaceutical themes with pharmaceutical examples. We argued that if a particular concept had never been used in a published pharmacy or pharmaceutical science paper, then it perhaps could be ignored. We have felt that the book served as a component of the *science of pharmacy*, as opposed to *science for pharmacy*.

The first edition was well received and a second and third followed, all published by the Macmillan Press. It was encouraging that the text was used widely throughout the world. Charles Fry in a previous existence encouraged us to publish the book. His career took him away from Macmillan Press, who published the first three editions, and in his former position at the Pharmaceutical Press he negotiated the rights of the book and reapplied the ever so gentle pressure for us to complete the fourth edition. This fifth edition is the result of considerable revision. There have of course been changes in pharmacy education since the first edition appeared. We have tried wherever possible to make links with real situations that occur with medicines or that might be important in pharmacy now and in the future. Some of the examples we have used are those in the original editions, because they have now become classic. New material has been added, always remembering that this is not a monograph on the latest advances, but a textbook for undergraduates and postgraduates. Nonetheless, we have added a completely new chapter on pharmaceutical nanotechnology given its growing importance. We have added key points at the end of sections or chapters, and changes have been made to the earlier chapters, for example by combining the chapter on gases with material in other chapters. All the editions of the book have made reference to clinical issues, but in this edition we have highlighted parts of the text that could be considered to be examples of clinical pharmaceutics. We strongly believe that clinical pharmacy practice must be based firmly in quantitative pharmaceutical science, otherwise it will not be distinguishable from other forms of clinical practice.

We hope that the book will continue to be used in undergraduate and postgraduate pharmacy courses in many parts of the world, and by students of pharmaceutical science and the increasing number of students of cognate disciplines interested in pharmaceutical formulation and the properties of medicines.

Alexander T Florence
Dundee
David Attwood
Manchester
December 2010

About the authors

Alexander Florence was Dean of The School of Pharmacy at the University of London from 1989 to 2006 and now is Professor Emeritus. He was previously James P. Todd Professor of Pharmaceutics at the University of Strathclyde. His research and teaching interests are in drug delivery and targeting, dendrimers, nanoparticles, nonaqueous emulsions, and general physical pharmaceutics. He is the author of *An Introduction to Clinical Pharmaceutics*, 2010, published by the Pharmaceutical Press.

David Attwood is Emeritus Professor of Pharmacy at the University of Manchester; he previously lectured at the University of Strathclyde. His research interests are in the physicochemical properties of drugs and surfactants, and in polymeric drug delivery systems. He has many years' experience in the teaching of physical pharmacy. He co-authored the book *Surfactant Systems: Their Chemistry, Pharmacy and Biology* with Alexander Florence and the FASTtrack book, *Physical Pharmacy*.

Introduction

Pharmacy has several component disciplines, all interlinked. Pharmaceutics or physical pharmacy or the physicochemical principles of pharmacy, as in the title of this book, is one of these. It comprises the study of drug formulations and their design, manufacture and delivery to the body. In brief, pharmaceutics is about the conversion of drug substances into medicines suitable for administration by or to patients. It is not a static discipline: the definition of pharmaceutics extends now into the targeting of drugs to specific sites in the body and the fabrication of nanoparticles and delivery devices as well as the monitoring of the behaviour of dose forms in the body. There are other vital component disciplines in pharmacy. The way drugs act in and on the body is the domain of pharmacology; the science of drug design and analysis belongs to medicinal and pharmaceutical chemistry. One cannot design formulations without a comprehensive knowledge of the chemistry of the drug substance, nor study how medicines behave in the laboratory or in patients without good analytical skills. An understanding of the pharmacology of a drug is crucial not only with respect to the optimal design of a delivery system, but also to the wider practice of pharmacy. There is certainly no dividing line in the sciences underlying these subjects: the physical chemistry that operates in the formulation laboratory is the same that holds within the human body. The forces acting between suspension particles and the walls of a container are the same as those acting on bacteria adsorbed onto a catheter or intestinal cell wall. The boundary conditions and the degree of complexity might differ, but the principles are the same. An understanding of the rules that govern what keeps drugs in solution in an infusion fluid allows us also to predict the extent to which a drug might precipitate in the renal tubules or in the blood after injection. Studying the solid-state properties of drugs should not only provide vital information for formulators but might also help us to understand the formation of crystals in joints or in the kidneys, and how to dissolve them or prevent their formation. There are many such examples in this book.

Physical chemistry and pharmacy

Undergraduates beginning their study of pharmacy are often surprised at the amount of physical chemistry they are expected to absorb, when they had expected perhaps a more biological flavour to their diet. It is sometimes still thought of as a subject only for those who will become formulators and industrial pharmacists, but this view neglects the fact that pharmacy is the guardian of this subject, as with pharmacognosy. The biological processes in the body do not operate and exist in some special non-physical world, although it is true that they are usually more complex than the processes we observe in the test tube. So in this book we not only try to give the physicochemical basis for understanding pharmaceutical formulation and drug delivery but we also stray into related areas, frequently referring to chemical structures and biological and clinical consequences. It is important that the underpinning sciences are used intelligently by pharmacy graduates, and not separated into compartments or silos.

Although in this edition of the book we have selected only key equations that illustrate key points, we do not derive all of them from first principles. The value in appreciating the way in which an equation is derived lies with the fact that one can better understand the limitations of the equation. Equations often apply only in certain conditions, for example, in extremely dilute solution, so the caveats in the derivations of equations must be heeded. Sometimes it is useful to be able to derive an equation from first principles. It would be sad if the modern pharmacist were an empiricist at a time when the science of drug development and drug therapy is becoming much more quantitative and predictable.

We have to admit that it is not always possible to apply precisely the equations in this book in the complex world of multicomponent medicines, especially after their administration, but rigorous physical chemistry is the starting point for better understanding. As an example, the knowledge of the way in which the solubility of a drug increases or decreases with change in the acidity of the stomach or the intestine is an essential starting point in the understanding of the complex process of drug absorption and of the stability of drugs in solution.

This book is not a complete survey of all the physical chemistry underlying pharmacy, but we have selected the most important in pharmaceutics and biopharmaceutics, without dealing with pharmacokinetics or with many aspects of pharmaceutical production, which are covered in specialised textbooks.

The clinical relevance of physical pharmacy: clinical pharmaceutics

To some it seems a long extrapolation from physical pharmacy to patient care. There are those who argue that with the increased emphasis on a clinical role for pharmacy, the importance of pharmaceutics diminishes. We certainly do not hold to this view. First we need products of high quality that are consistent and that work under a variety of circumstances. We need to understand the material in this book at a certain depth before embarking on a career in which medicines are central. But clinical pharmaceutics is more than biopharmaceutics: it is about applying knowledge of physical processes and phenomena, such as surface tension, rheology, precipitation and crystallisation, surface activity and diffusion, to events in patients. We have not introduced a special chapter to deal with these issues but rather each chapter provides selected examples where the physical chemistry assists in the understanding of adverse events, action of agents and so on. For a fuller account and more examples there is available an *Introduction to Clinical Pharmaceutics*, Pharmaceutical Press, London, 2010.

Pharmacists must be comfortable with the properties of dosage forms, conventional and otherwise, understand how they work, what features they have that can cause problems and which formulation might be better suited to one patient rather than another. More than that we need practitioners who can predict trends in medication, drug delivery and targeting, and the future use of biologicals. Graduates should be able to critically evaluate what pharmaceutical companies say about their products. The 'skeptical' pharmacist is needed more and more in health care.

Adjuvants or excipients

It is forgotten by many, patients included, that medicines contains much more than the drug. They contain the so-called inactive materials, excipients or adjuvants. In any medicine, the drug is central, whether we are dealing with its formulation, its delivery, its analysis or its activity. The formulation itself might simply be a means of delivering the dose conveniently to the patient, or it might have an influence on the site of delivery or the time over which the drug exerts its action, as with controlled-release products. Rational formulation requires a firm understanding of the physical mode of action of excipients in formulations. It is therefore vital that we understand the physical chemistry of materials used in formulations to control the rate of release or to solubilise insoluble molecules, to stabilise or to suspend drugs or to form microspheres and nanoparticles. These so-called adjuvants or excipients are generally regarded as inert, but few substances are totally inert and some, such as with a number of surfactants, may be biologically active and indeed harmful if used inappropriately. Surfactant toxicity has its roots in surface activity and hence membrane activity.

Arrangement of the book

How is the book arranged? In the first few chapters we examine the properties of drugs and excipients in the solid state and in solution. Gases are not neglected because of their importance in the design and use of therapeutic pressurised aerosols and implanted pumps. Special classes of materials and systems are also considered in separate chapters. Colloidal systems (which are those comprising particulates generally below 1 μm in diameter), including many suspensions and emulsions, have experienced a renaissance in pharmacy because of the use of microparticles and nanoparticles in drug targeting and controlled drug delivery. Polymers and macromolecules, used widely in pharmaceutical formulations as excipients in many forms, as hydrogels, lipogels, viscous solutions and solid matrices or membranes, are treated in one chapter. Proteins, peptides and oligonucleotides have a chapter devoted to the pharmaceutical challenges they pose because of their size, lability and physical properties.

Surface activity is a phenomenon that has widespread consequences. Surface-active substances are those that adsorb at surfaces and lower surface tension; these so-called surfactant materials have a wide applicability in pharmacy. In micellar form they can solubilise water-insoluble drugs and many at low concentrations can increase membrane permeability and aid the transport of drugs across biological barriers. Many drugs have surface-active properties and this might have consequences for their activity and behaviour. The topic is summarised in a chapter on surface activity and surfactants.

Crucial to the whole subject is the process of drug absorption, and how the physical properties of drugs and their formulation can influence the rate and extent (and sometimes site) of absorption. The basics of drug absorption and the oral route are now discussed in one chapter while the many alternative routes to achieving systemic levels of drugs are reviewed in a separate chapter. The emphasis is on the way in which the physiology of the route influences the design of formulations and the behaviour of drugs and dose forms.

Drugs are frequently given together and some interact with clinically important consequences. Often these interactions are pharmacological, but some have a basis in physical chemistry. Incompatibilities might arise from electrostatic interactions between oppositely charged drugs, or from complexation between drugs and ions or drugs and polymers; these and a variety of other interactions are discussed in the book.

It is not always possible to predict the behaviour of drugs and formulations in the complicated environments in which they find themselves *in vivo*, but this should not deter us from at least attempting to rationalise events once they have become known. In this way our predictive powers will be honed and will allow us to prevent adverse events in the future. Some unwanted effects are due to the degradation of drugs and drug formulations; the examination of stability is an important part of assessing the suitability of formulations. This requires a good understanding of the chemistry of the drug substance and reaction kinetics. This, too, is the subject of a chapter.

A new chapter on pharmaceutical aspects of nanotechnology has been added due to the increasing number of formulations and systems in the nanoscale (10^{-9}–10^{-7} m). Many drug targeting systems are nanoparticles; some liposomes have diameters below 200 nm and dendrimers can be as small as 5–6 nm in diameter. Issues of particle size, flocculation and aggregation are important when size can determine the fate in the body. With many biological agents one must also think of molecular size as a factor in restricting the diffusion and translocation of the molecules in question.

Objectives

Almost any of the topics discussed could be the subject of a complete textbook in its own right. The objective of this book is to present sufficient of the physical chemistry in context to illustrate the many and varied areas of pharmacy that the subject can illuminate. If one wishes to understand at more than a superficial level what makes modern delivery systems work, we would advocate close reading of all the pharmaceutical sciences, of which the topic of physical chemistry forms one important part. Examination of just one such delivery system (Fig. I.1), a simple transdermal patch, can bring into focus the diversity of physical phenomena that are involved in the design, use and action of delivery systems. One could list these in just this one example as: adsorption, the stability of suspensions, molecular transport through polymeric membranes, adhesion, the interaction of drugs with polymers, the physicochemical properties of the skin and the diffusional characteristics of drugs in the subsections of the skin, including crossing the capillary membrane into the blood. Perhaps enough, we hope, to convince you that reading the rest of the book is necessary.

Figure I.1 A drawing of a typical transdermal patch system to deliver drug into the systemic circulation by way of the skin. Drawn here is the system with (1) a reservoir containing the drug adsorbed to (2) lactose particles in (3) an oil; (4) the rate-controlling membrane, a copolymer whose thickness and composition are altered to achieve the desired rate of transport of the drug; and (5) the adhesive layer, also a polymer, although liquid, which attaches the patch to the skin. The basic structure of the skin (6) illustrates the routes of penetration of the drug through this barrier layer into the systemic circulation via the capillary blood supply (7).

'Reading' structures and formulae

Throughout this book you will come across two types of formulae: chemical (structural) formulae and physicochemical equations. 'Reading' and understanding formulae – of both kinds – is like learning a language. We often equate reading chemical formulae to reading Chinese characters. To a person without any knowledge of the components of Chinese pictograms, the beautiful shapes mean nothing: 化学结构. A physical equation, similarly, is possibly more akin to the first sight of Arabic: a jumble of unfamiliar letters to the unversed: المعادلات الرياضية. Before we delve into the book proper, we can rehearse how to see the important features of chemical structures and equations.

Chemical structures

It is not necessary always to understand how a drug was synthesised, but it is important to know about the chemistry of a drug as this determines so many features important in its formulation: its solubility in water, solubility in lipid phases, stability, interaction with excipients and of course absorption, not to mention ultimate metabolism.

There are of course classes of drugs with the same central 'core' to which are added substituents. It is important that we have a feel for the properties of the 'core' and the substituent groups, that is whether they are ionised or nonionised, polar or nonpolar, water-soluble or hydrophobic. A hydrophobic aromatic ring can have substituents that make the molecule water-soluble. Much of this is discussed in the text itself. This section simply asks that you look at the drug molecule (or an excipient or an additive molecule) in a certain way. Two drugs, meperidine (pethidine) (**I**) and procainamide (**II**) are shown below. Meperidine possesses an aromatic hydrocarbon ring and a piperidine ring and it is a carboxylic acid ester. The nitrogen is a tertiary amine and will be protonated at low pH; the ester is neutral. So one can predict something about the way the molecule will behave in solution and its relative hydrophobicity once the influence of substituent groups is realised. Also, a drug's name will often reveal something of its structure, hence the piperidine clue in meperidine. So too with procainamide (**II**), which is an amide with a primary amine group and a tertiary alkylamine as well. This drug will have two pK_a values (or pK_b values) and this will have consequences for its solubility and absorption.

Structure III Docetaxel

Structure IV Paclitaxel

Physical equations

One equation, which you will find on page 26, is the Noyes–Whitney equation, which relates the surface area of a drug powder to its rate of solution. Some equations are phenomenological (that is they are derived as a result of experiment and observation) and do not necessarily have a deep theoretical base, so there is no need to be frightened of them. These are often intuitive equations, quite logical, as this one is:

$$\frac{dw}{dt} = \frac{DA}{\delta}(c_s - c)$$

where dw is the increase of the mass of material going into solution with increase of time dt; D is the diffusion coefficient of the molecules escaping from the crystal surface; A is the surface area of the powder or of the crystal (if it is a single crystal); δ is the diffusion layer thickness; c_s is the saturation solubility of the drug; and c is the concentration of drug at any time point, t.

Structure I Meperidine

Structure II Procainamide

It is not so simple with larger drugs such as docetaxel (**III**) and paclitaxel (**IV**), but the relationships between drugs in a class can be identified at least.

It is quite logical that the rate of solution should increase as the available surface area for dissolution increases, so you would expect dw/dt to be directly proportional to A. D is a property of the drug molecule diffusing in concentrated drug solution. As the diffusion coefficient increases, one would expect the rate to increase. Diffusion takes place through a concentrated layer – the diffusion layer – and the thicker this is (i.e. the larger δ is), the further the drug has to diffuse to reach the bulk of the solution, hence dw/dt is proportional to $1/\delta$. Stirring reduces the thickness of the stationary layer, hence aids dissolution. The more soluble a compound is (i.e. the higher c_s is), the higher the rate of solution; it is clear that if $c_s = c$, then the dissolution stops.

So, by thinking of a process logically, one can almost formulate the equation. Noyes and Whitney did this for us, and precisely, although each equation operates only under certain boundary conditions. Nevertheless, from the Noyes–Whitney equation one can predict accurately what the effect on dissolution will be if the solubility of the drug in the medium is increased, for example, by a change in pH. There are other equations for calculating the effect of pH on the equilibrium solubility, so this helps us get a quantitative view of the world in question.

1

Solids

The physical properties of the solid state seen in crystals and powders of both drugs and pharmaceutical excipients are of interest because they can affect both the production of dosage forms and the performance of the finished product. Powders, as Pilpel[1] reminded us, 'can float like a gas or flow like a liquid' but when compressed can support a weight. Fine powders dispersed as suspensions in liquids are used in injections and aerosol formulations. Both liquid and dry powder aerosols are available and are discussed in Chapter 10. In this chapter we deal with the form and particle size of crystalline and amorphous drugs and the effect these characteristics have on drug behaviour, especially on drug dissolution and bioavailability.

Crystalline solids can exist in several subphases, such as polymorphs, solvates, hydrates, and co-crystals. Polymorphs are different crystalline forms (at different free energy states) of the same molecule or molecules. On the other hand, solvates, hydrates and co-crystals are similar in that they consist of more than one type of molecule, one of which is the drug while the other can be either an organic solvent (to form a solvate) or water (to form a hydrate), or another crystalline solid (to form co-crystals). Both types of molecules participate in the short-range and long-range orders of the crystal and therefore these subphases are regarded as single crystalline forms consisting of two types of molecules.

The nature of the crystalline form of a drug substance may affect its stability in the solid state, its solution properties and its absorption. It is with this topic that we start, to consider later other properties of the solid state that are important in production and formulation. Recently, nanocrystals of poorly soluble drugs have been produced to improve their dissolution and absorption.

1.1 Classification of solids

The solid phase can be classified into two major categories based on the order of molecular packing. The most common type of state is the crystalline state in which there is both short-range and long-range order; that is, there is a regular structure that extends throughout the crystal. This contrasts with amorphous solids in which the regularity of structure is limited to the immediate neighbours of any particular molecule within the solid. Crystalline solids can be further subdivided as shown in Fig. 1.1 into polymorphs, which result from different crystalline forms of the same molecule, and multicomponent crystals such as hydrates, solvates and co-crystals, which consist of more than one type of type of molecule.

1.2 Crystalline solids – structure and properties

1.2.1 Crystal structure

Crystals contain highly ordered arrays of molecules and atoms held together by non-covalent interactions. We can consider as a simple example the unit cell of an inorganic salt, sodium chloride. Figure 1.2 shows the ordered arrangement of Cl^- ions and Na^+ ions that make up the sodium chloride crystal structure. We can draw a square on one side connecting the chloride ions. Similar squares could be drawn on all the sides to form a cubic repeating unit, which we call the *unit cell*. Within a specific crystal, each unit cell is the same size and contains the same number of molecules or ions arranged in the same way. It

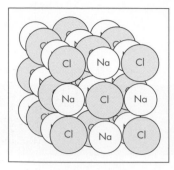

Figure 1.2 Space lattice of the sodium chloride crystal. Each sodium ion is octahedrally surrounded by six chloride ions and each chloride ion is octahedrally surrounded by six sodium ions.

is usually most convenient to think of the atoms or molecules as points and the crystal as a three-dimensional array of these points, or a *crystal lattice*.

For all possible crystals there are seven basic or primitive unit cells, which are shown in Fig. 1.3. We will represent the lengths of the sides as a, b and c and the angles as

α (between sides b and c)
β (between sides a and c)
γ (between sides a and b)

Figure 1.3 shows the characteristic side lengths and angles for these 'primitive' unit cells.

The structures in Fig. 1.3 have atoms or molecules only at each corner of the unit cell. It is possible to find unit cells with atoms or molecules also at the centre of the top or bottom faces (*end-centred*), at the centre of every face (*face-centred*) or with a single atom in the centre of the cell (*body-centred*), as in Fig. 1.4.

Note that these variations do not occur with every type of unit cell: we find

- End-centred monoclinic and orthorhombic
- Face-centred cubic and orthorhombic
- Body-centred, cubic, tetragonal and orthorhombic

Altogether there are 14 possible types of unit cell and we call these the *Bravais lattices*. For drugs there are three common types of unit cell: triclinic, monoclinic and orthorhombic.

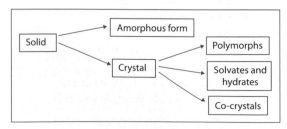

Figure 1.1 Classification of solids.

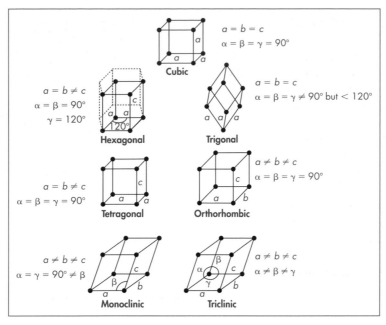

Figure 1.3 The seven possible primitive unit cells with atoms or molecules only at each corner of the unit cell. Drug molecules will typically form triclinic, monoclinic and orthorhombic unit cells.

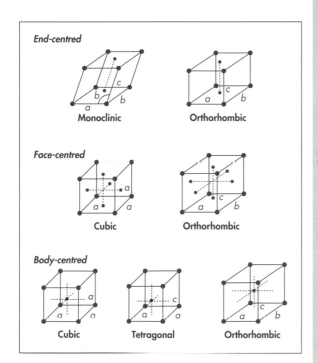

Figure 1.4 Variations on primitive cells.

Key points

- The crystal lattice is constructed from repeating units called unit cells; all unit cells in a specific crystal are the same size and contain the same number of molecules or ions arranged in the same way.
- There are seven primitive unit cells – cubic, trigonal, orthorhombic, triclinic, hexagonal, tetragonal and monoclinic which have molecules or ions arranged at each corner.
- In addition, monoclinic and orthorhombic unit cells may be end-centred; cubic and orthorhombic unit cells may be face-centred; and cubic, tetragonal and orthorhombic unit cells may be body-centred.
- There are therefore only 14 possible types – the Bravais lattices.
- Drug molecules usually have triclinic, monoclinic or orthorhombic unit cells.

Miller indices

We can identify the various planes of a crystal using the system of *Miller indices*. To understand how this system is used, let us consider the plane drawn through the cubic crystal shown in Fig. 1.5a. The plane cuts the *a* axis at one unit length and also the *c* axis at one unit length. It does not, however, cut the *b* axis, and hence the intercept to this axis is infinity. One way we could label planes is to denote each set by the distances along the axes to the point where the plane crosses the axis. So, for example, the planes marked in Fig. 1.5a would have intercept lengths of $a = 1, b = \infty, c = 1$. This system of labelling the faces is inconvenient because of the appearance of ∞. A way around this problem is to take the reciprocals of the numbers (since the reciprocal of $\infty = 0$). The plane shown then becomes 1/1, 1/∞, 1/1 for the *a*, *b* and *c* axes, i.e. 1, 0, 1. The Miller indices for this plane are then written as (101).

A second example is illustrated in Fig. 1.5b. This plane does not cut the *a* axis; it cuts the *b* axis at a unit cell length of $\frac{1}{2}$, and does not cut the *c* axis. The intercept lengths are therefore $a = \infty$, $b = \frac{1}{2}$, $c = \infty$, which on taking reciprocals become 0, 2, 0. A second rule of Miller indices is now applied, that is to reduce the numbers to the lowest terms – in this case by dividing them all by 2. The Miller indices for this plane are therefore (010).

Other rules for applying Miller indices are shown by the following examples, which for ease of illustration are shown using a two-dimensional array (the *c* axis can be imagined to be at right angles to the page). None of the sets of planes we will consider crosses the *c* axis, i.e. we consider them to intersect it at ∞. The plane X in Fig. 1.6 has *a*, *b* and *c* intercepts of 3, 2, and ∞, giving reciprocals of $\frac{1}{3}$, $\frac{1}{2}$ and 0. The procedure is now to clear the fractions, in this case by multiplying each term by 6, giving 2, 3, and 0. It is not possible to reduce these further, and the Miller indices are therefore (230). The plane Y in Fig. 1.6 shows an example of a negative intercept where the *a* axis is crossed. The reciprocals of the *a*, *b* and *c* intercepts are −1, 1, and 0. The procedure that is now used is to write the negative number using a bar above it, giving Miller indices for this plane of ($\bar{1}$10). We should notice that the smaller the number in the Miller index for a particular axis, the more parallel is the plane to that axis, a zero value indicating a plane exactly parallel to that axis. The larger a Miller index, the more nearly perpendicular a plane is to that axis.

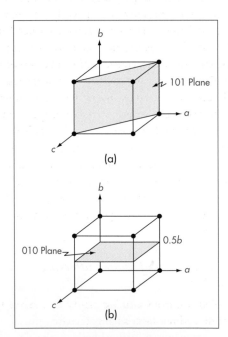

(a)

(b)

Figure 1.5 Cubic crystal showing planes with Miller indices of (a) (101) and (b) (010).

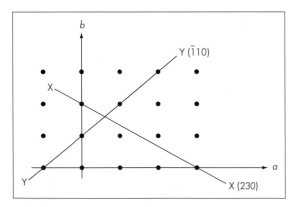

Figure 1.6 Planes in a two-dimensional array.

Key points

The general rules for expressing planes using the system of Miller indices:

- Determine the intercepts of the plane on the *a*, *b* and *c* axes in terms of unit cell lengths.
- Take the reciprocals of the intercepts.
- Clear the fractions by multiplying by the lowest common denominator.
- Reduce the numbers to the lowest terms.
- Indicate negative numbers with a bar above the number.

Example 1.1 Use of Miller indices

Draw a two-dimensional lattice array and indicate the planes with the following Miller indices: (i) (100); (ii) (010); (iii) (110); (iv) (120); (v) (230); and (vi) (410).

Answer

1.2.2 Crystal form

The solid state is important for a variety of reasons, summarised in Fig. 1.7: morphology, particle size, polymorphism, solvation or hydration can affect

filtration, flow, tableting, dissolution and bioavailability. These are described below. In addition, crystallisation can sometimes occur *in vivo*, often, as in the case of gout (see below), with painful consequences.

The crystals of a given substance may vary in size, the relative development of the given faces and the number and kind of the faces (or forms) present; that is, they may have different crystal *habits*. The habit describes the overall shape of the crystal in rather general terms and includes, for example, acicular (needle-like), prismatic, pyramidal, tabular, equant, columnar and lamellar types. Figure 1.8 shows the crystal habits of a hexagonal crystal.

Although there may not be significant differences in the bioavailability of drugs with different crystal habits, the crystal habit is of importance from a technological point of view. The ability to inject a suspension containing a drug in crystal form will be influenced by the habit: plate-like crystals are easier to inject through a fine needle than are needle-like crystals. The crystal habit can also influence the ease of compression of a powder and the flow properties of the drug in the solid state. The plate-like crystals of tolbutamide, for example, cause powder bridging in the hopper of the tablet machine and also capping problems during tableting. Neither of these problems occurs with tolbutamide in other crystal habits. The habits acquired depend on the conditions of crystallisation, such as the solvent used, the temperature, the concentration and presence of impurities. Ibuprofen crystallises from hexane as elongated needle-like crystals, which have been found to have poor flow properties; crystallisation from methanol produces equidimensional crystals with better flow properties and compaction characteristics, making them more suitable for tableting. The crystal morphology of the excipients (such as powdered cellulose) included in tablet formulations can also have a significant influence on the strength and disintegration time of tablets.

Crystallisation and factors affecting crystal form[2]

Crystallisation from solution can be considered to be the result of three successive processes:

- Supersaturation of the solution
- Formation of crystal nuclei
- Crystal growth round the nuclei

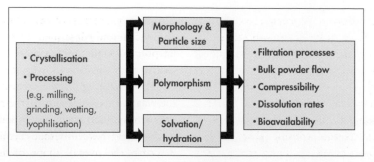

Figure 1.7 The solid state in pharmaceutical science: potential causes and effects of structural change (after A.J. Florence).

 Clinical point **Gout – a painful example of crystallisation**

Gout usually manifests itself as a sudden excruciating pain in the big toe (usually of men), although other joints such as the ankle, heel, instep, knee, wrist, elbow, fingers or spine may be affected. It is a consequence of the precipitation of needle-like crystals of uric acid, in the form of monosodium urate, on the articular cartilage of joints when the levels of uric acid in blood serum exceed a critical solubility level (approximately 6.7 mg/dL); the crystals inside the joint cause intense pain whenever the affected area is moved. Uric acid is a normal component of blood serum and is a product of the metabolism of purines, which are generated by the body via breakdown of cells in normal cellular turnover, and also are ingested as part of a normal diet in foods such as liver, sardines, anchovies and dried peas and beans. The uric acid is normally filtered out of the blood by the kidneys and excreted in the urine. Sometimes, however, too much uric acid is produced by the body or the kidneys are not sufficiently efficient at removing it and it accumulates in the blood, a condition known as hyperuricaemia. Precipitation of uric acid is also markedly enhanced when the blood pH is low (acidosis), a consequence of reduced solubility under such conditions. Patients with long-standing hyperuricaemia can have uric acid crystal deposits called tophi in other tissues such as the helix of the ear. High levels of uric acid in the urine can lead to uric acid crystals precipitating in the kidneys or bladder, forming uric acid kidney stones.

Supersaturation can be achieved by cooling, by evaporation, by the addition of a precipitant or by a chemical reaction that changes the nature of the solute. Supersaturation itself is insufficient to cause crystals to form; the crystal embryos must form by collision of molecules of solute in the solution, or sometimes by the addition of seed crystals, or dust particles, or even particles from container walls. Deliberate seeding is

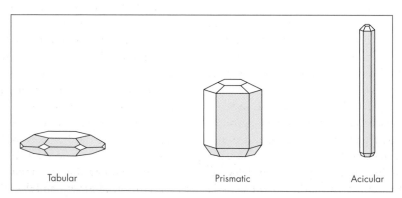

Tabular   Prismatic   Acicular

Figure 1.8 Crystal habits of a hexagonal crystal.

often carried out in industrial processes; seed crystals do not necessarily have to be of the substance concerned but may be isomorphous substances (i.e. of the same morphology). As soon as stable nuclei are formed, they begin to grow into visible crystals.

Crystal growth can be considered to be a reverse dissolution process and the diffusion theories of Noyes and Whitney, and of Nernst, consider that matter is deposited continuously on a crystal face at a rate proportional to the difference of concentration between the surface and the bulk solution. Thus an equation for crystallisation can be proposed in the form

$$\frac{dm}{dt} = Ak_m(c_{ss} - c_s) \qquad (1.1)$$

where m is the mass of solid deposited in time t, A is the surface area of the crystal, c_s is the solute concentration at saturation and c_{ss} is the solute concentration at supersaturation. As $k_m = D/\delta$ (D being the diffusion coefficient of the solute and δ the diffusion layer thickness; see Fig. 1.18), the degree of agitation of the system, which affects δ, also influences crystal growth. Crystals generally dissolve faster than they grow, so growth is not simply the reverse of dissolution. It has been suggested that there are two steps involved in growth in addition to those mentioned earlier, namely transport of the molecules to the surface and their arrangement in an ordered fashion in the lattice. Equation (1.1) turns out to be better written in a modified form:

$$\frac{dm}{dt} = Ak_g(c_{ss} - c_s)^n \qquad (1.2)$$

k_g being the overall crystal growth coefficient and n the 'order' of the crystal growth process. For more details reference 2 should be consulted.

Precipitation

Precipitation may be induced by altering the pH of the solution so that the saturation solubility is exceeded. Precipitation may be made to occur from a homogeneous solution by slowly generating the precipitating agent by means of a chemical reaction, a process likely to occur, for example, in intravenous infusion fluids and liquid pharmaceuticals. Precipitation by direct mixing of two reacting solutions sometimes does not bring about immediate nucleation and, as a result, the mixing stage may be followed by an appreciable lag time. The rate of precipitation is an important factor in determining habit, as might be imagined with a dynamic process such as crystallisation, involving nucleation and subsequent crystal growth. The form of phenylsalicylate, for example, depends on rate of crystal growth. Transition to an acicular shape occurs when the rate of growth increases. At low rates of growth, crystals of a more regular shape are obtained. In studies of the effect of solvents on habit it is generally found that less-viscous media favour the growth of coarse and more equidimensional crystal forms.

Habit modification

Crystal habit can be modified by adding impurities or 'poisons'; for example, sulfonic acid dyes alter the crystal habit of ammonium, sodium and potassium nitrates.

Surfactants in the solvent medium used for crystal growth (or, for example, in stabilisation or wetting of suspensions) can alter crystal form by adsorbing onto growing faces during crystal growth. This is best illustrated by the effect of anionic and cationic surfactants on the habit of adipic acid crystals.[3] X-ray analysis showed that the linear six-carbon dicarboxylic acid molecules were aligned end-to-end in a parallel array in the crystal with their long axis parallel to the (010) faces, so that the (001) face is made up entirely of −COOH groups while the (010) and (110) faces contain both −COOH and hydrocarbon (HC) portions of the molecule (Fig. 1.9). The cationic surfactant trimethyldodecylammonium chloride is twice as effective in hindering the growth of the (001) face as that of the (110) and (010) faces. In high concentrations it causes the formation of very thin plates or flakes. Conversely, the anionic surfactant sodium dodecylbenzene sulfonate at 55 ppm (parts per million) is three times as effective in reducing the growth rates of the (110) and (010) faces as of the (001) face. Higher levels of sodium dodecylbenzene sulfonate cause extreme habit modification, producing not hexagonal plates but long, thin rods or needles. The crystallographic faces whose growth rates are depressed most are those upon which surfactant adsorption is the greatest. Cationic additives adsorb on the face composed of carboxylic groups (001), and anionic additives on the (110) and (010) faces, which are hydrophobic. A coulombic interaction of the cationic head groups and the −COO− groups on the (001) faces has been suggested. The adsorption of

Figure 1.9 (a) Effect of anionic and cationic surfactants on the habit of adipic acid crystals. (b) A diagrammatic (not to scale) representation of the arrangement of molecules at the crystal surface.

the anionic surfactant, repelled from the anionic (001) faces, takes place amphipathically on the hydrophobic (110) faces and (010) faces (Fig. 1.9).

 Key points

- The crystal habit describes the external appearance of a crystal, i.e. its overall shape and the number and kind of faces. Common types of habit include acicular, prismatic, pyramidal, tabular, equant, columnar and lamellar.
- The crystal habit depends on the conditions of crystallisation and may affect the syringeability of suspensions of the drug, its ease of compression into tablets and its flow properties.
- The crystal habit can be modified by adding impurities (called poisons) or surfactants to the solvent used for crystallisation.

1.2.3 Polymorphism[4]

As we have seen, compounds can crystallise out of solution in a variety of different habits depending on the conditions of crystallisation. These crystal habits usually have the same internal structure and so have the same X-ray diffraction patterns. A more fundamental difference in properties may be found when the compounds crystallise as different *polymorphs*. When *polymorphism* occurs, the molecules arrange themselves in two or more different ways in the crystal; either they may be packed differently in the crystal lattice or there may be differences in the orientation or conformation of the molecules at the lattice sites. These variations cause differences in the X-ray diffraction patterns of the polymorphs and this technique is one of the main methods of detecting the existence of polymorphs. The polymorphs have different physical and chemical properties; for example, they may have different melting points and solubilities and they also usually exist in different habits.

We will consider two drugs that exhibit this phenomenon. Spironolactone (**I**), which is a diuretic steroidal aldosterone agonist, crystallises as two polymorphic forms and also as four solvated crystalline forms depending on the solvents and methods used for crystallisation.[5] We will consider the occurrence of solvated forms in section 1.2.4; at the moment we will concentrate on the two polymorphs only. Form 1 is produced when spironolactone powder is dissolved in acetone at a temperature very close to the boiling point and the solution is then cooled within a few hours down to 0°C. Form 2 is produced when the powder is dissolved in acetone, dioxane or chloroform at room temperature and the solvent is allowed to evaporate spontaneously over a period of several weeks. In both polymorphs the steroid nuclei (A, B, C and D rings) are almost planar and perpendicular to the E ring and to the 7α-acetothio side-chain. The packing of the molecules in the two polymorphs is compared in Fig. 1.10. Both unit cells are orthorhombic but they differ in their dimensions. The *a*, *b* and *c* axes of Form 1 were found to be 0.998, 3.557 and 0.623 nm, respectively, compared with equivalent lengths for Form 2 of 1.058, 1.900 and 1.101 nm. There are also differences in the crystal habits: Form 1 crystals are needle-like, while those of Form 2 are prisms (see Fig. 1.11). The melting points are slightly different: Form 1 melts at 205°C whereas Form 2 has a melting point of 210°C.

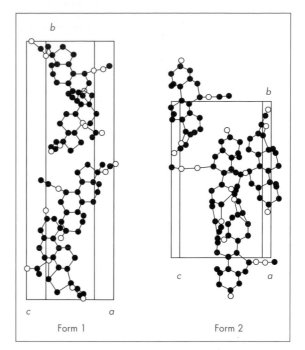

Figure 1.10 Unit cells of spironolactone.

Reproduced with permission from reference 5.

Structure I Spironolactone

Our second example of a drug exhibiting polymorphism is paracetamol (**II**). This drug is known to exist in two polymorphic forms, monoclinic (Form 1) and orthorhombic (Form 2), of which Form 1 is the more thermodynamically stable at room temperature and is the commercially used form.[6] However, this form is not suitable for direct compression into tablets and has to be mixed with binding agents before tableting, a procedure that is both costly and time-consuming. In contrast, Form 2 can readily undergo plastic deformation upon compaction and it has been suggested that this form may have distinct processing advantages over the

Figure 1.11 Crystal forms of spironolactone.

Reproduced with permission from reference 5.

monoclinic form. Monoclinic paracetamol is readily produced by crystallisation from aqueous solution and many other solvents; production of the orthorhombic form has proved more difficult but may be achieved, at least on a laboratory scale, by nucleating a supersaturated solution of paracetamol with seeds of Form 2 (from melt-crystallised paracetamol). Figure 1.12 shows scanning electron micrographs of the two polymorphic forms when crystallised from industrial methylated spirit (IMS). Form 1 is described as having a prismatic to plate-like habit that is elongated in the direction of the *c*-axis, while Form 2 crystallises as prisms that are elongated along the *c*-axis.

(a)

(b)

Figure 1.12 Scanning electron micrographs showing the crystal habit of (a) Form 1 and (b) Form 2 of paracetamol grown from supersaturated IMS. Note different scales.

Reproduced with permission from reference 6.

Structure II Paracetamol

Polymorphism is common with pharmaceutical compounds. Although we do not yet understand the process sufficiently well to predict which drugs are likely to exhibit this phenomenon, it is clear that certain classes of drug are particularly susceptible. Eight crystal modifications of phenobarbital have been isolated but 11 have been identified with melting points ranging from 112 to 176°C. Of the barbiturates used medicinally, about 70% exhibit polymorphism. The steroids frequently possess polymorphic modifications, testosterone having four: these are cases of true polymorphism and not pseudopolymorphism in which solvent is the cause (see section 1.2.4). Of the commercial sulfonamides, about 65% are found to exist in several polymorphic forms. Examples of the differing solubilities and melting points of polymorphic sulfonamides and steroids are given in Table 1.1.

Predictability of the phenomenon is difficult except by reference to past experience. Its pharmaceutical importance depends very much on the stability and solubility of the forms concerned. It is difficult, therefore, to generalise, except to say that where polymorphs of insoluble compounds occur there are likely to be biopharmaceutical implications. Table 1.2 is a partial listing of the drugs for which polymorphic and pseudopolymorphic states have been identified or for which an amorphous state has been reported.

Pharmaceutical implications of polymorphism

We have already considered the problems in tableting and injection that may result from differences in crystal habit (see section 1.2.2). Since polymorphs frequently have different habits, they too will be subject to these same problems. However, polymorphs also have different crystal lattices and consequently their energy contents may be sufficiently different to influence their stability and biopharmaceutical behaviour.

As the different polymorphs arise through different arrangement of the molecules or ions in the lattice, they will have different interaction energies in the solid

Table 1.1 Melting points of some polymorphic forms of steroids, sulfonamides and riboflavin[a]

Compound	Form and/or melting point (°C)			
Polymorphic steroids	(I)	(II)	(III)	(IV)
Corticosterone	180–186	175–179	163–168	155–160
β-Estradiol	178	169		
Estradiol	225	223		
Testosterone	155	148	144	143
Methylprednisolone	I (205, aqueous solubility 0.075 mg cm^{-3}) II (230, aqueous solubility 0.16 mg cm^{-3})			
Polymorphic sulfonamides				
Sulfafurazole	190–195	131–133		
Acetazolamide	258–260	248–250		
Tolbutamide	127	117	106	
Others				
Riboflavin	I (291, aqueous solubility 60 mg cm^{-3}) II (278, aqueous solubility 80 mg cm^{-3}) III (183, aqueous solubility 1200 mg cm^{-3})			

[a] Reproduced from Kuhnert-Brandstatter M, *Thermomicroscopy in the Analysis of Pharmaceuticals*, New York: Pergamon Press; 1971.

Table 1.2 Polymorphic and pseudopolymorphic drugs[a]

Compound	Number of forms		
	Polymorphs	**Amorphous**	**Pseudopolymorphs**
Ampicillin	1	—	1
Beclometasone dipropionate	—	—	2
Betamethasone	1	1	—
Betamethasone 21-acetate	1	1	—
Betamethasone 17-valerate	1	1	—
Caffeine	1	—	1
Cefaloridine	4	—	2
Chloramphenicol palmitate	3	1	—

(continued overleaf)

Table 1.2 *(continued)*

Compound	Number of forms		
	Polymorphs	Amorphous	Pseudopolymorphs
Chlordiazepoxide HCl	2	–	1
Chlorthalidone	2	–	–
Dehydropregnenolone	1	–	7
Dexamethasone acetate	3	–	1
Dexamethasone pivalate	4	–	7
Digoxin	–	1	–
Erythromycin	2	–	–
Fludrocortisone acetate	3	1	–
Fluprednisolone	3	–	2
Glutethimide	1	–	1
Hydrocortisone TBA[b]	1	–	3
Indometacin	3		
Mefenamic acid	2	–	–
Meprobamate	2	–	–
Methyl p-hydroxybenzoate	6	–	–
Methylprednisolone	2	–	–
Novobiocin	1	1	–
Prednisolone	2	–	–
Prednisolone TBA[b]	2	–	2
Prednisolone TMA[c]	3	–	–
Prednisolone acetate	2	–	–
Prednisone	1	–	1
Progesterone	2	–	–
Sorbitol	3	–	–
Testosterone	4	–	–
Theophylline	1	–	1
Triamcinolone	2	–	–

[a] Modified from Bouché R, Draguet-Brughmans M, *J Pharm Belg*, 1977; 32: 347 with additions.
[b] Tertiary butyl acetate (tebutate).
[c] Trimethyl acetate.

state. Under a given set of conditions the polymorphic form with the lowest free energy will be the most stable, and other polymorphs will tend to transform into it. The rate of conversion is variable and is determined by the magnitude of the energy barrier between the two polymorphs – the higher the energy barrier and the lower the storage temperature, the slower is the conversion rate. Occasionally, the most stable polymorph appears only several years after the compound was first marketed. We can determine which of two polymorphs is the more stable by a simple experiment in which the polymorphs are placed in a drop of saturated solution under the microscope. The crystals of the less-stable form will dissolve and those of the more stable form will grow until only this form remains. Figure 1.13 shows this process occurring with the two polymorphs of paracetamol discussed earlier. Figure 1.13a shows the presence of both forms of paracetamol at room temperature in saturated benzyl alcohol. Over a time interval of 30 minutes the less stable of the two forms, the orthorhombic Form 2, has completely converted to the more stable monoclinic Form 1 (Fig. 1.13b). For drugs with more than two polymorphs we need to carry out this experiment on successive pairs of the polymorphs of the drug until we eventually arrive at their rank order of stability.

Transformations

The transformation between polymorphic forms can lead to formulation problems. Phase transformations can cause changes in crystal size in suspensions and their eventual caking. Crystal growth in creams as a result of phase transformation can cause the cream to become gritty. Similarly, changes in polymorphic forms of vehicles, such as theobroma oil used to make suppositories, could cause products with different and unacceptable melting characteristics.

Analytical issues

For analytical work it is sometimes necessary to establish conditions whereby different forms of a substance, where they exist, might be converted to a single form to eliminate differences in the solid-state infrared spectra that result from the different internal structures of the crystal forms. As different crystal forms arise through different arrangements of the molecules or ions in a three-dimensional array, this implies different interaction energies in the solid state. Hence, one would expect different melting points and different

(a)

(b)

Figure 1.13 Photomicrographs showing the solution-phase polymorphic conversion of orthorhombic paracetamol (needles) to monoclinic paracetamol (prisms and plates). Micrograph (a) was taken at $t = 0$ and (b) was taken at $t = 30$ minutes. Scale bars $= 250 \, \mu m$.

Reproduced with permission from reference 6.

solubilities (and of course different infrared spectra). Changes in infrared spectra of steroids due to grinding with potassium bromide (KBr) have been reported; changes in the spectra of some substances have been ascribed to conversion of a crystalline form into an amorphous form (as in the case of digoxin), or into a second crystal form. Changes in crystal form can also be induced by solvent extraction methods used for isolation of drugs from formulations prior to examination by infrared spectroscopy. Difficulties in identification arise when samples that are thought to be the same substance give different spectra in the solid state; this can happen, for example, with cortisone acetate which exists in at least seven forms, or dexamethasone acetate which exists in four. Therefore, where there is a likelihood of polymorphism it is best where possible to record solution spectra if chemical identification only is required. The normal way to overcome the effects of polymorphism is to convert both samples into the same form by recrystallisation from the same solvent, although obviously this technique should not be used to hide the presence of polymorphs.

Consequences

The most important consequence of polymorphism is the possible difference in the bioavailability of different polymorphic forms of a drug; particularly when the drug is poorly soluble. The rate of absorption of such a drug is often dependent upon its rate of dissolution. The most stable polymorph usually has the lowest solubility and slowest dissolution rate and consequently often a lower bioavailability than the metastable polymorph. Fortunately, the difference in the bioavailability of different polymorphic forms of a drug is usually insignificant. It has been proposed that when the free energy differences between the polymorphs are small there may be no significant differences in their biopharmaceutical behaviour as measured by the blood levels they achieve. Only when the differences are large may they affect the extent of absorption. For example, $\Delta G_{B \rightarrow A}$ for the transition of chloramphenicol palmitate Form B to Form A is $-3.24 \, \text{kJ mol}^{-1}$; ΔH is $-27.32 \, \text{kJ mol}^{-1}$. For mefenamic acid $\Delta G_{II \rightarrow I}$ is $-1.05 \, \text{kJ mol}^{-1}$ and ΔH is $-4.18 \, \text{kJ mol}^{-1}$. Whereas differences in biological activity are shown by the palmitate polymorphs, no such differences are observed with the mefenamic acid polymorphs. When little energy is required to convert one polymorph into another, it is likely that the forms will interconvert *in vivo* and that the administration of one form in place of the other will be clinically unimportant.

Particle size reduction may lead to fundamental changes in the properties of the solid. Grinding of crystalline substances such as digoxin can lead to the formation of amorphous material (see section 1.3) that has an intrinsically higher rate of solution and therefore apparently greater activity. Such is the importance of the polymorphic form of poorly soluble drugs that it has to be controlled. For instance, there is a limit on the inactive polymorph of chloramphenicol palmitate. Of the three polymorphic forms of chloramphenicol palmitate, Form A has a low biological activity because it is so slowly hydrolysed *in vivo* to free chloramphenicol.[7] We can see from Fig. 1.14 that the maximum blood levels attained with 100% Form B polymorph

Figure 1.14 Comparison of serum levels (μg cm^{-3}) obtained with suspensions of chloramphenicol palmitate after oral administration of a dose equivalent to 1.5 g of chloramphenicol.

Redrawn from reference 8.

are about seven times greater than with 100% Form A polymorph, and that with mixtures of A and B the blood levels vary in proportion to the percentage of B in the suspension.[8]

During formulation development it is vital that sufficient care is taken to determine polymorphic tendencies of poorly soluble drugs. This is so that formulations can be designed to release drug at the correct rate and so that intelligent guesses can be made before clinical trial about possible influences of food and concomitant therapy on drug absorption. As will be seen later, particle characteristics (of nitrofurantoin, for example) can affect drug interaction as well as drug absorption. Above all, it is important that during toxicity studies care is given to the characterisation of the physical state of the drug, and that during development the optimal dosage form is attained. It is insufficient that drug is 'available' from the dosage form; on both economic and biological grounds, the maximum response must be achieved with the minimum amount of drug substance.

Key points

- The crystals of some drugs can crystallise in more than one polymorphic form characterised by differences in packing in the crystal lattice or in the orientation or conformation of the molecules at the lattice sites.
- Polymorphs of the same drug may have different melting points and solubilities and usually exist in different habits.
- Although polymorphism is common with pharmaceutical compounds, its likely occurrence cannot be predicted with confidence.
- The polymorphic form with the lowest free energy will be the most stable and other polymorphs will tend to transform into it over time.
- Polymorphism may cause problems in the formulation, analysis and bioavailability of drugs.

1.2.4 Multicomponent crystals

Crystal hydrates and solvates

When some compounds crystallise they may entrap solvent in the crystal. Crystals that contain solvent of crystallisation are called crystal *solvates*, or crystal *hydrates* when water is the solvent of crystallisation. Crystals that contain no water of crystallisation are termed *anhydrates*.

Crystal solvates exhibit a wide range of behaviour depending on the interaction between the solvent and the crystal structure. With some solvates the solvent plays a key role in holding the crystal together; for example, it may be part of a hydrogen-bonded network within the crystal structure. These solvates are very stable and are difficult to desolvate. When these crystals lose their solvent they collapse and recrystallise in a new crystal form. We can think of these as *polymorphic solvates*. In other solvates, the solvent is not part of the crystal bonding and merely occupies voids in the crystal. These solvates lose their solvent more readily and desolvation does not destroy the crystal lattice. This type of solvate has been called a *pseudopolymorphic solvate*.

By way of illustration of this phenomenon, we return to the case of spironolactone which we considered earlier. As well as the two polymorphs, this compound also possesses four solvates, depending on whether it is crystallised from acetonitrile, ethanol, ethyl acetate or methanol. Each of these solvates is transformed to the polymorphic Form 2 on heating, indicating that the solvent is involved in the bonding of the crystal lattice.

The stoichiometry of some of the solvates is unusual. Fludrocortisone pentanol solvate, for example, contains 1.1 molecules of pentanol for each steroid molecule, and its ethyl acetate solvate contains 0.5 molecules of ethyl acetate per steroid molecule. A succinylsulfathiazole solvate appears to have 0.9 moles of pentanol per mole of drug. Beclometasone dipropionate forms solvates with chlorofluorocarbon propellants.

Infrared measurements show that cefaloridine exists in α, β, δ, ε, ζ and μ forms (that is, six forms after recrystallisation from different solvents).[9] Proton magnetic resonance spectroscopy showed that although the μ form contained about 1 mole of methanol and the ε form about 1 mole of dimethyl sulfoxide, ethylene glycol or diethylene glycol (depending on the solvent), the α, β, anhydrous δ and ε forms contained less than 0.1 mole, that is nonstoichiometric amounts of solvent. The α form is characterised by containing about 0.05 mole of *N,N*-dimethylacetamide. This small amount of 'impurity', which cannot be removed by prolonged treatment under vacuum at 10^{-5}–10^{-6} torr, is apparently able to 'lock' the cefaloridine molecule in a particular crystal lattice.

Pharmaceutical consequences of solvate formation

Modification of the solvent of crystallisation may result in different solvated forms. This is of particular relevance because the hydrated and anhydrous forms of a drug can have melting points and solubilities sufficiently different to affect their pharmaceutical behaviour. For example, glutethimide exists in both an anhydrous form (m.p. 83°C, solubility 0.042% at 25°C) and a hydrated form (m.p. 68°C, solubility 0.026% at 25°C). Other anhydrous forms show similar higher solubilities than the hydrated materials and, as expected, the anhydrous forms of caffeine, theophylline, glutethimide and cholesterol show correspondingly higher dissolution rates than their hydrates.

One can assume that as the hydrate has already interacted intimately with water (the solvent), then the energy released for crystal break-up, on interaction of the hydrate with solvent, is less than for the anhydrous material. The nonaqueous solvates, on the other hand, tend to be more soluble in water than the non-solvates. The *n*-amyl alcohol solvate of fludrocortisone acetate

is at least five times as soluble as the parent compound, while the ethyl acetate solvate is twice as soluble.

The equilibrium solubility of the non-solvated form of a crystalline organic compound that does not dissociate in the solvent (for example, water) can be represented as

$$A_{(c)} \xrightleftharpoons{K_s} A_{(aq)}$$

where K_s is the equilibrium constant. This equilibrium will of course be influenced by the crystal form, as we have seen, as well as by temperature and pressure. For a hydrate $A \cdot xH_2O$, we can write

$$A \cdot xH_2O_{(c)} \xrightleftharpoons{K_{sh}} A_{(aq)} + xH_2O$$

K_{sh} is then the solubility of the hydrate. The process of hydration of an anhydrous crystal in water is represented by an equation of the type

$$\underset{\text{(anhydrate)}}{A_{(c)} + xH_2O_{liquid}} \xrightleftharpoons[K_{sh}]{K_s} \underset{\text{(hydrate)}}{A \cdot xH_2O_{(c)}}$$

and the free energy of the process is written

$$\Delta G_{trans} = RT \ln \frac{K_{sh}}{K_s} \tag{1.3}$$

ΔG_{trans} can be obtained from the solubility data of the two forms at a particular temperature, as for theophylline and glutethimide in Table 1.3.

Table 1.3 Solubility of theophylline and glutethimide forms at various temperatures[a]

	Temperature (°C)	Solubility	
		Hydrate (mg cm^{-3})	Anhydrate (mg cm^{-3})
Theophylline	25	6.25	12.5
	35	10.4	18.5
	45	17.6	27.0
	55	30	38
Glutethimide		(%w/v)	(%w/v)
	25	0.0263	0.042
	32	0.0421	0.0604
	40	0.07	0.094

[a] Reproduced from Eriksen SP, *Am J Pharm Educ*, 1964; 28: 47.

Table 1.4 Intrinsic dissolution rates of the crystal forms of oxyphenbutazone[a]

Sample	Intrinsic dissolution rate[b] ($\mu g \, min^{-1} \, cm^{-2}$)
Solvate C	21.05 ± 0.02
Solvate B	18.54 ± 0.47
Anhydrate	14.91 ± 0.47
Hemihydrate	17.01 ± 0.78
Monohydrate	9.13 ± 0.23

[a] Reproduced from Lotter AP, van der Walt JG, *J Pharm Sci*, 1988; 77: 1047.

[b] Mean $\pm$ range of uncertainty of two determinations.

The dissolution rates of solvates can vary considerably. Table 1.4 shows the range of intrinsic dissolution rates reported for solvates of oxyphenbutazone into a dissolution medium containing a surface active agent (to avoid wetting problems). The superior dissolution rates of the benzene and cyclohexane solvates (B and C respectively) are apparent but, of course, the possible use of these solvates is prohibited because of their likely toxicity.

Differences in solubility and dissolution rate between solvates can lead to measurable differences in their bioavailabilities. You can see in Table 1.5 the differences in *in vivo* absorption rates of solvates of prednisolone *t*-butyl acetate and hydrocortisone *t*-butyl acetate after implantation of pellets of these compounds. Note, for example, that the monoethanol solvate of prednisolone has an absorption rate *in vivo* that is nearly five times greater than that of the anhydrous *t*-butyl acetate. Differences in the absorption of ampicillin and its trihydrate can be observed (Fig. 1.15), but the extent of the difference is of doubtful clinical significance. The more soluble anhydrous form appears at a faster rate in the serum and produces higher peak serum levels.

Co-crystals

Pharmaceutical co-crystals are similar to crystal solvates in that the crystal is composed of the drug and another molecule; in co-crystals the other molecule is a crystalline solid rather than a liquid as in crystal hydrates. Co-crystals differ from solid dispersions (section 1.9), which are *physical* mixtures of drug and a highly water-soluble carrier molecule in microcrystalline form; the aim is nevertheless the same – to alter the physical properties of the drug, for example to increase solubility or reduce hygroscopicity. In selecting a suitable molecule to co-crystallise with the drug, consideration is made of the potential for hydrogen bonding between the two molecules. Figure 1.16 shows the molecular packing within the 1 : 1 co-crystals of carbamazepine and saccharin. The carbamazepine molecules hydrogen bond to each other to form a dimer and saccharin molecules form double hydrogen bonds to both N–H donor and O acceptor atoms on this dimer. Other drugs forming co-crystals include caffeine and theophylline, both of which form co-crystals with a range of dicarboxylic acids that have improved stability to high humidity.

Despite the successful application of co-crystallisation in manipulation of the physical properties of a drug, there are currently no marketed products utilising co-crystals. A possible reason for this may be a

Table 1.5 Absorption rate of hydrocortisone tertiary butyl acetate and prednisolone tertiary butyl acetate ($mg \, h^{-1} \, cm^{-2}$)[a]

Compound	Absorption rate ($mg \, h^{-1} \, cm^{-2}$)
Prednisolone tertiary butyl acetate	
Anhydrous	1.84 ± 10^{-3}
Monoethanol solvate	8.7 ± 10^{-3}
Hemiacetone solvate	2.2 ± 10^{-1}
Hydrocortisone tertiary butyl acetate	
Anhydrous	4.74 ± 10^{-3}
Monoethanol solvate	1.83 ± 10^{-3}
Hemichloroform solvate	7.40 ± 10^{-1}

[a] Modified from Ballard BE, Biles J, *Steroids*, 1964; 4: 273.

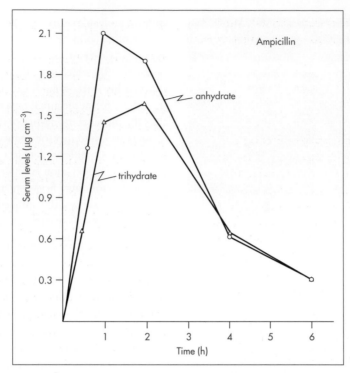

Figure 1.15 Serum levels ($\mu g\,cm^{-3}$) obtained after oral administration of a suspension containing 250 mg ampicillin as the anhydrate and as the trihydrate.

Reproduced from Poole JW *et al., Curr Ther Res*, 1968; 10: 292.

Figure 1.16 Packing of molecules in co-crystals of carbamazepine and saccharin. The dashed lines indicate hydrogen bonding of carbamazepine molecules to each other to form a dimer and the formation of double hydrogen bonds between saccharin and N—H donor and O acceptor atoms on the dimer.

Reproduced from Fleischman SG *et al., Cryst Growth Des*, 2003; 3: 909.

concern that these metastable crystal forms may change their form during storage, necessitating recall of the product.

1.3 Amorphous solids

Solids in which there is no long-range ordering of the molecules are said to be *amorphous*. These disordered systems differ in solubility, stability, dissolution properties and compression characteristics from the more traditionally used crystalline counterparts and provide attractive alternatives to them in drug delivery formulations. In principle, most classes of material can be prepared in the amorphous state if the rate at which they are solidified is faster than that at which their molecules can align themselves into a crystal lattice with three-dimensional order. It is also possible to inadvertently convert crystalline material to amorphous when supplying mechanical or thermal energy, for example during grinding, compression and milling the solid or during drying processes. Some materials, notably polymers such as poly(lactic acid), polyvinylpyrrolidone and polyethylene glycol are inherently amorphous. Even at slow solidification rates, large molecules such as these are often unable to form perfect crystals because of the difficulty in arranging the chains of these flexible molecules in an ordered manner; such materials are frequently *semicrystalline*, with areas of a crystalline nature surrounded by amorphous regions as shown in Fig 1.17.

Unlike crystals, amorphous or semicrystalline materials do not have sharp melting points, but instead there is a change in the properties of the material at a characteristic temperature called the *glass transition temperature*, T_g. Below T_g, the material is said to be in its glassy state and is brittle; as the temperature is increased above T_g, the molecules become more mobile and the material is said to become rubbery. The transition temperature may be lowered by the addition of plasticisers, which are generally small molecules that are able to fit between the glassy molecules, so increasing their mobility. Water, for example, is used as a plasticiser for a wide range of polymers used in film coating.

Amorphous solids, because they exhibit a higher energy state than crystalline solids, are inherently less stable and have the potential for converting to the thermodynamically more stable crystalline form over time. In addition, because of their higher molecular mobility they often show stronger chemical reactivity and hence a faster rate of chemical degradation.

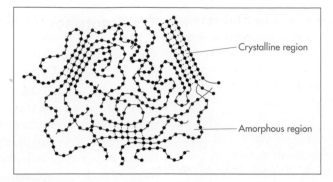

Figure 1.17   Diagrammatic representation of a solid polymer showing regions of crystallinity and regions that are amorphous.

Nevertheless, the amorphous form of a drug often has a higher solubility than its crystalline form and the use of the amorphous form of a drug may provide an opportunity to enhance its bioavailability in the case of poorly water-soluble drugs.

1.4 Dissolution of solid drugs

Whether the solution process takes place in the laboratory or *in vivo*, there is one law that defines the rate of solution of solids when the process is diffusion controlled and involves no chemical reaction. This is the *Noyes–Whitney equation*, which may be written

$$\frac{dw}{dt} = kA(c_s - c) \tag{1.4}$$

where $k = D/\delta$. The equation is the analogue of equation (1.1) discussed previously. Figure 1.18 shows the model on which this equation is based. The terms of the equation are: dw/dt, the rate of increase of the amount of material in solution dissolving from a solid; k, the rate constant of dissolution; c_s, the saturation solubility of the drug in solution in the diffusion layer; and c the concentration of the drug in the bulk solution. A is the area of the solvate particles exposed to the solvent, δ is the thickness of the diffusion layer, and D is the diffusion coefficient of the dissolved solute.

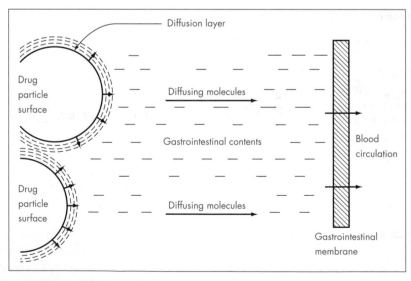

Figure 1.18   Schematic diagram of dissolution from a solid surface.

The relevance of polymorphism and solid-state properties to this equation lies in the fact that A is determined by particle size. Particle size reduction, if it leads to a change in polymorph, results in a change in c_s, and if dissolution is the rate-limiting step in absorption then bioavailability is affected. In more general terms, one can use the equation to predict the effect of solvent change or other parameters on the dissolution rate of solid drugs. These factors are listed in Table 1.6.

Example 1.2 Use of Noyes–Whitney equation

A preparation of drug granules weighing 5.5 g and having a total surface area of $2.8 \times 10^3 \, cm^2$ dissolves in 500 mL of water at 25°C. The quantity of drug dissolved after the first minute is 0.76 g. The saturated solubility of the drug is $15 \, mg \, mL^{-1}$ and the diffusion layer thickness is $5 \times 10^{-3} \, cm$. Calculate (a) the dissolution rate constant, (b) the diffusion coefficient and (c) the effect on the dissolution rate of an increase of surface area to $5 \times 10^3 \, cm^2$.

Answer

(a) Converting the mass of drug dissolved into mg gives the rate of dissolution at $t = 60 \, s$ as

$$dw/dt = 0.76 \times 1000/60 = 12.67 \, mg \, s^{-1}$$

The concentration of the drug in the bulk solution is

$$c = 0.76 \times 1000/500 = 1.52 \, mg \, cm^{-3}$$

$$c_s - c = 15 - 1.52 = 13.48 \, mg \, cm^{-3}$$

Therefore, from equation (1.4),

$$k = (12.67/2.8 \times 10^3) \times (1/13.48) = 3.36 \times 10^{-4} \, cm \, s^{-1}$$

(b) The diffusion coefficient D can be calculated from

$$D = k\delta = 3.36 \times 10^{-4} \times 5 \times 10^{-3} = 1.68 \times 10^{-6} \, cm^2 \, s^{-1}$$

(c) When the surface area is increased to $5 \times 10^3 \, cm^2$,

$$dw/dt = 3.36 \times 10^{-4} \times 5 \times 10^3 \times 13.48 = 22.65 \, mg \, s^{-1}$$

i.e. the increase in surface area has caused an increase of the rate of dissolution from 12.67 to $22.65 \, mg \, s^{-1}$.

Note the importance of ensuring that the parameters are converted to the appropriate units when substituting in equation (1.4) or indeed in any equation. If you are in doubt about units then it is easy to carry out a check to ensure that the units balance on both sides of the equation. In the particular example of equation (1.4) we have:

$$mg \, s^{-1} = cm \, s^{-1} \times cm^2 \times mg \, cm^{-3} = mg \, s^{-1}$$

Table 1.6 How the parameters of the dissolution equation can be changed to increase (+) or decrease (−) the rate of solution

Equation parameter	Comments	Effect on rate of solution
D (diffusion coefficient of drug)	May be decreased in presence of substances which increase viscosity of the medium	(−)
A (area exposed to solvent)	Increased by micronisation and in 'amorphous' drugs	(+)
δ (thickness of diffusion layer)	Decreased by increased agitation in gut or flask	(+)
c_s (solubility in diffusion layer)	That of weak electrolytes altered by change in pH, by use of appropriate drug salt or buffer ingredient	(−)(+)
c (concentration in bulk)	Decreased by intake of fluid in stomach, by removal of drug by partition or absorption	(+)

1.5 Importance of particle size in the formulation and manufacture of solid dosage forms

We have seen in the previous section that particle size has an important influence on dissolution rate, the larger surface exposed to the solvent increasing significantly the dissolution rate of smaller particles. Particle size also influences the uniformity of dosage of very potent drugs formulated as a solid dosage form, and is greater with smaller particles because of the larger number of particles constituting the dose. As discussed in Chapter 10, control of particle size is important in pulmonary delivery because only very fine particles are able to penetrate the alveolar regions of the respiratory tract. But there is an optimum. Indeed, if the particle size is reduced too far, particles may be exhaled and not deposited. Particle size also has important effects on the *bulk properties* of a powder, particularly those that influence powder flow during manufacturing processing when large quantities of material are handled. It is important that pharmaceutical powders are able to flow freely into storage containers or hoppers of tablet and capsule-filling equipment so that a uniform packing of the particles and hence a uniform tablet or capsule weight is achieved. Uneven particle flow can also cause excessive entrapment of air within the powders, which may promote capping of tablets. Particle size influences the bulk properties of powders mainly through its effect on the *cohesivity* of the particles.

Cohesive forces between particles arise from short-range van der Waals forces, electrostatic forces from frictional charging during handling or surface tension forces between adsorbed liquid layers on the particle surface. These are all related to the surface area of the particle and increase as the particle size decreases. Particles larger than about 250 μm are usually relatively free flowing, but flow problems are likely to be observed when the size falls below 100 μm because of cohesion. Very fine particles (below 10 μm) are usually extremely cohesive and have a high resistance to flow. We should, however, note when making these generalisations that particle shape also influences flow properties and particles of similar sizes but different shapes can have markedly different flow properties because of differences in interparticulate contact areas. The cohesion of particles or the adhesion of particles to a substrate can be determined by a variety of experimental methods including, for example, by measurement of the tensile or shear strength of the powder bed or the angle of repose assumed by a cone-like pile of the powder formed on a horizontal surface when the powder is allowed to fall under gravity from a nozzle. Details of these methods are given in national pharmacopoeias.

1.6 Biopharmaceutical importance of particle size

It has generally been believed that only substances in the molecularly dispersed form (that is, in solution) are transported across the intestinal wall and absorbed into the systemic circulation. This is the premise on which much thinking on bioavailability from pharmaceutical dosage forms is based. Although this is generally true, it has been shown that very small particles in the nanometre size range can also be transported through enterocytes by way of pinocytosis, and that solid particles of starch, for example, in the micrometre size range enter by a mechanism involving passage of particles between the enterocytes.[10] Submicrometre particulate uptake by the M-cells of the gut-associated lymphoid tissue (GALT) is a phenomenon of increasing importance.[11] Because of the much greater absorptive area available to molecules, however, the opportunity for molecules to penetrate the cell membrane is obviously higher than that for particles.

The rate of absorption of many slightly soluble drugs from the gastrointestinal tract and other sites is limited by the rate of dissolution of the drug. The particle size of a drug is therefore of importance if the substance in question has a low solubility. In some cases, notably that of griseofulvin, there is pharmacopoeial control of particle size; the British Pharmacopoeia (2010) specifies for this drug 'a microfine powder, the particles of which generally have a maximum dimension of up to 5 μm, although larger particles that may exceed 30 μm may occasionally be present.' The control exercised over the particle size is due to its very low solubility; the experience is that if the solubility of a drug substance is about 0.3% or less then the dissolution rate *in vivo* may be the rate-controlling step in absorption.

The Noyes–Whitney equation demonstrates that solubility is one of the main factors determining rate of solution. When the rate of solution is less than the rate of absorption, the solution process becomes rate limiting. Generally speaking, it should become so only when the drug is of low solubility at the pH of the stomach and intestinal contents. The rate of absorption, the speed of onset of effect and the duration of therapeutic response can all be determined by particle size for most routes of administration. Figure 1.19 shows the effect of particle size of phenobarbital suspensions on the drug's bioavailability after intramuscular

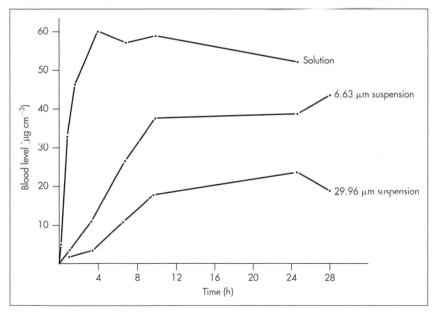

Figure 1.19 Blood levels (μg cm^{-3}) of phenobarbital versus time after intramuscular injection of three formulations.
Redrawn from Miller LG, Fincher JH, *J Pharm Sci*, 1971; 60: 1733.

injection compared with a solution of the drug, which probably precipitates in fine crystal form at the site of injection. The rate of solution of the drug crystals controls the extent of absorption from the intramuscular site.

The vital influence (for mainly aerodynamic reasons) of particle size and density in the activity of inhaled drug particles is discussed in Chapter 10, section 10.7.

The effect of particle size reduction on dissolution rate is one of exposure of increasing amounts of surface of the drug to the solvent. It is only when comminution reduces particle size below 0.1 μm that there is an effect on the intrinsic solubility of the substance (see Chapter 4), and thus on its intrinsic dissolution rate. Very small particles have a very high surface/bulk ratio. If the surface layer has a higher energy than the bulk, as is the case with these small particles, they will interact more readily with solvent to produce higher degrees of solubility.

It was with the action of phenothiazine that the importance of particle size was first recognised, in 1939, in relation to its toxicity to codling moth larvae, and in 1940 in relation to its anthelmintic effect, in both of which it was shown that reduction in particle size increased activity. The improvement in biological response to griseofulvin on micronisation is well known; similar blood levels of the drug were obtained with half the dose of micronised drug compared with those of non-micronised griseofulvin.[12] The influence of particle size on the bioavailability of digoxin[13] and dicoumarol (bishydroxycoumarin)[14] has also been investigated. In both cases, plasma levels of drug are of high significance in clinical and toxic responses.

In the case of digoxin there is evidence that milling to reduce particle size can produce an amorphous modification of the drug with enhanced solubility and hence increased bioavailability. The possibility of changing the crystal structure during processing is therefore important: comminution, recrystallisation and drying can all affect crystal properties.

During the pharmacological and toxicological testing of drugs before formal formulation exercises have been carried out, insoluble drugs are frequently administered in suspension form, often routinely in a vehicle containing gum arabic or methylcellulose. Without adequate control of particle size or adequate monitoring, the results of these tests must sometimes be in doubt, as both pharmacological activities and toxicity generally result from absorption of the drug. In a few cases particle size influences side-effects such as gastric bleeding or nausea. Gastric bleeding may in part be the direct result of contact of acidic particles of aspirin or nonsteroidal anti-inflammatory agents with the mucosal wall. The influence of drug form on the LD_{50} of pentobarbital in mice is shown in Table 1.7. A twofold range of LD_{50} values is obtained by the use of different, simple formulations of the barbiturate. Even in solution form, sodium carboxymethylcellulose affects the LD_{50} by mechanisms that are not confirmed. Adsorption of the polymer at the intestinal surface may retard absorption, or some of the drug may be adsorbed onto the polymer.

The deliberate manipulation of particle size leads to a measure of control of activity and side-effects. Rapid solution of nitrofurantoin from tablets of fine particulate material led to a high incidence of nausea

Table 1.7 Influence of formulation on the potency ratios of pentobarbital in the form of the sodium salt and the free acid[a]

Pentobarbital form	Dosage form	Vehicle	Particle size (μm)	LD_{50}	Potency ratio[b]
Sodium salt	Solution	Water	–	132	1
Sodium salt	Solution	1% NaCMC[c]	–	170	0.78
Free acid	Suspension	1% NaCMC[c]	< 44	189	0.70
Free acid	Suspension	1% NaCMC[c]	297–420	288	0.46

[a] Reproduced from Ritschel WA *et al.*, *Arzneim Forsch*, 1975; 25: 853.

[b] Relative to aqueous solution of the sodium salt.

[c] Aqueous solution of sodium carboxymethylcellulose.

in patients, as local high concentrations of the drug produce a centrally mediated nausea. Development of macrocrystalline nitrofurantoin (as in Macrodantin) has led to the introduction of a form of therapy in which the incidence of nausea is reduced. Capsules are used to avoid compression of the large crystals during manufacture. Although the urinary levels of the antibacterial are also lowered by the use of a more slowly dissolving form of the drug, levels are still adequate to produce efficient antibacterial effects.[15]

 Key points

The size of drug particles has important effects on:

- The dissolution rate, because the rate at which the drug dissolves is proportional to the surface area exposed to the solvent (see the Noyes–Whitney equation), which increases as the particle size is reduced.
- The uniformity of dosage of very potent drugs formulated as a solid dosage form; this is greater with smaller particles because of the larger number of particles constituting the dose.
- Pulmonary delivery of drugs, because only very fine particles are able to remain dispersed and thus penetrate to and deposit in the alveolar regions of the respiratory tract.
- The ability of powders to flow mainly because of its effect on the cohesivity of the particles, which increases as the particle size decreases. Particles larger than about 250 µm are usually relatively free flowing, but very fine particles (below 10 µm) are usually extremely cohesive and have a high resistance to flow.
- The rate of absorption, the speed of onset of effect and the duration of therapeutic response of slightly soluble drugs, because of its effect on their rate of dissolution.

1.7 Wetting of powders

Penetration of water into tablets or into granules precedes dissolution. The wettability of the powders, as measured by the contact angle (θ) of the substance with water (Fig. 1.20), therefore determines the contact of solvent with the particulate mass. The measurement of the contact angle gives an indication of the nature of the surface. The behaviour of crystalline materials can be related to the chemical structure of the materials concerned, as is shown by the results in Table 1.8 on a series of substituted barbiturates. The more hydrophobic the individual barbiturate molecules, the more hydrophobic the crystal that forms, although this would not be necessarily a universal finding but one dependent on the orientation of the drug molecules in the crystal and the composition of the faces, as we have already seen with adipic acid. Thus, hydrophobic drugs have dual problems: they are not readily wetted, and even when wetted they have low solubility. On the other hand, because they are lipophilic, absorption across lipid membranes is facilitated.

1.7.1 Contact angle and wettability of solid surfaces

There are many situations in which the wetting of surfaces is important, not only in the action of surfactants in aqueous media wetting hydrophobic drugs discussed above, but also in the case of polymer solution droplets spreading on tablet cores during spray coating (see Chapter 7). Tear fluids wet the cornea, and dewetting results in dry eye syndrome (see Chapter 10). A representation of the several forces acting on a drop of liquid placed on a flat, solid surface is shown in Fig. 1.20a. The surface tension of the solid, $\gamma_{S/A}$, will favour spreading of the liquid, but this is opposed by the solid–liquid interfacial tension, $\gamma_{S/L}$, and the horizontal component of the surface tension of the liquid $\gamma_{L/A}$ in the plane of the solid surface, that is $\gamma_{L/A} \cos \theta$. Equating these forces gives

$$\gamma_{S/A} = \gamma_{S/L} + \gamma_{L/A} \cos \theta \qquad (1.5)$$

Equation (1.5) is generally referred to as *Young's equation*. The angle θ is termed the *contact angle*. The condition for complete wetting of a solid surface

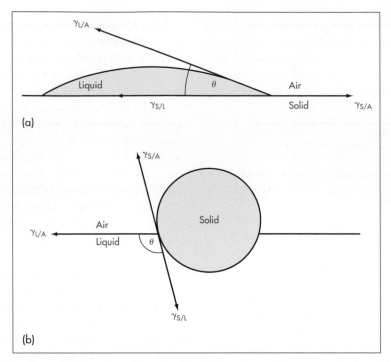

Figure 1.20 Equilibrium between forces acting on (a) a drop of liquid on a solid surface, and (b) a partially immersed solid.

Table 1.8 Relationship between chemical structure of barbiturates and contact angle (θ) with water[a]

R¹	R²	θ (deg)
Et	Et	70
Et	Bu	78
Et	$CH_2CH_2CH(CH_3)_2$	102
$-CH-CH_3$ $\ CH_3$	$CH_2-CH=CH_2$	75
$-CH_2-CHCH_3$ $\ CH_3$	$CH_2-CH=CH_2$	87

[a] Reproduced from Lerk CF *et al.*, *J Pharm Sci*, 1977; 66: 1480.

is that the contact angle should be zero. This condition is fulfilled when the forces of attraction between the liquid and solid are equal to or greater than those between liquid and liquid.

The type of wetting in which a liquid spreads over the surface of the solid is referred to as *spreading wetting*. The tendency for spreading may be quantified in terms of the spreading coefficient S, where $S = \gamma_{S/A} - (\gamma_{S/L} + \gamma_{L/A})$. The surface tension at the solid–air interface is not a readily measured parameter, but this term may be replaced by substitution from equation (1.5) giving

$$S = \gamma_{L/A}(\cos \theta - 1) \qquad (1.6)$$

If the contact angle is larger than $0°$, the term ($\cos \theta - 1$) will be negative, as will the value of S. The condition for complete, spontaneous wetting is thus a *zero* value for the contact angle.

A useful indicator of the wettability of a solid surface is its *critical surface tension for spreading*, γ_c. This parameter is determined from measurements of the contact angle θ of drops of a series of liquids of known surface tension when placed on a flat nonporous surface of the chosen solid. Extrapolation of a plot of $\cos \theta$ against surface tension (a Zisman plot) to a value of $\cos \theta = 1$ (i.e. to $\theta = 0$) (see Fig. 1.21) provides a value of γ_c.

Figure 1.21 Determination of critical surface tension for wetting, γ_c, from a plot of the cosine of the contact angle against surface tension.

Only those liquids or solutions having a surface tension less than γ_c will wet the surface. γ_c is a characteristic property of a solid and is determined by the polarity; solid hydrocarbons and waxes have a low critical surface tension and will be wetted only by solutions of low surface tension, more polar solids such as those of nylon and cellulose have higher γ_c values and consequently are more easily wetted. Human skin has a γ_c of between 22 and 30 mN m^{-1} and it is usual to add surfactants to lotions for application to the skin to ensure adequate wetting. Similarly, insecticide sprays have to be formulated to wet the surfaces of leaves.

The measurement of γ_c values for tablet surfaces can provide useful information for use in developing an adequate film coating for the tablets. For example, pure acetylsalicylic acid tablets present a surface with a γ_c value of about 31 mN m^{-1}. The addition of a lubricant such as magnesium stearate decreases the γ_c value because of the surface is richer in $-CH_3$ and $-CH_2$ groups, whereas the inclusion in the tablet of excipients such as starch, cellulose and talc results in surface richer in $=O$ and $-OH$, causing an increase in γ_c value. Increased γ_c values result in increased wetting by the coating solution and an increased bonding force between the tablet surface and the polymer film coating after the solvent has evaporated.

1.7.2 Wettability of powders

When a solid is immersed in a liquid, the initial wetting process is referred to as *immersional wetting*. The effectiveness of immersional wetting may be related to the contact angle that the solid makes with the liquid–air interface (see Fig. 1.20b). The condition for complete immersion of the solid in the liquid is that there should be a decrease in surface free energy as a result of the immersion process. Once the solid is submerged in the liquid, the process of spreading wetting (see the previous section) becomes important.

Table 1.9 gives the contact angles of a series of pharmaceutical powders. These values were determined using compacts of the powder (produced by compressing the powder in a large-diameter tablet die) and a saturated aqueous solution of each compound as the test liquid. Many of the powders are slightly hydrophobic (for example, indometacin and stearic acid), or even strongly hydrophobic (for example, magnesium stearate, phenylbutazone and chloramphenicol palmitate). Formulation of these drugs as suspensions (for example, Chloramphenicol Palmitate Oral Suspension USP) presents wetting problems. Table 1.9 shows that θ can be affected by the crystallographic structure, as for chloramphenicol palmitate. Surface modification or changes in crystal structure are clearly not routine methods of lowering the contact angle and the normal method of improving wettability is by the inclusion of surfactants in the formulation. The surfactants not only reduce $\gamma_{L/A}$ but also adsorb onto the surface of the powder, thus reducing $\gamma_{S/L}$. Both of these effects reduce the contact angle and improve the dispersibility of the powder.

Key points

- The type of wetting that occurs when a liquid spreads over a solid surface is referred to as spreading wetting. The tendency for spreading is described by the spreading coefficient, which for spontaneous spreading should be positive or zero. The value of the spreading coefficient depends on the contact angle; complete wetting occurs when the contact angle is zero.
- Solid surfaces may be characterised by their critical surface tension for wetting, γ_c; low γ_c values indicate poor wetting properties.
- The process of initial wetting when a powder is immersed in a liquid is referred to as immersional wetting. Wetting problems occur when the contact angle is greater than 90°; several pharmaceutical powders have been identified that, because of their high contact angle, present wetting problems.
- Wettability may be improved by the inclusion of surfactants in the formulation.

Table 1.9 Contact angles of some pharmaceutical powders[a]

Material	Contact angle θ (deg)	Material	Contact angle θ (deg)
Acetylsalicylic acid (aspirin)	74	Lactose	30
Aluminium stearate	120	Magnesium stearate	121
Aminophylline	47	Nitrofurantoin	69
Ampicillin (anhydrous)	35	Phenylbutazone	109
Ampicillin (trihydrate)	21	Prednisolone	43
Caffeine	43	Prednisone	63
Calcium carbonate	58	Salicyclic acid	103
Calcium stearate	115	Stearic acid	98
Chloramphenicol	59	Succinylsulfathiazole	64
Chloramphenicol palmitate (α form)	122	Sulfadiazine	71
Chloramphenicol palmitate (β form)	108	Sulfamethazine	48
Diazepam	83	Sulfathiazole	53
Digoxin	49	Theophylline	48
Indometacin	90	Tolbutamide	72
Isoniazid	49		

[a] Selected values from Lerk CF *et al.*, *J Pharm Sci*, 1976; 65: 843; *J Pharm Sci*, 1977; 66: 1481.

1.8 Sublimation

Sublimation, i.e. the direct transition from the solid to the vapour phase, forms the basis of the widely used technique of *freeze drying* for the drying of heat-sensitive materials such as proteins and blood products. The process may be understood by reference to the phase diagram for water (Fig. 1.22) which shows the changes in the melting point of ice and the boiling point of water as the external pressure above the water is decreased from atmospheric pressure. Also shown is the equilibrium between ice and vapour when the external pressure has been reduced below the *triple point*, when all the liquid water has been solidified. The triple point is the unique point at which all three phases co-exist. In the process of freeze drying, an aqueous solution of the heat-sensitive material is frozen and its pressure is reduced to below the triple point; a small amount of heat is then supplied to increase the temperature to the sublimation curve at which the ice changes directly to vapour without passing through the liquid phase. The pressure is prevented from increasing above the triple point during the freeze drying process by removing the vapour as it is formed. Removal of water, i.e. drying, is therefore achieved at temperatures well below room temperature, so preventing decomposition of the thermolabile product.

The handling and storage of some drugs in their solid state can pose problems arising from the sublimation of the drug. Evidence for a transition from solid to vapour is seen from the haze developed on the inner walls of the glass vials containing solid

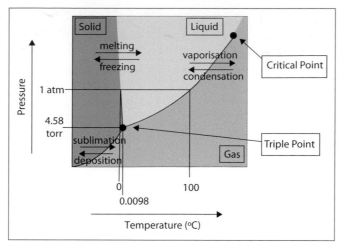

Figure 1.22 Phase diagram of water (not to scale) showing the boundaries between liquid, solid and vapour phases.

Box 1.1 The Clausius–Clapeyron equation

The Clausius–Clapeyron, which concerns the variation of vapour pressure with temperature, is usually derived from a consideration of the equilibrium between vapour and liquid phases, although in its generalised form it is equally applicable to solid–liquid equilibria. The increased motion of the molecules of the liquid following an increase of temperature leads to a greater tendency for escape of molecules into the vapour phase, with a consequent increase of vapour pressure. The variation of vapour pressure with temperature may be expressed in terms of the molar enthalpy of vaporisation of the liquid, ΔH_{vap}, using the Clapeyron equation:

$$\frac{dP}{dT} = \frac{\Delta H_{vap}}{T \Delta V} \tag{1.7}$$

In this equation ΔV is the difference in molar volumes of the two phases. Since the molar volume of the vapour, V_v, is very much larger than that of the liquid, ΔV may be approximately equated with V_v. If it is also assumed that the vapour obeys the ideal gas equation, so that V_v may be replaced by RT/P, equation (1.7) reduces to

$$\frac{dP}{dT} = \frac{P \Delta H_{vap}}{RT^2}$$

or

$$\frac{d \ln P}{dT} = \frac{\Delta H_{vap}}{RT^2} \tag{1.8}$$

Equation (1.8) is the Clausius–Clapeyron equation. General integration, assuming ΔH_{vap} to be constant, gives

$$\log P = \frac{-\Delta H_{vap}}{2.303 RT} + \text{constant} \tag{1.9}$$

A plot of log vapour pressure versus reciprocal temperature should be linear with a slope of $-\Delta H_{vap}/2.303R$, from which values of enthalpy of vaporisation may be determined.

ibuprofen when these are stored at 40°C.[16] The Clausius–Clapeyron equation describes the variation of vapour pressure with temperature (see Box 1.1). Over the temperature range 23–64°C ibuprofen vapour pressure–temperature data obey a generalised form of the Clausius–Clapeyron equation:

$$\log P = \frac{-\Delta H_{vap}}{2.303RT} + \text{constant}$$

where P is the vapour pressure and ΔH_{vap} is the molar enthalpy of vaporisation of ibuprofen (121 kJ mol^{-1}). Figure 1.23 shows that although the vapour pressure exerted at 25°C is negligible (9×10^{-6} torr), the value increases by several orders of magnitude as the temperature is increased and as a result the rate of loss of ibuprofen becomes significant at higher temperatures. For example, the measured weight loss at 55°C is 4.15 mg day^{-1}. Weight losses of this magnitude are significant during drying and coating processes and during accelerated stability testing procedures.

Two factors – the vapour pressure of the drug and the particle size – are influential in determining the rate of evaporation of the drug in powdered form. Table 1.10 shows the significantly higher evaporation times calculated for several widely used antineoplastic agents when the mean particle size is 1 μm compared with those of 100 μm particles and emphasises the greatly increased risks involved when handling fine powder.

Clinical point

A further example of the applicability of the Clausius–Clapeyron equation is in the assessment of risk associated with the handling of hazardous drugs, particularly by personnel who are potentially exposed to cytostatic agents routinely used for cancer chemotherapy. Most of the contamination detected with cytostatics occurs because of spillage, inhalation of aerosolised liquid (which can occur for example when a needle is withdrawn from a drug vial) or direct contact with contaminated material such as gloves. There is, however, also evidence that cytotoxic agents evaporate and form a vapour during normal handling, which presents a risk to personnel from inhalation of this vapour.[17]

The influence of temperature on the vapour pressure of these drugs is plotted according to equation (1.9) in Fig. 1.24. The vapour above the drugs behaves as an ideal gas because of the low quantity of drug transferred to the gaseous phase and the Clausius–Clapeyron equation is obeyed in all cases. The vapour pressure of carmustine is about 10–100 times greater than that of the other antineoplastic agents and approaches that of mercury (1.0 Pa at 40°C) at elevated temperature, with implications for occupational safety when handling this drug.

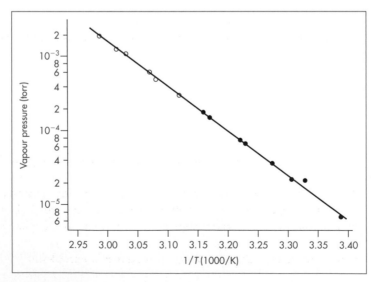

Figure 1.23 Ibuprofen vapour pressure data plotted according to the Clausius–Clapeyron equation (equation 1.9).

Reproduced with permission from reference 16.

Table 1.10 Vapour pressure and evaporation time for drug particles of diameter, d^a

Compound	Measured vapour pressure (Pa)		Calculated evaporation time (s)	
	20°C	40°C	$d = 1\mu m$	$d = 100\ \mu m$
Carmustine	0.019	0.530	12	1.2×10^5
Cisplatin	0.0018	0.0031	110	11.0×10^5
Cyclophosphamide	0.0033	0.0090	44	4.4×10^5
Etoposide	0.0026	0.0038	51	5.1×10^5
Fluorouracil	0.0014	0.0039	210	21.0×10^5

[a] Reproduced from reference 17.

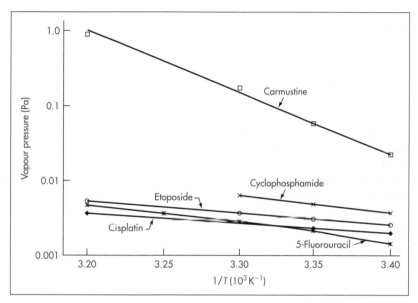

Figure 1.24 The vapour pressures of antineoplastic agents plotted according to the Clausius–Clapeyron equation.
Redrawn from reference 17.

Key points

- The process by which solids pass directly from the solid phase to the vapour phase is referred to as sublimation.
- Sublimation forms the basis of the technique of freeze drying for the drying of thermolabile materials.
- Sublimation can cause weight loss of some drugs when they are stored in the solid state. The rate of weight loss increases with temperature according to the Clausius–Clapeyron equation.
- Sublimation of some toxic drugs during handling can present safety problems.

1.9 Solid dispersions

Over the past few years interest has been shown in *solid solutions* of drugs in attempts to change the biopharmaceutical properties of drugs that are poorly soluble or difficult to wet. The object is usually to provide a system in which the crystallinity of the drug is so altered as to change its solubility and solution rate, and to surround the drug intimately with water-soluble material. A solid solution comprises solute and solvent – a solid solute molecularly dispersed in a solid solvent. These systems are sometimes termed *mixed crystals* because the two components crystallise together in a homogeneous one-phase system. They should, however, be distinguished from co-crystals (see section 1.2.4) which are *single* crystalline forms consisting of two types of molecule. For understanding of the systems and their potential use, an arbitrary system might be considered.

In Fig. 1.25, the melting temperature of mixtures of A and B is plotted against mixture composition. On addition of B to A or of A to B, melting points are reduced. At a particular composition the *eutectic point* is reached, the eutectic mixture (the composition at that point) having the lowest melting point of any mixture of A and B. Below the eutectic temperature, no liquid phase exists. The phenomenon is important because of the change in the crystallinity at this point.

If we cool a solution of A and B that is richer in A than the eutectic mixture (see M in Fig. 1.25), crystals of pure A will appear. As the solution is cooled further, more and more A crystallises out and the solution becomes richer in B. When the eutectic temperature is reached, however, the remaining solution crystallises out, forming a microcrystalline mixture of pure A and pure B, differing markedly at least in superficial characteristics from either of the pure solids. This has obvious pharmaceutical possibilities. This method of obtaining microcrystalline dispersions for administration of drugs involves the formation of a eutectic mixture composed of drug and a substance readily soluble in water. The soluble 'carrier' dissolves, leaving the drug in a fine state of solution *in vivo*, usually in a state that predisposes to rapid solution.

This technique has been applied to several poorly soluble drugs such as griseofulvin. A griseofulvin–succinic acid (soluble carrier) system has a eutectic point at 0.29 mole fraction of drug (55% w/w griseofulvin) (Fig. 1.26a). The eutectic mixture consists here of two physically separate phases; one is almost pure griseofulvin, while the other is a saturated solid solution of griseofulvin in succinic acid. The solid solution contains about 25% griseofulvin; the eutectic mixture, which has a fixed ratio of drug to carrier, thus comprises 60% solid solution and 40% almost pure griseofulvin. As can be seen from Fig. 1.26b,

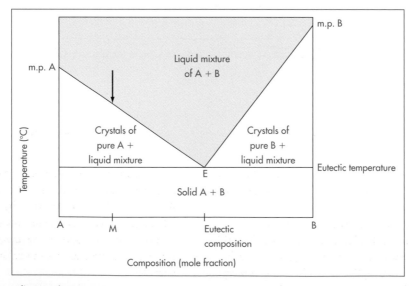

Figure 1.25 Phase diagram (temperature versus composition) showing boundaries between liquid and solid phases, and the eutectic point, E.

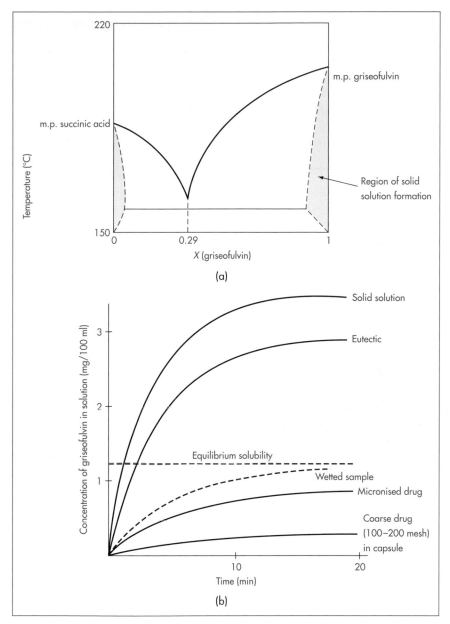

Figure 1.26 (a) Griseofulvin–succinic acid phase diagram. (b) Rate of solution of griseofulvin solid solutions, eutectic and crystalline material.

which shows the solution profiles of the different forms, the solid solution dissolves 6–7 times faster than pure griseofulvin.

The simplest eutectic mixtures are usually prepared by the rapid solidification of the fused liquid mixture of components that show complete miscibility in the liquid state and negligible solid–solid solubility. In addition to the reduction in crystalline size, the following factors may contribute to faster dissolution rate of drugs in eutectic mixtures:

- An increase in drug solubility because of the extremely small particle size of the solid
- A possible solubilisation effect by the carrier, which may operate in the diffusion layer immediately surrounding the drug particle
- Absence of aggregation and agglomeration of the particles
- Improved wettability in the intimate drug–carrier mixture
- Crystallisation in metastable forms

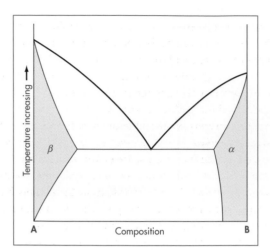

Figure 1.27 Melting point–composition plot for a system in which α and β are regions of solid solution formation. Each component dissolves the other component to some extent above the eutectic temperature. As the temperature is lowered, the solid solution regions become narrower.

Where more complex solubility patterns emerge, as with the griseofulvin and succinic acid phase, the phase diagram becomes correspondingly more complex. Figure 1.27 shows one example of a system in which each component dissolves in the other above and below the eutectic temperature.

Other systems that form eutectic mixtures are chloramphenicol–urea, sulfathiazole–urea, and niacinamide–ascorbic acid. The solid solution of chloramphenicol in urea was found to dissolve twice as rapidly as a physical mixture of the same composition and about four times as rapidly as the pure drug. *In vivo*, however, the system failed to display improved bioavailability. On the other hand, the eutectic mixture of sulfathiazole–urea did give higher blood levels than pure sulfonamide.

1.9.1 Eutectics and drug identification

As the eutectic temperature of a substance in mixtures with other compounds is, as a rule, different even when the other substances have the same melting point, this parameter can be used for identification purposes. Benzanilide (m.p. 163°C), phenacetin (m.p. 134.5°C) and salophen (m.p. 191°C) are often used as test substances. The eutectic temperatures of mixtures of benzanilide with various drugs are shown in Table 1.11. Substances of identical melting points can be distinguished by measurement of the eutectic temperature with another suitable compound.

Ternary eutectics are also possible. The binary eutectic points of three mixtures are as follows: for aminophenazone–phenacetin 82°C; for aminophenazone–caffeine 103.5°C; and for phenacetin–caffeine 125°C. The ternary eutectic temperature of aminophenazone–phenacetin–caffeine is 81°C. In this mixture the presence of aminophenazone and phenacetin can be detected by the mixed melting point test, but the caffeine causes little depression of the eutectic given by the other two components.

The possibility of determining eutectic temperatures of multicomponent mixtures has practical value

Table 1.11 Eutectic temperatures of drugs with benzanilide[a]

Compound	Melting point (°C)	Eutectic temperature (°C)
Allobarbital	173	144
Ergotamine	172–174	135
Imipramine HCl	172–174	109

[a] Reproduced from Kuhnert-Brandstatter M, *Thermomicroscopy in the Analysis of Pharmaceuticals*, New York: Pergamon Press; 1971.

 Clinical point **A formulation containing a eutectic**

A topical preparation is available for intradermal anaesthesia to reduce the pain of venepuncture. The cream, Emla (Eutectic Mixture of Local Anaesthetics) (AstraZeneca), contains a eutectic of procaine and lidocaine.[18] The eutectic mixture (50 : 50 mixture) is an oil, which is then formulated as an oil-in-water emulsion. This allows much higher concentrations than would have been possible by using the individual drugs dissolved in an oil.

in another respect. During tableting, for example, heat is generated in the punch and die and in the powder compact; measurement of the eutectic temperature can give information on whether this rise in temperature is likely to cause problems of melting and fusion.

 Key points

- A solid solution comprises a solid solute molecularly dispersed in a solid solvent and is designed to provide a system in which the drug is surrounded intimately with water-soluble material (carrier) and its crystallinity is so altered as to increase its solubility and solution rate.
- Mixing of the drug with a soluble carrier reduces the freezing point; the lowest temperature at which the system freezes/melts is called the eutectic point and below this point the mixture is composed of a microcrystalline dispersion of pure drug and carrier.
- Pharmaceutical examples of solid dispersions include griseofulvin–succinic acid, chloramphenicol–urea, sulfathiazole–urea, and niacinamide–ascorbic acid.
- Substances having identical melting points can be distinguished by measurement of the eutectic temperature with another suitable compound.

Summary

In this chapter we have examined those aspects of the structure of crystalline and amorphous solids that influence their formulation and the properties, both physical and pharmacological, of the formulated product. We have seen that crystal lattices are constructed from repeating units called unit cells of which there are 14 possible types (Bravais lattices) and which, for any particular compound, are all of the same size and contain the same number of molecules or ions arranged in the same way. The external

appearance of the crystal, that is its habit, is affected by the rate of crystallisation and by the presence of impurities, particularly surfactants. The habit of a crystal is of pharmaceutical importance, since it affects the compression characteristics and flow properties of the drug during tableting and also the ease with which the suspensions of insoluble drugs will pass through syringe needles. Many high-molecular-weight materials, particularly polymers, are unable to form crystals and exist as amorphous or semicrystalline solids. These materials do not have sharp melting points but change their properties at a glass transition temperature, T_g, from a glassy state below T_g to a more mobile or rubbery state as the temperature is increased.

Problems arising from the occurrence of drug polymorphs – a largely unpredictable phenomenon – have been discussed. The various polymorphs of a particular drug have different physical and chemical properties and usually exist in different habits. The transformation between polymorphic forms can cause formulation problems; phase transformations can cause changes in crystal size, which in suspensions can eventually cause caking, and in creams can cause detrimental changes in the feel of the cream. Changes in polymorphic form of vehicles, such as theobroma oil used to make suppositories, can result in unacceptable melting characteristics. Problems may also result from phase transformation when attempting to identify drugs using infrared spectroscopy. The most significant consequence of polymorphism is the possible difference in the bioavailability of the different polymorphic forms of a drug as, for example, in the case of polymorphs of chloramphenicol palmitate. The entrapment of solvent during crystallisation can result in polymorphic solvates in which the entrapped solvent becomes an integral part of the crystal structure, or pseudopolymorphic solvates, in which the solvent is not part of the crystal bonding and merely occupies voids in the crystal. Similarly, co-crystals may be formed in which a solid is hydrogen bonded to the drug. The formation of crystal solvates and co-crystals can significantly affect the aqueous solubility and also the dissolution characteristics of the drug.

The rate of absorption of many slightly soluble drugs from the gastrointestinal tract and other sites is limited by the rate of dissolution of the drug. The particle size of a drug is therefore of importance if the substance in question has a low solubility. The rate of dissolution of a solid can be increased by reduction in the particle size, providing that this does not induce changes in polymorphic form, which could alter the drug's solubility. The reduction of particle size of some drugs to below 0.1 μm can cause an increase in the intrinsic solubility. This is the basis of a method for increasing the rate of dissolution and solubility of poorly soluble drugs such as griseofulvin, by forming a eutectic mixture or solid dispersion with a highly soluble carrier compound. The cohesivity of particles increases with decrease of the particle size, with consequences for the flow properties of powders; particles larger than about 250 μm are usually relatively free flowing, but very fine particles (below 10 μm) are usually extremely cohesive and have a high resistance to flow. Penetration of water into tablets or into granules precedes dissolution. The wettability of the powders, as measured by the contact angle (θ) of the substance with water, therefore determines the contact of solvent with the particulate mass.

The contact angle is an indicator of the ability of a liquid to wet a solid surface; for complete, spontaneous wetting the contact angle should be zero. There are two types of wetting – spreading wetting, in which a liquid spreads over the surface of a solid, and immersional wetting, which is the initial wetting process that occurs when a solid is immersed in a liquid. Several pharmaceutical powders have been identified that, because of their high contact angle, present wetting problems.

References

1. Pilpel N. Powders – gaseous, liquid and solid. *Endeavour (NS)* 1982;6:183–188.

2. Mullin JW. Crystallization 4th edn London: Butterworth-Heinemann, 2001.
3. Michaels AS, Colville AR. The effect of surface-active agents on crystal growth rate and crystal habit. *J Phys Chem* 1960;64:13–19.
4. Vippagunta SR *et al.* Crystalline solids. *Adv Drug Deliv Rev* 2001;48:3–26.
5. Agafonov V *et al.* Polymorphism of spironolactone. *J Pharm Sci* 1991;80:181–185.
6. Nichols G, Frampton CS. Physicochemical characterization of the orthorhombic polymorph of paracetamol crystallized from solution. *J Pharm Sci* 1998;87:684–693.
7. Koda A *et al.* Characterization of chloramphenicol palmitate form C and absorption assessments of chloramphenicol palmitate polymorphs. *J Pharm Sci Technol Jpn* 2000;60:43–52.
8. Aiguiar AJ, Zelmer JE. Dissolution behaviour of polymorphs of chloramphenicol palmitate and mefanamic acid. *J Pharm Sci* 1969;58:983–987.
9. Chapman JH *et al.* Polymorphism of cephaloridine. *J Pharm Pharmacol* 1968;20:418–429.
10. Volkheimer G. Persorption of particles: physiology and pharmacology. *Adv Pharmacol Chemother* 1977;14: 163–187.
11. Florence AT. The oral absorption of micro- and nanoparticulates: neither exceptional nor unusual. *Pharm Res* 1997;14:259–266.
12. Atkinson RM *et al.* Effect of particle size on blood griseofulvin levels in man. *Nature* 1962;193: 588–589.
13. Shaw TRD *et al.* Particle size and absorption of digoxin. *Lancet* 1973;2:209–210.
14. Nash JF *et al.* Relation between the particle size of dicoumarol and its bioavailability in dogs. I. Capsules. *Drug Dev Commun* 1975;1:443–457.
15. Fincher JH. Particle size of drugs and its relationship to absorption and activity. *J Pharm Sci* 1968;57: 1825–1835.
16. Ertel KD *et al.* Determination of ibuprofen vapor pressure at temperatures of pharmaceutical interest. *J Pharm Sci* 1990;79:552.
17. Kiffmeyer TK *et al.* Vapour pressures, evaporation behaviour and airborne concentrations of hazardous drugs: implications for occupational safety. *Pharm J* 2002;268:331–337.
18. Broberg, Evers HCA. *Local anaesthetic emulsion cream.* Eur Pat 0 002 425 (1981).

2

Physicochemical properties of drugs in solution

In this chapter we examine some of the important physicochemical properties of drugs in aqueous solution that are of relevance to such liquid dosage forms as injections, solutions and eye drops. Some basic thermodynamic concepts will be introduced, particularly that of thermodynamic activity, an important parameter in determining drug potency. It is important that parenteral solutions are formulated with osmotic pressure close to that of blood serum; in this chapter we will see how to adjust the tonicity of the formulation to achieve this aim. Most drugs are at least partially ionised at physiological pH and many studies have suggested that the charged group is essential for biological activity. We look at the influence of pH on the ionisation of several types of drug in solution and consider equations that allow the calculation of the pH of solutions of these drugs.

First, however, we recount the various ways to express the strength of a solution, since it is of fundamental importance that we are able to interpret the various units used to denote solution concentration and to understand their interrelationships, not least in practice situations.

2.1 Concentration units

A wide range of units is commonly used to express solution concentration, and confusion often arises in the interconversion of one set of units to another. Wherever possible throughout this book we have used the SI system of units. Although this is the currently recommended system of units in Great Britain, other more traditional systems are still widely used. Some useful conversions between concentration units are given in Box 2.1.

Box 2.1 Conversion into SI units

- *Volume* is commonly expressed in litres (L) and millilitres (mL) rather than the SI unit of cubic metres (m^3).

$$1\,L = 1\,dm^3 = 10^{-3}\,m^3$$
$$1\,mL = 1\,cm^3 = 10^{-6}\,m^3$$

- *Concentration* is often given in grams per litre ($g\,L^{-1}$) rather than kilograms per cubic metre ($kg\,m^{-3}$).

$$1\,g\,L^{-1} = 1\,g\ dm^{-3} = 1\,kg\,m^{-3}$$

Note also that $1\,mg\,mL^{-1}$ is therefore also equal to $1\,kg\,m^{-3}$.

- *Molarity* is commonly expressed as $mol\,L^{-1}$ and often written using the symbol M or M; its conversion to SI units is

$$1\,mol\,L^{-1}(or\ 1\,M) = 1\,mol\,dm^{-3}$$
$$= 10^3\,mol\,m^{-3}$$

2.1.1 Weight or volume concentration

Concentration is often expressed as the weight of solute in a unit volume of solution; for example, $g\,dm^{-3}$, or as % w/v, which is the number of grams of solute in 100 mL of solution. When the solute is a liquid, the concentration may also be expressed as the volume of solute in a unit volume of solution, for example as % v/v, which is the number of mL of solute in 100 mL of solution. These are not exact methods when working at a range of temperatures, since the volume of the solution is temperature dependent and hence the weight or volume concentrations also change with temperature.

Whenever a hydrated compound is used it is important to use the correct state of hydration in the calculation of weight concentration. Thus, 10% w/v $CaCl_2$ (anhydrous) is approximately equivalent to 20% w/v $CaCl_2 \cdot 6H_2O$ and consequently the use of the vague statement '10% calcium chloride' could result in gross error.

When very dilute solutions are involved the concentration may be expressed as parts per million (or ppm), which is the number of grams in 10^6 grams of solution (which equals the number of mg per kg of solution) or, if the solute is a liquid, the number of mL in 10^6 mL (1000 litres) of solution. Since the density of very dilute aqueous solutions at room temperature approximates to $1\,g\,mL^{-1}$, a concentration of 1 ppm is approximately 1 mg of solute per litre of solution (i.e. 1 g in 10^6 mL).

2.1.2 Molarity and molality

These two similar-sounding terms should not be confused. The *molarity* of a solution is the number of moles (gram molecular weights) of solute in 1 litre ($1\,dm^3$) of *solution*. The *molality* is the number of moles of solute in 1 kg of *solvent*. Molality has the unit, $mol\,kg^{-1}$, which is an accepted SI unit. Molarity may be converted to SI units as shown in Box 2.1; interconversion between molarity and molality requires knowledge of the density of the solution.

Of the two units, molality is preferable for a precise expression of concentration because, unlike molarity, it does not depend on the solution temperature; also, the molality of a component in a solution remains unaltered by the addition of a second solute, whereas the molarity of the first component decreases because the total volume of solution increases following the addition of the second solute.

2.1.3 Milliequivalents

These units are commonly used clinically in expressing the concentration of an ion in solution. The term 'equivalent' or 'gram equivalent weight' is analogous to the mole or gram molecular weight. When monovalent ions are considered, these two terms are identical. A 1 molar ($1\,mol\,L^{-1}$) solution of sodium bicarbonate (sodium hydrogen carbonate), $NaHCO_3$, contains 1 mol or 1 Eq of Na^+ and 1 mol or 1 Eq of HCO_3^- per litre of solution. With multivalent ions, attention must be paid to the valency of each ion; for example, 10% w/v $CaCl_2 \cdot 2H_2O$ contains 6.8 mmol or 13.6 mEq of Ca^{2+} in $10\,cm^3$.

The Pharmaceutical Codex[1] gives a table of milliequivalents for various ions and also a simple

Box 2.2 Calculation of milliequivalents

The number of milliequivalents in 1 g of substance is given by

$$mEq = \frac{\text{valency} \times 1000 \times \text{no. of specified units in 1 atom/molecule/ion}}{\text{atomic, molecular or ionic weight}}$$

For example, $CaCl_2 \cdot 2H_2O$ (mol wt $= 147.0$ Da):

> $mEq\ Ca^{2+}$ in 1 g $CaCl_2 \cdot 2H_2O$
> $= (2 \times 1000 \times 1)/147.0 = 13.6\ mEq$

and

> $mEq\ Cl^-$ in 1 g $CaCl_2 \cdot 2H_2O$
> $= (1 \times 1000 \times 2)/147.0 = 13.6\ mEq$

that is, each gram of $CaCl_2 \cdot 2H_2O$ represents 13.6 mEq of calcium and 13.6 mEq of chloride.

---

formula for the calculation of milliequivalents per litre (see Box 2.2).

In analytical chemistry, a solution that contains 1 Eq per litre is referred to as a *normal* solution. Unfortunately the term 'normal' is also used to mean physiologically normal with reference to saline solution. In this usage, a physiologically normal saline solution contains 0.9 g NaCl in 100 cm^3 aqueous solution and not 1 equivalent (58.44 g) per litre.

2.1.4 Mole fraction

The mole fraction of a component of a solution is the number of moles of that component divided by the total number of moles present in solution. In a two-component (binary) solution, the mole fraction of solvent, x_1, is given by $x_1 = n_1/(n_1 + n_2)$, where n_1 and n_2, are respectively the number of moles of solvent and solute present in solution. Similarly, the mole fraction of solute, x_2, is given by $x_2 = n_2/(n_1 + n_2)$. The sum of the mole fractions of all components is, of course, unity, i.e. for a binary solution, $x_1 + x_2 = 1$.

Example 2.1 Units of concentration

Isotonic saline contains 0.9% w/v of sodium chloride (mol wt $= 58.5$ Da). Express the concentration of this solution as: (a) molarity; (b) molality; (c) mole fraction and (d) milliequivalents of Na^+ per litre. Assume that the density of isotonic saline is 1 g cm^{-3}.

Answer $9g/58.5 = 0\ 154$

(a) 0.9% w/v solution of sodium chloride contains 9 g dm^{-3} $= 0.154$ mol dm^{-3}.

(b) 9 g of sodium chloride are dissolved in 991 g of water (assuming density $= 1$ g cm^{-3}). Therefore, 1000 g of water contains 9.08 g of sodium chloride $= 0.155$ mol, i.e. molality $= 0.155$ mol kg^{-1}.

(c) Mole fraction of sodium chloride, x_1, is given by

> $x_1 = n_1/(n_1 + n_2)$
> $= 0.154/(0.154 + 55.06)$
> $= 2.79 \times 10^{-3}$

(Note: 991 g of water contains 991/18 moles, i.e. $n_2 = 55.06$.)

(d) Since Na^+ is monovalent, the number of milliequivalents of $Na^+ =$ number of millimoles. Therefore, the solution contains 154 mEq dm^{-3} of Na^+.

2.2 Thermodynamics – a brief introduction

The importance of thermodynamics in the pharmaceutical sciences is apparent when it is realised that such processes as the partitioning of solutes between immiscible solvents, the solubility of drugs, micellisation and drug–receptor interaction can all be treated in thermodynamic terms. This brief section merely introduces some of the concepts of thermodynamics that are referred to throughout the book. Readers requiring a greater depth of treatment should consult standard texts on this subject.[2]

2.2.1 Energy

Energy is a fundamental property of a system. Some idea of its importance may be gained by considering its role in chemical reactions, where it determines what reactions may occur, how fast the reaction may proceed, and in which direction the reaction will occur. Energy takes several forms: *kinetic energy* is that which a body possesses as a result of its motion; *potential energy* is the energy a body has due to its position, whether gravitational potential energy or coulombic potential energy associated with charged particles at a given distance apart. All forms of energy are related, but in converting between the various types it is not possible to create or destroy energy. This forms the basis of the *law of conservation of energy*.

The *internal energy* U of a system is the sum of all the kinetic and potential energy contributions to the energy of all the atoms, ions and molecules in that system. In thermodynamics we are concerned with *change* in internal energy, ΔU, rather than the internal energy itself. (Notice the use of Δ to denote a finite change.) We may change the internal energy of a closed system (one that cannot exchange matter with its surroundings) in only two ways: by transferring energy as *work* (w) or as *heat* (q). An expression for the change in internal energy is

$$\Delta U = w + q \tag{2.1}$$

If the system releases its energy to the surroundings, ΔU is negative, i.e. the total internal energy has been reduced. Where heat is absorbed (as in an endothermic process), the internal energy will increase and consequently q is positive. Conversely, in a process that releases heat (an exothermic process) the internal energy is decreased and q is negative. Similarly, when energy is supplied to the system as work, w is positive and when the system loses energy by doing work, w is negative.

It is frequently necessary to consider infinitesimally small changes in a property; we denote these by the use of d rather than Δ. Thus, for an infinitesimal change in internal energy we write equation (2.1) as

$$\mathrm{d}u = \mathrm{d}w + \mathrm{d}q \tag{2.2}$$

We can see from this equation that it does not really matter whether energy is supplied as heat or as work or as a mixture of the two: the change in internal energy is the same. Equation (2.2) thus expresses the principle of the law of conservation of energy but is much wider in its application since it involves changes in heat energy, which were not encompassed in the conservation law.

It follows from equation (2.2) that a system that is completely isolated from its surroundings, such that it cannot exchange heat or interact mechanically to do work, cannot experience any change in its internal energy. In other words, *the internal energy of an isolated system is constant* – this is the *first law of thermodynamics*.

2.2.2 Enthalpy

When a change occurs in a system at *constant pressure* as, for example, in a chemical reaction in an open vessel, the increase in internal energy is not equal to the energy supplied as heat because some energy will have been lost by the work done (against the atmosphere) during the expansion of the system. It is convenient, therefore, to consider the heat change in isolation from the accompanying changes in work. For this reason we consider a property that is equal to the heat supplied at constant pressure: this property is called the *enthalpy* (H). We can define enthalpy by

$$\Delta H = q \text{ at constant pressure} \tag{2.3}$$

ΔH is positive when heat is supplied to a system that is free to change its volume and negative when the system releases heat (as in an exothermic reaction). Enthalpy is related to the internal energy of a system by the relationship

$$H = U + pV \tag{2.4}$$

where p and V are the pressure and volume of the system, respectively.

Enthalpy changes accompany such processes as the dissolution of a solute, the formation of micelles, chemical reaction, adsorption on to solids, vaporisation of a solvent, hydration of a solute, neutralisation of acids and bases, and the melting or freezing of solutes.

2.2.3 Entropy

The first law, as we have seen, deals with the conservation of energy as the system changes from one state to another, but it does not specify which particular changes will occur spontaneously. The reason why some changes have a natural tendency to occur is not that the system is moving to a lower-energy state but that there are changes in the randomness of the system. This can be seen by considering a specific example: the diffusion of one gas into another occurs without any external intervention – i.e. it is spontaneous – and yet there are no differences in either the potential or kinetic energies of the system in its equilibrium state and in its initial state where the two gases are segregated. The driving force for such spontaneous processes is the tendency for an increase in the chaos of the system – the mixed system is more disordered than the original.

A convenient measure of the randomness or disorder of a system is the *entropy* (S). When a system becomes more chaotic, its entropy increases in line with the degree of increase in disorder caused. This concept is encapsulated in the *second law of thermodynamics*, which states that *the entropy of an isolated system increases in a spontaneous change*.

The second law, then, involves entropy change, ΔS, and this is defined as the heat absorbed in a *reversible process*, q_{rev}, divided by the temperature (in kelvins) at which the change occurred.

For a finite change,

$$\Delta S = q_{rev}/T \tag{2.5}$$

and for an infinitesimal change,

$$dS = dq_{rev}/T \tag{2.6}$$

By a 'reversible process' we mean one in which the changes are carried out infinitesimally slowly, so that the system is in equilibrium with its surroundings. In this case we infer that the temperature of the surroundings is infinitesimally higher than that of the system and consequently the heat changes are occurring at an infinitely slow rate, so that the heat transfer is smooth and uniform.

We can see the link between entropy and disorder by considering some specific examples. For instance, the entropy of a perfect gas changes with its volume V according to the relationship

$$\Delta S = nR \ln \frac{V_f}{V_i} \tag{2.7}$$

where the subscripts f and i denote the final and initial states. Note that if $V_f > V_i$ (i.e. if the gas expands into a larger volume) the logarithmic (ln) term will be positive and the equation predicts an increase of entropy. This is expected since expansion of a gas is a spontaneous process and will be accompanied by an increase in the disorder because the molecules are now moving in a greater volume.

Similarly, increasing the temperature of a system should increase the entropy because at higher temperature the molecular motion is more vigorous and hence the system is more chaotic. The equation that relates entropy change to temperature change is

$$\Delta S = C_V \ln \frac{T_f}{T_i} \tag{2.8}$$

where C_V is the molar heat capacity at constant volume. Inspection of equation (2.8) shows that ΔS will be positive when $T_f > T_i$, as predicted.

The entropy of a substance will also change when it undergoes a phase transition, since this too leads to a change in the order. For example, when a crystalline solid melts, it changes from an ordered lattice to a more chaotic liquid (see Fig. 2.1) and consequently an increase in entropy is expected. The entropy change accompanying the melting of a solid is given by

$$\Delta S = \Delta H_{fus}/T \tag{2.9}$$

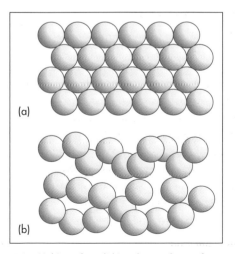

Figure 2.1 Melting of a solid involves a change from an ordered arrangement of molecules, represented by (a), to a more chaotic liquid, represented by (b). As a result, the melting process is accompanied by an increase in entropy.

where ΔH_{fus} is the enthalpy of fusion (melting) and T is the melting temperature. Similarly, we may determine the entropy change when a liquid vaporises from

$$\Delta S = \Delta H_{vap}/T \qquad (2.10)$$

where ΔH_{vap} is the enthalpy of vaporisation and T now refers to the boiling point. Entropy changes accompanying other phase changes, such as change of the polymorphic form of crystals (see section 1.2.3), may be calculated in a similar manner.

At absolute zero all the thermal motions of the atoms of the lattice of a crystal will have ceased and the solid will have no disorder and hence a zero entropy. This conclusion forms the basis of the *third law of thermodynamics*, which states that *the entropy of a perfectly crystalline material is zero when* $T = 0$.

2.2.4 Free energy

The free energy is derived from the entropy and is, in many ways, a more useful function to use. The free energy referred to when we are discussing processes at constant pressure is the *Gibbs free energy* (G). This is defined by

$$G = H - TS \qquad (2.11)$$

The change in the free energy at constant temperature arises from changes in enthalpy and entropy and is

$$\Delta G = \Delta H - T\Delta S \qquad (2.12)$$

Thus, at constant temperature and pressure,

$$\Delta G = -T\Delta S \qquad (2.13)$$

from which we can see that the change in free energy is another way of expressing the change in overall entropy of a process occurring at constant temperature and pressure.

In view of this relationship, we can now consider changes in free energy that occur during a spontaneous process. From equation (2.13) we can see that ΔG will decrease during a spontaneous process at constant temperature and pressure. This decrease will occur until the system reaches an equilibrium state when ΔG becomes zero. This process can

be thought of as a gradual using up of the system's ability to perform work as equilibrium is approached. Free energy can therefore be looked at in another way in that it represents the maximum amount of work, w_{max} (other than the work of expansion) that can be extracted from a system undergoing a change at constant temperature and pressure; i.e.

$$\Delta G = w_{max} \text{ at constant temperature and pressure} \qquad (2.14)$$

This non-expansion work can be extracted from the system as electrical work, as in the case of a chemical reaction taking place in an electrochemical cell, or the energy can be stored in biological molecules such as adenosine triphosphate (ATP).

When the system has attained an equilibrium state, it no longer has the ability to reverse itself. Consequently *all spontaneous processes are irreversible*. The fact that all spontaneous processes taking place at constant temperature and pressure are accompanied by a negative free energy change provides a useful criterion of the spontaneity of any given process.

By applying these concepts to chemical equilibria we can derive (see Box 2.3) the following simple relationship between free energy change and the equilibrium constant of a reversible reaction, K:

$$\Delta G^{\ominus} = -RT \ln K$$

where the standard free energy $G^{\ominus}$ is the free energy of 1 mole of gas at a pressure of 1 bar.

A similar expression may be derived for reactions in solutions using the *activities* (see section 2.3.1) of the components rather than the partial pressures. $\Delta G^{\ominus}$ values can readily be calculated from the tabulated data and hence equation (2.19) is important because it provides a method of calculating the equilibrium constants without resort to experimentation.

A useful expression for the temperature dependence of the equilibrium constant is the *van't Hoff equation* (equation 2.23), which may be derived as outlined in Box 2.4.

Box 2.3 Relationship between free energy change and the equilibrium constant

Consider the following reversible reaction taking place in the gaseous phase:

$$aA + bB \rightleftharpoons cC + dD$$

According to the law of mass action, the equilibrium constant, K, can be expressed as

$$K = \frac{(p'_C)^c \, (p'_D)^d}{(p'_A)^a \, (p'_B)^b} \tag{2.15}$$

where p' represents the partial pressures of the components of the reaction at equilibrium. The relationship between the free energy of a perfect gas and its partial pressure is given by

$$\Delta G = G - G^{\ominus} = RT \ln p \tag{2.16}$$

where $G^{\ominus}$ is the free energy of 1 mole of gas at a pressure of 1 bar.
Applying equation (2.16) to each component of the reaction gives

$$aG_A = a(G_A^{\ominus} + RT \ln p_A)$$
$$bG_B = b(G_B^{\ominus} + RT \ln p_B)$$

etc.

As

$$\Delta G = \sum G_{prod} - \sum G_{react}$$

so

$$\Delta G = \Delta G^{\ominus} + RT \ln \frac{(p_C)^c (p_D)^d}{(p_A)^a (p_B)^b} \tag{2.17}$$

$\Delta G^{\ominus}$ is the standard free energy change of the reaction, given by

$$\Delta G^{\ominus} = cG_C^{\ominus} + dG_D^{\ominus} - aG_A^{\ominus} - bG_B^{\ominus}$$

As we have noted previously, the free energy change for systems at equilibrium is zero, and hence equation (2.17) becomes

$$\Delta G^{\ominus} = -RT \ln \frac{(p'_C)^c (p'_D)^d}{(p'_A)^a (p'_B)^b} \tag{2.18}$$

Substituting from equation (2.15) gives

$$\Delta G^{\ominus} = -RT \ln K \tag{2.19}$$

Substituting equation (2.19) into equation (2.17) gives

$$\Delta G = -RT \ln K + RT \ln \frac{(p_C)^c (p_D)^d}{(p_A)^a (p_B)^b} \tag{2.20}$$

Equation (2.20) gives the change in free energy when a moles of A at a partial pressure p_A and b moles of B at a partial pressure p_B react together to yield c moles of C at a partial pressure p_C and d moles of D at a partial pressure p_D. For such a reaction to occur spontaneously, the free energy change must be negative, and hence equation (2.20) provides a means of predicting the ease of reaction for selected partial pressures (or concentrations) of the reactants.

Box 2.4 Derivation of the van't Hoff equation

From equation (2.19),

$$-\Delta G^{\ominus}/RT = \ln K$$

Since

$$\Delta G^{\ominus} = \Delta H^{\ominus} - T\Delta S^{\ominus}$$

then at a temperature T_1

$$\ln K_1 = -\Delta G^{\ominus}/RT_1 \\ = -\Delta H^{\ominus}/RT_1 + \Delta S^{\ominus}/R \quad (2.21)$$

and at temperature T_2

$$\ln K_2 = -\Delta G^{\ominus}/RT_2 \\ = -\Delta H^{\ominus}/RT_2 + \Delta S^{\ominus}/R \quad (2.22)$$

If we assume that the standard enthalpy change $\Delta H^{\ominus}$ and the standard entropy change $\Delta S^{\ominus}$ are independent of temperature, then subtracting equation (2.21) from equation (2.22) gives

$$\ln K_2 - \ln K_1 = -\frac{\Delta H^{\ominus}}{R}\left(\frac{1}{T_2} - \frac{1}{T_1}\right)$$

or

$$\log\frac{K_2}{K_1} = \frac{\Delta H^{\ominus}}{2.303R}\frac{(T_2 - T_1)}{T_1 T_2} \quad (2.23)$$

Equation (2.23), which is often referred to as the *van't Hoff equation*, is useful for the prediction of the equilibrium constant K_2 at a temperature T_2 from its value K_1 at a second temperature T_1.

A more general form of this equation is

$$\log K = \frac{-\Delta H^{\ominus}}{2.303RT} + \text{constant} \quad (2.24)$$

Plots of $\log K$ against $1/T$ should be linear with a slope of $-\Delta H^{\ominus}/2.303R$, from which $\Delta H^{\ominus}$ may be calculated.

Equations (2.19) and (2.24) are fundamental equations that find many applications in the broad area of the pharmaceutical sciences: for example, in the determination of equilibrium constants in chemical reactions and for micelle formation; in the treatment of stability data

Key points

- All forms of kinetic and potential energy can be interconverted provided that in so doing energy is neither created or destroyed (law of conservation of energy). The internal energy change ΔU of a closed system is the sum of the changes in energy resulting from the heat q absorbed (endothermic process) or released (exothermic process) and the work w done by or on the system. When the system is completely isolated from its surrounding so that there are no changes in heat or work, then its internal energy is constant (first law of thermodynamics).
- The enthalpy H of a system is the heat supplied at constant pressure. The enthalpy change ΔH is positive when heat is supplied and negative when heat is released.
- The entropy S is related to the disorder of the system and increases when the system becomes more chaotic. Such processes are spontaneous (i.e. occur without external intervention). The entropy of an isolated system therefore increases when a reaction or change of state is spontaneous (second law of thermodynamics).
- The change in the Gibbs free energy ΔG of a system is related to changes in enthalpy and entropy by the equation,
  $\Delta G = \Delta H - \Delta S$.

  ΔG decreases during a spontaneous change at constant temperature and pressure until the system reaches equilibrium, when ΔG becomes zero. The free energy is a measure of the work that a system can do and therefore at equilibrium the system no longer has the ability to perform any further work. Consequently, all spontaneous processes are irreversible.

for some solid dosage forms (see section 3.4.3); and for investigations of drug–receptor binding.

2.3 Activity and chemical potential

2.3.1 Activity and standard states

The term *activity* is used in the description of the departure of the behaviour of a solution from ideality. In any real solution, interactions occur between the components which reduce the *effective concentration* of the solution. The activity is a way of describing this effective concentration. In an ideal solution or in a real solution at infinite dilution, there are no interactions between components and the activity equals the concentration. Nonideality in real solutions at higher concentrations causes a divergence between the values of activity and concentration. The ratio of the activity to the concentration is called the *activity coefficient*, γ; that is,

$$\gamma = \text{activity/concentration} \qquad (2.25)$$

Depending on the units used to express concentration we can have either a *molal* activity coefficient, γ_m, a *molar* activity coefficient, γ_c, or, if mole fractions are used, a *rational* activity coefficient, γ_x.

In order to be able to express the activity of a particular component numerically, it is necessary to define a reference state in which the activity is arbitrarily unity. The activity of a particular component is then the ratio of its value in a given solution to that in the reference state. For the solvent, the reference state is invariably taken to be the pure liquid, and, if this is at a pressure of 1 atmosphere and at a definite temperature, it is also the *standard state*. Since the mole fraction as well as the activity is unity: $\gamma_x = 1$.

Several choices are available in defining the standard state of the solute. If the solute is a liquid that is miscible with the solvent (as, for example, in a benzene–toluene mixture) then the standard state is again the pure liquid. Several different standard states have been used for solutions of solutes of limited solubility. In developing a relationship between drug activity and thermodynamic activity, the pure substance has been used as the standard state. The activity of the drug in solution was then taken to be the ratio of its concentration to its saturation solubility. The use of a pure substance as the standard state is of course of limited value since a different state is used for each compound. A more feasible approach is to use the infinitely dilute solution of the compound as the reference state. Since the activity equals the concentration in such solutions, however, it is not equal to unity as it should be for a standard state. This difficulty is overcome by defining the standard state as a hypothetical solution of unit concentration possessing, at the same time, the properties of an infinitely dilute solution. Some workers[3] have chosen to define the standard state in terms of an alkane solvent rather than water; one advantage of this solvent is the absence of specific solute–solvent interactions in the reference state that would be highly sensitive to molecular structure.

2.3.2 Activity of ionised drugs

A large proportion of the drugs that are administered in aqueous solution are salts which, on dissociation, behave as electrolytes. Simple salts such as ephedrine hydrochloride ($C_6H_5CH(OH)CH(NHCH_3)CH_3HCl$) are 1:1 (or uni-univalent) electrolytes; that is, on dissociation each mole yields one cation, $C_6H_5CH(OH)CH(N^+H_2CH_3)CH_3$, and one anion, Cl^-. Other salts are more complex in their ionisation behaviour; for example, ephedrine sulfate is a 1:2 electrolyte, each mole giving two moles of the cation and one mole of SO_4^{2-} ions.

The activity of each ion is the product of its activity coefficient and its concentration, that is,

$$a_+ = \gamma_+ m_+ \quad \text{and} \quad a_- = \gamma_- m_-$$

The anion and cation may each have a different ionic activity in solution and it is not possible to determine individual ionic activities experimentally. It is therefore necessary to use combined terms; for example, the combined activity term is the *mean ionic activity*, $a_\pm$. Similarly, we have the *mean ion activity coefficient*, $\gamma_\pm$, and the *mean ionic molality*, $m_\pm$. The relationship between the mean ionic parameters is then

$$\gamma_\pm = a_\pm / m_\pm$$

More details of these combined terms are given in Box 2.5.

Values of the mean ion activity coefficient may be determined experimentally using several methods, including electromotive force measurement, solubility determinations and colligative properties. It is possible, however, to calculate $\gamma_\pm$ in very dilute solution using a theoretical method based on the Debye–Hückel theory. In this theory each ion is considered to be surrounded by

Box 2.5 Mean ionic parameters

In general, we will consider a strong electrolyte that dissociates according to

$$C_{v+}A_{v-} \rightarrow v_+ C^{z+} + v_- A^{z-}$$

where v_+ is the number of cations, C^{z+}, of valence z_+, and v_- is the number of anions, A^{z-}, of valence z_-.

The activity, a, of the electrolyte is then

$$a = a_+^{v+} a_-^{v-} = a_\pm^v \tag{2.26}$$

where $v = v_+ + v_-$

In the simple case of a solution of the 1:1 electrolyte sodium chloride, the activity will be

$$a = a_{Na^+} \times a_{Cl^-} = a_\pm^2$$

whereas, for morphine sulfate, which is a 1:2 electrolyte,

$$a = a_{morph^+}^2 \times a_{SO_4^{2-}} = a_\pm^3$$

Similarly, we may also define a mean ion activity coefficient, $\gamma_\pm$, in terms of the individual ionic activity coefficients γ_+ and γ_-:

$$\gamma_\pm^v = \gamma_+^{v+} \gamma_-^{v-} \tag{2.27}$$

or

$$\gamma_\pm = (\gamma_+^{v+} \gamma_-^{v-})^{1/v} \tag{2.28}$$

For a 1:1 electrolyte equation (2.28) reduces to

$$\gamma_\pm = (\gamma_+ \gamma_-)^{1/2} \tag{2.29}$$

Finally, we define a *mean ionic molality*, $m_\pm$, as

$$m_\pm^v = m_+^{v+} m_-^{v-} \tag{2.30}$$

or

$$m_\pm = (m_+^{v+} m_-^{v-})^{1/v} \tag{2.31}$$

For a 1:1 electrolyte, equation (2.31) reduces to

$$m_\pm = (m_+ m_-)^{1/2} = m \tag{2.32}$$

that is, mean ionic molality may be equated with the molality of the solution.

The activity of each ion is the product of its activity coefficient and its concentration:

$$a_+ = \gamma_+ m_+ \quad \text{and} \quad a_- = \gamma_- m_-$$

so that

$$\gamma_+ = a_+/m_+ \quad \text{and} \quad \gamma_- = a_-/m_-$$

Expressed as the mean ionic parameters, we have

$$\gamma_\pm = a_\pm/m_\pm \tag{2.33}$$

Substituting for $m_\pm$ from equation (2.31) gives

$$\gamma_\pm = a_\pm/(m_+^{v+} m_-^{v-})^{1/v} \tag{2.34}$$

This equation applies in any solution, whether the ions are added together as a single salt or separately as a mixture of salts. For a solution of a single salt of molality, m:

$$m_+ = \nu_+ m \quad \text{and} \quad m_- = \nu_- m$$

Equation (2.34) reduces to

$$\gamma_\pm = \frac{a_\pm}{m(\nu_+{}^{\nu+} \, \nu_-{}^{\nu-})^{1/\nu}} \tag{2.35}$$

For example, for morphine sulfate, $\nu_+ = 2$, $\nu_- = 1$, and thus

$$\gamma_\pm = \frac{a_\pm}{(2^2 \times 1)^{1/3} \, m} = \frac{a_\pm}{4^{1/3} \, m}$$

an 'atmosphere' in which there is a slight excess of ions of opposite charge. The electrostatic energy due to this effect is related to the chemical potential of the ion to give a limiting expression for dilute solutions:

$$-\log \gamma_\pm = z_+ z_- \, A \sqrt{I} \tag{2.36}$$

where z_+ and z_- are the valencies of the ions, A is a constant whose value is determined by the dielectric constant of the solvent and the temperature ($A - 0.509$ in water at 298 K), and I is the total ionic strength defined by

$$I = \tfrac{1}{2} \sum (mz^2) = \tfrac{1}{2}(m_1 z_1{}^2 + m_2 z_2{}^2 + \cdots) \tag{2.37}$$

where the summation is continued over all the different species in solution. It can readily be shown from equation (2.37) that for a 1 : 1 electrolyte the ionic strength is equal to its molality; for a 1 : 2 electrolyte $I = 3m$; and for a 2 : 2 electrolyte $I = 4m$.

The Debye–Hückel expression as given by equation (2.36) is valid only in dilute solution ($I < 0.02 \text{ mol kg}^{-1}$). At higher concentrations a modified expression has been proposed:

$$\log \gamma_\pm = \frac{-A \, z_+ z_- \sqrt{I}}{1 + a_i \, \beta \sqrt{I}} \tag{2.38}$$

where a_i is the mean distance of approach of the ions or the mean effective ionic diameter, and β is a constant whose value depends on the solvent and temperature. As an approximation, the product $a_i \beta$ may be taken to be unity, thus simplifying the equation. Equation (2.38) is valid for $I < 0.1 \text{ mol kg}^{-1}$.

2.3.3 Solvent activity

Although the phrase 'activity of a solution' usually refers to the activity of the *solute* in the solution as in the preceding section, we also can refer to the activity of the *solvent*. Experimentally, solvent activity a_1 may be determined as the ratio of the vapour pressure p_1 of the solvent in a solution to that of the pure solvent $p_1^\ominus$, that is,

$$a_1 = p_1/p_1^\ominus = \gamma_1 x_1 \tag{2.39}$$

where γ_1 is the solvent activity coefficient and x_1 is the mole fraction of solvent.

The relationship between the activities of the components of the solution is expressed by the Gibbs–Duhem equation:

$$x_1 \, \mathrm{d}(\ln a_1) + x_2 \, \mathrm{d}(\ln a_2) = 0 \tag{2.40}$$

which provides a way of determining the activity of the solute from measurements of vapour pressure. An example of the role of water activity in inhibiting bacterial growth in wounds is given below.

Water activity and inhibition of bacterial growth

When the aqueous solution in the environment of a microorganism is concentrated by the addition of solutes such as sucrose, the consequences for microbial growth result mainly from the change in water activity a_w. Every microorganism has a limiting a_w below which it will not grow. The minimum a_w levels for growth of human bacterial pathogens such as streptococci, *Klebsiella*, *Escherichia coli*, *Corynebacterium*, *Clostridium perfringens* and other clostridia, and

Example 2.2 Calculation of mean ionic activity coefficient

Calculate: (a) the mean ionic activity coefficient and the mean ionic activity of $0.002 \, \text{mol kg}^{-1}$ aqueous solution of ephedrine sulfate; (b) the mean ionic activity coefficient of an aqueous solution containing $0.002 \, \text{mol kg}^{-1}$ ephedrine sulfate and $0.01 \, \text{mol kg}^{-1}$ sodium chloride. Both solutions are at 25°C.

Answer

(a) Ephedrine sulfate is a 1:2 electrolyte and hence the ionic strength is given by equation (2.37) as

$$I = {}^{1}\!/_{2}[(0.002 \times 2 \times 1^{2}) + (0.002 \times 2^{2})] = 0.006 \, \text{mol kg}^{-1}$$

From the Debye–Hückel equation (equation 2.36),

$$-\log \gamma_{\pm} = 0.509 \times 1 \times 2 \times \sqrt{0.006}$$

$$\log \gamma_{\pm} = -0.0789$$

$$\gamma_{\pm} = 0.834$$

The mean ionic activity may be calculated from equation (2.35):

$$a_{\pm} = 0.834 \times 0.002 \times (2^{2} \times 1)^{{}^{1}\!/_{3}} = 0.00265$$

(b) Ionic strength of $0.01 \, \text{mol kg}^{-1} \, \text{NaCl} = {}^{1}\!/_{2}(0.01 \times 1^{2}) + (0.01 \times 1^{2}) = 0.01 \, \text{mol kg}^{-1}$

Total ionic strength $= 0.006 + 0.01 = 0.016 \, \text{mol kg}^{-1}$

$$-\log \gamma_{\pm} = 0.509 \times 2 \times \sqrt{0.016}$$

$$\log \gamma_{\pm} = -0.1288$$

$$\gamma_{\pm} = 0.743$$

Pseudomonas is 0.91.[4] *Staphylococcus aureus* can proliferate at an a_w as low as 0.86. Figure 2.2 shows the influence of a_w, adjusted by the addition of sucrose, on the growth rate of this microorganism at 35°C and pH 7.0. The control medium, with a water activity value of $a_w = 0.993$, supported the rapid growth of the test organism. Reduction of a_w of the medium by addition of sucrose progressively increased generation times and lag periods and lowered the peak cell counts. Complete growth inhibition was achieved at an a_w of 0.858 (195 g sucrose per 100 g water) with cell numbers declining slowly throughout the incubation period.

Clinical point

These results explain why the old remedy of treating infected wounds with sugar, honey or molasses is successful. When the wound is filled with sugar, the sugar dissolves in the tissue water, creating an environment of low a_w, which inhibits bacterial growth. However, the difference in water activity between the tissue and the concentrated sugar solution causes migration of water out of the tissue, hence diluting the sugar and raising a_w. Further sugar must then be added to the wound to maintain growth inhibition. Sugar may be applied as a paste with a consistency appropriate to the wound characteristics; thick sugar paste being suitable for cavities with wide openings, a thinner paste with the consistency of thin honey being more suitable for instillation into cavities with small openings.

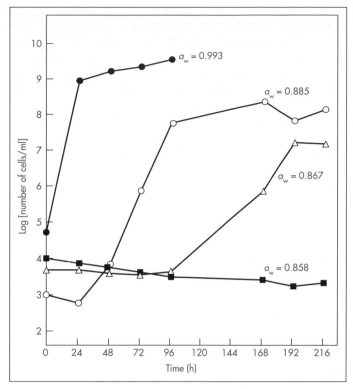

Figure 2.2 Staphylococcal growth at 35°C in medium alone ($a_w = 0.993$) and in media with a_w values lowered by additional sucrose. Reproduced with permission from Chirife J *et al.*, *Lancet,* 1982; 319: 560–561.

An *in vitro* study has been reported[5] of the efficacy of thick sugar pastes, and also of those prepared using xylose as an alternative to sucrose, in inhibiting the growth of bacteria commonly present in infected wounds. Polyethylene glycol was added to the pastes as a lubricant and hydrogen peroxide was included in the formulation as a preservative. To simulate the dilution that the pastes invariably experience as a result of fluid being drawn into the wound, serum was added to the formulations in varying amounts. Figure 2.3 illustrates the effects of these sucrose pastes on the colony-forming ability of *Proteus mirabilis* and shows the reduction in efficiency of the pastes as a result of dilution and the consequent increase of their water activity (see Fig. 2.4). It is clear that *P. mirabilis* was susceptible to the antibacterial activity of the pastes, even when they were diluted by 50%. It was reported that although a_w may not be maintained at less than 0.86 (the critical level for inhibition of growth of *S. aureus*) for more than 3 h after packing of the wound, nevertheless clinical experience had shown that twice-daily dressing was adequate to

remove infected slough from dirty wounds within a few days.

2.3.4 Chemical potential

Properties such as volume, enthalpy, free energy and entropy that depend on the quantity of substance are called *extensive* properties. In contrast, properties such as temperature, density and refractive index that are independent of the amount of material are referred to as *intensive* properties. The quantity denoting the rate of increase in the magnitude of an extensive property with increase in the number of moles of a substance added to the system at constant temperature and pressure is termed a *partial molar quantity*. Such quantities are distinguished by a bar above the symbol for the particular property. For example:

$$\left(\frac{\partial V}{\partial n_2}\right)_{T, P, n_1} = \overline{V}_2 \tag{2.41}$$

Note the use of the symbol ∂ to denote a partial change, which, in this case, occurs under conditions

Figure 2.3 The effects of sucrose pastes diluted with serum on the colony-forming ability of *P. mirabilis*.
Reproduced with permission from reference 5.

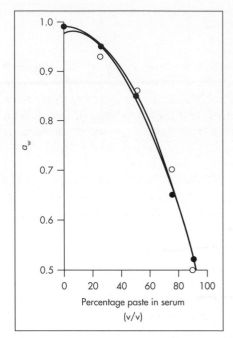

Figure 2.4 Effects on a_w of adding xylose (solid symbols) and sucrose paste (open symbols) to serum.
Reproduced with permission from reference 5.

of constant temperature, pressure and number of moles of solvent (denoted by the subscripts outside the brackets).

In practical terms the partial molar volume, $\overline{V}$, represents the change in the total volume of a large amount of solution when one additional mole of solute is added – it is the effective volume of 1 mole of solute in solution.

Of particular interest is the partial molar free energy, $\overline{G}$, which is also referred to as the *chemical potential*, μ, and is defined for component 2 in a binary system by

$$\left(\frac{\partial G}{\partial n_2}\right)_{T,P,n_1} = \overline{G}_2 = \mu_2 \qquad (2.42)$$

Partial molar quantities are of importance in the consideration of open systems, that is those involving transference of matter as well as energy. For an open system involving two components,

$$dG = \left(\frac{\partial G}{\partial T}\right)_{P,n_1,n_2} dT + \left(\frac{\partial G}{\partial P}\right)_{T,n_1,n_2} dP$$

$$+ \left(\frac{\partial G}{\partial n_1}\right)_{T,P,n_2} dn_1 + \left(\frac{\partial G}{\partial n_2}\right)_{T,P,n_1} dn_2 \qquad (2.43)$$

At constant temperature and pressure equation (2.43) reduces to

$$dG = \mu_1\, dn_1 + \mu_2\, dn_2 \qquad (2.44)$$

Thus,

$$G = \int dG = \mu_1 n_1 + \mu_2 n_2 \qquad (2.45)$$

The chemical potential therefore represents the contribution per mole of each component to the total free energy. It is the effective free energy per mole of each component in the mixture and is always less than the free energy of the pure substance.

It can be readily shown (see Box 2.6) that the chemical potential of a component in a two-phase system (for example, oil and water) at equilibrium at a fixed temperature and pressure is identical in both phases. Because of the need for equality of chemical potential at equilibrium, a substance in a system that is

Box 2.6 Chemical potential in two-phase systems

Consider a system of two phases, a and b, in equilibrium at constant temperature and pressure. If a small quantity of substance is transferred from phase a to phase b, then, because the overall free energy change is zero, we have

$$dG_a + dG_b = 0 \qquad (2.46)$$

where dG_a and dG_b are the free energy changes accompanying the transference of material for each phase.

From equation (2.44),

$$dG_a = \mu_a \, dn_a \quad \text{and} \quad dG_b = \mu_b \, dn_b$$

and thus

$$\mu_a \, dn_a + \mu_b \, dn_b = 0 \qquad (2.47)$$

A decrease of dn moles of component in phase a leads to an increase of exactly dn moles of this component in phase b; that is,

$$dn_a = -dn_b \qquad (2.48)$$

Substitution of equation (2.48) into equation (2.47) leads to the result

$$\mu_a = \mu_b \qquad (2.49)$$

In general, the chemical potential of a component is identical in all the phases of a system at equilibrium at a fixed temperature and pressure.

where

$$\mu^\ominus = \mu_2^\ominus + RT \ln M_1 - RT \ln 1000$$

and M_1 is the molecular weight of the solvent.

In the case of *strong electrolytes*, the chemical potential is the sum of the chemical potential of the ions. For the simple case of a $1:1$ electrolyte, the chemical potential is given by

$$\mu_2 = \mu_2^\ominus + 2RT \ln m\gamma_\pm$$

The derivations of these equations are given in Box 2.7.

Key points

- The activity a of an *ideal* solution is equal to the solution concentration. The activity is reduced when there are interactions between the components of the solution (a *nonideal* or real solution). The degree of nonideality is expressed by the activity coefficient γ which is the ratio of the activity to the concentration. In an electrolyte solution each ion has an activity and the mean ion activity coefficient of the solution is the ratio of the mean ion activity to the mean ion molality.

- The chemical potential of a component of a mixture is its effective free energy per mole when in the mixture, which, because of interactions in the mixture, is less than its molar free energy in its pure state. The chemical potential of a component in a two-phase system (for example, oil and water) is identical in both phases of the system when it is at equilibrium at a fixed temperature and pressure. A component in a two-phase system that is not at equilibrium will have a tendency to diffuse spontaneously from a phase in which it has a high chemical potential to another in which it has a low chemical potential. The difference in chemical potential is the driving force for diffusion between the two phases.

not at equilibrium will have a tendency to diffuse spontaneously from a phase in which it has a high chemical potential to another in which it has a low chemical potential. In this respect, the chemical *potential* resembles electrical *potential* and hence its name is an apt description of its nature.

Chemical potential of a component in solution

Where the component of the solution is a *nonelectrolyte*, its chemical potential in dilute solution at a molality m can be calculated from

$$\mu_2 = \mu^\ominus + RT \ln m$$

Box 2.7 Chemical potential of a component in solution

Non-electrolytes

In dilute solutions of non-volatile solutes the chemical potential of the solute is given by equation (2.50):

$$\mu_2 = \mu_2^\ominus + RT \ln x_2 \tag{2.50}$$

It is usually more convenient to express solute concentration as molality, m, rather than mole fraction using

$$x_2 = mM_1/1000$$

where M_1 = molecular weight of the solvent. Thus

$$\mu_2 = \mu^\ominus + RT \ln m \tag{2.51}$$

where

$$\mu^\ominus = \mu_2^\ominus + RT \ln M_1 - RT \ln 1000$$

At higher concentrations, the solution generally exhibits significant deviations from ideality and mole fraction must be replaced by activity

$$\mu_2 = \mu_2^\ominus + RT \ln a_2 \tag{2.52}$$

or

$$\mu_2 = \mu_2^\ominus + RT \ln \gamma_2 + RT \ln x_2 \tag{2.53}$$

Electrolytes

The chemical potential of a strong electrolyte, which may be assumed to be completely dissociated in solution, is equal to the sum of the chemical potentials of each of the component ions. Thus

$$\mu_+ = \mu_+^\ominus + RT \ln a_+ \tag{2.54}$$

and

$$\mu_- = \mu_-^\ominus + RT \ln a_- \tag{2.55}$$

and therefore

$$\mu_2 = \mu_2^\ominus + RT \ln a \tag{2.56}$$

where $\mu_2^\ominus$ is the sum of the chemical potentials of the ions, each in their respective standard state, i.e.

$$\mu_2^\ominus = v_+ \mu_+^\ominus + v_- \mu_-^\ominus$$

where v_+ and v_- are the number of cations and anions, respectively, and a is the activity of the electrolyte as given in section 2.3.2.

For example, for a 1 : 1 electrolyte, from equation (2.26) $a = a_\pm^2$. Therefore,

$$\mu_2 = \mu_2^\ominus + 2RT \ln a_\pm$$

From equation (2.33), $a_\pm = m \gamma_\pm$. Therefore,

$$\mu_2 = \mu_2^\ominus + 2RT \ln m\gamma_\pm$$

2.4 Osmotic properties of drug solutions

A nonvolatile solute added to a solvent affects not only the magnitude of the vapour pressure above the solvent but also the freezing point and the boiling point to an extent that is proportional to the relative number of solute molecules present, rather than to the weight concentration of the solute. Properties that are dependent on the number of molecules in solution in this way are referred to as *colligative* properties, and the most important of such properties from a pharmaceutical viewpoint is the osmotic pressure.

2.4.1 Osmotic pressure

Whenever a solution is separated from a solvent by a membrane that is permeable only to solvent molecules (referred to as a *semipermeable membrane*), there is a passage of solvent across the membrane into the solution. This is the phenomenon of *osmosis*. If the solution is totally confined by a semipermeable membrane and immersed in the solvent, a pressure differential develops across the membrane, which is referred to as the *osmotic pressure*. Solvent passes through the membrane because of the inequality of the chemical potentials on either side of the membrane. Since the chemical potential of a solvent molecule in solution is less than that in pure solvent, solvent will spontaneously enter the solution until this inequality is removed. The equation that relates the osmotic pressure of the solution, Π, to the solution concentration is the *van't Hoff equation*:

$$\Pi V = n_2 RT \tag{2.57}$$

On application of the van't Hoff equation to the drug molecules in solution, consideration must be made of any ionisation of the molecules, since osmotic pressure, being a colligative property, will be dependent on the total number of particles in solution (including the free counterions). To allow for what was at the time considered to be anomalous behaviour of electrolyte solutions, van't Hoff introduced a correction factor, i. The value of this factor approaches a number equal to that of the number of ions, ν, into which each molecule dissociates as the solution is progressively diluted. The ratio i/ν is termed the *practical osmotic coefficient*, ϕ.

For nonideal solutions, the activity and osmotic pressure are related by the expression

$$\ln a_1 = \frac{-\nu m M_1}{1000} \phi \tag{2.58}$$

where M_1 is the molecular weight of the solvent and m is the molality of the solution. The relationship between the osmotic pressure and the osmotic coefficient is thus

$$\Pi = \left(\frac{RT}{\overline{V}_1}\right) \frac{\nu m M_1}{1000} \phi \tag{2.59}$$

where $\overline{V}_1$ is the partial molal volume of the solvent.

2.4.2 Osmolality and osmolarity

The experimentally derived osmotic pressure is frequently expressed as the *osmolality* ξ_m, which is the mass of solute that when dissolved in 1 kg of water will exert an osmotic pressure, Π', equal to that exerted by a mole of an ideal un-ionised substance dissolved in 1 kg of water. The unit of osmolality is the osmole (abbreviated as osmol), which is the amount of substance that dissociates in solution to form one mole of osmotically active particles, thus 1 mole of glucose (not ionised) forms 1 osmole of solute, whereas 1 mole of NaCl forms 2 osmoles (1 mole of Na^+ and 1 mole of Cl^-). In practical terms, this means that a 1 molal solution of NaCl will have (approximately) twice the osmolality (osmotic pressure) as a 1 molal solution of glucose.

According to the definition, $\xi_m = \Pi/\Pi'$. The value of Π' may be obtained from equation (2.59) by noting that for an ideal un-ionised substance $\nu = \phi = 1$, and since m is also unity, equation (2.59) becomes

$$\Pi' = \left(\frac{RT}{\overline{V}_1}\right) \frac{M_1}{1000}$$

Thus

$$\xi_m = \nu m \phi \tag{2.60}$$

Example 2.3 Calculation of osmolality

A 0.90% w/w solution of sodium chloride (mol wt = 58.5 Da) has an osmotic coefficient of 0.928. Calculate the osmolality of the solution.

Answer

Osmolality is given by equation (2.60) as

$$\xi_m = \nu m \phi$$

so

$$\xi_m = 2 \times (9.0/58.5) \times 0.928$$
$$= 286 \,\mathrm{mosmol\,kg^{-1}}$$

Pharmaceutical labelling regulations sometimes require a statement of the osmolarity; for example, the USP 27 requires that sodium chloride injection should be labelled in this way. *Osmolarity* is defined as the mass of solute which, when dissolved in 1 litre of solution, will exert an osmotic pressure equal to that exerted by a mole of an ideal un-ionised substance dissolved in 1 litre of solution. The relationship between osmolality and osmolarity has been discussed by Streng *et al.*[6]

Table 2.1 Tonicities (osmolalities) of intravenous fluids

Solution	Tonicity (mosmol kg^{-1})
Vamin 9	700
Vamin 9 Glucose	1350
Vamin 14	1145
Vamin 14 Electrolyte-free	810
Vamin 18 Electrolyte-free	1130
Vaminolact	510
Vitrimix KV	1130
Intralipid 10% Novum	300
Intralipid 20%	350
Intralipid 30%	310
Intrafusin 22	1400
Hyperamine 30	1450
Gelofusine	279[a]
Lipofundin MCT/LCT 10%	345[a]
Lipofundin MCT/LCT 20%	380[a]
Nutriflex 32	1140[a]
Nutriflex 48	1400[a]
Nutriflex 70	2100[a]
Sodium Bicarbonate Intravenous Infusion BP	
8.4% w/v	2000[a]
4.2% w/v	1000[a]

[a] Osmolarity (mosmol dm^{-3}).

Table 2.1 lists the osmolalities of commonly used intravenous fluids.

2.4.3 Clinical relevance of osmotic effects

Tonicity

Osmotic effects are particularly important from a physiological viewpoint since biological membranes, notably the red blood cell membrane, behave in a manner similar to that of semipermeable membranes. Consequently, when red blood cells are immersed in a solution of greater osmotic pressure than that of their contents, they shrink as water passes out of the cells in an attempt to reduce the chemical potential gradient across the cell membrane. Conversely, on placing the cells in an aqueous environment of lower osmotic pressure, the cells swell as water enters and eventually lysis may occur. It is an important consideration, therefore, to ensure that the *effective* osmotic pressure of a solution for injection is approximately the same as that of blood serum. This effective osmotic pressure, which is termed the *tonicity*, is not always identical to the osmolality because it is concerned only with those solutes in solution that can exert an effect on the passage of water through the biological membrane. Solutions that have the same tonicity as blood serum are said to be *isotonic* with blood. Solutions with a higher tonicity are *hypertonic* and those with a lower tonicity are termed *hypotonic* solutions. Similarly, in order to avoid discomfort on administration of solutions to the delicate membranes of the body, such as the eyes, these solutions are made isotonic with the relevant tissues.

The osmotic pressures of many of the products in Table 2.1 are in excess of that of plasma (291 mosmol dm^{-3}). It is generally recommended that any fluid with an osmotic pressure above 550 mosmol dm^{-3} should not be infused rapidly as this would increase the incidence of venous damage. The rapid infusion of marginally hypertonic solutions (in the range 300–500 mosmol dm^{-3}) would appear to be clinically practicable; the higher the osmotic pressure of the solution within this range, the slower should be its rate of infusion to avoid damage. Patients with centrally inserted lines are not normally affected by limits on tonicity as infusion is normally slow and dilution is rapid.

Clinical point

Certain oral medications commonly used in the intensive care of premature infants have very high osmolalities. The high tonicity of enteral feedings has been implicated as a cause of necrotising enterocolitis (NEC). A higher frequency of gastrointestinal illness including NEC has been reported[7] among premature infants fed undiluted calcium lactate than among those fed no supplemental calcium or calcium lactate eluted with water or formula. White and Harkavy[8] have discussed a similar case of the development of NEC following medication with calcium glubionate elixir.

White and Harkavy[8] have measured osmolalities of several medications by freezing point depression and compared these with the osmolalities of analogous intravenous (IV) preparations (see Table 2.2). Except in the case of digoxin, the osmolalities of the IV preparations were very much lower than those of the corresponding oral preparations despite the fact that the IV preparations contained at least as much drug per millilitre as did the oral forms. This striking difference may be attributed to the additives such as ethyl alcohol, sorbitol and propylene glycol, which make a large contribution to the osmolalities of the oral preparations. The vehicle for the IV digoxin consists of 40% propylene glycol and 10% ethyl alcohol with calculated osmolalities of 5260 and 2174 mosmol kg^{-1} respectively, thus explaining the unusually high osmolality of this IV preparation. These authors have recommended that extreme caution should be exercised in paediatric and neonatal therapy in the administration of these oral preparations and perhaps any medication in a syrup or elixir form when the infant is at risk from necrotising enterocolitis.

Table 2.2 Measured and calculated osmolalities of drugs[a]

Drug (route)	Concentration of drug	Mean measured osmolality (mosmol kg^{-1})	Calculated available milliosmoles in 1kg of drug preparation[b]
Theophylline elixir (oral)	80 mg/15 cm^3	>3000	4980
Aminophylline (i.v.)	25 mg cm^{-3}	116	200
Calcium glubionate (oral)	115 mg/5 cm^3	>3000	2270
Calcium gluceptate (i.v.)	90 mg/5 cm^3	507	950
Digoxin elixir	25 mg dm^{-3}	>3000	4420
Digoxin (i.v.)	100 mg dm^{-3}	>3000	9620
Dexametasone elixir (oral)	0.5 mg/5 cm^3	>3000	3980
Dexametasone sodium phosphate (i.v.)	4 mg cm^{-3}	284	312

[a] Reproduced from reference 8.

[b] This would be the osmolality of the drug if the activity coefficient were equal to 1 in the full-strength preparation. The osmolalities of serial dilutions of the drug were plotted against the concentrations of the solution, and a least-squares regression line was drawn. The value for the osmolality of the full-strength solution was then estimated from the line. This is the 'calculated available milliosmoles'.

Clinical point

The osmolarity of preparations for oral administration to premature infants should be less than 400–500 mosmol dm^{-3} to limit stress imposed on the gastrointestinal system, which could lead to *pneumatosis intestinalis*.[9] Many drugs administered to preterm infants, however, have osmolarities greatly exceeding this limit; for example, paracetamol (acetaminophen) drugs have osmolarities of $10\,000$–$16\,000$ mosmol dm^{-3}.

Where no suitable alternative drugs are available, it may be possible to reduce osmolarity by administering the drugs by mixing with an infant formula. In such cases the final osmolarity of the mixture (OM) is calculated from

$$OM = \frac{(OD \times VD) + (OF \times VF)}{VD + VF} \quad (2.61)$$

where OD and OF are the osmolarities of drug and infant formula, respectively, and VD and VF are the volumes of drug solution and infant formula, respectively. Example 2.4 (taken from reference 9) illustrates the use of this equation.

Example 2.4 Reduction of osmolarity by mixing with an infant formula

A 0.25 mL solution of Ferinsol drops has an approximate osmolarity of 5010 mosmol dm^{-3}; calculate the final osmolarity of the preparation obtained when this dose is added to 15 mL of Premature Enfamil Formula (osmolarity 305 mosmol dm^{-3}).

Answer

Substitution in equation (2.61) gives

$$OM = \frac{(5010 \times 0.00025) + (305 \times 0.015)}{0.00025 + 0.015}$$
$$= 382 \text{ mosmol } dm^{-3}$$

Note that the volumes are converted to litres (dm^{-3}) before substitution

Table 2.3 Osmolalities of drug-infant formula mixtures[a]

Drug (dose)	Volume of drug (cm^3) + volume of formula (cm^3)	Mean measured osmolality (mosmol kg^{-1})
Infant formula	–	292
Theophylline elixir, 1 mg kg^{-1}	0.3 + 15	392
	0.3 + 30	339
Calcium glubionate syrup, 0.5 mmol kg^{-1}	0.5 + 15	378
	0.5 + 30	330
Digoxin elixir, 5 µg kg^{-1}	0.15 + 15	347
	0.15 + 30	322
Dexamethasone elixir, 0.25 mg kg^{-1}	3.8 + 15	1149
	3.8 + 30	791

[a] Reproduced from reference 8.

In some cases the osmolality of the elixir is so high that even mixing with infant formula does not reduce the osmolality to a tolerable level. For example, when a clinically appropriate dose of dexametasone elixir was mixed in volumes of formula appropriate for a single feeding for a 1500 g infant, the osmolalities of the mixes increased by at least 300% compared to formula alone (see Table 2.3).

Volatile anaesthetics

The aqueous solubilities of several volatile anaesthetics can be related to the osmolarity of the solution.[10] The inverse relationship between solubility (expressed as the liquid/gas partition coefficient) of those anaesthetics and the osmolarity is shown in Table 2.4.

These findings have practical applications for the clinician. Although changes in serum osmolarity within the physiological range (209–305 mosmol dm^{-3}) have only a small effect on the liquid/gas partition coefficient, changes in the serum osmolarity and the concentration of serum constituents at the extremes of the physiological range may significantly decrease the liquid/gas partition coefficient. For

Table 2.4 Liquid/gas partition coefficients of anaesthetics in four aqueous solutions at 37°C[a]

Solution	Osmolarity (mosmol dm^{-3})	Partition coefficient			
		Isoflurane	Enflurane	Halothane	Methoxyflurane
Distilled H_2O	0	0.626 ± 0.05	0.754 ± 0.06	0.859 ± 0.02	4.33 ± 0.5
Normal saline	308	0.590 ± 0.01	0.713 ± 0.01	0.825 ± 0.02	4.22 ± 0.30
Isotonic heparin (1000 U cm^{-3})	308	0.593 ± 0.01	0.715 ± 0.01	–	4.08 ± 0.22
Mannitol (20%)	1098	0.476 ± 0.023	0.575 ± 0.024	0.747 ± 0.03	3.38 ± 0.14

[a] Reproduced from reference 10.

example, the blood/gas partition coefficient of isoflurane decreases significantly after an infusion of mannitol. This decrease may be attributed to both a transient increase in the osmolarity of the blood and a more prolonged decrease in the concentration of serum constituents caused by the influx of water due to the osmotic gradient.

Rehydration solutions

An interesting application of the osmotic effect has been in the design of rehydration solutions. During the day the body moves many litres of fluid from the blood into the intestine and back again. The inflow of water into the intestine, which aids the breakdown of food, is an osmotic effect arising from the secretion of Cl^- ions by the crypt cells of the intestinal lining (see section 9.2.2) into the intestine. Nutrients from the food are taken up by the villus cells in the lining of the small intestine. The villus cells also absorb Na^+ ions, which they pump out into the extracellular spaces, from where they return to the circulation. As a consequence of this flow of Na^+, water and other ions follow by osmotic flow and hence are also transferred to the blood. This normal functioning is disrupted by diarrhoea-causing microorganisms, which either increase the Cl^--secreting activity of the crypt cells or impair the absorption of Na^+ by the villus cells, or both. Consequently, the fluid that is normally returned to the blood across the intestinal wall is lost in watery stool. If untreated, diarrhoea can eventually lead to a severe decline in the volume of the blood, the

circulation may become dangerously slow, and death may result.

Oral rehydration therapy

Treatment of dehydration by oral rehydration therapy (ORT) is based on the discovery that the diarrhoea-causing organisms do not usually interfere with the carrier systems that bring sodium and glucose simultaneously into the villus cells from the intestinal cavity. This 'co-transport' system only operates when both sodium and glucose are present. The principle behind ORT is that if glucose is mixed into an electrolyte solution it activates the co-transport system, causing electrolyte and then water to pass through the intestinal wall and to enter the blood, so minimising the dehydration.

Oral rehydration therapy requires administration to the patient of small volumes of fluid throughout the day (to prevent vomiting); it does not reduce the duration or severity of the diarrhoea, it simply replaces lost fluid and electrolytes. Let us examine, using the principles of the osmotic effect, two possible methods by which the process of fluid uptake from the intestine might be speeded up. It might seem reasonable to suggest that more glucose should be added to the formulation in an attempt to enhance the co-transport system. If this is done, however, the osmolarity of the glucose will become greater than that of normal blood, and water would now flow from the blood to the intestine and so exacerbate the problem. An alternative is to substitute starches for simple glucose in the ORT. When these polymer molecules are broken down in the intestinal lumen, they release many hundreds of glucose molecules, which are immediately taken up by the co-transport system and removed from the lumen. The effect is therefore as if a high concentration of glucose were administered, but because osmotic pressure is a *colligative* property (dependent on the *number* of molecules rather than the mass of substance), there is no associated problem of a high osmolarity when starches are used. The process is summarised in Fig. 2.5. A similar effect is achieved by the

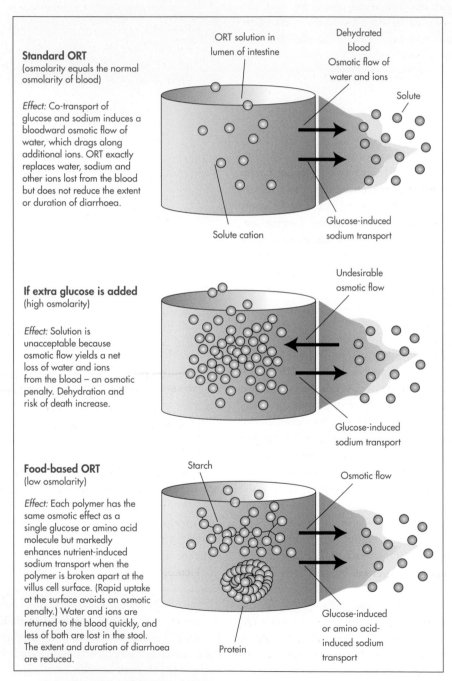

Figure 2.5　How osmosis affects the performance of solutions used in oral rehydration therapy (ORT).

addition of proteins, since there is also a co-transport mechanism whereby amino acids (released on breakdown of the proteins in the intestine) and Na^+ ions are simultaneously taken up by the villus cells.

This process of increasing water uptake from the intestine has an added appeal since the source of the starch and protein can be cereals, beans and rice, which are likely to be available in the parts of the world where problems arising from diarrhoea are most prevalent. Food-based ORT offers additional advantages: it can be made at home from low cost ingredients and can be cooked, which kills the pathogens in the water.

2.4.4 Preparation of isotonic solutions

Since osmotic pressure is not a readily measurable quantity, it is usual to make use of the relationship between the colligative properties and to calculate the osmotic pressure from a more easily measured property such as the freezing point depression. In so doing, however, it is important to realise that the red blood cell membrane is not a perfect semipermeable membrane and allows through small molecules such as urea and ammonium chloride. Therefore, although the quantity of each substance required for an isotonic solution may be calculated from freezing point depression values, these solutions may cause cell lysis when administered.

It has been shown that a solution that is isotonic with blood has a freezing point depression, ΔT_f, of 0.52°C. One has therefore to adjust the freezing point of the drug solution to this value to give an isotonic solution. Freezing point depressions for a series of compounds are given in reference texts[1,11] and it is a simple matter to calculate the concentration required for isotonicity from these values. For example, a 1% NaCl solution has a freezing point depression of 0.576°C. The percentage concentration of NaCl required to make isotonic saline solution is therefore $(0.52/0.576) \times 1.0 = 0.90\%$ w/v.

With a solution of a drug, it is of course not possible to alter the drug concentration in this manner, and an adjusting substance must be added to achieve isotonicity. The quantity of adjusting substance can be calculated as shown in Box 2.8

Box 2.8 Preparation of isotonic solutions

If the drug concentration is x g per 100 cm³ solution, then

$$\Delta T_f \text{ for drug solution}$$
$$= x \times (\Delta T_f \text{ of 1\% drug solution})$$
$$= a$$

Similarly, if w is the weight in grams of adjusting substance to be added to 100 cm³ of drug solution to achieve isotonicity, then

$$\Delta T_f \text{ for adjusting solution}$$
$$= w \times (\Delta T_f \text{ of 1\% adjusting substance})$$
$$= w \times b$$

For an isotonic solution, $a + (w \times b) = 0.52$. Therefore,

$$w = \frac{0.52 - a}{b} \qquad (2.62)$$

 Example 2.5 Isotonic solutions

Calculate the amount of sodium chloride that should be added to 50 cm³ of a 0.5% w/v solution of lignocaine hydrochloride to make a solution isotonic with blood serum.

Answer

From reference lists, the values of b for sodium chloride and lignocaine hydrochloride are 0.576°C and 0.130°C, respectively.
From equation (2.62) we have

$$a = 0.5 \times 0.13 = 0.065$$

Hence,

$$w = (0.52 - 0.065)/0.576 = 0.790 \, g$$

Therefore, the weight of sodium chloride to be added to 50 cm³ of solution is 0.395 g.

Key points

- Parenteral solutions should be of approximately the same tonicity as blood serum. The amount of adjusting substance which must be added to a formulation to achieve isotonicity can be calculated from

$$w = \frac{0.52 - a}{b}$$

where w is the weight in grams of adjusting substance to be added to 100 mL of drug solution to achieve isotonicity, a is the number of grams of drug in 100 mL of solution multiplied by the freezing point depression ΔT_f of a 1% drug solution, b is ΔT_f of 1% adjusting substance.

2.5 Ionisation of drugs in solution

Many drugs are either weak organic acids (for example, acetylsalicylic acid (aspirin)), or weak organic bases (for example, procaine), or their salts (for example, ephedrine hydrochloride). The degree to which these drugs are ionised in solution is highly dependent on the pH. The exceptions to this general statement are the nonelectrolytes, such as the steroids, and the quaternary ammonium compounds, which are completely ionised at all pH values and in this respect behave as strong electrolytes.

2.5.1 Clinical relevance of drug ionisation

The extent of ionisation of a drug has an important effect on its absorption, distribution and elimination and there are many examples of the alteration of pH to change these properties. The pH of urine may be adjusted (for example by administration of ammonium chloride or sodium bicarbonate) in cases of overdosing with amfetamines, barbiturates, narcotics and salicylates, to ensure that these drugs are completely ionised and hence readily excreted. Conversely, the pH of the urine may be altered to prevent ionisation

Table 2.5 Nominal pH values of some body fluids and sites[a]

Site	Nominal pH
Aqueous humour	7.21
Blood, arterial	7.4
Blood, venous	7.39
Blood, maternal umbilical	7.25
Cerebrospinal fluid	7.35
Duodenum	5.5
Faeces[b]	7.15
Ileum, distal	8.0
Intestine, microsurface	5.3
Lacrimal fluid (tears)	7.4
Milk, breast	7.0
Muscle, skeletal[c]	6.0
Nasal secretions	6.0
Prostatic fluid	6.45
Saliva	6.40
Semen	7.2
Stomach	1.5
Sweat	5.4
Urine, female	5.8
Urine, male	5.7
Vaginal secretions, premenopause	4.5
Vaginal secretions, postmenopause	7.0

[a] Reproduced from Newton DW, Kluza RB, *Drug Intell Clin Pharm*, 1978; 12: 547.
[b] Value for normal soft, formed stools; hard stools tend to be more alkaline, whereas watery, unformed stools are acidic.
[c] Studies conducted intracellularly in the rat.

of a drug in cases where reabsorption is required for therapeutic reasons. Sulfonamide crystalluria may also be avoided by making the urine alkaline. An understanding of the relationship between pH and drug ionisation is of use in the prediction of the causes of precipitation in admixtures, in the calculation of the solubility of drugs, and in the attainment of optimum bioavailability by maintaining a certain ratio of ionised to un-ionised drug. Table 2.5 shows the nominal pH values of some body fluids and sites, which are useful in the prediction of the percentage ionisation of drugs *in vivo*.

2.5.2 Dissociation of weakly acidic and basic drugs and their salts

According to the Lowry–Brønsted theory of acids and bases, an acid is a substance that will donate a proton and a base is a substance that will accept a proton. Thus the dissociation of acetylsalicylic acid, a weak acid, could be represented as in Scheme 2.1. In this equilibrium, acetylsalicylic acid acts as an acid because it donates a proton, and the acetylsalicylate ion acts as a base because it accepts a proton to yield an acid. An acid and base represented by such an equilibrium is said to be a *conjugate acid–base pair*.

Scheme 2.1

Scheme 2.1 is not a realistic expression, however, since protons are too reactive to exist independently and are rapidly taken up by the solvent. The proton-accepting entity, by the Lowry–Brønsted definition, is a base, and the product formed when the proton has been accepted by the solvent is an acid. Thus a second acid–base equilibrium occurs when the solvent accepts the proton, and this may be represented by

$$H_2O + H^+ \rightleftharpoons H_3O^+$$

The overall equation on summing these equations is shown in Scheme 2.2, or, in general,

$$HA + H_2O \rightleftharpoons A^- + H_3O^+$$

Scheme 2.2

By a similar reasoning, the dissociation of benzocaine, a weak base, may be represented by the equilibrium

$$\underset{\text{base 1}}{NH_2\,C_6H_5\,COOC_2H_5} + \underset{\text{acid 2}}{H_2O}$$
$$\rightleftharpoons \underset{\text{acid 1}}{NH_3^+\,C_6H_5\,COOC_2H_5} + \underset{\text{base 2}}{OH^-}$$

or, in general,

$$B + H_2O \rightleftharpoons BH^+ + OH^-$$

Comparison of the two general equations shows that H_2O can act as either an acid or a base. Such solvents are called *amphiprotic* solvents.

Salts of weak acids or bases are essentially completely ionised in solution. For example, ephedrine hydrochloride (salt of the weak base ephedrine, and the strong acid HCl) exists in aqueous solution in the form of the conjugate acid of the weak base, $C_6H_5CH(OH)CH(CH_3)N^+H_2CH_3$, together with its Cl^- counterions. In a similar manner, when sodium salicylate (salt of the weak acid salicylic acid, and the strong base NaOH) is dissolved in water, it ionises almost entirely into the conjugate base of salicylic acid, $HOC_6H_5COO^-$, and Na^+ ions.

The conjugate acids and bases formed in this way are, of course, subject to acid–base equilibria described by the general equations above.

2.5.3 The effect of pH on the ionisation of weakly acidic or basic drugs and their salts

If the ionisation of a weak acid is represented as described above, we may express an equilibrium constant as follows:

$$K_a = \frac{a_{H_3O^+} \times a_{A^-}}{a_{HA}} \tag{2.63}$$

Assuming the activity coefficients approach unity in dilute solution, the activities may be replaced by concentrations:

$$K_a = \frac{[H_3O^+]\,[A^-]}{[HA]} \tag{2.64}$$

K_a is variously referred to as the *ionisation constant*, *dissociation constant*, or *acidity constant* for the weak acid. The negative logarithm of K_a is referred to as

pK_a, just as the negative logarithm of the hydrogen ion concentration is called the pH. Thus

$$pK_a = -\log K_a \qquad (2.65)$$

Similarly, the *dissociation constant* or *basicity constant* for a weak base is

$$K_b = \frac{a_{OH^-} \times a_{BH^+}}{a_B} \approx \frac{[OH^+][BH^+]}{[B]} \qquad (2.66)$$

and

$$pK_b = -\log K_b \qquad (2.67)$$

The pK_a and pK_b values provide a convenient means of comparing the strengths of weak acids and bases. The lower the pK_a, the stronger the acid; the lower the pK_b, the stronger is the base. The pK_a values of a series of drugs are given in Table 2.6. pK_a and pK_b values of conjugate acid–base pairs are linked by the expression

$$pK_a + pK_b = pK_w \qquad (2.68)$$

where pK_w is the negative logarithm of the dissociation constant for water, K_w. K_w is derived from consideration of the equilibrium

$$H_2O + H_2O \rightleftharpoons H_3O^+ + OH^-$$

Table 2.6 pK_a values of some medicinal compounds[a]

Compound	pKa		Compound	pKa	
	Acid	Base		Acid	Base
Acebutolol		9.4	Apomorphine	8.9	7.0
Acetazolamide		7.2, 9.0	Atenolol		9.6
Acetylsalicylic acid	3.5		Ascorbic acid	4.2, 11.6	
Aciclovir		2.3, 9.3	Astemizole		8.4
Adrenaline	9.9	8.5	Atropine		9.9
Adriamycin		8.2	Azapropazone	<1.8	6.6
Allopurinol	10.2		Azathioprine	8.2	
Alphaprodine		8.7	Azelastine		9.5
Alprazolam		2.4	Benazepril	3.1	5.3
Alprenolol		9.6	Benzylpenicillin	2.8	
Amikacin		8.1	Benzocaine		2.8
p-Aminobenzoic acid	4.9	2.4	Bupivacaine		8.1
Aminophylline		5.0	Bupropion		7.9
p-Aminosalicylic acid	3.2		Captopril	3.5	
Amitriptyline		9.4	Carteolol		9.7
Amiodorone		6.6 (5.6)[b]	Cefadroxil	7.6	2.7
Amoxicillin	2.4	7.4, 9.6	Cefalexin	7.1	2.3
Amoxapine		7.6	Cefaclor	7.2	2.7
Ampicillin	2.7	7.2	Celiprolol		9.7

(continued overleaf)

Table 2.6 *(continued)*

Compound	pK_a Acid	pK_a Base	Compound	pK_a Acid	pK_a Base
Cetirizine	2.9	2.2, 8.0	Diltiazem		8.0
Chlorambucil	4.5 (4.9)[b]	2.5	Diphenhydramine		9.1
Chloramphenicol		5.5	Dithranol		9.4
Chlorcyclizine		8.2	Doxepin		8.0
Chlordiazepoxide		4.8	Doxorubicin		8.2, 10.2
Chloroquine		8.1, 9.9	Doxycycline	7.7	3.4, 9.3
Chlorothiazide	6.5	9.5	Enalapril		5.5
Chlorphenamine		9.0	Enoxacin	6.3	8.6
Chlorpromazine		9.3	Epirubicin		8.1
Chlorpropamide		4.9	Ergometrine		6.8
Chlorprothixene		8.8	Ergotamine		6.4
Cilazapril		6.4	Erythromycin		8.8
Cimetidine		6.8	Famotidine		6.8
Cinchocaine		8.3	Fenoprofen	4.5	
Clarithromycin		8.3	Flucloxacillin	2.7	
Clindamycin		7.5	Flufenamic acid	3.9	
Cocaine		8.5	Flumequine	6.5	
Codeine		8.2	Fluopromazine		9.2
Cyclopentolate		7.9	Fluorouracil	8.0, 13.0	
Daunomycin		8.2	Fluphenazine		3.9, 8.1
Desipramine		10.2	Flurazepam	8.2	1.9
Dextromethorphan		8.3	Flurbiprofen	4.3	
Diamorphine		7.6	Furosemide	3.9	
Diazepam		3.4	Glibenclamide	5.3	
Dibucaine		8.3	Guanethidine		11.9
Diclofenac	4.0		Guanoxan		12.3
Diethylpropion		8.7	Halofantrine		9.7

(continued overleaf)

Table 2.6 *(continued)*

Compound	pK_a		Compound	pK_a	
	Acid	Base		Acid	Base
Haloperidol		8.3	Naltrexone	9.5	8.1
Hexobarbital	8.3		Naproxen	4.3	
Hydralazine		0.5, 7.1	Nitrofurantoin		7.2
Ibuprofen	4.4		Nitrazepam	10.8	3.2 (3.4)[b]
Imipramine		9.5	Norfloxacin	6.2	8.6
Indometacin	4.5		Nortriptyline		9.7
Ketoprofen	4.0		Novobiocin	4.3, 9.1	
Labetalol	7.4	9.4	Ofloxacin	6.1	8.3
Levamisole		8.0	Oxolinic acid	6.6	
Levodopa	2.3, 9.7, 13.4		Oxprenolol		9.5
Lidocaine		7.94 (26°C), 7.55 (36°C)	Oxybutynin		6.9
Lincomycin		7.5	Oxycodone		8.9
Loxoprofen	4.2		Oxytetracycline	7.3	3.3, 9.1
Maprotiline		10.2	Paroxetine		9.9
Meclofenamic acid	4.0		Penbutolol		9.3
Metoprolol		9.7	Pentazocine		8.8
Methadone		8.3	Pethidine		8.7
Methotrexate	3.8, 4.8	5.6	Phenazocine		8.5
Metronidazole		2.5	Phenytoin	8.3	
Minocycline	7.8	2.8, 5.0, 9.5	Physostigmine		2.0, 8.1
Minoxidil		4.6	Pilocarpine		1.6, 7.1
Morphine	8.0 (phenol)	9.6 (amine)	Pindolol		8.8
Nadolol		9.7	Piperazine		5.6, 9.8
Nafcillin	2.7		Piroxicam	2.3	
Nalidixic acid	6.4		Polymyxin B		8.9
Nalorphine		7.8	Prazocin		6.5
Naloxone		7.9	Procaine		8.8

(continued overleaf)

Table 2.6 *(continued)*

Compound	pKa		Compound	pKa	
	Acid	**Base**		**Acid**	**Base**
Prochlorperazine		3.7, 8.1	Terazosin		7.1
Promazine		9.4	Terfenadine		9.5 (8.6)[b]
Promethazine		9.1	Tetracaine		8.4
Propofol	11.0		Tetracycline	7.7	3.3, 9.5
Propranolol		9.5	Theophylline	8.6	3.5
Quinapril		2.8, 5.4	Thiopental	7.5	
Quinidine		4.2, 8.3	Ticlopidine		7.6
Quinine		4.2, 8.8	Timolol		9.2 (8.8)[b]
Ranitidine		2.7, 8.2	Tolrestat	3.0	
Sotalol	8.3	9.8	Tolbutamide	5.3	
Sulfadiazine	6.5	2.0	Triflupromazine		9.2
Sulfaguanidine	12.1	2.8	Trimethoprin		7.3
Sulfamerazine	7.1	2.3	Triprolidine		9.3
Sulfathiazole	7.1	2.4	Valproate	5.0	
Tamoxifen		8.9	Verapamil		8.8
Temazepam		1.6	Warfarin	5.1	
Tenoxicam	1.1	5.3	Zidovudine		9.7

[a] For a more complete list see: Dollery C, ed., *Therapeutic Drugs*, Vols 1, 2, Suppl. 1, 2, Edinburgh: Churchill Livingstone; 1991, 1994. Newton DW, Kluza RB, *Drug Intell Clin Pharm*, 1978; 12: 547. Raymond GC, Born JL, *Drug Intell Clin Pharm*, 1986; 20: 683. Jack DB, *Handbook of Clinical Pharmacokinetic Data*, London: Macmillan; 1992. *The Pharmaceutical Codex*, 12th edn. London: Pharmaceutical Press; 1994.
[b] Values in parenthesis represent alternative values from the literature.

where one molecule of water is behaving as the weak acid or base and the other is behaving as the solvent. Then

$$K = \frac{a_{H_3O^+} \times a_{OH^-}}{a_{H_2O}^2} \approx \frac{[H_3O^+][OH^-]}{[H_2O]^2} \quad (2.69)$$

The concentration of molecular water is considered to be virtually constant for dilute aqueous solutions.

Therefore,

$$K_w = [H_3O^+][OH^-] \quad (2.70)$$

where the dissociation constant for water (the *ionic product*) now incorporates the term for molecular water and has the values given in Table 2.7.

When the pH of an aqueous solution of the weakly acidic or basic drug approaches the pKa or pKb, there is a very pronounced change in the ionisation of that

Box 2.9 The degree of ionisation of weak acids and bases

Weak acids

Taking logarithms of the expression for the dissociation constant of a weak acid (equation 2.64),

$$-\log K_a = -\log[H_3O^+] - \log\frac{[A^-]}{[HA]}$$

which can be rearranged to

$$pH = pK_a + \log\frac{[A^-]}{[HA]} \qquad (2.71)$$

Equation (2.71) may itself be rearranged to facilitate the direct determination of the molar percentage ionisation as follows:

$$[HA] = [A^-]\, antilog\,(pK_a - pH)$$

Therefore,

$$percentage\ ionisation = \frac{[A^-]}{[HA]+[A^-]} \times 100$$

$$percentage\ ionisation$$
$$= \frac{100}{1 + antilog(pK_a - pH)} \qquad (2.72)$$

Weak bases

An analogous series of equations for the percentage ionisation of a weak base may be derived as follows. Taking logarithms of equation (2.66) and rearranging gives

$$-\log K_b = -\log[OH^-] - \log\frac{[BH^+]}{[B]}$$

Therefore,

$$pH = pK_w - pK_b - \log\frac{[BH^+]}{[B]} \qquad (2.73)$$

Rearranging to facilitate calculation of the percentage ionisation leads to

$$percentage\ ionisation$$
$$= \frac{100}{1 + antilog(pH - pK_w + pK_b)} \qquad (2.74)$$

Table 2.7 Ionic product for water

Temperature (°C)	$K_w \times 10^{14}$	pK_w
0	0.1139	14.94
10	0.2920	14.53
20	0.6809	14.17
25	1.008	14.00
30	1.469	13.83
40	2.919	13.54
50	5.474	13.26
60	9.614	13.02
70	15.1	12.82
80	23.4	12.63

 e.g.

Example 2.6 Calculation of percentage ionisation

Calculate the percentage of cocaine existing as the free base in a solution of cocaine hydrochloride at pH 4.5, and at pH 8.0. The pK_b of cocaine is 5.6.

Answer

From equation (2.74):

At pH 4.5:

Percentage ionisation

$$= \frac{100}{1 + antilog\,(4.5 - 14.0 + 5.6)}$$
$$= 100/1.000126$$
$$= 99.99\%$$

Thus the percentage existing as cocaine base = 0.01%.

At pH 8.0:

Percentage ionisation

$$= \frac{100}{1 + antilog\,(8.0 - 14.0 + 5.6)}$$
$$= 100/1.398$$
$$= 71.53\%$$

Thus the percentage existing as cocaine base = 28.47%

drug. An expression that enables predictions of the pH dependence of the degree of ionisation to be made can be derived as shown in Box 2.9. The influence of pH on the percentage ionisation may be determined for drugs of known pK_a using Table 2.8.

Table 2.8 Percentage ionisation of anionic and cationic compounds as a function of pH

	At pH above pK_a			At pH below pK_a	
pH – pK_a	If anionic	If cationic	pK_a – pH	If anionic	If cationic
6.0	99.999 90	0.000 099 9	0.1	44.27	55.73
5.0	99.999 00	0.000 999 9	0.2	38.68	61.32
4.0	99.990 0	0.009 999 0	0.3	33.39	66.61
–	–	–	0.4	28.47	71.53
–	–	–	0.5	24.03	75.97
3.5	99.968	0.031 6	–	–	–
3.4	99.960	0.039 8	–	–	–
3.3	99.950	0.050 1	0.6	20.07	79.93
3.2	99.937	0.063 0	0.7	16.63	83.37
3.1	99.921	0.079 4	0.8	13.70	86.30
–	–	–	0.9	11.19	88.81
–	–	–	1.0	9.09	90.91
3.0	99.90	0.099 9	–	–	–
2.9	99.87	0.125 7	–	–	–
2.8	99.84	0.158 2	1.1	7.36	92.64
2.7	99.80	0.199 1	1.2	5.93	94.07
2.6	99.75	0.250 5	1.3	4.77	95.23
–	–	–	1.4	3.83	96.17
–	–	–	1.5	3.07	96.93
2.5	99.68	0.315 2	–	–	–
2.4	99.60	0.396 6	–	–	–
2.3	99.50	0.498 7	1.6	2.450	97.55
2.2	99.37	0.627 0	1.7	1.956	98.04
2.1	99.21	0.787 9	1.8	1.560	98.44
–	–	–	1.9	1.243	98.76
–	–	–	2.0	0.990	99.01
2.0	99.01	0.990	–	–	–
1.9	98.76	1.243	–	–	–

(continued overleaf)

Table 2.8 *(continued)*

	At pH above pK_a			At pH below pK_a	
pH − pK_a	If anionic	If cationic	pK_a − pH	If anionic	If cationic
1.8	98.44	1.560	2.1	0.787 9	99.21
1.7	98.04	1.956	2.2	0.627 0	99.37
1.6	97.55	2.450	2.3	0.498 7	99.50
–	–	–	2.4	0.396 6	99.60
–	–	–	2.5	0.315 2	99.68
1.5	96.93	3.07	–	–	–
1.4	96.17	3.83	–	–	–
1.3	95.23	4.77	2.6	0.250 5	99.75
1.2	94.07	5.93	2.7	0.199 1	99.80
1.1	92.64	7.36	2.8	0.158 2	99.84
			2.9	0.125 7	99.87
1.0	90.91	9.09	3.0	0.099 9	99.90
0.9	88.81	11.19	–	–	–
0.8	86.30	13.70	3.1	0.079 4	99.921
0.7	83.37	16.63	3.2	0.063 0	99.937
0.6	79.93	20.07	3.3	0.050 1	99.950
–	–	–	3.4	0.039 8	99.960
0.5	75.97	24.03	3.5	0.031 6	99.968
0.4	71.53	28.47	–	–	–
0.3	66.61	33.39	4.0	0.009 999 0	99.990 0
0.2	61.32	38.68	5.0	0.000 999 9	99.999 00
0.1	55.73	44.27	6.0	0.000 099 9	99.999 90
0	50.00	50.00	–	–	–

If we carry out calculations such as those of Example 2.6 over the whole pH range for both acidic and basic drugs, we arrive at the graphs shown in Fig. 2.6. Notice from this figure that

- A basic drug is virtually completely ionised at pH values up to 2 units below its pK_a, and virtually completely un-ionised at pH values greater than 2 units above its pK_a.
- An acidic drug is virtually completely un-ionised at pH values up to 2 units below its pK_a and virtually completely ionised at pH values greater than 2 units above its pK_a.

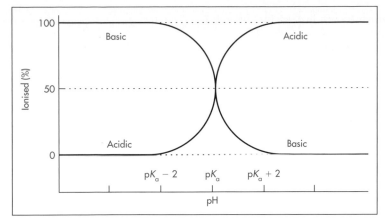

Figure 2.6 Percentage ionisation of weakly acidic and weakly basic drugs as a function of pH.

• Both acidic and basic drugs are exactly 50% ionised at their pK_a values.

2.5.4 Ionisation of amphoteric drugs

Ampholytes (amphoteric electrolytes) can function as either weak acids or weak bases in aqueous solution and have pK_a values corresponding to the ionisation of each group. They may be conveniently divided into two categories – ordinary ampholytes and zwitterionic ampholytes – depending on the relative acidity of the two ionisable groups.[12,13]

Ordinary ampholytes

In this category of ampholytes, the pK_a of the acidic group, pK_a^{acidic}, is higher than that of the basic group, pK_a^{basic}, and consequently the first group that loses its proton as the pH is increased is the basic group. Table 2.6 includes several examples of this type of ampholyte. We will consider, as a simple example, the ionisation of *m*-aminophenol (**I**), which has $pK_a^{acidic} = 9.8$ and $pK_a^{basic} = 4.4$.

OH

NH₂

Structure I *m*-Aminophenol

The steps of the ionisation on increasing pH are shown in the following equilibria:

$$NH_3^+C_6H_4OH \rightleftharpoons NH_2C_6H_4OH \rightleftharpoons NH_2C_6H_5O^-$$

This compound can exist as a cation, as an un-ionised form, or as an anion depending on the pH of the solution, but because the difference between pK_a^{acidic} and pK_a^{basic} is > 2, there will be no simultaneous ionisation of the two groups and the distribution of the species will be as shown in Fig. 2.7. The ionisation pattern will become more complex, however, with drugs in which the difference in pK_a of the two groups is much smaller because of overlapping of the two equilibria.

Zwitterionic ampholytes

This group of ampholytes is characterised by the relation $pK_a^{acidic} < pK_a^{basic}$. The most common examples of zwitterionic ampholytes are the amino acids, peptides and proteins. There are essentially two types of

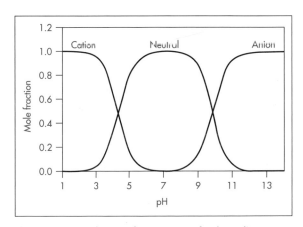

Figure 2.7 Distribution of ionic species for the ordinary ampholyte *m*-aminophenol.

Redrawn from Pagliara A *et al.*, *Chem. Rev.*, 1997; 97: 3385.

zwitterionic electrolyte depending on the difference ΔpK_a between the pK_a^{acidic} and pK_a^{basic} values.

Large ΔpK_a

The simplest type to consider is that of compounds having two widely separated pK_a values, for example glycine. The pK_a values of the carboxylate and amino groups on glycine are 2.34 and 9.6, respectively and the changes in ionisation as the pH is increased are described by the following equilibria:

$$HOOCCH_2 \cdot NH_3^+ \leftrightharpoons {}^-OOCCH_2\,NH_3^+ \leftrightharpoons$$
$${}^-OOCCH_2\,NH_2$$

Over the pH range 3–9, glycine exists in solution predominantly in the form ${}^-OOCCH_2\,NH_3^+$. Such a structure, having both positive and negative charges on the same molecule, is referred to as a zwitterion and can react as an acid,

$${}^-OOCCH_2\,NH_3^+ + H_2O \leftrightharpoons {}^-OOCCH_2\,NH_2 + H_3O^+$$

or as a base,

$${}^-OOCCH_2\,NH_3^+ + H_2O \leftrightharpoons$$
$$HOOCCH_2\,NH_3^+ + OH^-$$

This compound can exist as a cation, a zwitterion, and an anion depending on the pH of the solution. The two pK_a values of glycine are >2 pH units apart and hence the distribution of the ionic species will be similar to that shown in Fig. 2.7.

At a particular pH, known as the *isoelectric pH* or *isoelectric point*, pH_i, the effective net charge on the molecule is zero. pH_i can be calculated from

$$pH_i = \frac{pK_a^{\text{acidic}} + pK_a^{\text{basic}}}{2}$$

Small ΔpK_a

In cases where the two pK_a values are $\ll 2$ pH units apart there is overlap of the ionisation of the acidic and basic groups, with the result that the zwitterionic electrolyte can exist in four different electrical states – the cation, the un-ionised form, the zwitterion, and the anion (Scheme 2.3).

$$(ABH_2)^+ \xrightleftharpoons{K_a^{\text{acidic}}} \begin{bmatrix} (ABH)^{\pm} \\ (ABH) \end{bmatrix} \xrightleftharpoons{K_a^{\text{basic}}} (AB)^-$$

Scheme 2.3

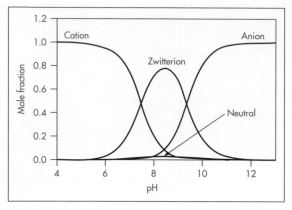

Figure 2.8 Distribution of ionic species for the zwitterionic ampholyte labetalol.

Redrawn from Pagliara A *et al.*, *Chem. Rev.*, 1997; 97: 3385.

In Scheme 2.3, $(ABH)^{\pm}$ is the zwitterion and, although possessing both positive and negative charges, is essentially neutral. The un-ionised form, (ABH), is of course also neutral and can be regarded as a tautomer of the zwitterion. Although only two dissociation constants K_a^{acidic} and K_a^{basic} (*macrodissociation constants*) can be determined experimentally, each of these is composed of individual *microdissociation constants* because of simultaneous ionisation of the two groups (see section 2.5.6). These microdissociation constants represent equilibria between the cation and zwitterion; the anion and the zwitterion; the cation and the un-ionised form; and the anion and the un-ionised form. At pH_i, the un-ionised form and the zwitterion always coexist, but the ratio of the concentrations of each will vary depending on the relative magnitude of the microdissociation constants. The distribution of the ionic species for labetalol which has $pK_a^{\text{acidic}} = 7.4$ and $pK_a^{\text{basic}} = 9.4$ is shown in Fig. 2.8.

Examples of zwitterionic drugs with both large and small ΔpKa values are given in Box 2.10; others can be noted in Table 2.6.

2.5.5 Ionisation of polyprotic drugs

In the examples we have considered so far, the acidic drugs have donated a single proton. There are several acids, for example citric, phosphoric and tartaric acids, that are capable of donating more than one proton; these compounds are referred to as *polyprotic* or *polybasic* acids. Similarly, a polyprotic base is one

Box 2.10 Chemical structures and pKₐ values of some zwitterionic drugs

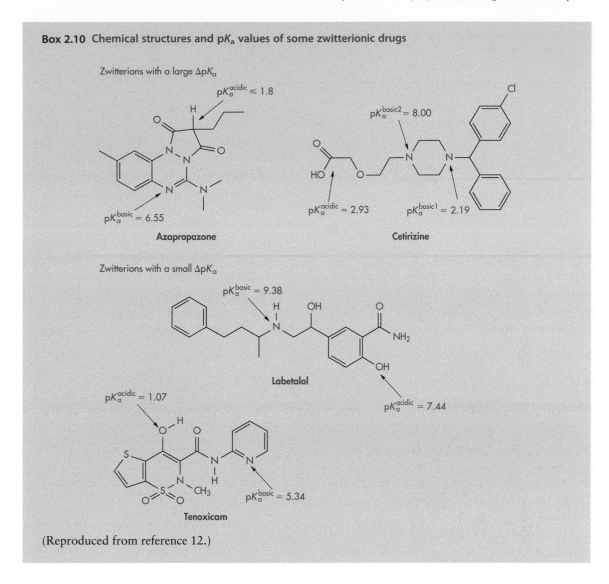

Zwitterions with a large ΔpK_a

$pK_a^{acidic} \leqslant 1.8$

$pK_a^{basic} = 6.55$

Azapropazone

$pK_a^{basic2} = 8.00$

$pK_a^{acidic} = 2.93$ $pK_a^{basic1} = 2.19$

Cetirizine

Zwitterions with a small ΔpK_a

$pK_a^{basic} = 9.38$

Labetalol

$pK_a^{acidic} = 7.44$

$pK_a^{acidic} = 1.07$

$pK_a^{basic} = 5.34$

Tenoxicam

(Reproduced from reference 12.)

capable of accepting two or more protons. Many examples of both types of polyprotic drugs can be found in Table 2.6, including the polybasic acids amoxicillin and fluorouracil, and the polyacidic bases pilocarpine, doxorubicin and aciclovir. Each stage of the dissociation may be represented by an equilibrium expression and hence each stage has a distinct pK_a or pK_b value. The dissociation of phosphoric acid, for example, occurs in three stages; thus:

$$H_3PO_4 + H_2O \rightleftharpoons H_2PO_4^- + H_3O^+ \quad K_1 = 7.5 \times 10^{-3}$$

$$H_2PO_4^- + H_2O \rightleftharpoons HPO_4^{2-} + H_3O^+ \quad K_2 = 6.2 \times 10^{-8}$$

$$HPO_4^{2-} + H_2O \rightleftharpoons PO_4^{3-} + H_3O^+ \quad K_3 - 2.1 \times 10^{-13}$$

2.5.6 Microdissociation constants

The experimentally determined dissociation constants for the various stages of dissociation of polyprotic and zwitterionic drugs are referred to as macroscopic values. However, it is not always easy to assign macroscopic dissociation constants to the ionisation of specific groups of the molecule, particularly when the pK_a values are close together, as discussed in section 2.5.5. The diprotic drug morphine has macroscopic pK_a values of 8.3 and 9.5, arising from ionisation of amino and phenolic groups. Experience suggests that the first pK_a value is probably associated with the ionisation of the amino group and the second with that of the phenolic group; but it is not possible to assign the values of these groups unequivocally, and for a more complete picture of the dissociation it is necessary to take into account all possible ways in which the molecule may be ionised and all the possible species present in solution. We may represent the most highly protonated form of morphine, $^+$HMOH, as $+O$, where the '+' refers to the protonated amino group and the O refers to the uncharged phenolic group. Dissociation of the amino proton only produces an uncharged form MOH, represented by OO, while dissociation of the phenolic proton gives a zwitterion $^+$HMO$^-$ represented by '+−'. The completely dissociated form MO$^-$ is represented as O−. The entire dissociation scheme is given in Scheme 2.4.

Scheme 2.4

The constants K_1, K_2, K_{12}, and K_{21} are termed microdissociation constants and are defined by

$$k_1 = \frac{[+-][H_3O^+]}{[+O]} \qquad k_2 = \frac{[OO][H_3O^+]}{[+O]}$$

$$k_{12} = \frac{[O-][H_3O^+]}{[+-]} \qquad k_{21} = \frac{[O-][H_3O^+]}{[OO]}$$

The micro- and macrodissociation constants are related by the following expressions:

$$K_1 = k_1 + k_2 \tag{2.75}$$

$$\frac{1}{K_2} = \frac{1}{k_{12}} + \frac{1}{k_{21}} \tag{2.76}$$

$$K_1 K_2 = k_1 k_{12} = k_2 k_{21} \tag{2.77}$$

Various methods have been proposed whereby the microdissociation constants for the morphine system may be evaluated.[14] Other drugs for which microdissociation constants have been derived include the tetracyclines,[15] doxorubicin,[16] cephalosporin,[17] dopamine[18] and the group of drugs shown in Box 2.10.

2.5.7 pK_a values of proteins

The pK_a values of ionisable groups in proteins and other macromolecules can be significantly different from those of the corresponding groups when they are isolated in solution. The shifts in pK_a values between native and denatured states or between bound and free forms of a complex can cause changes in binding constants or stability of the protein due to pH effects. For example, the acid denaturation of proteins may be a consequence of anomalous shifts of the pK_a values of a small number of amino acids in the native protein.[19] Several possible causes of such shifts have been proposed. They may arise from interactions between ionisable groups on the protein molecule; for example, an acidic group will have its pK_a lowered by interactions with basic groups. Other suggested cases of shifts of pK_a include hydrogen-bonding interactions with nonionisable groups and the degree of exposure to the bulk solvent; for example, an acidic group will have its pK_a increased if it is fully or partially removed from solvent, but the effect may be reversed by strong hydrogen-bonding interactions with other groups.

The calculation of pK_a values of protein molecules thus requires a detailed consideration of the environment of each ionisable group, and is consequently highly complex. An additional complication is that a protein with N ionisable residues has 2^N possible ionisation states; the extent of the problem is apparent when it is realised that a moderately sized protein may contain as many as 50 ionisable groups.

2.5.8 Calculation of the pH of drug solutions

We have considered above the effect on the ionisation of a drug of buffering the solution at given pH values. When these weakly acidic or basic drugs are dissolved in water they will, of course, develop a pH value in their own right. In this section we examine how the pH of drug solutions of known concentration can be simply calculated from a knowledge of the pK_a of the drug. We will consider the way in which one of these expressions may be derived from the expression for the ionisation in solution; the derivation of the other expressions follows a similar route and you may wish to derive these for yourselves.

Weakly acidic drugs

The pH of a solution of a weakly ionised acidic drug is given by

$$pH = \tfrac{1}{2}\, pK_a - \tfrac{1}{2}\log c$$

The derivation of this expression is given in Box 2.11.

Box 2.11 Derivation of an expression for the pH of a solution of a weakly acidic drug

We saw above that the dissociation of these types of drugs may be represented by equation (2.64). We can now express the concentrations of each of the species in terms of the degree of dissociation, α, which is a number with a value between 0 (no dissociation) and 1 (complete dissociation):

$$HA + H_2O \rightleftharpoons A^- + H_3O^+$$
$$(1-\alpha)c \qquad \alpha c \qquad \alpha c$$

where c is the initial concentration of the weakly acidic drug in $mol\,dm^{-3}$.

Because the drugs are weak acids, α will be very small and hence the term $(1-\alpha)$ can be approximated to 1. We may therefore write

$$K_a = \frac{\alpha^2 c^2}{(1-\alpha)c} \approx \alpha^2 c \qquad (2.78)$$

Therefore,

$$\alpha^2 = \left(\frac{K_a}{c}\right)^{1/2}$$

To introduce pH into the discussion we note that

$$\alpha c = [H_3O^+] = [H^+]$$
$$\therefore [H^+] = (K_a c)^{1/2}$$
$$\therefore -\log[H^+] = -\tfrac{1}{2}\log K_a - \tfrac{1}{2}\log c$$
$$pH = \tfrac{1}{2}\, pK_a - \tfrac{1}{2}\log c$$

$$(2.79)$$

We now have an expression that enables us to calculate the pH of any concentration of the weakly acidic drug provided that its pK_a value is known.

Example 2.7 Calculation of the pH of a weak acid

Calculate the pH of a $50\,mg\,cm^{-3}$ solution of ascorbic acid (mol wt $= 176.1\,Da; pK_a = 4.17$).

Answer

For a weakly acidic drug,

$$pH = \tfrac{1}{2}\, pK_a - \tfrac{1}{2}\log c$$
$$c = 50\,mg\,cm^{-3} = 50\,g\,dm^{-3}$$
$$= 0.2839\,mol\,dm^{-3}$$
$$\therefore pH = 2.09 + 0.273 = 2.36$$

Weakly basic drugs

We can show by a similar derivation to that of Box 2.11 that the pH of aqueous solutions of weakly basic drugs will be given by

$$pH = \tfrac{1}{2}\, pK_w + \tfrac{1}{2}\, pK_a + \tfrac{1}{2}\log c \quad (2.80)$$

Example 2.8 Calculation of the pH of a weakly basic drug

Calculate the pH of a saturated solution of codeine monohydrate (mol wt $= 317.4$) given that its pK_a is 8.2 and its solubility at room temperature is 1 g in $120\,cm^3$ water.

Answer

Codeine is a weakly basic drug and hence its pH will be given by

$$pH = \tfrac{1}{2}\, pK_w + \tfrac{1}{2}\, pK_a + \tfrac{1}{2}\log c$$

where $c = 1\,g$ in $120\,cm^3 = 8.33\,g\,dm^{-3} = 0.02633\,mol\,dm^{-3}$.

$$\therefore pH = 7.0 + 4.1 - 0.790 = 10.31$$

Drug salts

Because of the limited solubility of many weak acids and weak bases in water, drugs of these types are commonly used as their salts; for example, sodium salicylate is the salt of a weak acid (salicylic acid) and a strong base (sodium hydroxide). The pH of a solution of this type of salt is given by $\rightarrow$ *basic*

$$pH = {}^1/_2\,pK_w + {}^1/_2\,pK_a + {}^1/_2\log c \quad (2.81)$$

Alternatively, a salt may be formed between a weak base and a strong acid; for example, ephedrine hydrochloride is the salt of ephedrine and hydrochloric acid. Solutions of such drugs have a pH given by $\rightarrow$ *acidic*

$$pH = {}^1/_2\,pK_a - {}^1/_2\log c \quad (2.82)$$

Finally, a salt may be produced by the combination of a weak base and a weak acid, as in the case of codeine phosphate. Solutions of such drugs have a pH given by

$$pH = {}^1/_2\,pK_w + {}^1/_2\,pK_a - {}^1/_2\,pK_b \quad (2.83)$$

Note that this equation does not include a concentration term and hence the pH is independent of concentration for such drugs.

Example 2.9 Calculation of the pH of drug salts

Calculate the pH of the following solutions:
(a) 5% oxycodone hydrochloride ($pK_a = 8.9$, mol wt = 405.9 Da).
(b) 600 mg of benzylpenicillin sodium ($pK_a = 2.76$, mol wt = 356.4 Da) in 2 cm^3 of water for injection.
(c) 100 $mg\,cm^{-3}$ chlorphenamine maleate (mol wt = 390.8 Da) in water for injection (pK_b chlorphenamine = 5.0, pK_a maleic acid = 1.9).

Answer

(a) Oxycodone hydrochloride is the salt of a weak base and a strong acid, hence

$$pH = {}^1/_2\,pK_a - {}^1/_2\log c$$

where $c = 50\,g\,dm^{-3} = 0.1232\,mol\,dm^{-3}$.

$$\therefore pH = 4.45 + 0.45 = 4.90$$

(b) Benzylpenicillin sodium is the salt of a weak acid and a strong base, hence

$$pH = {}^1/_2\,pK_w + {}^1/_2\,pK_a + {}^1/_2\log c$$

where $c = 600\,mg$ in 2 $cm^3 = 0.842\,mol\,dm^{-3}$.

$$\therefore pH = 7.00 + 1.38 - 0.037 + 8.34$$

(c) Chlorphenamine maleate is the salt of a weak acid and a weak base, hence

$$pH = {}^1/_2\,pK_w + {}^1/_2\,pK_a - {}^1/_2\,pK_b$$
$$\therefore pH = 7.00 + 0.95 - 2.5 = 5.45$$

Key points

- While some drugs such as tadalafil have no ionisable groups, many drugs are either weak organic acids (for example, acetylsalicylic acid (aspirin)), or weak organic bases (for example, procaine), or their salts (for example, ephedrine hydrochloride); the degree to which these drugs are ionised in solution is highly dependent on the pH. The exceptions to this general statement are the nonelectrolytes, such as the steroids, and the quaternary ammonium compounds, which are completely ionised at all pH values and in this respect behave as strong electrolytes.

- The negative logarithm of the dissociation constant K_a of a weakly acidic drug is the pK_a and that of a weakly basic drug is the pK_b; the sum of pK_a and pK_b values of conjugate acid–base pairs is equal to the negative logarithm of the dissociation constant for water, pK_w (see Table 2.7 for values).

- *Acidic drugs* are completely un-ionised at pH values up to 2 units below their pK_a and completely ionised at pH values greater than 2 units above their pK_a. Conversely, *basic drugs* are completely ionised at pH values up to 2 units below their pK_a and completely un-ionised when the pH is more than 2 units above their pK_a. Both types of drug are exactly 50% ionised at their pK_a values.

- *Salts of weak acids or bases* are essentially completely ionised in solution; for example, when sodium salicylate (salt of the weak acid, salicylic acid, and the strong base NaOH) is dissolved in water, it ionises almost entirely into the conjugate base of salicylic acid, $HOC_6H_5COO^-$, and Na^+ ions. The conjugate acids or bases formed in this way are subject to the usual acid–base equilibria.

- *Amphoteric drugs* can function as either weak acids or weak bases in aqueous solution depending on the pH and have pK_a values corresponding to the ionisation of each group. Depending on the relative acidity of the two ionisable groups, they may be ordinary ampholytes (when the pK_a of the acidic group, pK_a^{acidic}, is higher than that of the basic group, pK_a^{basic}), or zwitterionic ampholytes (when $pK_a^{acidic} < pK_a^{basic}$). Ordinary ampholytes exist in solution as a cation, an un-ionised form, and an anion. Zwitterionic ampholytes exist in solution as a cation, a zwitterion (having both positive and negative charges), and an anion depending on the pH of the solution.

- Several acids, for example citric, phosphoric and tartaric acid, are capable of donating more than one proton and these compounds are referred to as *polyprotic* or *polybasic* acids. Similarly, polyprotic bases are capable of accepting two or more protons. Each stage of the dissociation of the drug may be represented by an equilibrium expression and hence each stage has a distinct pK_a or pK_b value. In cases where the dissociation constants of each dissociation stage are less than about 2 pH units apart, it is necessary to take into account all possible ways in which the molecule may be ionised and all the possible species present in solution. In this case the constants are called *microdissociation constants*.

- The pH of aqueous solutions of each of these types of drug and their salts can be calculated from their pK_a and the concentration c of the drug:
  - *Weakly acidic drugs:* $pH = \frac{1}{2}pK_a - \frac{1}{2}\log c$
  - *Weakly basic drugs:* $pH = \frac{1}{2}pK_w + \frac{1}{2}pK_a + \frac{1}{2}\log c$
  - *Drug salts:*
    - Salts of a weak acid and a strong base: $pH = \frac{1}{2}pK_w + \frac{1}{2}pK_a + \frac{1}{2}\log c$
    - Salts of a weak base and a strong acid: $pH = \frac{1}{2}pK_a - \frac{1}{2}\log c$
    - Salts of a weak acid and a weak base: $pH = \frac{1}{2}K_w + \frac{1}{2}pK_a - \frac{1}{2}pK_b$ (Note that there is no concentration term in this equation meaning that the pH does not vary with concentration.)

2.5.9 Buffer solutions

A mixture of a weak acid and its salt (that is, a conjugate base) or of a weak base and its conjugate acid has the ability to reduce the large changes in pH that would otherwise result from the addition of small amounts of acid or alkali to the solution. The reason for the buffering action of a weak acid HA and its ionisable salt (for example, NaA) is that the A^- ions from the salt combine with the added H^+ ions,

removing them from solution as an undissociated weak acid:

$$A^- + H_3O^+ \rightleftharpoons H_2O + HA$$

Added OH^- ions are removed by combination with the weak acid to form undissociated water molecules:

$$HA + OH^- \rightleftharpoons H_2O + A^-$$

The buffering action of a mixture of a weak base and its salt arises from a removal of H^+ ions by the base B to form the salt and removal of OH^- ions by the salt to form undissociated water:

$$B + H_3O^+ \rightleftharpoons H_2O + BH^+$$
$$BH^+ + OH^- \rightleftharpoons H_2O + B$$

The concentration of buffer components required to maintain a solution at the required pH may be calculated using equation (2.71). Since the acid is weak and therefore only very slightly ionised, the term [HA] in this equation may be equated with the total acid concentration. Similarly, the free A^- ions in solution may be considered to originate entirely from the salt and the term $[A^-]$ may be replaced by the salt concentration.

Equation (2.71) now becomes

$$pH = pK_a + \log \frac{[\text{salt}]}{[\text{acid}]} \qquad (2.84)$$

By a similar reasoning, equation (2.73) may be modified to facilitate the calculation of the pH of a solution of a weak base and its salt, giving

$$pH = pK_w - pK_a + \log \frac{[\text{base}]}{[\text{salt}]} \qquad (2.85)$$

Equations (2.84) and (2.85) are often referred to as the *Henderson–Hasselbalch equations*.

Example 2.10 Buffer solutions

Calculate the amount of sodium acetate to be added to $100 \, cm^3$ of a $0.1 \, mol \, dm^{-3}$ acetic acid solution to prepare a buffer of pH 5.20.

Answer

The pK_a of acetic acid is 4.76. Substitution in equation (2.84) gives

$$5.20 = 4.76 + \log \frac{[\text{salt}]}{[\text{acid}]}$$

The molar ratio of [salt]/[acid] is 2.754. Since $100 \, cm^3$ of $0.1 \, mol \, dm^{-3}$ acetic acid contains 0.01 mol, we would require 0.02754 mol of sodium acetate (2.258 g), ignoring dilution effects.

Equations (2.84) and (2.85) are also useful in calculating the change in pH that results from the addition of a specific amount of acid or alkali to a given buffer solution, as seen from the calculation in Example 2.11.

Example 2.11 Calculation of the pH change in buffer solutions

Calculate the change in pH following the addition of $10 \, cm^3$ of $0.1 \, mol \, dm^{-3}$ NaOH to the buffer solution described in Example 2.10.

Answer

The added $10 \, cm^3$ of $0.1 \, mol \, dm^{-3}$ NaOH (equivalent to 0.001 mol) combines with 0.001 mol of acetic acid to produce 0.001 mol of sodium acetate. Reapplying equation (2.84) using the revised salt and acid concentrations gives

$$pH = 4.76 + \log \frac{(0.02754 + 0.001)}{(0.01 - 0.001)}$$
$$= 5.26$$

The pH of the buffer has been increased by only 0.06 units following the addition of the alkali.

Buffer capacity

The effectiveness of a buffer in reducing changes in pH is expressed as the buffer capacity, β. The buffer capacity is defined by the ratio

$$\beta = \frac{dc}{d(pH)} \qquad (2.86)$$

where dc is the number of moles of alkali (or acid) needed to change the pH of 1 litre of solution by an amount $d(pH)$. If the addition of 1 mol of alkali to 1 litre of buffer solution produces a pH change of 1 unit, the buffer capacity is unity.

The capacity of a buffer of total initial concentration c_0 can be readily calculated from the pK_a value of the component weak acid using equation (2.90), the derivation of which is given in Box 2.12.

Box 2.12 Derivation of an equation for buffer capacity

Equation (2.71) may be rewritten in the form

$$pH = pK_a + \frac{1}{2.303} \ln \left[\frac{c}{c_0 - c} \right] \quad (2.87)$$

where c_0 is the total initial buffer concentration and c is the amount of alkali added. Rearrangement and subsequent differentiation yields

$$c = \frac{c_0}{1 + \exp[-2.303(pH - pK_a)]} \quad (2.88)$$

Therefore,

$$\beta = \frac{dc}{d(pH)}$$
$$= \frac{2.303\, c_0 \exp[2.303\,(pH - pK_a)]}{1 + \exp[2.303 \exp(pH - pK_a)]^2} \quad (2.89)$$

$$\beta = \frac{2.303 c_0 K_a [H_3O^+]}{([H_3O^+] + K_a)^2} \quad (2.90)$$

Example 2.12 Calculation of buffer capacity

Calculate the buffer capacity of the acetic acid–acetate buffer of Example 2.10 at pH 4.0.

Answer

The total amount of buffer components in $100\,cm^3$ of solution $= 0.01 + 0.02754 = 0.03754$ mol. Therefore,

$$c_0 = 0.3754\,mol\,dm^{-3}$$

The pK_a of acetic acid $= 4.76$. Therefore,

$$K_a = 1.75 \times 10^{-5}$$

The pH of the solution $= 4.0$. Therefore,

$$[H_3O^+] = 10^{-4}\,mol\,dm^{-3}$$

Substituting in equation (2.90):

$$\beta = \frac{2.303 \times 0.3754 \times 1.75 \times 10^{-5} \times 10^{-4}}{(10^{-4} + 1.75 \times 10^{-5})^2}$$
$$= 0.1096$$

The buffer capacity of the acetic acid–acetate buffer is $0.1096\,mol\,dm^{-3}$ per pH unit.

Figure 2.9 shows the variation of buffer capacity with pH for the acetic acid–acetate buffer used in the numerical examples above ($c_0 = 0.3754\,mol\,dm^{-3}$) as calculated from equation (2.90). It should be noted that β is at a maximum when $pH = pK_a$ (that is, at pH 4.76). When selecting a weak acid for the preparation of a buffer solution, therefore, the chosen acid should have a pK_a as close as possible to the pH required. Substituting $pH = pK_a$ into equation (2.90) gives the useful result that the maximum buffer capacity, β_{max}, is

$$\beta_{Max} = 0.576 c_0 \quad (2.91)$$

where c_0 is the total buffer concentration.

Buffer solutions are widely used in pharmacy to adjust the pH of aqueous solutions to that required for maximum stability or that needed for optimum physiological effect. Solutions for application to delicate

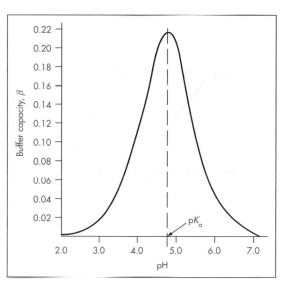

Figure 2.9 Buffer capacity of acetic acid–acetate buffer (initial concentration $= 0.3754\,mol\,dm^{-3}$) as a function of pH.

tissues, particularly the eye, should also be formulated at a pH not too far removed from that of the appropriate tissue fluid, as otherwise irritation may be caused on administration. The pH of tears lies between 7 and 8, with an average value of 7.4. Fortunately, the buffer capacity of tears is high, and provided that the solutions to be administered have a low buffer capacity, a reasonably wide range of pH may be tolerated, although there is a difference in the irritability of the various ionic species that are commonly used as buffer components. As explained below, the pH of blood is maintained at about 7.4 by primary buffer components in the plasma (carbonic acid–carbonate and the acid–sodium salts of phosphoric acid) and secondary buffer components in the erythrocytes. Values of 0.025 and 0.039 mol dm^{-3} per pH unit have been quoted for the buffer capacity of whole blood. Parenteral solutions are not normally buffered, or alternatively are buffered at a very low capacity, since the buffers of the blood are usually capable of bringing them within a tolerable pH range.

 Clinical point

The normal pH of arterial blood is 7.4, while that of venous blood and of interstitial fluids is about 7.35, because of extra quantities of carbon dioxide that form carbonic acid in these fluids. A person is considered to have *acidosis* whenever the pH of blood plasma falls below 7.35; in this state the central nervous system becomes depressed, causing symptoms such as confusion, disorientation and coma. If the pH rises above 7.45 the person is said to have *alkalosis*, a condition characterised by over stimulation of the skeletal muscles causing muscle spasms, convulsion or respiratory paralysis. The importance of control of the pH of arterial blood is apparent when it is realised that the lower pH limit at which a person can survive for more than a few hours is about 7.0 and the upper limit approximately 7.7; the situation quickly becomes fatal if pH falls below 6.8 or rises above 8.0.

Physiological regulation of acid-base balance

Several control mechanisms are available to prevent acidosis and alkalosis. All the body fluids are supplied with acid–base buffer systems that immediately combine with any acid or alkali and thereby prevent excessive changes in hydrogen ion concentration. These *chemical* buffer systems are discussed in more detail below. In addition, if the hydrogen ion concentration does change measurably, two *physiological* buffer mechanisms – the respiratory and urinary systems – come into operation. These systems are appreciably slower to react to changes in pH than the chemical buffers, which can respond within a fraction of a second. The basis of the buffering action of the *respiratory* system is an immediate alteration of the rate of pulmonary ventilation and consequently the rate of removal of carbon dioxide from the body fluids; a process that takes two to three minutes to restore the pH to normal. The *urinary* buffer system operates differently from the other buffering systems in that the hydrogen ions are actually expelled from the body in the urine, thereby readjusting their concentration in body fluids to normal. Although the kidneys are more effective in restoring pH than the other buffering mechanisms, the process is considerably slower, taking several hours to readjust the hydrogen ion concentration.

The three major *chemical* buffers are the bicarbonate, phosphate and protein systems. Each of these performs major buffering functions under different conditions.

The *bicarbonate* buffer system consists of a solution of the weak acid carbonic acid (pK_a 6.1) and its salt sodium bicarbonate.

$$H_2CO_3 \rightleftharpoons HCO_3^- + H^+$$

An acidic substance added to the blood would be neutralised by the bicarbonate ions and the carbon dioxide produced excreted by the lungs.

$$HCO_3^- + H^+ \rightleftharpoons H_2CO_3 \rightleftharpoons H_2O + CO_2$$

A base added to the blood would be neutralised by the reaction

$$H_2CO_3 + OH^- \rightleftharpoons HCO_3^- + H_2O$$

This might seem, at first sight, to be a rather ineffective system for two reasons. Firstly, the buffer is operating at a pH (7.4) well away from its maximum buffering capacity which, as we have already discussed, is at the pK_a (6.1). Secondly, the concentrations of the bicarbonate buffer are relatively low. The buffer system is, however, extremely efficient because it is self-regulating; carbonic acid is replenished by carbon dioxide from respiration, and bicarbonate ions by the kidneys.

The *phosphate* buffer system operates in the internal fluid of all cells and consists of dihydrogenphosphate ions ($H_2PO_4^-$) as hydrogen-ion donor (acid) and hydrogenphosphate ions (HPO_4^{2-}) as hydrogen-ion acceptor (base). These two ions are in equilibrium with each other as indicated by the chemical equation

$$H_2PO_4^- \rightleftharpoons H^+ + HPO_4^{2-}$$

If additional hydrogen ions enter the cellular fluid, they are consumed in the reaction with HPO_4^{2-}, and the equilibrium shifts to the left. If additional hydroxide ions enter the cellular fluid, they react with $H_2PO_4^-$, producing HPO_4^{2-}, and shifting the equilibrium to the right. The pK_a of this equilibrium, 7.2, is closer to the physiological pH than that of the bicarbonate buffer, but its concentration in the extracellular fluids is only one sixth of this buffer.

The *protein* buffer system accounts for about 75% of all chemical buffering ability of the body fluids. The buffering ability of proteins is due to the dissociation of the acidic –COOH groups of the amino acid residues to –COO$^-$ and H$^+$, and the dissociation of the basic –NH$_3$OH groups of the amino acids into NH$_3$ and OH$^-$. Furthermore, the pK_a values of the amino acids are not far from 7.4, making the protein buffering systems by far the most powerful of the body.

Universal buffers

We have seen from Fig. 2.9 that the buffer capacity is at a maximum at a pH equal to the pK_a of the weak acid used in the formulation of the buffer system and decreases appreciably as the pH extends more than 1 unit either side of this value. If, instead of a single weak monobasic acid, a suitable mixture of polybasic and monobasic acids is used, it is possible to produce a buffer that is effective over a wide pH range. Such solutions are referred to as *universal buffers*. A typical example is a mixture of citric acid ($pK_{a1} = 3.06$, $pK_{a2} = 4.78$, $pK_{a3} = 5.40$), Na$_2$HPO$_4$ (pK_a of

conjugate acid, $H_2PO_4^- = 7.2$), diethylbarbituric acid ($pK_{a1} = 7.43$) and boric acid ($pK_{a1} = 9.24$). Because of the wide range of pK_a values involved, each associated with a maximum buffer capacity, this buffer is effective over a correspondingly wide pH range (pH 2.4 – 12).

Key points

- Buffers are usually mixtures of a weak acid and its salt (conjugate base), or a weak base and its conjugate acid.
- The concentration of buffer components required to maintain a solution at the required pH may be calculated from the *Henderson–Hasselbalch equations*:
  - Weak acid and its salt:
    $$pH = pK_a + \log \frac{[salt]}{[acid]}$$
  - Weak base and its salt:
    $$pH = pK_w - pK_b + \log \frac{[base]}{[salt]}$$
- The effectiveness of a buffer in reducing changes in pH is greatest at a pH equal to the pK_a of the weak acid component of the buffer; the maximum buffer capacity, β_{max}, is $0.576c_0$ where c_0 is the total initial buffer concentration.
- Mixtures of polybasic and monobasic acids with a wide range of pK_a values act as universal buffers that are effective over a wide pH range.

2.6 Diffusion of drugs in solution

Diffusion is the process by which a concentration difference is reduced by a spontaneous flow of matter. Consider the simplest case of a solution containing a single solute. The solute will spontaneously diffuse from a region of high concentration to one of low concentration. Strictly speaking, the driving force for diffusion is the gradient of chemical potential, but it is more usual to think of the diffusion of solutes in terms of the gradient of their concentration. Imagine the solution to be divided into volume elements. Although no individual solute particle in a particular volume element shows a preference for motion in any particular direction, a definite fraction of the molecules in this element may be considered to be moving in, say, the x direction. In an adjacent volume element, the same fraction may be moving in the reverse direction. If the concentration in the first volume element is greater than that in the second, the overall effect is that more particles are leaving the first element for the second and hence there is a net flow of solute in the x direction, the direction of decreasing concentration. The expression that relates the flow of material to the concentration gradient (dc/dx) is referred to as *Fick's first law*:

$$J = -D(dc/dx) \qquad (2.92)$$

where J is the flux of a component across a plane of unit area and D is the diffusion coefficient (or diffusivity). The negative sign indicates that the flux is in the direction of decreasing concentration. J is in units of $mol\,m^{-2}\,s^{-1}$, c is in $mol\,m^{-3}$ and x is in metres; therefore, the units of D are $m^2\,s^{-1}$.

The relationship between the radius, a, of the diffusing molecule and its diffusion coefficient (assuming spherical particles or molecules) is given by the *Stokes–Einstein equation* as

$$D = \frac{RT}{6\pi\eta a N_A} \qquad (2.93)$$

Table 2.9 shows diffusion coefficients of some p-hydroxybenzoate (paraben) preservatives and typical proteins in aqueous solution. Although the trend for a decrease of D with increase of molecular size (as predicted by equation 2.93) is clearly seen from the data of this table, it is also clear that other factors such as branching of the p-hydroxybenzoate molecules (as with the isoalkyl derivatives) and the shape of the protein molecules also affect the diffusion coefficients. The diffusion coefficients of more complex molecules such as proteins will also be affected by the shape of the molecule,

Table 2.9 Effect of molecular weight on diffusion coefficient (25°C) in aqueous media

Compound	Molecular weight	D $(10^{-10}\,m^2\,s^{-1})$
p-Hydroxybenzoates[a]		
Methyl hydroxybenzoate	152.2	8.44
Ethyl hydroxybenzoate	166.2	7.48
n-Propyl hydroxybenzoate	180.2	6.81
Isopropyl hydroxybenzoate	180.2	6.94
n-Butyl hydroxybenzoate	194.2	6.31
Isobutyl hydroxybenzoate	194.2	6.40
n-Amyl hydroxybenzoate	208.2	5.70
Proteins[b]		
Cytochrome c (horse)	12 400	1.28
Lysozyme (chicken)	14 400	0.95
Trypsin (bovine)	24 000	1.10
Albumin (bovine)	66 000	0.46

[a] From reference 20.
[b] From reference 21; see also Chapter 12 for further values of therapeutic peptides and proteins.

more asymmetric molecules having a greater resistance to flow.

The diffusional properties of a drug have relevance in pharmaceutical systems in consideration of such processes as the dissolution of the drug and transport through artificial (e.g. polymer) or biological membranes. Diffusion in tissues such as the skin or in tumours is a process that relies on the same criteria as discussed above, even though the diffusion takes place in complex media. Diffusion is discussed in several other chapters.

Summary

This chapter has dealt with several physicochemical properties of drugs of relevance to their formulation in aqueous solution and their biological activity. Of primary importance is their ionisation in solution since this influences such important physicochemical properties as their osmolarity, solubility and activity, and their *in vivo* absorption, distribution and elimination. We have seen how the extent of ionisation of the large number of drugs that are weak acids or bases or salts of acids or bases is dependent on pH and can be predicted from the pK_a value. Acidic drugs are completely un-ionised at pH values up to 2 units below their pK_a and completely ionised at pH values greater than 2 units above their pK_a. Conversely, basic drugs are completely ionised at pH values up to 2 units below their pK_a and completely un-ionised when the pH is more than 2 units above their pK_a. Both types of drug are exactly 50% ionised at their pK_a values.

The pH of liquid formulations may be confined to within narrow limits through the use of buffers consisting of mixtures of weak acids or bases and their salts and we have seen how to formulate buffer systems effective at a chosen pH or, in the case of universal buffers, over a wide range of pH values. In a clinical setting, drug ionisation may be altered by adjustment of, for example, the pH of urine with the aim of increasing the excretion of toxic substances.

Osmotic effects are important from a physiological viewpoint since the red blood cell membrane acts as a semipermeable membrane, with implications for the integrity of red blood cells when immersed in solutions of osmotic pressures which differ from that of their contents. A simple equation (the Henderson–Hasselbalch equation), for the calculation of the amount of adjusting substance required to ensure the isotonicity of a drug solution has been proposed. Additives, such as ethyl alcohol, sorbitol and propylene glycol make a large contribution to the osmolarities of oral formulations, which must be recognised when these are administered to infants at risk from necrotising enterocolitis. Applications of the osmotic effect in the design of rehydration solutions and in oral rehydration therapy have been discussed.

The driving force for the spontaneous diffusion of drugs in solution is the difference in concentration, or more precisely, the chemical potential gradient between different regions of the system. For example, a drug will transfer between two immiscible phases until its chemical potential is the same in both phases, when a state of equilibrium will be reached. The diffusional properties of a drug are relevant to processes such as the dissolution of the drug and its membrane transport.

References

1. *The Pharmaceutical Codex*, 12th edn. London: Pharmaceutical Press, 1994.
2. Atkins PW, de Paula J. *Atkins' Physical Chemistry*. 8th edn. Oxford: Oxford University Press; 2006.
3. Rytting JH *et al.* Suggested thermodynamic standard state for comparing drug molecules in structure-activity studies. *J Pharm Sci* 1972;61:816–818.
4. Christian JHB. In: Rockland LB, Stewart GF, eds. *Water Activity: Influences on Food Quality*. New York: Academic Press; 1981: 825
5. Ambrose U *et al. In vitro* studies of water activity and bacterial growth inhibition of sucrose-polyethylene glycol 400-hydrogen peroxide and xylose-polyethylene glycol 400-hydrogen peroxide pastes used to treat infected wounds. *Antimicrob Agents Chemother* 1991; 35:1799–1803.
6. Streng WH *et al.* Relationship between osmolality and osmolarity. *J Pharm Sci* 1978;67:384–386.
7. Willis DM *et al.* Unsuspected hyperosmolality of oral solutions contributing to necrotizing enterocolitis in very-low-birth-weight infants. *Pediatrics* 1977;60: 535–538.
8. White KC, Harkavy KL. Hypertonic formula resulting from added oral medications. *Am J Dis Child* 1982;136:931–933.
9. Luedtke SA. Pediatric and neonatal therapy. In: Helms RA, Quan DJ, eds. *Textbook of Therapeutics: Drug and Disease Management*. 8th edn. Philadelphia: Lippincott, Williams and Wilkins; 2006: 325–340.
10. Lerman J *et al.* Osmolarity determines the solubility of anesthetics in aqueous solutions at $37°C$. *Anesthesiology* 1983;59:554–558.
11. *The Merck Index*. 12th edn. Rahway, NJ: Merck; 1996
12. Pagliara A *et al.* Lipophilicity profiles of ampholytes. *Chem Rev* 1997;97:3385–3400.
13. Bouchard G *et al.* Theoretical and experimental exploration of the lipophilicity of zwitterionic drugs in 1,2-dichloroethane/water system. *Pharm Res* 2002;19:1150–1159.
14. Niebergall PJ *et al.* Spectral determination of microdissociation constants. *J Pharm Sci* 1972;61, 232.
15. Leeson LJ *et al.* Structural assignment of the second and third acidity constants of tetracycline antibiotics. *Tetrahedron Lett* 1963;18:1155–1160.
16. Sturgeon RJ, Schulman SG. Electronic absorption spectra and protolytic equilibriums of doxorubicin: direct

spectrophotometric determination of microconstants. *J Pharm Sci* 1977;66:958–961.

17. Streng W.H. *et al*. Ionization constants of cephalosporin zwitterionic compounds. *J Pharm Sci*, 65, 1034 (1976); 66, 1357 (1977).

18. Ishimitsu T *et al*. Microscopic acid dissociation constants of 3, 4-dihydroxyphenethylamine (dopamine). *Chem Pharm Bull* 1978;26:74–78.

19. Honig B, Nicholls A. Classical electrostatics in biology and chemistry. *Science* 1995;268:1144–1149.

20. Seki T *et al*. Measurement of diffusion coefficients of parabens by the chromatographic broadening method. *J Pharm Sci Technol Jpn* 2000;60:114–117.

21. Baden N, Terazima M. A novel method for measurement of diffusion coefficients of proteins and DNA in solution. *Chem Phys Lett* 2004;393:539–545.

3

Drug stability

Many drugs are susceptible to some form of chemical decomposition when formulated in either liquid or even solid dosage forms. Such degradation can lead to rejection of a drug product for one or more of the following reasons.

- Chemical degradation of the active drug can lead to a substantial lowering of the quantity of the therapeutic agent in the dosage form. Many drugs, including for example digoxin and theophylline, have narrow therapeutic indices, and they need to be carefully titrated in individual patients so that serum levels are neither so high that they are potentially toxic, nor so low that they are ineffective. For these drugs, it is important that the dosage form reproducibly delivers the same amount of drug.
- Although chemical degradation of the active drug may not be extensive, a toxic product may be formed in the decomposition process. There are several examples in which the products of degradation are significantly more toxic than the original therapeutic agent. For example, the conversions of tetracycline to epianhydrotetracycline, of arsphenamine to oxophenarsine of and p-aminosalicylic acid to m-aminophenol in dosage forms give rise to potentially toxic agents that, when ingested, can cause undesirable effects.
- A substantial lowering in the therapeutic efficacy of the dosage form, may occur as a consequence of physical or chemical changes in the excipients present in the dosage form, irrespective of any changes in the active drug.
- There may be noticeable changes in the physical appearance of the dosage form, for example, discoloration following the photochemical decomposition of the drug; mottling of tablets; creaming of emulsions and caking of suspensions. Although such changes may not affect therapeutic efficacy, they may lead to a loss of confidence by the patient in the product.

In this chapter we will identify those classes of drugs that are particularly susceptible to chemical breakdown and examine some of the precautions that can be taken to minimise the loss of activity. It is important to be able to determine a time interval over which the drug retains sufficient potency for it to be used. Usually the shelf-life is assumed to be the time taken for the concentration of the drug to be reduced to 95% of its value when originally prepared. To be able to make shelf-life predictions we should first understand the kinetics of the decomposition process. We will look at how reactions can be classified into various 'orders', and how we can calculate the rate constant for a reaction under a given set of environmental conditions. Methods for accelerating the drug breakdown using elevated temperatures will be examined and we will see how it is possible to estimate the stability of the drug for the required storage conditions from these measurements. Although such experiments cannot replace the rigorous stability testing procedures on the product in the form in which it is finally to be marketed, they do lead to considerable saving of time at the product development stage when it is necessary to identify rapidly a formulation in which the stability is at an acceptable level.

3.1 The chemical decomposition of drugs

In this section we examine various ways in which drugs in both liquid and solid formulations can lose their activity, so that we can be aware of those chemical groups that when present in drug molecules can cause stability problems. We will later see how to prevent or minimise the chemical breakdown for each type of decomposition process. Although each decomposition scheme is considered separately, it should be noted that with some drug molecules more than one type of decomposition may be occurring at the same time; this, of course, complicates the analysis of the system.

3.1.1 Hydrolysis

Drugs susceptible to hydrolytic degradation

How can we tell whether a drug is likely to be susceptible to this type of degradation? If the drug is a derivative of carboxylic acid or contains functional groups based on this moiety, for example, an ester, amide, lactone, lactam, and imide or carbamate (see Scheme 3.1), then we are dealing with a drug that is liable to undergo hydrolytic degradation. We will consider some examples.

Drugs that contain ester linkages include acetylsalicylic acid, physostigmine, methyldopa, tetracaine and procaine. Ester hydrolysis is usually a bimolecular reaction involving acyl-oxygen cleavage. For example, the hydrolysis of procaine is shown in Scheme 3.2.

The hydrolysis of amides involves the cleavage of the amide linkage as, for example, in the breakdown of the local anaesthetic cinchocaine (Scheme 3.3). This type of link is also found in drugs such as chloramphenicol, ergometrine and benzylpenicillin sodium.

As examples of lactam ring hydrolysis we can consider the decomposition of nitrazepam and chlordiazepoxide, which is discussed in more detail later (section 3.2.7). Other drugs, apart from the benzodiazepines, which are susceptible to lactam-ring hydrolysis include the penicillins and cephalosporins.

Structure	Chemical class
O O $\parallel$ H $\parallel$ $RC-N-CR$	Imide
$RCH---CO$ $\backslash$ $\vert$ $(CH_2)_n-NH$	Lactam
$RCH---CO$ $\backslash$ $\vert$ $(CH_2)_n-O$	Lactone
O $\parallel$ $RC-OR'$	Ester
O $\parallel$ $RC-NH_2$	Amide

Scheme 3.1 Examples of chemical groups susceptible to hydrolysis.

Scheme 3.2 Hydrolysis of the ester group of procaine.

Scheme 3.3 Hydrolysis of the amide linkage of cinchocaine.

The lactones pilocarpine and spironolactone are susceptible to hydrolysis, as are the imides glutethimide and ethosuximide.

A recent review by LePree and Connors[1] gives a detailed account of the mechanisms involved in the hydrolytic degradation of drugs.

Controlling drug hydrolysis in solution

Optimisation of formulation

Hydrolysis is frequently catalysed by hydrogen ions (specific acid-catalysis) or hydroxyl ions (specific base-catalysis) and also by other acidic or basic species that are commonly encountered as components of buffers. This latter type of catalysis is referred to as general acid–base catalysis. Both types of catalysis will be dealt with in greater depth in section 3.4.1. Several methods are available to stabilise a solution of a drug that is susceptible to acid–base catalysed hydrolysis. The usual method is to determine the pH of maximum stability from kinetic experiments at a range of pH values and to formulate the product at this pH (section 3.4.1). Alteration of the dielectric constant by the addition of nonaqueous solvents such as alcohol, glycerin or propylene glycol may in many cases reduce hydrolysis (section 3.4.1).

Since only that portion of the drug which is in solution will be hydrolysed, it is possible to suppress degradation by making the drug less soluble. The stability of penicillin in procaine penicillin suspensions was significantly increased by reducing its solubility by using additives such as citrates, dextrose, sorbitol and gluconate. Adding a compound that forms a complex with the drug can increase stability. The addition of caffeine to aqueous solutions of benzocaine, procaine and tetracaine was shown to decrease the base-catalysed hydrolysis of these local anaesthetics in this way. In many cases, solubilisation of a drug by surfactants protects against hydrolysis, as discussed in section 3.4.1.

Modification of chemical structure of drug

The control of drug stability by modifying chemical structure using appropriate substituents has been suggested for drugs for which such a modification does not reduce therapeutic efficiency. The *Hammett linear*

free energy relationship for the effect of substituents on the rates of aromatic side-chain reactions, such as the hydrolysis of esters, is given by

$$\log k = \log k_0 + \sigma\rho \qquad (3.1)$$

where k and k_0 are the rate constants for the reaction of the substituted and unsubstituted compounds, respectively, σ is the Hammett substituent constant (which is determined by the nature of the substituents and is independent of the reaction), and ρ is the reaction constant, which is dependent on the reaction, the conditions of reaction and the nature of the side-chains undergoing reaction. Thus, a plot of $\log k$ against the Hammett constant (values are readily available in the literature[2]) is linear if this relationship is obeyed, with a slope of ρ. This concept has been used, for example, in the production of the best substituents for allylbarbituric acids to obtain optimum stability.[3]

3.1.2 Oxidation[4]

After hydrolysis, oxidation is the next most common pathway for drug breakdown. However, whereas the hydrolytic degradation of drugs has been thoroughly studied, their oxidative degradation has received comparatively little attention. Indeed, in cases where simultaneous hydrolytic and oxidative degradation can occur, the oxidative process has usually been eliminated by storage under anaerobic conditions without an investigation of the oxidative mechanism.

Oxidation processes

Oxidation involves the removal of an electropositive atom, radical or electron, or the addition of an electronegative atom or radical. Oxidative degradation can occur by *autoxidation*, in which reaction is uncatalysed and proceeds quite slowly under the influence of molecular oxygen, or may involve *chain processes* consisting of three concurrent reactions – initiation, propagation and termination. Initiation can be via free radicals formed from organic compounds by the action of light, heat or transition metals such as copper and iron that are present in trace amounts in almost every buffer. The propagation stage of the reaction involves the combination of molecular oxygen with the free radical R• to form a peroxy radical ROO•, which then removes H from a molecule of the organic compound to form a hydroperoxide, ROOH, and in so doing creates a new free radical (Scheme 3.4).

Initiation: $X^• + RH \longrightarrow R^• + XH$

Propagation: $R^• + O_2 \longrightarrow ROO^•$

$ROO^• + RH \longrightarrow ROOH + R^•$

Termination: $ROO^• + ROO^• \longrightarrow$ stable product

$ROO^• + R^• \longrightarrow$ stable product

$R^• + R^• \longrightarrow$ stable product

Scheme 3.4 Simplified oxidation scheme involving a chain process.

The reaction proceeds until the free radicals are destroyed by inhibitors or by side-reactions that eventually break the chain. The rancid odour that is a characteristic of oxidised fats and oils is due to aldehydes, ketones and short-chain fatty acids, which are the breakdown products of the hydroperoxides. Peroxides (ROOR') and hydroperoxides (ROOH) are photolabile, breaking down to hydroxyl (HO•) and/or alkoxyl (RO•) radicals, which are themselves highly oxidising species. The presence of residual peroxides in polyoxyethylene glycols (PEGs) is a cause for concern when these excipients are used in formulation, as for example in the case of fenprostalene.[5]

Drugs susceptible to oxidation

We will consider some examples of drugs and excipients that are subject to oxidative degradation owing to the possession of functional groups that are particularly sensitive to oxidation.

Steroids and sterols represent an important class of drugs that are subject to oxidative degradation through the possession of carbon–carbon double bonds (alkene moieties) to which peroxyl radicals can readily add. Similarly, *polyunsaturated fatty acids*, commonly used in drug formulations, are particularly susceptible to oxidation and care must be exercised to minimise degradation in formulations containing high concentrations of, for example, vegetable oils.[6] For drugs such as the cholesterol-lowering agent *simvastatin* (**I**) that contain conjugated double bonds, addition of peroxyl radicals may lead to the formation of polymeric peroxides (simvastatin polymerises up to a pentamer[7]), cleavage of which produces epoxides which may further degrade into aldehydes or ketones.

Structure I Simvastatin

Polyene antibiotics, such as amphotericin B (**II**) which contains seven conjugated double bonds (heptaene moiety), are subject to attack by peroxyl radicals leading to aggregation and loss of activity.[8]

Structure II Amphotericin B

Scheme 3.5 Oxidation of phenothiazines.

The oxidation of *phenothiazines* to the sulfoxide involves two single-electron transfer reactions involving a radical cation intermediate as shown in Scheme 3.5. The sulfoxide is subsequently formed by reaction of the cation with water.

The ether group in drugs such as *econazole nitrate* (**III**) and *miconazole nitrate* (**IV**) is susceptible to oxidation. The process involves removal of hydrogen from the C–H bonds in the α-position to the oxygen to produce a radical, which further degrades to α-hydroperoxides and eventually to aldehydes, ketones, alcohols and carboxylic acids.

Structure III   Econazole nitrate

Structure IV   Miconazole nitrate

Stabilisation against oxidation

Various precautions should be taken during manufacture and storage to minimise oxidation. The oxygen in pharmaceutical containers should be replaced with nitrogen or carbon dioxide; contact of the drug with heavy-metal ions such as iron, cobalt or nickel that catalyse oxidation should be avoided; and storage should be at reduced temperatures.

Antioxidants

It is very difficult to remove all of the oxygen from a container and even traces of oxygen are sufficient to initiate the oxidation chain. The propagation of the chain reaction may be prevented or delayed by adding low concentrations of compounds that act as inhibitors. Such compounds are called *antioxidants* and interrupt the propagation by interaction with the free radical. The antioxidant free radical so formed is not sufficiently reactive to maintain the chain reaction and is eventually annihilated. The structures of some commonly used antioxidants are given in Scheme 3.6. Reducing agents such as sodium metabisulfite may also be added to formulations to prevent oxidation. These compounds are more readily oxidised than the drug and so protect it from oxidation by consuming the oxygen. They are particularly effective in closed systems in which the oxygen cannot be replaced once it has been consumed. Chelating agents, such as ethylenediaminetetraacetic acid (EDTA) derivatives, may also protect the drug from autooxidation. These act by forming complexes with the heavy metal ions that are often required to initiate oxidation reactions. Oxidation is catalysed by unprotonated amines such as aminophylline, and hence admixture of susceptible drugs with such compounds should be avoided.

3.1.3 Isomerisation

Isomerisation is the process of conversion of a drug into its optical or geometric isomers. Since the various isomers of a drug are frequently of different activities, such a conversion may be regarded as a form of degradation, often resulting in a serious loss of therapeutic activity. For example, the appreciable loss of activity of solutions of adrenaline at low pH has been attributed to *racemisation* – the conversion of the therapeutically active form, in this case the levorotary form, into its less-active isomer.

In acidic conditions the tetracyclines undergo epimerisation at carbon atom 4 to form an equilibrium mixture of tetracycline and the epimer, 4-epi-tetracycline

Butylated hydroxyanisole (BHA)   Butylated hydroxytoluene (BHT)   Propyl gallate

Vitamin E
α-Tocopherol ($R^1 = R^2 = R^3 = Me$)
β-Tocopherol ($R^1 = R^3 = Me$, $R^2 = H$)
γ-Tocopherol ($R^1 = R^2 = Me$, $R^3 = H$)
δ-Tocopherol ($R^1 = Me$, $R^2 = R^3 = H$)

Ascorbic acid (vitamin C)   Ascorbyl palmitate   Thioglycerol   Thioglycolic acid

Sodium bisulfite   Sodium sulfite   Sodium metabisulfite

Scheme 3.6 Structures of some common antioxidants.

Partial structure of 4-epi-tetracycline   Partial structure of natural tetracycline

Scheme 3.7 Epimerisation of tetracyclines.

(Scheme 3.7). The 4-epi-tetracycline is toxic and its content in medicines is restricted to not more than 3%. The epimerisation follows the kinetics of a first-order reversible reaction (see equation 3.24). The degradation rate is pH-dependent (maximum epimerisation occurring at pH 3.2) and is also catalysed by phosphate and citrate ions.

Cephalosporin esters are widely used as intermediates in cephalosporin synthesis and as prodrugs for oral administration of parenteral cephalosporins. These esters undergo reversible base-catalysed isomerisation

Scheme 3.8 Proposed mechanism for the base-catalysed isomerisation of cephalosporin esters.
Reproduced from Richter WF et al., J Pharm Sc., 1990; 79: 185.

Scheme 3.9 Isomerisation of vitamin A.

according to the mechanism shown in Scheme 3.8. A proton in the 2-position is abstracted by a base (B) and the resulting carbanion can be reprotonated in the 4-postion, giving a Δ^2-ester. On hydrolysis, Δ^2-cephalosporin esters yield Δ^2-cephalosporins, which are biologically inactive.

Cis-trans isomerisation may be a cause of loss of potency of a drug if the two geometric isomers have different therapeutic activities. Vitamin A (all-*trans*-retinol) is enzymatically oxidised to the aldehyde and then isomerised to yield 11-*cis*-retinal (Scheme 3.9), which has a decreased activity compared with the all-*trans* molecule.

3.1.4 Photochemical decomposition[9]

Many pharmaceutical compounds, including the phenothiazine tranquillisers, hydrocortisone, prednisolone, riboflavin, ascorbic acid and folic acid, degrade when exposed to light. As a result there will be a loss of potency of the drug, often accompanied by changes in the appearance of the product, such as discoloration or formation of a precipitate. Photodecomposition might occur not only during storage but also during usage of the product. For example, sunlight is able to penetrate the skin to a sufficient depth to cause photodegradation of drugs circulating in the surface capillaries or in the eyes of patients receiving the drug.

Primary photochemical reaction occurs when the wavelength of the incident light is within the wavelength range of absorption of the drug (usually within the ultraviolet range, unless the drug is coloured), so that the drug molecule itself absorbs radiation and degrades. Photodegradation may also occur with drugs that do not directly absorb the incident radiation, as a consequence of absorption of radiation by excipients in the formulation (*photosensitisers*) that transfer the absorbed energy to the drug, causing it to degrade. In assessing the photostability of a product it is therefore necessary to consider the final formulation rather than simply the drug itself. The rate of the photodegradation is dependent on the rate at which light is absorbed by the system and also the efficiency of the photochemical process. In formulations that contain low drug concentrations, the primary photochemical reaction follows first-order kinetics; the kinetics are more complicated at higher concentrations and in the solid state because most of the light is then absorbed near the surface of the product.

Although it is difficult to predict which drugs are likely to be prone to photodegradation, there are certain chemical functions that are expected to introduce photoreactivity, including carbonyl, nitroaromatic and N-oxide functions, aryl halides, alkenes, polyenes, and sulfides.[10] The mechanisms

Scheme 3.10 The effect of ultraviolet light on chlorpromazine (CLP).
The first step of the photodegradation is the loss of an electron to yield the semiquinone free radical R. Further stages in the degradation yield the phenazathonium ion P, which is thought to react with water to yield chlorpromazine sulfoxide (CPO). The chlorpromazine sulfoxide is itself photolabile and further decomposition occurs. Other products of the photooxidation include chlorpromazine N-oxide and hydroxychlorpromazine.

Reproduced from Merkle FH, Discher CA, *J Pharm Sci*, 1964; 53: 620.

of photodegradation are of such complexity as to have been fully elucidated in only a few cases. We will consider two examples – chlorpromazine and ketoprofen.

The phenothiazine *chlorpromazine* (CLP) is rapidly decomposed under the action of ultraviolet light, the decomposition being accompanied by discoloration of the solutions (Scheme 3.10).

Structure V   Polymer produced by the ultraviolet irradiation of chlorpromazine under anaerobic conditions.

Scheme 3.11 Photodegradation of ketoprofen.
Photodegradation of ketoprofen by decarboxylation (reaction 1) and subsequent reduction (reaction 2), and also by dimerisation of the ketoprofen (reaction 3).
Reproduced from Tønnesen HH, *Int J Pharm*, 2001: 225; 1.

Chlorpromazine behaves differently towards ultraviolet irradiation under anaerobic conditions. A polymerisation process has been proposed[11] that involves the liberation of HCl in its initial stages. The polymer (**V**) was isolated and upon intracutaneous injection produced a bluish-purple discoloration typical of that observed in some patients receiving prolonged chlorpromazine medication. It was suggested that the skin irritation that accompanies the discoloration may be a result of the HCl liberation during photodecomposition.

The photodegradation of *ketoprofen* can involve decarboxylation to form an intermediate that then undergoes reduction, or dimerisation of the ketoprofen itself as illustrated in Scheme 3.11.

Stabilisation against photochemical decomposition

Pharmaceutical products can be adequately protected from photoinduced decomposition by the use of coloured glass containers and storage in the dark. Amber glass excludes light of wavelength <470 nm and so affords considerable protection of compounds sensitive to ultraviolet light. Coating tablets with a polymer film containing ultraviolet absorbers has been suggested as an additional method for protection from light. In this respect, a film coating of vinyl acetate containing oxybenzone as an ultraviolet absorber has been shown[12] to be effective in minimising the discoloration and photolytic degradation of sulfasomidine tablets.

3.1.5 Polymerisation

Polymerisation is the process by which two or more identical drug molecules combine together to form a complex molecule. It has been demonstrated that a polymerisation process occurs during the storage of concentrated aqueous solutions of aminopenicillins, such as ampicillin sodium. The reactive β-lactam bond of the ampicillin molecule is opened by reaction with the side-chain of a second ampicillin molecule and a dimer is formed (Scheme 3.12). The process can continue to form higher polymers. Such polymeric substances have been shown to be highly antigenic in animals and they are considered to play a part in eliciting penicilloyl-specific allergic reactions to ampicillin in humans. The dimerising tendency of the aminopenicillins increases with the increase in the basicity of the side-chain group, the order in terms of increasing rates being cyclacillin ≪ ampicillin < epicillin < amoxycillin.

The hydrate of formaldehyde, $HOCH_2OH$, may under certain conditions polymerise in aqueous solution to form paraformaldehyde, $HOCH_2(OCH_2)_n OCH_2OH$, which appears as a white deposit in the solution. The polymerisation may be prevented by adding to the solution 10–15% of methanol.

Scheme 3.12 Dimerisation and hydrolysis of ampicillin.

Reproduced from Bundgaard H, *Acta Pharm Suec*, 1976; 13: 9.

Key points

- The most common cause of degradation of drugs in aqueous systems is hydrolysis and the most susceptible drugs are those containing ester, amide, lactone, lactam, imide or carbamate groups. Hydrolytic breakdown is catalysed by hydrogen and/or hydroxyl ions and consequently the extent of hydrolysis may be reduced by formulating the product at the pH of maximum stability. The inclusion into the formulation of nonaqueous solvents may, in some cases, reduce hydrolysis by alteration of the dielectric constant. It may also be possible to achieve stability by modification of the chemical structure of the drug.

- Oxidative degradation is the second most common cause of drug breakdown and can occur by autoxidation, in which the reaction is uncatalysed and proceeds quite slowly under the influence of molecular oxygen, or may involve chain processes consisting of three concurrent reactions: initiation, propagation and termination. Oxidative degradation is a problem with drugs possessing carbon–carbon double bonds such as the steroids, polyunsaturated fatty acids and polyene antibiotics. Such drugs can be stabilised by replacing the oxygen in the system with inert gases such as nitrogen; by avoiding contact with metals such as iron, cobalt and nickel; and by adding antioxidants or reducing agents to the solution. Some oxidative reactions are pH-dependent, in which case the product can be stabilised by buffering the system.

- Loss of activity of solutions of some drugs such as the tetracyclines can occur because of epimerisation of the drug molecule while others such as vitamin A lose activity because of geometrical isomerisation.

- Photochemical decomposition can be a problem with drugs such as the phenothiazine tranquillisers and can cause discoloration of the solution and loss of activity. Formulations containing light-sensitive drugs have to be stored in amber glass containers, which remove the ultraviolet components of light.

3.2 Kinetics of chemical decomposition in solution

Before we can predict the shelf-life of a dosage form it is essential to determine the kinetics of the breakdown of the drug under carefully controlled conditions. Unfortunately, drug decomposition often does not follow simple reaction schemes and in this section we will look not only at the traditional ways of classifying reactions but also at some of the complications that can arise with pharmaceutical preparations, which confuse this simple classification.

3.2.1 Classifying reactions: the order of reaction

Reactions are classified according to the number of reacting species whose concentration determines the rate at which the reaction occurs, i.e. the *order of reaction*. We will concentrate mainly on *zero-order* reactions, in which the breakdown rate is independent of the concentration of any of the reactants; *first-order* reaction, in which the reaction rate is determined by one concentration term, and *second-order* reactions, in which the rate is determined by the concentrations of two reacting species.

Experimentally we can monitor the rate of breakdown of the drug either by its decrease in concentration with time or alternatively by the rate of appearance of one of the breakdown products. If we represent the initial concentration of drug A as a mol dm^{-3} and if we find experimentally that x mol dm^{-3} of the drug has reacted in time t, then the amount of drug remaining at a time t is $(a - x)$ mol dm^{-3} and the rate of reaction is

$$\frac{-d[A]}{dt} = \frac{-d(a-x)}{dt} = dx/dt \tag{3.2}$$

Notice that the term a is a constant and therefore disappears during differentiation. We will use dx/dt to describe the reaction rate in this section.

If we assume that a typical reaction between a drug molecule A and a reactant B occurs when two molecules are in collision, then we might expect that the number of collisions, and hence the reaction rate,

would be proportional to the concentration of the two reacting molecules, i.e.

Rate $\propto$ [A][B]

or

$$\frac{dx}{dt} = k[A][B] \tag{3.3}$$

where the proportionality constant, k, is called the *rate constant*. The order of reaction is the sum of the exponents of the concentration terms in the rate equation and so this is an example of a *second-order* reaction. As we will see (section 3.4.1), many hydrolysis reactions are catalysed by H$^+$, OH$^-$ or buffer components and so we can write equation (3.3) as, for example,

$$\frac{dx}{dt} = k_2[A][H^+] \tag{3.4}$$

k_2 is a second-order rate constant and has units of (concentration)$^{-1}$(time)$^{-1}$, for example (mol dm^{-3})$^{-1}$ min^{-1}. When the solution is buffered at constant pH, [H$^+$] is now constant and we can write equation (3.4) as

$$\frac{dx}{dt} = k_1[A] = k_1(a - x) \tag{3.5}$$

where $k_1 = k_2[H^+]$. Since the rate of reaction now effectively depends on one concentration term it is a *first-order* reaction or, more correctly in this case, a *pseudo first-order* reaction (see section 3.2.3). The majority of decomposition reactions involving drugs fall into this category, either because the species reacting with the drug is maintained constant by buffering or because, as in the case of uncatalysed hydrolysis reactions, the water is in such large excess that any change in its concentration is negligible.

If as well as maintaining a constant amount of water in a reaction, we also maintain a fixed drug concentration, then equation (3.3) becomes

$$\frac{dx}{dt} = k_0 \tag{3.6}$$

where $k_0 = k_1[A] = k_2[A][B]$.

This type of reaction, which is called a *zero-order* reaction, can often occur in suspensions of poorly soluble drugs. In these systems the suspended drug slowly dissolves as the drug decomposes and so a constant drug concentration in solution is maintained.

We will now examine the ways in which we can determine the rate constants for these three types of reaction.

3.2.2 Zero-order reactions

In this type of reaction the decomposition proceeds at a constant rate and is independent of the concentrations of any of the reactants. The rate equation is given by equation (3.6) as

$$\frac{\mathrm{d}x}{\mathrm{d}t} = k_0$$

Integration of this equation (see Box 3.1) gives equation (3.8)

$$x = k_0 t$$

A plot of the amount remaining (as ordinate) against time (as abscissa) is linear with a slope of k_0 (concentration $\times$ time^{-1}).

Many decomposition reactions in the solid phase (section 3.3), or in suspensions, apparently follow zero-order kinetics. Figure 3.1 shows the hydrolysis of a suspension of acetylsalicylic acid.

Figure 3.1 Hydrolysis of a suspension of acetylsalicylic acid at 34°C.

Reproduced with permission from James KC, *J Pharm Pharmacol*, 1958; 10: 363.

3.2.3 First-order reactions

The rate of first-order reactions is determined by one concentration term and may be written using equation (3.5) as

$$\frac{\mathrm{d}x}{\mathrm{d}t} = k_1(a - x)$$

Integration of this equation (see Box 3.1) gives equation (3.11)

$$t = \frac{2.303}{k_1}\log a - \frac{2.303}{k_1}\log (a - x)$$

According to equation (3.11), a plot of the logarithm of the amount of drug remaining (as ordinate) as a function of time (as abscissa) is linear if the decomposition follows first-order kinetics. The first-order rate constant may be obtained from the gradient of the plot (gradient $= -k_1/2.303$). k_1 has the dimensions of time^{-1}.

The time taken for half of the reactant to decompose is referred to as the *half-life* of the reaction, $t_{0.5}$. The half-life of a first-order reaction may be calculated from equation (3.13) (Box 3.1)

$$t_{0.5} = \frac{0.693}{k_1}$$

The half-life is therefore independent of the initial concentration of reactants.

Even in the case of a reaction involving more than one reacting species, the rate may still follow first-order kinetics. The most common example of this occurs when one of the reactants is in such a large excess that any change in its concentration is negligible compared with changes in the concentration of the other reactants. This type of reaction is termed a *pseudo first-order reaction*. Such reactions are often met in stability studies of drugs that hydrolyse in solution, the water being in such excess that changes in its concentration are negligible and hence the rate of reaction is dependent solely on the drug concentration.

Example 3.1 Calculation of first-order rate constant and half-life

The following data were obtained for the hydrolysis of homatropine in 0.226 mol dm^{-3} HCl at 90°C:

Percentage homatropine remaining	93.4	85.2	75.9	63.1	52.5	41.8
Time (h)	1.38	3.0	6.0	8.6	12	17

Show that the hydrolysis follows first-order kinetics and calculate (a) the rate constant, and (b) the half-life.

Answer

(a) The reaction will be first-order if a plot of the logarithm of the amount of homatropine remaining against time is linear.

Log percentage remaining	1.97	1.93	1.88	1.80	1.72	1.62
Time (h)	1.38	3.0	6.0	8.6	12	17

Figure 3.2 shows a linear plot with a gradient $= -(1.96 - 1.55)/(20 - 2) = -2.278 \times 10^{-2}\,h^{-1}$.

Gradient $= -k_1/2.303$

Therefore,

$$k_1 = 5.25 \times 10^{-2}\,h^{-1}$$

(b) From equation (3.13),

$$t_{0.5} = 0.693/k_1 = 13.2\,h$$

The half-life of the reaction is 13.2 h.

Figure 3.2 First-order plot for hydrolysis of homatropine in hydrochloric acid (0.226 mol dm^{-3}) at 90°C.

Data from Krasowska MH *et al.*, *Dansk Tidsskr Farm*, 1968; 42: 170 with permission.

3.2.4 Second-order reactions

The rate of a second-order reaction is determined by the concentrations of two reacting species. The general rate equation is given by equation (3.3) as

$$\frac{dx}{dt} = k_2[A][B]$$

In most second-order reactions the reactants have different initial concentrations, in which case the rate equation is given by equation (3.15) (Box 3.1):

$$\frac{dx}{dt} = k_2(a - x)(b - x)$$

Integration of this equation as shown in Box 3.1, yields equation (3.17):

$$t = \frac{2.303}{k_2(a-b)}\log\frac{b}{a} + \frac{2.303}{k_2(a-b)}\log\frac{(a-x)}{(b-x)}$$

from which it is seen that k_2 can then be obtained from the gradient, $2.303/k_2(a-b)$, of a plot of t (as ordinate) against $\log[(a-x)/(b-x)]$ (as abscissa).

An examination of equation (3.17) shows that the second-order rate constant is dependent on the units used to express concentration; the units of k_2 are concentration^{-1} time^{-1}.

For second-order reactions in which both concentration terms refer to the same reactant or in which the initial concentrations of the two reactants are the same we may write

$$\frac{-d[A]}{dt} = k_2[A]^2 \quad \text{and} \quad \frac{dx}{dt} = k_2(a - x)^2$$

Integration as shown in Box 3.1 yields equation (3.20):

$$t = \frac{1}{k_2}\left[\frac{1}{a-x} - \frac{1}{a}\right] = \frac{x}{k_2a(a-x)}$$

from which it is seen that a plot of t (ordinate) against $x/[a(a-x)]$ (abscissa) yields a linear plot of gradient $1/k_2$.

The half-life of a reaction that follows equation (3.20) is given by

$$t_{0.5} = 1/(k_2a) \tag{3.21}$$

Unlike $t_{0.5}$ for first-order reactions, the half-life of the second-order reaction is dependent on the initial concentration of reactants. It is not possible to derive a simple expression for the half-life of a second-order reaction with unequal initial concentrations.

3.2.5 Third-order reactions

Third-order reactions are only rarely encountered in drug stability studies involving, as they do, the simultaneous collision of three reactant molecules. The overall rate of ampicillin breakdown by simultaneous hydrolysis and polymerisation may be represented by an equation of the form

$$\frac{-d[A]}{dt} = k_a[A] + k_b[A]^2 + k_c[A]^3 \tag{3.22}$$

where k_a, k_b and k_c are the pH-dependent apparent rate constant for hydrolysis, uncatalysed polymerisation and the general acid–base catalysed polymerisation of ampicillin, respectively.[13] As seen from equation (3.22) the decomposition rate shows both second-order and third-order dependency on the total ampicillin concentration [A].

3.2.6 Determination of the order of reaction

The most obvious method of determining the order of a reaction is to determine the amount of drug decomposed after various intervals and to substitute the data into the integrated equations for zero-, first- and second-order reactions. The equation giving the most consistent value of k for a series of time intervals is that corresponding most closely to the order of the reaction. Alternatively, the data may be displayed graphically according to the linear equations for the various orders of reactions until a straight line plot is obtained. Thus, for example, if the data yield a linear graph when plotted as t against $\log(a - x)$ the reaction is then taken to be first-order.

Fitting data to the standard rate equations may, however, produce misleading results if a fractional order of reaction applies. An alternative method of determining the order of reaction, which avoids this problem, is based on equation (3.23):

$$\log t_{0.5} = \log\left[\frac{2^{n-1} - 1}{k(n-1)}\right] + (1-n)\log C_0 \tag{3.23}$$

The half-life of the reaction is determined for a series of initial drug concentrations, C_0, and the order, n, is calculated from the slope of plots of $\log t_{0.5}$ as a function of $\log C_0$.

University Of Sunderland
The Murray Library
Tel (0191) 515 3691

Customer name: Mr Joseph Arul Finney
Abraham
Customer ID: ******02673

Title: Physicochemical principles of pharmacy
ID: 11112584013
Due: 08/05/2013 23:55

Total Items: 1
10/04/2013 18:38

Please Retain This Receipt To Ensure You
Return Items On Time

Need Help?
Try our new 'Live Chat' service.
For further information see the library web
pages at https://my.sunderland.ac.uk

MLI2a

Box 3.1 Derivations of rate equations for zero-, first- and second-order reactions

Zero-order reactions

The rate equation is

$$dx/dt = k_0$$

Integration, noting that $x = 0$ at $t = 0$, gives

$$\int_0^x dx = k_0 \int_0^t dt \qquad (3.7)$$

i.e.

$$x = k_0 t \qquad (3.8)$$

First-order reactions

The rate equation is

$$dx/dt = k_1(a - x)$$

Since $x = 0$ at the start of the measurements (that is, when $t = 0$),

$$\int_0^x \frac{dx}{(a-x)} = k_1 \int_0^t dt \qquad (3.9)$$

$$k_1 = \frac{2.303}{t} \log \frac{a}{a-x} \qquad (3.10)$$

Or, rearranging into a linear form,

$$t = \frac{2.303}{k_1} \log a - \frac{2.303}{k_1} \log(a - x) \qquad (3.11)$$

An expression for the half-life $t_{0.5}$ may be derived from equation (3.10), noting that when $t = t_{0.5}$, $x = a/2$:

$$t_{0.5} = \frac{2.303}{k_1} \log \frac{a}{a/2} \qquad (3.12)$$

Thus,

$$t_{0.5} = \frac{2.303}{k_1} \log 2 = \frac{0.693}{k_1} \qquad (3.13)$$

Second-order reactions

The rate equation is

$$dx/dt = k_2[A][B] \qquad (3.14)$$

If the initial concentrations of reactants A and B are a and b, respectively, equation (3.14) may be written

$$dx/dt = k_2(a - x)(b - x) \qquad (3.15)$$

where x is the amount of A and B decomposed in time t. Integration of equation (3.15) by the method of partial fractions yields

$$k_2 = \frac{2.303}{t(a-b)} \log \frac{b(a-x)}{a(b-x)} \tag{3.16}$$

Rearranging into a linear form suitable for plotting gives

$$t = \frac{2.303}{k_2(a-b)} \log \frac{b}{a} + \frac{2.303}{k_2(a-b)} \log \frac{(a-x)}{(b-x)} \tag{3.17}$$

For reactions in which both concentration terms refer to the same reactant we may write

$$-d[A]/dt = k_2[A]^2 \tag{3.18}$$

and

$$dx/dt = k_2(a-x)^2 \tag{3.19}$$

A similar equation applies to second-order reactions in which the initial concentrations of the two reactants are the same.

Integration of equation (3.19) between the limits of t from 0 to t and of x from 0 to x yields

$$t = \frac{1}{k_2}\left[\frac{1}{a-x} - \frac{1}{a}\right] = \frac{x}{k_2 a(a-x)} \tag{3.20}$$

Example 3.2 Determination of the order of reaction

The kinetics of decomposition of a drug in aqueous solution were studied using a series of solutions of different initial drug concentrations, C_0. For each solution the time taken for half the drug to decompose (that is, $t_{0.5}$) was determined with the following results:

C_0 (mol dm^{-3})	4.625	1.698	0.724	0.288
$t_{0.5}$ (min)	87.17	240.1	563.0	1414.4

Determine the order of reaction and calculate the rate constant.

Answer

Application of equation (3.23) requires values for $\log C_0$ and $\log t_{0.5}$; thus

$\log C_0$	0.665	0.230	-0.140	-0.540
$\log t_{0.5}$	1.94	2.38	2.75	3.15

A plot of $\log t_{0.5}$ against $\log C_0$ is linear (Figure 3.3) with gradient $(1-n) = -1.01$. Hence $n = 2.01$, i.e. the reaction is second-order.

The intercept of the graph (that is, the value of $\log t_{0.5}$ at $\log C_0 = 0$) is 2.60. Thus, from equation (3.23),

$$\log[(2-1)/k] = 2.60$$

and

$$k = 2.51 \times 10^{-3} (\text{mol dm}^{-3})^{-1}\,\text{min}^{-1}$$

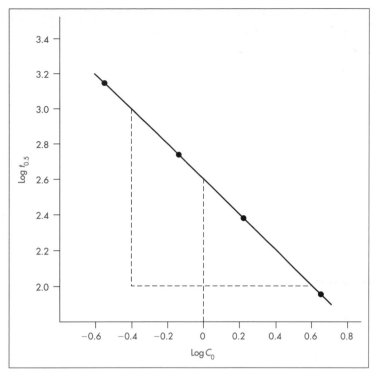

Figure 3.3 Example 3.2: Plot of log of half-life ($t_{0.5}$) against log of initial drug concentration (C_0).

3.2.7 Complex reactions

There are many examples of drugs in which decomposition occurs simultaneously by two or more pathways, or involves a sequence of decomposition steps or a reversible reaction. Indeed, the degradative pathways of some drugs include examples of each of these types of complex reactions. Modification of the rate equations is necessary whenever such reactions are encountered.

Reversible reactions

Treatment of the kinetics of a reversible reaction involves two rate constants; one, k_f, to describe the rate of the forward reaction and the other k_r to describe the rate of the reverse reaction. For the simplest example in which both of these reactions are first-order, that is

$$ A \underset{k_f}{\overset{k_r}{\rightleftharpoons}} B $$

the rate of decomposition of reactant is given by equation (3.24) (Box 3.2):

$$ \frac{-d[A]}{dt} = k_f[A] - k_r[B] $$

As explained in Box 3.2, values of the equilibrium constants k_f and k_r may be evaluated separately from plots of t (as ordinate) against $\log[([A]_0 - [A]_{eq})/([A] - [A]_{eq})]$, and from the ratio R of the concentration of products formed by each reaction at equilibrium using equation (3.26).

The epimerisation of tetracycline (see section 3.1.3) is an example of a first-order reversible decomposition reaction.

Parallel reactions

The decomposition of many drugs involves two or more pathways, the preferred route of reaction being dependent on reaction condition. Nitrazepam (**VI**) decomposes in two pseudo first-order parallel reactions giving different breakdown products in solution and in

Box 3.2 Derivations of equations for complex reactions

Reversible reactions

The rate of decomposition of reactant is given by

$$- d[A]/dt = k_f[A] - k_r[B] \tag{3.24}$$

Equation (3.24) may be integrated noting that $[A_0] - [A] = [B]$ and introducing the equilibrium condition $k_f[A]_{eq} = k_r[B]_{eq}$ to yield

$$t = \frac{2.303}{(k_f + k_r)} \log \frac{[A]_0 - [A]_{eq}}{[A] - [A]_{eq}} \tag{3.25}$$

where $[A]_0$, $[A]$ and $[A]_{eq}$ represent the initial concentration, the concentration at time t and the equilibrium concentration of reactant A, respectively. Equation (3.25) indicates that a plot of t (as ordinate) against $\log[([A]_0 - [A]_{eq})/([A] - [A]_{eq})]$ should be linear with a gradient of $2.303/(k_f + k_r)$. k_f and k_r may be calculated separately if the equilibrium constant K is also determined, since

$$K = \frac{[B]_{eq}}{[A]_{eq}} = \frac{1 - [A]_{eq}}{[A]_{eq}} = \frac{k_f}{k_r} \tag{3.26}$$

where $[B]_{eq}$ is the equilibrium concentration of product B.

Parallel reactions

The rate equation is

$$- d[X]/dt = (k_A + k_B)[X] = k_{exp}[X] \tag{3.27}$$

where k_A and k_B are the rate constants for the formation of A and B, respectively, and k_{exp} is the experimentally determined rate constant.

Values of the rate constants k_A and k_B may be evaluated separately if it is possible to monitor the concentration of drug X and those of the breakdown products A and B as a function of time. The rate of formation of A can be expressed as

$$\frac{d[A]}{dt} = k_A[X] = k_A[X]_0 e^{-k_{exp}t} \tag{3.28}$$

where $[A]$ is the concentration of the prod-uct A at time t, and $[X]_0$ is the initial concentration of the drug. It is reasonable to assume that the initial concentration of product A is zero and therefore integration of equation (3.28) gives

$$[A] = \frac{k_A}{k_{exp}} [X]_0 (1 - e^{-k_{exp}t}) \tag{3.29}$$

Similarly, for product B,

$$[B] = \frac{k_B}{k_{exp}} [X]_0 (1 - e^{-k_{exp}t}) \tag{3.30}$$

Plots of [A] or [B] against $(1 - e^{-k_{exp}t})$ should be linear with gradients $k_A[X]_0/k_{exp}$ and $k_B[X]_0/k_{exp}$ respectively, from which values of the rate constants k_A and k_B may be determined. Alternatively, values of the rate constants k_A and k_B may be evaluated from the ratio R of the concentration of products formed by each reaction at equilibrium. From equations (3.29) and (3.30)

$$R = \frac{[A]_{eq}}{[B]_{eq}} = \frac{k_A}{k_B} \tag{3.31}$$

Since

$$k_{exp} = k_A + k_B \tag{3.32}$$

$$k_{exp} = k_A + k_A/R \tag{3.33}$$

Solving for k_A gives

$$k_A = k_{exp} \frac{R}{(R+1)} \tag{3.34}$$

Similarly,

$$k_B = \frac{k_{exp}}{(R+1)} \tag{3.35}$$

Consecutive reactions

The rate of decomposition of A is

$$-d[A]/dt = k_A[A] \tag{3.36}$$

The rate of change of concentration of B is

$$d[B]/dt = k_A[A] - k_B[B] \tag{3.37}$$

and that of C is

$$d[C]/dt = k_B[B] \tag{3.38}$$

Integration of the rate equation (equation 3.36) yields

$$[A] = [A]_0 e^{-k_A t} \tag{3.39}$$

Substitution of equation (3.39) into equation (3.37) gives

$$d[B]/dt = k_A[A]_0 e^{-k_A t} - k_B[B] \tag{3.40}$$

which upon integration gives

$$[B] = \frac{k_A[A_0]}{(k_B - k_A)}[e^{-k_A t} - e^{-k_B t}] \tag{3.41}$$

At any time,

$$[A]_0 = [A] + [B] + [C] \tag{3.42}$$

so that

$$
\begin{aligned}
[C] &= [A]_0 - [A] - [B] \\
&= [A]_0 \left[1 + \frac{1}{k_A - k_B}(k_B e^{-k_A t} - k_A e^{-k_B t}) \right]
\end{aligned}
\tag{3.43}
$$

the solid state as illustrated in Scheme 3.13. Decomposition of nitrazepam tablets in the presence or moisture will occur by both routes, the ratio of the two products being dependent on the amount of water present.

In other cases decomposition may occur simultaneously by two different processes, as in the simultaneous hydrolysis and epimerisation of pilocarpine (see Example 3.3).

Scheme 3.13 Simplified decomposition scheme for nitrazepam (**VI**) in the solid state and aqueous solution. The main decomposition product is 2-amino-5-nitrobenzophenone (**VII**) in aqueous solution and 3-amino-6-nitro-4-phenyl-2(1*H*)-quinolone (**VIII**) in the solid state.

Reproduced from Meyer W *et al.*, *Pharmazie* 1972; 27: 32.

Example 3.3 Calculation of rate constants of parallel reactions

Pilocarpine has been shown to undergo simultaneous hydrolysis and epimerisation in aqueous solution. The experimentally determined rate constant, k_{exp}, at 25°C is 6.96×10^2 $(mol\,dm^{-3})^{-1}\,h^{-1}$. Analysis has shown that at equilibrium the percentage of the epimerised form of pilocarpine (isopilocarpine) at 25°C is 20.6%. Calculate the rate constants for hydrolysis, k_H, and epimerisation, k_E.

Answer

The ratio R of pilocarpine to isopilocarpine is

$$R = 79.38/20.62 = 3.85$$

From equation (3.34),

$$k_H = (6.96 \times 10^2)(3.85/4.85)$$

i.e.

$$k_H = 5.48 \times 10^2 (mol\,dm^{-3})^{-1}\,h^{-1}$$

From equation (3.35),

$$k_E = (6.96 \times 10^2)/4.85$$

i.e.

$$k_E = 1.44 \times 10^2\,(mol\,dm^{-3})^{-1}\,h^{-1}$$

The rate constants for hydrolysis and epimerisation are 5.48×10^2 and 1.44×10^2 $(mol\,dm^{-3})^{-1}\,h^{-1}$, respectively.

The overall rate equation for a parallel reaction is the sum of the constants for each pathway. For example, for a decomposition of a drug X involving two pathways, each of which is first-order,

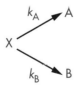

the rate equation is given by equation (3.27) (Box 3.2)

$$\frac{-d[X]}{dt} = (k_A + k_B)[X] = k_{exp}[X]$$

where k_A and k_B are the rate constants for the formation of A and B, respectively, and k_{exp} is the experimentally determined rate constant. Values of the rate constants k_A and k_B may be evaluated separately from plots of [A] or [B] against $(1 - e^{-k_{exp}t})$ using

equations (3.29) and (3.30) as explained in Box 3.2, or from the ratio R of the concentration of products formed by each reaction at equilibrium using equations (3.34) and (3.35).

Consecutive reactions

The simplest example of a consecutive reaction is that described by a sequence

$$A \xrightarrow{k_A} B \xrightarrow{k_B} C$$

where each step is a nonreversible first-order reaction. The hydrolysis of chlordiazepoxide follows a first-order decomposition scheme similar to that described in this equation (Scheme 3.14).

Equations (3.39), (3.41) and (3.43) (see Box 3.2) may be used to estimate the rate constants k_A and k_B and also the concentration of the breakdown product C.

Scheme 3.14 Decomposition scheme for chlordiazepoxide.

The neutral or cationic chlordiazepoxide (**IX** or **IXH**$^+$) is transformed to the lactam (**X**) and, finally, in acidic solutions, to the yellow benzophenone (**XI**).

Reproduced from Maudling HV *et al.*, *J Pharm Sci*, 1975; 64: 278.

Key points

- Reactions may be classified according to the order of reaction, which is the number of reacting species whose concentrations determine the rate at which the reaction occurs.
- The most important orders of reaction are zero-order (breakdown rate is independent of the concentration of any of the reactants), first-order (reaction rate is determined by one concentration term) and second-order (rate is determined by the concentrations of two reacting species). In solutions containing two reactants, the reaction rate may still follow first-order kinetics if one of the reactants (usually water) is in such large excess that changes in its concentration are negligible; such reactions are called pseudo first-order reactions. The breakdown of drugs in the majority of preparations in which the drug is dissolved in aqueous solution follows first-order or pseudo first-order kinetics.
- The rate constant of a reaction is determined graphically by substitution of experimental data in the linear equations for the appropriate order of reaction:
  - Zero-order: $x = k_0 t$

  - First-order: $t = \dfrac{2.303}{k_1} \log a - \dfrac{2.303}{k_1} \log (a - x)$

  - Second-order: $t = \dfrac{2.303}{k_2(a-b)} \log \dfrac{b}{a} + \dfrac{2.303}{k_2(a-b)} \log \dfrac{(a-x)}{(b-x)}$

- The order of reaction is usually determined by plotting data according to the equations for each of the main types of reaction, linearity of the plot being indicative of the applicability of that order of reaction. This method is not suitable if decomposition follows fractional-order kinetics and in such cases an alternative method in which the half-life is plotted as a function of initial drug concentration may be used.
- The half-life of a reaction is the time taken for half of the reactant to decompose; the half-life of a first-order reaction is given by $t_{0.5} = 0.693/k_1$.
- The decomposition of many drugs can occur simultaneously by two or more pathways (parallel reactions), or may involve a sequence of decomposition steps (consecutive reactions) or may be a reversible reaction.

3.3 Solid dosage forms: kinetics of chemical decomposition

In spite of the importance of solid dosage forms, there have been relatively few attempts to evaluate the detailed kinetics of decomposition. Most of the earlier work was carried out with the sole objective of predicting stability, and data were treated using the rate equations derived for reaction in solution. More recently, the mechanisms that were developed to describe the kinetics of decomposition of pure solids have been applied to pharmaceutical systems and some rationalisation of decomposition behaviour has been possible. A comprehensive account of this topic has been presented by Carstensen[14,15] on which the following summary is based.

It is convenient to divide single-component systems into two categories – those solids that decompose to a solid product and a gas, and those that decompose to give a liquid and a gas.

Solids that decompose to give a solid and a gas

An example of this category is p-aminosalicylic acid, which decomposes to a solid (p-aminophenol) and a gas (carbon dioxide):

$$NH_2C_6H_3(OH)COOH \rightarrow NH_2C_6H_4OH + CO_2$$

The decomposition curves that result from such a reaction show either (a) an initial rapid decomposition followed by a more gradual decomposition rate, or (b) an initial lag period, giving a sigmoidal appearance. The shape produced by (a) can usually be accounted for by *topochemical* (or contracting geometry) reactions and that produced in (b) by *nucleation* theories.

The model used in the treatment of topochemical decomposition is that of a cylinder or sphere (Fig. 3.4) in which it is assumed that the radius, r, of the intact chemical substance decreases linearly with time, t, i.e., $r = r_0 - kt$, where r_0 is the initial radius. For the contracting cylinder model, the mole fraction x decomposed at time t is given by

$$(1-x)^{1/2} = 1 - (k/r_0)t \tag{3.44}$$

For the contracting sphere model,

$$(1-x)^{1/3} = 1 - (k/r_0)t \tag{3.45}$$

There are a few pharmaceutical examples of compounds that decompose by topochemical reaction.

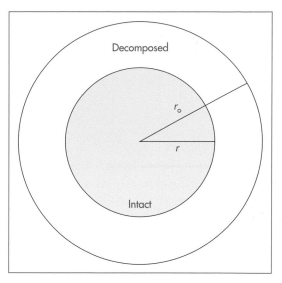

Figure 3.4 Model of sphere or cylinder used in theoretical treatment of topochemical reactions.

Reproduced from Carstensen JT, *J Pharm Sci*, 1974; 63: 1.

Thus, the decomposition of aspirin at elevated temperatures has been shown to conform to equation (3.44) (Fig. 3.5).

A similarity between equations (3.44) and (3.45) and the first-order rate equations was pointed out by Carstensen[14], who suggested that this similarity might account for the fact that many decompositions in solid dosage forms appear to follow first-order kinetics.

The sigmoidal decomposition curves can be interpreted using the Prout and Tompkins model. This model assumes that the decomposition is governed by the formation and growth of active nuclei that occur on the surface as well as inside the crystals. The formation of product molecules sets up further strains in the crystal since the surface array of product molecules has a different unit cell from the original substance. The strains are relieved by the formation of cracks. Reaction takes place at the mouth of these cracks owing to lattice imperfections and spreads down into the crevices. Decomposition on these surfaces produces further cracking and so the chain reaction spreads.

The equation proposed to describe decomposition by this process is of the form

$$\ln\left[\frac{x}{(1-x)}\right] = \frac{k}{r_0}t + C \tag{3.46}$$

where C is a lag-time term.

The decomposition curves of p-aminosalicylic acid are sigmoidal (see Fig. 3.6) and linear plots are

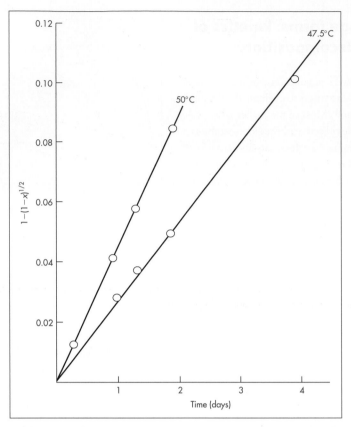

Figure 3.5 Decomposition of aspirin at elevated temperatures in tablets containing sodium bicarbonate, plotted according to equation (3.44).

Reproduced with permission from Nelson E *et al.*, *J Pharm Sci*, 1974; 63: 755.

produced when the data are plotted according to equation (3.46). Stability measurements made inadvertently in the lag periods of this type of decomposition would suggest zero-order kinetics.

Solids that decompose to give a liquid and a gas

An example of a solid in this category is *p*-aminobenzoic acid, which decomposes into aniline and carbon dioxide. Decomposition causes a layer of liquid to form around the solid, which dissolves the solid. The decomposition curves show an initial lag period (Fig. 3.7) that corresponds to the establishment of the liquid layer. Beyond this region, the plot represents first-order decomposition of the solid in solution in its liquid decomposition products. There are thus two rate constants, that for the initial decomposition of the solid itself, and that for the decomposition of the solid in solution.

3.4 Factors influencing drug stability

Before we can suggest ways in which we might prevent the decomposition of drugs, we should first consider the various factors that accelerate the decomposition processes. For convenience we will consider liquid and solid dosage forms separately, although, as we will see, there are similarities in the influence of several factors on drug breakdown in both.

3.4.1 Liquid dosage forms

pH

pH is perhaps the most important parameter that affects the hydrolysis rate of drugs in liquid formulations; it is certainly the one that has been most widely examined.

Figure 3.6 Degradation of powdered *p*-aminosalicylic acid in a dry atmosphere at elevated temperatures.

Reproduced with permission from Kornblum SS, Sciarrone BJ, *J Pharm Sci*, 1964; 53: 935.

Figure 3.7 Decomposition curves of *p*-aminobenzoic acid at temperatures in the range 130–145°C showing the initial lag phase in *p*-aminobenzoic acid decomposition.

Reproduced from Carstensen JT, Musa MN, *J Pharm Sci*, 1972; 61: 1113.

Studying the influence of pH on degradation rate is not as simple as might at first be imagined. If the hydrolysis rate of the drug in a series of solutions buffered to the required pH is measured and the hydrolytic rate constant is then plotted as a function of pH, a pH–rate profile will be produced, but this will almost certainly be influenced by the buffers used to prepare the solutions. It is probable that a different pH–rate profile would be obtained using a different buffer. To understand why this should be, we have to consider not only the catalytic effect of hydrogen and hydroxyl ions, which is called *specific acid–base catalysis*, but also the possible accelerating effect of the components of the buffer system, which we refer to as *general acid–base catalysis*. These two types of acid–base catalysis can be combined together in a general expression as follows:

$$k_{obs} = k_0 + k_{H^+}[H^+] + k_{OH^-}[OH^-]$$
$$+ k_{HX}[HX] + k_{X^-}[X^-] \qquad (3.47)$$

In this equation, k_{obs} is the experimentally determined hydrolytic rate constant, k_0 is the uncatalysed or solvent catalysed rate constant, k_{H^+} and k_{OH^-} are the specific acid- and base-catalysis rate constants respectively, k_{HX} and k_{X^-} are the general acid- and base-catalysis rate constants, respectively, and [HX] and [X⁻] denote the concentrations of protonated and unprotonated forms of the buffer.

For a complete evaluation of the stability of the drug we need to evaluate the catalytic coefficients for specific acid- and base-catalysis and also to determine the catalytic coefficients of possible buffers that we might wish to use in the formulation.

First we will examine how to achieve a buffer-independent pH–rate profile, since this will show us at which pH the stability is greatest. By way of illustration we can consider a specific example of a stability study that has been reported for the antihypertensive vasodilator ciclosidomine. Experiments carried out at constant temperature and constant ionic strength using a series of different buffers over the pH range 3–6 produced the graphs shown in Fig. 3.8. These plots

Figure 3.8 Effect of buffer concentration on the hydrolytic rate constant for ciclosidomine at 60°C as a function of pH.

Reproduced with permission from Carney CF, *J Pharm Sci*, 1987; 76: 393.

show that an increase of buffer concentration, particularly at pH 3, had a marked effect on the hydrolysis rate. The effect of the phosphate buffer on this system became less pronounced with increase of pH and was found to have a negligible effect above pH 7.5.

To remove the influence of the buffer, the reaction rate should be measured at a series of buffer concentrations at each pH and the data extrapolated back to zero concentration as shown in Fig. 3.8. If these extrapolated rate constants are plotted as a function of pH, the required buffer-independent pH–rate profile will be obtained. Figure 3.9 illustrates the simple type of pH–rate profile that is obtained with codeine sulfate.

As we can see from Fig. 3.9, this drug is very stable in unbuffered solution over a wide pH range but degrades relatively rapidly in the presence of strong acids or bases. Since the influence of buffer components has been removed, this plot allows us to calculate the rate constants for specific acid and base catalysis. Removing the terms for the effect of buffer from equation (3.47) we have

$$k_{obs} = k_0 + k_{H^+}[H^+] + k_{OH^-}[OH^-] \qquad (3.48)$$

and consequently a plot of measured rate constant k_{obs} against the hydrogen ion concentration $[H^+]$ at low pH will have a gradient equal to the rate constant for acid catalysis. Similarly, of course, if we plot k_{obs} against $[OH^-]$ at high pH, the gradient will be the rate constant for base-catalysed hydrolysis. Example 3.4 illustrates the calculation of these catalytic coefficients.

Figure 3.9 Log rate–pH profile for the degradation of codeine sulfate in buffer-free solutions at 60°C.

Reproduced with permission from Powell MF, *J Pharm Sci*,1986; 75: 901.

Example 3.4 Calculation of rate constants for base-catalysed hydrolysis

The following data were obtained for the hydrolytic rate constant, k_{obs} of codeine sulfate in aqueous buffer-free solution at 80°C:

$10^7 k_{obs}$ (s^{-1})	5.50	4.40	2.30	1.25	0.70
pH	11.63	11.53	11.23	10.93	10.63

Determine graphically (a) the catalytic coefficient for base-catalysis, k_{OH^-}, and also (b) the coefficient for solvent catalysis, k_0.

Answer

At high pH,

$$k_{obs} = k_0 + k_{OH^-}[OH^-]$$

where $[OH^-]$ is calculated from

$$p[OH^-] = -\log[OH^-] = 12.63 - pH$$

(Note: $pK_w = 12.63$ at 80°C.)

A plot of k_{obs} against $[OH^-]$ has a gradient of k_{OH^-} and an intercept of k_0.

From a graph of the above data,

$$k_0 = 2.0 \times 10^{-8}\,s^{-1}$$
$$k_{OH^-} = 5.2 \times 10^{-6}\,(mol\,dm^{-3})^{-1}\,s^{-1}$$

The degradation of codeine is particularly susceptible to the effects of buffers. Its hydrolysis rate in 0.05 mol dm^{-3} phosphate buffer at pH 7 is almost 20 times faster than in unbuffered solution at this pH, so this is a good drug to use as an example of the determination of the influence of buffer components on the breakdown rate.

In phosphate buffers of neutral pH, the major buffer species are $H_2PO_4^-$ and HPO_4^{2-}, either of which may act as a catalyst for codeine degradation. To find out which of these is the stronger catalyst, we can treat the experimental data in the following way. In neutral pH solutions we can write the following expression for the observed rate constant,

$$k_{obs} = k_0 + k_{H_2PO_4^-}[H_2PO_4^-] + k_{HPO_4^{2-}}[HPO_4^{2-}] \tag{3.49}$$

or

$$k_{obs} = k_0 + k' B_T$$

where $k_{H_2PO_4^-}$ and $k_{HPO_4^{2-}}$ are the rate constants for catalysis by $H_2PO_4^-$ and HPO_4^{2-} ions, respectively, and B_T is the total concentration of phosphate buffer. Notice that the terms for specific acid- and base-catalysis have little effect at this pH and we need not consider them in this treatment.

From equation (3.49), a plot of k_{obs} against B_T will have an intercept k_0 and a gradient k'. To find values for the catalytic coefficients, we rearrange the equation into the following linear form:

$$\begin{aligned} k' &= \frac{(k_{obs} - k_0)}{B_T} \\ &= \frac{k_{H_2PO_4^-}[H_2PO_4^-]}{B_T} + k_{HPO_4^{2-}}\left(\frac{B_T - [H_2PO_4^-]}{B_T}\right) \end{aligned} \tag{3.50}$$

We can now see that a second plot of the apparent rate constant k' against the fraction of the acid buffer component present, i.e. $[H_2PO_4^-/B_T]$, will have an intercept at $[H_2PO_4^-/B_T] = 0$ equal to $k_{HPO_4^{2-}}$. Furthermore, the k' value at $[H_2PO_4^-/B_T] = 1$ is the other catalytic coefficient, $k_{H_2PO_4^-}$.

The relationship between the ability of a buffer component to catalyse hydrolysis, denoted by the catalytic coefficient, k, and its dissociation constant, K, may be expressed by the Brønsted catalysis law as

$$k_A = aK_A^\alpha \quad \text{for a weak acid} \tag{3.51}$$

and

$$k_B = bK_B^\beta \quad \text{for a weak base} \tag{3.52}$$

where a, b, α and β are constants characteristic of the solvent and temperature. α and β are positive and vary between 0 and 1.

Example 3.5 Calculation of the catalytic coefficients for buffer species

The following data were obtained for the hydrolytic rate constant k of codeine sulfate at 100°C in phosphate buffers of varying total concentration B_T at pH values of 6 and 8:

B_T (mol dm^{-3})	0.03	0.06	0.09	0.12
$10^7 k$ (s^{-1}) at pH 6	6.1	11.2	16.3	21.4
$10^7 k$ (s^{-1}) at pH 8	12.9	25.0	37.0	49.0

If the fraction of $[H_2PO_4^-]$ present in buffer solutions at pH 6 is 0.74 and at pH 8 is 0.23, determine graphically the catalytic coefficients for the buffer species (a) $H_2PO_4^-$ and (b) HPO_4^{2-}.

Answer

From equation (3.49), a plot of k_{obs} against B_T has an intercept k_0 and a gradient k'.

Therefore, plot k_{obs} against B_T from the given data at each pH and measure the gradient of the graph.

From the graph:

$$k' \text{ at pH 6} = 1.7 \times 10^{-5} (\text{mol dm}^{-3})^{-1} \text{s}^{-1}$$

$$k' \text{ at pH 8} = 4.0 \times 10^{-5} (\text{mol dm}^{-3})^{-1} \text{s}^{-1}$$

From equation (3.50), a plot of k' against the fraction of acidic buffer component, $[H_2PO_4^-]/B_T$, has an intercept of $k_{HPO_4^{2-}}$.

Also when $[H_2PO_4^-]/B_T = 1$,

$$k' = k_{H_2PO_4^-}$$

From the graph:

$$k_{HPO_4^{2-}} = 5.1 \times 10^{-5} (\text{mol dm}^{-3})^{-1} \text{s}^{-1}$$

$$k_{H_2PO_4^-} = 0.5 \times 10^{-5} (\text{mol dm}^{-3})^{-1} \text{s}^{-1}$$

In our treatment of the degradation of codeine sulfate we have not yet considered any effect that changes in its ionisation might have on its stability. Codeine has a pK_a of 8.2 at 25°C and so its ionisation state will change over the pH range 6–10. With this particular drug, the stability was not affected by any such changes. This is not the case with many drugs, however, and complex pH–rate profiles are often produced because of the differing susceptibility of the un-ionised and ionised forms of the drug molecule to hydrolysis.

By way of illustration we will look at the case of the hydrolysis of mecillinam (**XII**), which is an antimicrobially active amidopenicillamic acid. This amphoteric drug can exist as a cation, which we can write as MH_2^+, a zwitterion $MH^\pm$ or an anion M^-. Figure 3.10 shows the pH–rate profile at zero buffer concentration. The reason this plot is so much more complex than that of codeine sulfate is that each of the species present in solution can undergo specific acid–base catalysis to varying extents and so each contributes to the overall profile shown in Fig. 3.10.

Structure XII   Mecillinam

The various reactions thought to occur are

$$MH_2^+ + H^+ \xrightarrow{k_H} \text{products} \quad 1$$
$$MH + H^+ \xrightarrow{k_H'} \text{products} \quad 2$$
$$MH + H_2O \xrightarrow{k_0} \text{products} \quad 3$$
$$MH + OH^- \xrightarrow{k_{OH}'} \text{products} \quad 4$$
$$M^- + OH^- \xrightarrow{k_{OH}} \text{products} \quad 5 \qquad (3.53)$$

The part of the pH–rate profile at very low pH (below pH 1.5) is given entirely by reaction (1). This is because the mecillinam exists as the cation MH_2^+, the hydrolysis of which will be acid-catalysed over this pH range. The shoulder in the pH-rate profile at around pH 2 coincides approximately with the first pK_a value of mecillinam and indicates an increased acid-catalysis of the zwitterion relative to the cationic species. The decrease of hydrolysis rate constant with increasing pH up to pH 4 can be explained by assuming that both reactions (1) and (2) are occurring. We can see from Fig. 3.10 that the hydrolysis rate is almost constant between pH 4 and 6, and this suggests that the hydrolysis is water-

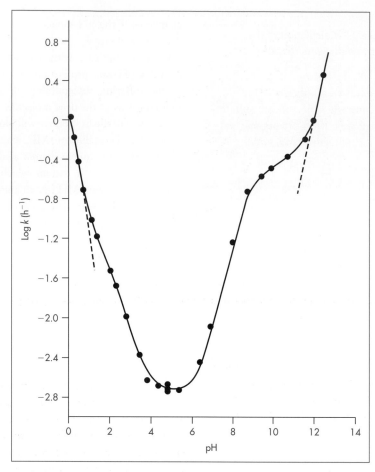

Figure 3.10 Log k–pH profile for the degradation of mecillinam in aqueous solution at 35°C (ionic strength = 0.5), where k is the apparent first-order rate constant for degradation in buffer-free solutions or in buffers showing no effect on rate of degradation.
Reproduced from Larsen C, Bundgaard H, *Arch Pharm Chem*, 1977; 5: 66.

catalysed (reaction 3) over this pH region. The hydrolysis rate now starts to increase with increasing pH, which indicates that base-catalysis is now the dominating factor. Between pH 6.5 and the pK_a for ionisation of the amidino side-chains (pK_{a2} = 8.79), it is reaction (4) that describes the hydrolysis rate. The plot changes slope at around pH 8 because it is affected by the changes that are occurring in the state of ionisation of the amidino side-chain. Above pH 12, the mecillinam exists in solution as the anion and this final part of the graph is described entirely by the base-catalysis of this species (reaction 5).

Even though we may not always be able to explain the pH–rate profile as completely as we can for mecillinam, we can still, of course, choose the pH at which to buffer the drug solution for maximum stability. In the case of mecillinam this would be between pH 4 and 6.

We should also note that the *oxidative degradation* of some drugs in solution may be pH-dependent; for example, the oxidation of prednisolone is base-catalysed. Similarly, the oxidation of morphine occurs more rapidly in alkaline or neutral solution than in acid solution. The reason for this may be the effect of pH on the oxidation–reduction potential, E_0, of the drug.

The *photodegradation* of several drugs is also pH-dependent. For example, the photochemical decomposition of the benzodiazepine derivative

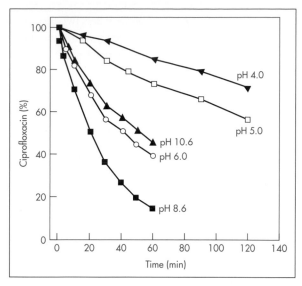

Figure 3.11 The effect of pH on the photodegradation of ciprofloxacin. Radiation source: mercury lamp at wavelength 313 nm.
Reproduced from Torniainen K et al., Int J Pharm, 1996; 132, 53.

midazolam (**XIII**) increases with pH,[16] and ciproflox-acin (**XIV**) is most sensitive to photodegradation at slightly basic pH at which the drug is in zwitterionic form, the stability increasing when the pH is lowered to 3–4[17] (Fig. 3.11).

Structure XIII Midazolam

Structure XIV Ciprofloxacin

Temperature

Increase in temperature usually causes a very pro-nounced increase in the hydrolysis rate of drugs in solu-tion, a fact which is used to good effect in the experimental studies of drug stability described above. Such studies are usually carried out at high tempera-tures, say 60 or 80°C, because the hydrolysis rate is greater at these temperatures and can therefore be mea-sured more easily. Of course, if a formulation has to be heat sterilized then its stability will, in any case, have to be measured at elevated temperatures. Figure 3.12 shows the pH–rate profiles for the degradation of codeine sulfate at several temperatures and also the calculated values at 25°C. We will now see how these calculated values can be obtained.

The equation that describes the effect of tempera-ture on decomposition, and which shows us how to calculate the rate of breakdown at room temperature from measurements at much higher temperatures, is the *Arrhenius equation*.

$$\log k = \log A - \frac{E_a}{2.303\,RT} \qquad (3.54)$$

In this equation, E_a is the activation energy, which is the energy barrier that has to be overcome if reaction is to

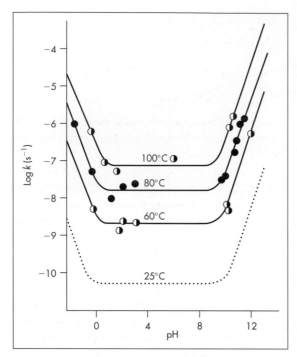

Figure 3.12 Log rate–pH profiles for the degradation of codeine sulfate in buffer-free solutions at several temperatures. The dashed line is the log rate–pH profile calculated from the Arrhenius equation.

Reproduced from Powell MF, *J Pharm Sci*, 1986; 75: 901.

occur when two reactant molecules collide. A is the frequency factor and this is assumed to be independent of temperature for a given reaction. R is the gas constant $(8.314\,J\,mol^{-1}\,K^{-1})$ and T is the temperature in kelvins. We can see from equation (3.54) that a plot of the log rate constant, k, against the reciprocal of the temperature should be linear with a gradient of $-E_a/2.303R$. Therefore, assuming that there is not a change in the form of the reaction as the temperature is changed, we can extrapolate plots of $\log k$ against $1/T$ to any required temperature and so determine the rate of breakdown at that temperature. We can also, of course, calculate the activation energy from the gradient of this plot. Figure 3.13 shows Arrhenius plots for the breakdown of the drug ciclosidomine at several pH values.

When it is clear from stability determinations that a drug is particularly unstable at room temperature, then of course it will need to be labelled with instructions to store in a cool place. This is the case, for example, with injections of penicillin, insulin, oxytocin and vasopressin.

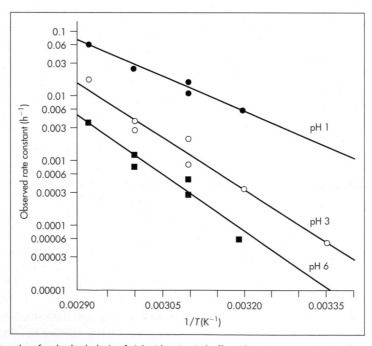

Figure 3.13 Arrhenius plots for the hydrolysis of ciclosidomine in buffer solutions at several pH values.

Reproduced from Carney CF, *J Pharm Sci*, 1987; 76: 393.

Example 3.6 Calculation using the Arrhenius equation

The following values were determined for the specific acid-catalytic constants k_{H+} for an anti-inflammatory drug:

Temperature(°C)	95	90	85	75	65
$10^3 k_{H+}$ $(mol\,dm^{-3})^{-1}\,s^{-1}$		8.15	4.85	2.76	1.02	0.29

Determine graphically (a) the rate constant for acid-catalysis at 25°C, (b) the activation energy.

Answer

According to the Arrhenius equation, a plot of $\log k$ against $1/T$ has a gradient of $-E_a/2.303R$. From the graph:

(a) At $1/T = 3.356 \times 10^{-3}\,K^{-1}$, $\log k = -5.85$. Therefore, k at 25°C $= 1.41 \times 10^{-6}$ $(mol\,dm^{-3})^{-1}\,s^{-1}$.

(b) Gradient $= -5.91 \times 10^3\,K$. Therefore $E_a = 113\,kJ\,mol^{-1}$.

Ionic strength

We often need to add electrolytes to drug solutions, for example to control their tonicity. Consequently we must pay particular attention to any effect they may have on stability. In fact, the stability experiments that we considered earlier in this section should all be carried out at constant electrolyte concentration to avoid any confusion arising from possible differences in electrolyte effects between different systems.

The equation that describes the influence of electrolyte on the rate constant is the *Brønsted–Bjerrum equation*,

$$\log k = \log k_0 + 2Az_A z_B \mu^{1/2} \qquad (3.55)$$

In this equation, z_A and z_B are the charge numbers of the two interacting ions and A is a constant for a given solvent and temperature (see equation 2.36). μ is the ionic strength of the solution, which we can calculate from

$$\mu = \frac{1}{2}\sum(mz^2)$$
$$= \frac{1}{2}(m_A z_A^2 + m_B z_B^2 + \cdots) \qquad (3.56)$$

For example, if we have a monovalent drug ion of concentration $0.01\,mol\,kg^{-1}$ in the presence of $0.001\,mol\,kg^{-1}$ of Ca^{2+} ions then the ionic strength of the solution will be

$$\mu = \frac{1}{2}[(0.01 \times 1^2) + (0.001 \times 2^2)]$$
$$= 0.007\,mol\,kg^{-1}$$

If the drug ion and the electrolyte ion are both monovalent, then the ionic strength will be equal to the total molality of the solution.

We can see from equation (3.55) that if we determine the rate constant of a reaction in the presence of a series of different concentrations of the same electrolyte and plot $\log k$ against $\mu^{1/2}$, then the plot should be linear with an intercept of $\log k_0$ and a gradient of $2Az_A z_B$. This is frequently found to be the case even in solutions of high ionic strength, although equation (3.55) is strictly valid only for ionic strengths of less than $0.01\,mol\,kg^{-1}$. At higher ionic strengths (up to about $0.1\,mol\,kg^{-1}$) it is preferable to use the following modified form of the Brønsted–Bjerrum equation in which we plot $\log k$ against $\mu^{1/2}/(1 + \mu^{1/2})$.

$$\log k = \log k_0 + 2Az_A z_B \left[\frac{\mu^{1/2}}{(1 + \mu^{1/2})} \right] \qquad (3.57)$$

Figure 3.14 shows the degradation of phentolamine hydrochloride at two different pH values plotted according to equation (3.57). The gradients of these plots should be proportional to the product of the charge carried by the reactive species. Whether or not the gradient is positive or negative depends on the reaction involved. Reactions between ions of similar charge, for example the acid-catalysed hydrolysis of a cationic drug ion, will produce plots of positive slope, (i.e. the reaction rate will be increased by electrolyte addition), whereas the base-catalysed hydrolysis of positively charged drug species will produce negative gradients. Investigations of the influence of ionic strength on reaction rate may therefore be used to provide confirmation of the type of reaction that is occurring. For example, the gradients of the two plots of Fig. 3.14 are 0.260 and -1.759 at pH 3.1 and 7.2, respectively. Since the value of $2A$ at 90°C is 1.174, we can calculate values of the product $z_A z_B$ of 0.221 and -1.498 at pH 3.1 and 7.2, respectively. These values are not integers as they should be if the reactions involved were simple acid- and base-catalysed reactions. This has been explained by suggesting complex reactions between the buffer species and the phentolamine at each pH.

Figure 3.14 The effect of ionic strength, μ, on the hydrolytic rate constant, k, for phentolamine hydrochloride in buffer solutions of pH 3.1 and 7.2 at 90°C.

Example 3.7 Calculation using the Brønsted–Bjerrum equation

The following values of the rate constant, k, were obtained at 60°C for the hydrolysis of penicillin in phosphate buffer at pH 8.8 in a series of solutions of varying ionic strength, μ:

$k(h^{-1})$	0.078	0.068	0.056	0.049
μ (mol kg^{-1})	0.49	0.38	0.27	0.20

Plot the data in accordance with the modified Brønsted–Bjerrum equation (equation 3.57) and determine the gradient of the plot. Comment on whether this value would be expected for the acid-catalysis of the protonated penicillin ion. (Note: Assume a value of unity for A at this temperature.)

Answer

The gradient of the plot of $\log k$ against $\mu^{1/2}/(1+\mu^{1/2})$ is +2.0. As expected for a reaction between ions of like charge (acid and protonated penicillin ion), the gradient is positive.

Solvent effects

Since we are considering the hydrolysis of drugs it might seem that an obvious way to reduce the breakdown would be to replace some or all of the water in the system with a solvent such as alcohol or propylene glycol. As we will see in this section, however, this is effective only in certain systems and in others it can, in fact, increase the rate of breakdown. The equation that allows us to predict the effect of the solvent on the hydrolysis rate is

$$\log k = \log k_{\varepsilon=\infty} - \frac{Kz_A z_B}{\varepsilon} \tag{3.58}$$

In this equation, K is a constant for a given system at a given temperature. We can see that a plot of $\log k$ as a function of the reciprocal of the dielectric constant, ε, of the solvent should be linear with a gradient of $-Kz_A z_B$ and an intercept equal to the logarithm of the rate constant in a theoretical solvent of infinite dielectric constant. If the charges on the drug ion and the interacting species are the same, then we can see that the gradient of the line will be negative. In this case, if we replace the water with a solvent of lower dielectric constant then we will achieve the desired effect of reducing the reaction rate. If the drug ion and the interacting ion are of opposite signs, however, then the slope will be positive and the choice of a nonpolar solvent will only result in an increase of decomposition.

Oxygen

Since molecular oxygen is involved in many oxidation schemes, we could use oxygen as a challenge to find out whether a particular drug is likely to be affected by oxidative breakdown. We would do this by storing solutions of the drug in ampoules purged with oxygen and then comparing their rate of breakdown with similar solutions stored under nitrogen. Formulations that are shown to be susceptible to oxidation can be stabilised by replacing the oxygen in the storage containers with nitrogen or carbon dioxide, by avoiding contact with heavy metal ions, and by adding antioxidants (see section 3.1.2).

Light

Photolabile drugs are usually stored in containers that exclude ultraviolet light, since exposure to light in this wavelength range is the most usual cause of photodegradation (see section 3.1.4) Amber glass is particularly effective in this respect because it excludes light of wavelength of less than about 470 nm. As an added precaution, it is always advisable to store photolabile drugs in the dark.

Surfactants

As might be expected, the presence of surfactants in micellar form has a modifying effect on the rate of hydrolysis of drugs. The magnitude of the effect depends on the difference in the rate constant when the drug is in aqueous solution and when it is solubilised within the micelle, and also on the extent of solubilisation. Thus

$$k_{obs} = k_m f_m + k_w f_w \qquad (3.59)$$

where k_{obs}, k_m and k_w are the observed, micellar and aqueous rate constants, respectively, and f_m and f_w are the fractions of drug associated with the micelles and aqueous phase, respectively. The value of k_m is dependent on the location of the drug within the micelle. A solubilisate may be incorporated into the micelle in a variety of locations. Nonpolar compounds are thought to be solubilised within the lipophilic core and, as such, are likely to be more effectively removed from the attacking species than those compounds that are located close to the micellar surface. Where the drug is located near to the micellar surface, and therefore still susceptible to attack, the ionic nature of the surfactant is an important influence on decomposition rate. For base-catalysed hydrolysis, solubilisation into anionic micelles affords an effective stabilisation due to repulsion of OH^- by the micelles. Conversely, solubilisation into cationic micelles might be expected to cause an enhanced base-catalysed hydrolysis.

Many drugs associate to form micelles in aqueous solution (see section 5.3) and several studies have been reported of the effect of this self-association on stability. In micellar solutions of benzylpenicillin (500 000 units cm^{-3}) the apparent rate of the hydrogen-ion-catalysed degradation was increased 2-fold, but that of water- and hydroxide-ion-catalysed hydrolysis was decreased 2- to 3-fold.[18] Consequently, the pH profile was shifted to higher pH values and the pH of minimum degradation was found to be 7.0 compared with 6.5 for monomeric solution (8000 units cm^{-3}). When compared at the respective pH-rate profile minima, micellar benzylpenicillin was reported to be 2.5 times as stable as the monomeric solutions under conditions of constant pH and ionic strength.

3.4.2 Semisolid dosage forms

The chemical stability of active ingredients incorporated into ointments or creams is frequently dependent on the nature of the ointment or cream base used in the formulation. Hydrocortisone in a series of commercially available bases exhibits maximum decomposition in polyethylene glycol base.[19,20] The reported shelf-life was only 6 months in this base, which makes manufacture on a commercial basis an unreasonable proposition, considering the length of time involved in distribution of the drug from wholesaler to patient.

Not only should possible stability problems be borne in mind in the choice of ointment base at the formulation stage, but also similar care should be exercised if the ointment is diluted at a later stage. Such dilution is, unfortunately, common practice in cases where the practitioner wishes to reduce the potency of highly active topical preparations, particularly steroids. The pharmaceutical and biopharmaceutical dangers of this procedure have been stressed.[21] Of particular interest here are the problems of drug stability, which can occur through the use of unsuitable diluents. An example has been cited of the dilution of betamethasone valerate cream with a cream base having a neutral to alkaline pH. Under such conditions, conversion of the 17-ester to the less-active betamethasone 21-ester can occur. Similarly, diluents containing oxidising agents could cause chemical degradation of fluocinolone acetate to less-active compounds.

Incorporation of drugs into gel structures frequently leads to a change in their stability, such as increased degradation of benzylpenicillin sodium in hydrogels of various natural and semisynthetic polymers.[22] At pH 6 in Carbopol hydrogels, the percentage of undecomposed pilocarpine at equilibrium is a simple function of the apparent viscosity of the medium.[23] The rate constant for degradation was not, however, significantly affected by changes in viscosity. Little influence of viscosity on the rate of oxidation of ascorbic acid in gels of polysorbate 80 has been noted.[24]

3.4.3 Solid dosage forms

Moisture

Water-soluble drugs present in a solid dosage form will dissolve in any moisture that has adsorbed on the solid surface. The drug will now be in an aqueous environment and its decomposition could be influenced by many of the factors we have already discussed when dealing with liquid dosage forms. For example, decomposition could now occur by hydrolytic cleavage of ester or amide linkages in the drug molecule and hence will be affected by the pH of the adsorbed moisture film. It is not surprising, therefore, that moisture is considered to be one of the most important factors that must be controlled in order to minimise decomposition.

We can get an idea of the extent to which moisture adsorption affects stability from the results shown in Fig. 3.15. We can see from this figure that an increase in the water vapour pressure (and therefore an increase in the amount of moisture associated with the drug) greatly increases the percentage decomposition at any given time. The problem is even more pronounced with drugs that are hygroscopic or that

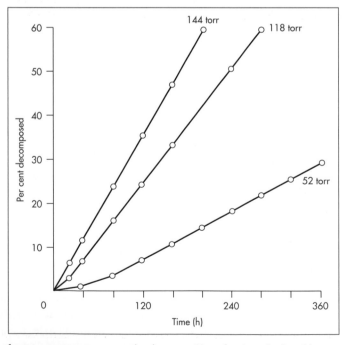

Figure 3.15 The effect of water vapour pressure on the decomposition of aminosalicylic acid.

Reproduced from Kornblum SS, Sciarrone BJ, *J Pharm Sci*, 1964; 53: 935.

decompose to give hygroscopic products. In such cases it is worth trying to prepare a less hygroscopic salt of the drug.

In all cases it is important to minimise access of moisture during manufacture and storage. The correct selection of packaging is obviously important, although this is not as straightforward as you might at first think. For example, tablets containing a water-labile drug were found to be more stable in a water-permeable blister package at 50°C than in a sealed glass bottle and yet the situation was reversed at room temperature and 70% relative humidity.[25] The reason for this behaviour was attributed to the loss of considerable amounts of water through the film at 50°C, so improving stability, and the reverse diffusion at room temperature, so decreasing stability.

Excipients

One of the main ways in which the excipients of the solid dosage form can affect the degradation of drugs is by increasing the moisture content of the preparation. Excipients such as starch and povidone have particularly high water contents (povidone contains about 28% equilibrium moisture at 75% relative humidity). However, whether this high moisture level has an effect on stability depends on how strongly it is bound and whether the moisture can come into contact with the drug. Magnesium trisilicate causes increased hydrolysis of aspirin in tablet form because, it is thought, of its high water content.

Many examples of the effects of tablet excipients on drug decompositions are reported in the pharmaceutical literature. Chemical interaction between components in solid dosage forms may lead to increased decomposition. Replacement of the phenacetin in compound codeine and APC tablets by paracetamol in NHS formulations in Australia in the 1960s (because of the undesirable side-effects of phenacetin), led to an unexpected decreased stability of the tablets. The cause was later attributed to a transacetylation reaction between aspirin and paracetamol and also a possible direct hydrolysis of the paracetamol (Scheme 3.15).

Figure 3.16 shows the increased generation of free salicylic acid at 37°C in the tablets containing paracetamol. It is interesting to note from this figure the effect on stability of tablet excipients. Addition of 1% talc caused only a minimal increase in the decomposition, while 0.5% magnesium stearate increased the breakdown rate dramatically.

Other studies on the influence of tablet excipients on drug decomposition have identified problems with stearate salts and it has been suggested that these

Scheme 3.15 Reactions showing the postulated transacetylation between aspirin and paracetamol and the direct hydrolysis of paracetamol.

Reproduced from Boggianno BG *et al., Aust J Pharm*, 1970; 51: S14.

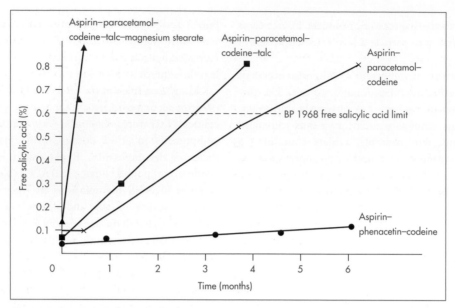

Figure 3.16 Development of free salicylic acid in aspirin–paracetamol–codeine and aspirin–phenacetin–codeine tablets at 37°C.
Reproduced from Boggianno BG *et al. Aust J Pharm*, 1970; 51: S14.

salts should be avoided as tablet lubricants if the active component is subject to hydroxide-ion-catalysed degradation. The degradative effect of the alkali stearates is inhibited in the presence of malic, hexamic or maleic acid owing, it is thought, to competition for the lubricant cation between the drug and the additive acid.

The base used in the formulation of suppositories can often affect the rate of decomposition of the active ingredients. Aspirin decomposes in several polyoxyethylene glycols that are often incorporated into suppository bases.[26] Degradation was shown to be due in part to transesterification, giving the decomposition products salicylic acid and acetylated polyethylene glycol. The rate of decomposition, which followed pseudo first-order kinetics, was considerably greater than when a fatty base such as cocoa butter was used.[27] Analysis of commercial batches of 100 mg indometacin–polyethylene glycol suppositories[28] showed that approximately 2%, 3.5% and 4.5% of the original amount of indometacin was esterified with polyoxyethylene glycol 300 (**XV**) after storage times of 1, 2 and 3 years, respectively.

Excipients present in tablet formulations can have an impact on the photostability of the product, the effect arising in many cases from impurities present in the excipients.[9] For example, free radical reactions

Structure XV Polyethylene glycol esters of indometacin identified in stored suppositories (n = number of ethylene oxide units)

involving phenolic impurities in tablet binding agents such as povidone, disintegrants such as crospovidone, and viscosity-modifying agents such as alginates can lead to photodegradation. Similarly, coloured products may be formed by the reaction of aldehydes formed during spray-drying or autoclaving of lactose with primary amine groups in the product.

Temperature

Investigation of the effect of temperature change on the stability of solid dosage forms can be complicated for many possible reasons. The drug or one of the excipients may, for example, melt or change its polymorphic form as temperature is increased, or it may contain loosely bound water that is lost at higher temperatures. We should also remember that the relative humidity will change with temperature and so we must take care to keep this at a constant value.

Despite these possible complications, many authors have found that the effect of temperature on decomposition rate can be described by an Arrhenius-type equation; i.e. plots of $\log k$ against $1/T$ are linear. This then enables the stability to be predicted at room temperature from measurements made at elevated temperatures. Although we can calculate an apparent activation energy, E_a, from the gradient of the plots, we must remember that this does not have the same meaning as the activation energy for reactions in solution. The E_a value in the solid state is affected, for example, by changes not only in the solubility of the drug in the moisture layer but also in the intrinsic rate of reaction. We cannot, however, use the Arrhenius equation in cases where decomposition shows an approach to equilibrium. Examples of such systems include vitamin A in gelatin beadlets and vitamin E

in lactose base tablets. In these cases we can often use the van't Hoff equation to describe the effect of temperature on breakdown. We determine the equilibrium concentrations of products and reactants at a series of temperatures and then plot the logarithm of the equilibrium constant, K, against the reciprocal of the temperature (see Fig. 3.17) according to the equation

$$\ln K = \frac{-\Delta H}{RT} + \text{constant} \qquad (3.60)$$

Light and oxygen

We have examined above the stability problems that arise with drugs that are susceptible to photodecomposition or oxidation. We will not reconsider them here but merely re-emphasise that we should take all the necessary precautions to exclude light or oxygen when storing these drugs. In this respect we should remember that water contains dissolved oxygen and so the presence of moisture on the surface of solid preparations may increase the oxidation of susceptible drugs; such drugs must, therefore, be stored under dry conditions.

Figure 3.17 Van't Hoff plot for vitamin E succinate decomposition in lactose base tablets.

Reproduced with permission from Carstensen JT et al., J Pharm Sci, 968: 57: 23.

Key points

- The rate of hydrolysis of drugs in liquid dosage forms is strongly influenced by the pH of the solution and can be catalysed not only by H^+ and OH^- ions (specific acid–base catalysis) but also by the components of the buffer used (general acid–base catalysis). To remove the influence of the buffer, the reaction rate is measured at a series of buffer concentrations at each pH and the data extrapolated back to zero concentration. These extrapolated rate constants are then plotted as a function of pH to give a buffer-independent pH-rate profile from which the pH of maximum stability of the solution can be determined and the rate constants for specific acid–base catalysis calculated.

- Temperature increase usually causes a pronounced increase of hydrolytic degradation. The hydrolytic rate constant at room temperature is determined by extrapolation of data at elevated temperatures using the Arrhenius equation,

$$\log k = \log A - \frac{E_a}{2.303RT}$$

- The effect of addition of electrolyte on the hydrolysis rate is determined from the Brønsted–Bjerrum equation, $\log k = \log k_0 + 2Az_A z_B \mu^{1/2}$. The reaction will be increased by electrolyte addition when it involves the interaction of the drug ion with an ion of the same charge and decreased when reaction is between ions of opposite charge.

- The effect of solvent on hydrolysis rate is determined by the equation $\log k = \log k_{\varepsilon = \infty} - K z_A z_B / \varepsilon$; a change of solvent to one of lower dielectric constant will only stabilise reaction between ions of the same charge.

- Formulations that are shown to be susceptible to oxidation can be stabilised by replacing the oxygen in the storage containers with nitrogen or carbon dioxide, by avoiding contact with heavy metal ions, and by adding antioxidants. Photolabile drugs should be stored in containers that exclude ultraviolet light.

- The bases used for the preparation of ointments and creams should be chosen carefully to avoid possible drug stability problems. Care should also be taken with the choice of bases if it is necessary to dilute these semisolid dosage forms.

- In solid dosage forms containing drugs that are susceptible to hydrolysis, decomposition of the drug can occur if moisture is allowed to adsorb on the surface of the dosage form. Careful selection of packaging is important to reduce this possibility. The stability of drugs that dissolve in this surface layer will be affected by many of the factors that influence their decomposition in liquid dosage forms. Excipients of the solid dosage form can affect the drug breakdown by increasing the moisture content of the dosage form.

- Temperature increase causes an increase in the rate of breakdown of drugs in solid dosage forms, which can often be described by the Arrhenius equation, although the effect of temperature change is usually far more complicated than for simple liquid formulations. This equation cannot be used for systems that show an approach to equilibrium. The van't Hoff equation, $\ln K = -\Delta H / RT + \text{constant}$, is often useful to describe the effect of temperature on the decomposition of these systems.

3.5 Stability testing and prediction of shelf-life

It is clearly most important to be able to ensure that a particular formulation when packaged in a specific container will remain within its physical, chemical, microbiological, therapeutic and toxicological specifications on storage for a specified period. In order to make such an assurance, we obviously need to conduct a rigorous stability testing programme on the product in the form that is finally to be marketed. Since the testing period can be as long as two years, it has become essential to devise a more rapid technique that can be used during product development to speed up the identification of the most suitable formulation. In this section we shall examine ways of predicting the chemical stability of a formulation during preformulation studies using accelerated storage tests. We will not be considering the toxicological or microbiological studies or the determination of physical stability, all of which are essential elements in the overall stability testing of the formulation but which are outside the scope of this chapter. Although most of this section will be concerned with the prediction of the effect of temperature on drug decomposition, other environmental factors will also be briefly considered.

3.5.1 Effect of temperature on stability

We have already considered the basic method of accelerating the chemical decomposition by raising the temperature of the preparations. We shall briefly reconsider essential steps in the process. The order of reaction can be determined by plotting stability data at several elevated temperatures according to the equations relating decomposition to time for each of the orders of reaction, until linear plots are obtained. We can now calculate values of rate constant at each temperature from the gradient of these plots, and plot the logarithm of k against reciprocal temperature according to the Arrhenius equation

$$\log k = \log A - \frac{E_a}{2.303RT} \tag{3.61}$$

The required value of k can be interpolated from this plot at room temperature, and the activation energy E_a calculated from the gradient, which is $-E_a/2.303R$.

Values of E_a are usually within the range $50-96 \, \text{kJ mol}^{-1}$.

A convenient, approximate method that is useful for estimation of decomposition rates at room temperature makes use of the ratio of rate constants at room temperature (T_1) and a higher temperature (T_2). If we subtract the Arrhenius equations at temperatures T_1 and T_2, assuming that the $\log A$ term is the same at each temperature, we obtain

$$\log \left[\frac{k_2}{k_1}\right] = -\frac{E_a}{2.303R}\left[\frac{1}{T_2} - \frac{1}{T_1}\right] \tag{3.62}$$

or

$$\log \left[\frac{k_2}{k_1}\right] = \frac{E_a(T_2 - T_1)}{2.303RT_2T_1} \tag{3.63}$$

We must, of course, have a value of E_a in order to be able to use these equations for the calculation of the room temperature rate constant k_1. If we only require a rough estimation of k_1 then we can assume a mid-range value of E_a, say $75 \, \text{kJ mol}^{-1}$, for these calculations.

 Example 3.8 Application of the Arrhenius equation

The first-order rate constant for the hydrolysis of sulfacetamide at 120°C is $9 \times 10^{-6} \, \text{s}^{-1}$ and the activation energy is $94 \, \text{kJ mol}^{-1}$. Calculate the rate constant at 25°C.

Answer

Using equation (3.63) with an E_a value of $94 \, \text{kJ mol}^{-1}$ we have

$$\log \left[\frac{k_{120}}{k_{25}}\right] = \frac{94 \times 10^3 \times (393 - 298)}{2.303 \times 8.314 \times (393 \times 298)}$$

$$= 3.98$$

Removing the logarithms, $k_{120}/k_{25} = 9.55 \times 10^3$.

Therefore, $k_{25} = 9 \times 10^{-6}/9.55 \times 10^3 = 9.4 \times 10^{-10} \, \text{s}^{-1}$.

An alternative method of data treatment is to plot the logarithm of the half-life, $t_{0.5}$, as a function of reciprocal temperature. From equation (3.13), $t_{0.5} = 0.693/k$. Therefore,

$$\log k = \log 0.693 - \log t_{0.5} \qquad (3.64)$$

and substituting into equation (3.54) gives

$$\log t_{0.5} = \log 0.693 \\ - \log A + (E_a/2.303RT) \qquad (3.65)$$

Once the rate constant is known at the required storage temperature it is a simple matter to calculate a shelf-life for the product based on an acceptable degree of decomposition. The equations we can use for 10% loss of activity are obtained by substituting $x = 0.1a$ in the zero- and first-order equations (equations 3.8 and 3.10), giving

$$t_{0.9} = 0.1 \frac{[D]_0}{k_0} \qquad \text{(zero order)} \qquad (3.66)$$

and

$$t_{0.9} = \frac{0.105}{k_1} \qquad \text{(first order)} \qquad (3.67)$$

where $[D_0]$ is the initial concentration of drug. Although $t_{0.9}$ is usually used as an estimate of shelf life, other percentage decompositions may be required, for example when the decomposition products produce discoloration or have undesirable side-effects. The required equations for these may be derived by substituting in the relevant rate equations.

Example 3.9 Calculation of expiry date

The initial concentration of active principle in an aqueous preparation was $5.0 \times 10^{-3}\,\text{g cm}^{-3}$. After 20 months the concentration was shown by analysis to be $4.2 \times 10^{-3}\,\text{g cm}^{-3}$. The drug is known to be ineffective after it has decomposed to 70% of its original concentration. Assuming that decomposition follows first-order kinetics, calculate the nominal expiry date of the drug preparation.

Answer

Substituting into the first-order equation (equation 3.10)

$$k = (2.303/20) \\ \times \log\left[(5 \times 10^{-3})/(4.2 \times 10^{-3})\right]$$

$$k = 8.719 \times 10^{-3}\,\text{month}^{-1}$$

70% of the initial concentration $= 3.5 \times 10^{-3}\,\text{g cm}^{-3}$.

$$t = (2.303/8.719 \times 10^{-3}) \\ \times \log\left[(5 \times 10^{-3})/(3.5 \times 10^{-3})\right]$$

$$t = 40.9\,\text{months}$$

The nominal expiry date is thus 40.9 months after initial preparation (although in practice the shelf-life would probably be calculated for a decomposition to 95% of its value).

Although accelerated storage testing based on the use of the Arrhenius equation has resulted in a very significant saving of time, it still involves the time-consuming step of the initial determination of the order of reaction for the decomposition. While most investigators have emphasised the need for a knowledge of the exact kinetic pathway of degradation, some have bypassed this initial step by assuming a particular decomposition model. At less than 10% degradation and within the limits of experimental error involved in stability studies, it is not possible to distinguish between zero-, first- or simple second-order kinetics using curve-fitting techniques; consequently the assumption of first-order kinetics for any decomposition reaction should involve minimum error. In fact, it was shown that there was a linear relationship between the logarithm of $t_{0.9}$ (the time taken for the concentration of the reactant to decompose to 90% of its original value) and the reciprocal temperature, which was independent of the order of reaction for the decomposition of a series of drugs.[29] On the basis of these findings it was suggested that the use of such linear plots to determine $t_{0.9}$ at the required temperature would provide a rapid, and yet sufficiently accurate, means of studying decomposition rate during the development stage.

Even with the modifications suggested above, the method of stability testing based on the Arrhenius equation is still time-consuming, involving as it does the separate determination of rate constants at a series of elevated temperatures. Experimental techniques have been developed[30,31] that enable the decomposition rate to be determined from a single experiment. Such methods involve raising the temperature of the product in accordance with a predetermined temperature–time programme and are consequently referred to as nonisothermal stability studies. Any suitable temperature–time programme may be used; Box 3.3 illustrates the method proposed by Rogers[30] in which the rise of temperature was programmed so that the reciprocal of the temperature varied logarithmically with time.

The advantages of the method shown in Box 3.3 over the conventional method of stability testing are that (a) the data required to calculate the stability are obtained in a single one-day experiment rather than from a series of experiments that might last for several weeks; (b) no preliminary experiments are required to determine the optimum temperatures for the accelerated storage test; and (c) the linearity of the plot of $\log f(c)$ against $\log(1 + t)$ confirms that the correct order of reaction has been assumed.

Several improvements on the original nonisothermal stability testing methods have been suggested. Rather than subjecting the drug formulation to a predetermined fixed time–temperature profile, the temperature may be changed during the course of the experiment at a rate consistent with the analytical results from the experiment.[31] The resultant time–temperature data are fitted to a polynomial expression of sufficient degree to describe the changes. This relationship and the experimental data are then combined and used to compute a series of degradation pathways corresponding to a series of values of activation energy. The curves are matched with the experimental analytical data to obtain the correct activation energy for the reaction. Using this activation energy and the analytical data, the reaction rate and stability may be calculated. Computational procedures whereby the activation energy and frequency factor of the Arrhenius equation may be determined from simple nonisothermal experiments with a fixed temperature-time profile have been described.[32,33]

An improvement in the design of stability tests has been suggested that avoids the difficulties inherent in the nonlinear curve-fitting procedures outlined above.[34] The experimental procedure involves changing the temperature of the samples being studied until degradation is rapid enough to proceed at a convenient rate for isothermal studies to be carried out. The analytical information obtained during the nonisothermal and isothermal portions of the experiment is used in calculating the activation energy and determining the order of reaction and the reaction rate and predicting stability at any required temperature.

Box 3.3 Nonisothermal methods for determination of drug stability

In the method proposed by Rogers[30] the rise of temperature was programmed so that the reciprocal of the temperature varied logarithmically with time according to

$$(1/T_0) - (1/T_t) = 2.303\, b \log(1 + t) \tag{3.68}$$

where T_0 and T_t are the temperatures at zero time and at time t, respectively, and b is any suitable proportionality constant. Applying the Arrhenius equation at both temperatures and subtracting gives

$$\log k_t = \log k_0 + \frac{E_a}{2.303R}\left(\frac{1}{T_0} - \frac{1}{T_t}\right) \tag{3.69}$$

Substituting equation (3.68) into equation (3.69) gives

$$\log k_t = \log k_0 + \frac{E_a b}{R}\log(1 + t) \tag{3.70}$$

Therefore,

$$k_t = k_0(1 + t)^{E_a b/R} \tag{3.71}$$

For first-order reactions $-dc/dt = kc$, where c is concentration. Substituting for k from equation (3.71) and integrating gives

$$-\int_{c_0}^{c_t} \frac{dc}{c} = k_0 \int_0^t (1 + t)^{E_a b/R} dt \tag{3.72}$$

where c_0 and c_t are the concentrations at zero time and at time t, respectively. Therefore,

$$\log f(c) = \log k_0 - \log\left(1 + \frac{E_a b}{R}\right) + \left(1 + \frac{E_a b}{R}\right)\log(1 + t) + \log\left[1 - \left(\frac{k_0}{k_t}\right)^{1 + R/E_a b}\right] \tag{3.73}$$

where

$$f(c) = 2.303 \log(c_0/c_t) \tag{3.74}$$

A similar equation applies to second-order reactions with

$$\log f(c) = \frac{2.303}{a_0 - b_0}\log\frac{a_t}{b_t} + \frac{2.303}{a_0 - b_0}\log\frac{b_0}{a_0} \tag{3.75}$$

where a_0 and b_0 are the concentrations of the reactants at the beginning of the experiment, and a_t and b_t their concentrations at time t. The value of the final term of equation (3.73) rapidly tends to zero as k_t becomes greater than k_0. Thus a graph of $\log f(c)$ against $\log(1 + t)$ will be linear from that time after which k_0 is negligible in comparison with k_t. The gradient of the line is $(1 + E_a b/R)$, enabling E_a to be determined. The rate constant k_0 may then be calculated from the intercept when $\log(1 + t) = 0$, which is equal to $\log k_0 - \log(1 + E_a b/R)$. The rate constant at any other temperature may be calculated from k_0 and E_a.

Example 3.10 Accelerated storage testing using temperature–time programme

In a study of the first-order decomposition of riboflavine in $0.05 \ mol \ dm^{-3}$ NaOH using accelerated storage techniques, the temperature was programmed to rise from 12.5 to 55 °C using a programme constant, b, of $2.171 \times 10^{-4} \ K^{-1}$. The initial concentration, c_0, of riboflavine was $10^{-4} \ mol \ dm^{-3}$, and the concentration remaining at time t, c_t, was as follows:

t (h)	0.585	0.996	1.512	2.163	2.982	4.013	5.312	6.946
$10^5 \ c_t \ (mol \ dm^{-3})$	9.881	9.763	9.532	9.109	8.371	6.902	4.931	2.435

Calculate the activation energy and the rate constant at 20°C.

Answer

For first-order reactions the data are plotted according to equations (3.73) and (3.74).

t	$\log(1+t)$	$\log[2.303 \log(c_0/c_t)]$
0.585	0.2	−1.94
0.996	0.3	−1.62
1.512	0.4	−1.32
2.163	0.5	−1.03
2.982	0.6	−0.75
4.013	0.7	−0.43
5.321	0.8	−0.15
6.946	0.9	+0.15

A plot of $\log[2.303 \log(c_0/c_t)]$ against $\log(1+t)$ is linear (see Fig. 3.18) with a gradient of 2.95. From equation (3.73),

$$\text{Gradient} = 1 + \frac{E_a b}{R}$$

Therefore,

$$E_a = (1.95 \times 8.314)/(2.171 \times 10^{-4})$$
$$= 74.68 \ kJ \ mol^{-1}$$

Intercept at $\log(1+t) = 0$ is −2.55. From equation (3.73),

$$\text{Intercept} = \log k_0 - \log\left[1 + \frac{E_a b}{R}\right]$$

where the final term on the right of equation (3.73) is neglected. Therefore,

$$\log k_0 = -2.55 + \log 2.95 = -2.08$$

and

$$k_0 = 0.0083 \ h^{-1}$$

That is, the rate constant at temperature T_0 (12.5°C) is $0.0083 \ h^{-1}$.

The rate constant at 20°C may then be calculated from the Arrhenius equation in the form of equation (3.69):

$$\log k_t = -2.08 + [74\,680/(2.303 \times 8.314)][(1/285.5) - (1/293)]$$
$$= -2.08 + 0.3497 = -1.730$$

and

$$k_t = 1.86 \times 10^{-2} \ h^{-1}$$

The rate constant at 20°C is thus $0.0186 \ h^{-1}$.

Figure 3.18 Example 3.10: Accelerated storage plot for the decomposition of riboflavin in 0.05 mol dm^{-3} NaOH using data from reference 30.

Although accelerated storage testing has proved invaluable in the development of stable formulations, it is important that we consider some of the limitations of this technique. We must take care that the order of reaction is not different at the higher temperatures from that which occurs at room temperature. There are several cases where this might be so. For example, with complex decomposition processes involving parallel or consecutive reactions, there may be a change in the relative contributions of the component reactions as the temperature is increased.

Suspensions

One complication that arises when we are carrying out stability testing of suspensions is the changes in the solubility of the suspended drug with increase in temperature. With suspensions, the concentration of the drug in solution usually remains constant because, as the decomposition reaction proceeds, more of the drug dissolves to keep the solution saturated. As we have seen, this situation usually leads to zero-order release kinetics. If the actual decomposition of dissolved drug is first-order, then we can express the decrease of concentration, c, with time, t, as

$$-\frac{dc}{dt} = k_0 \qquad (3.76)$$

where $k_0 = k_1 S$ and S is the solubility of the drug.

The problem that arises with these systems is that an increase of temperature causes not only the usual increase in rate constant, but also an increase in solubility. Application of the Arrhenius equation to the data involves the measurement of the changes in solubility of the drug over the temperature range involved. An alternative method that does not necessitate the determination of solubility uses the relationship between solubility and temperature:

$$\log S = -\frac{\Delta H_f}{2.303RT} + \text{constant} \qquad (3.77)$$

Since $k_0 = k_1 S$,

$$\log k_0 = \log k_1 + \log S$$

If we substitute for $\log k_1$, using the Arrhenius equation, we obtain

$$\log k_0 = \frac{(-E_a + \Delta H_f)}{2.303RT} + \text{constant} \qquad (3.78)$$

where ΔH_f is the molar heat of fusion. You can now see that we can plot $\log k_0$ against $1/T$ and extrapolate to give a room temperature value of k_0. It is important we remember that this treatment assumes that drug degradation in solution follows first-order kinetics and that the kinetics are not limited by the dissolution rate.

Solid state

The main problems arising in stability testing of solid dosage forms are[25] (a) that the analytical results tend to have more scatter because tablets and capsules are distinct dosage units rather than the true aliquots encountered with stability studies on drugs in solution, and (b) that these dosage forms are heterogeneous systems often involving a gas phase (air and water vapour), a liquid phase (adsorbed moisture) and the solid phase itself. The compositions of all of these phases can vary during an experiment.

The first of these problems can be overcome by ensuring uniformity of the dosage form before commencing the stability studies. The problems arising from the heterogeneity are more difficult to overcome. The main complicating factor is associated with the presence of moisture. As we have seen in section 3.4.3, moisture can have a significant effect on the kinetics of decomposition and this may produce many experimental problems during stability testing. For example, with gelatin capsules the water in the capsule shell

must equilibrate with that in the formulation and surrounding air and this may require an appreciable time. The prediction of stability is difficult in solid dosage forms in which there is chemical interaction between components, or chemical equilibrium phenomena. In fact, the data for stability studies involving the latter are often plotted using a van't Hoff plot rather than an Arrhenius plot.

To reduce some of these problems, particularly those associated with moisture, during stability testing, the following have been suggested:[25] (a) the use of tightly sealed containers, except where the effect of packaging is to be investigated; (b) that the amount of water present in the dosage form should be determined, preferable at each storage temperature, and (c) that a separate, sealed ampoule should be taken for each assay point and water determination, thus avoiding disturbance of water equilibrium on opening the container.

As has been discussed above, we can often use the Arrhenius equation to predict stability in the solid state, even though the kinetics of breakdown are different from those in solution. The exception to this is when equilibrium reactions occur, in which case we can often use the van't Hoff equation (equation 3.60) to predict room-temperature stability.

3.5.2 Other environmental factors affecting stability

Light

Photostability testing of drug substances usually involves the initial stress testing of the drug to determine its overall photostability and the identification of any degradation products. In this process the sample is irradiated at all absorbing wavelengths using a broad-spectrum light source. Those drugs or formulations that are shown to be photosensitive are then subjected to more formal photostability testing in which they are challenged with light of wavelength comparable to that to which the formulations are exposed in practical situations. During their shelf-life it is most likely that the products will be exposed

Figure 3.19 Logarithm of the nitrazepam decomposition constant, k, as a function of relative humidity at various temperatures.
Reproduced with permission from Genton D, Kesselring UW, *J Pharm Sci*, 1977; 66: 676.

to fluorescent light, direct daylight and daylight filtered through window glass, and the stability testing procedures are designed to cover these possibilities. A specific protocol for testing the photostability of new drugs and products is described in the ICH Guideline.[35]

Oxygen

The stability of an oxidisable drug in a liquid dosage form is generally a function of the efficiency of any antioxidant included in the formulation. Exaggeration of the effect of oxygen on stability may be achieved by an increase in the partial pressure of oxygen in the system. It is not often easy, however, to make decisions on what would be the normal access of oxygen during storage and a meaningful extrapolation of the acquired data may be difficult.

Moisture content

The stability of solid dosage forms is usually very susceptible to the moisture content of the atmosphere in the container in which they are stored (see section 3.4.3) A linear relationship between $\log k$ and the water vapour pressure for vitamin A palmitate beadlets in sugar-coated tablets has been found.[36] Similarly, a linear relationship has been established between the logarithm of the rate constant for the decomposition of nitrazepam in the solid state and the relative humidity (Fig. 3.19). The need for consideration of the effect of moisture on stability has been stressed by Carstensen,[14] who stated that stability programmes should always include samples that have been artificially stressed by addition of moisture. One purpose of a stability programme should be to define the stability of the dosage form as a function of moisture content.

Key points

- It is most important to be able to ensure that a particular formulation when packaged in a specific container will remain within its physical, chemical, microbiological, therapeutic and toxicological specifications on storage for a specified time period. In order to make such an assurance we need to conduct a rigorous stability testing programme on the product in the form that is finally to be marketed.
- To calculate the shelf-life it is necessary to know the rate constant at the storage temperature. However, the rate of breakdown of most pharmaceutical products is so slow that it would take many months to determine this at room temperature and it has become essential to devise a more rapid technique that can be used during product development to speed up the identification of the most suitable formulation.
- The method that is used for accelerated storage testing is based on the Arrhenius equation, $\log k = \log A - (E_a/2.303RT)$.
- The shelf-life for first-order reactions assuming 10% loss of activity, i.e. $t_{0.9}$, is calculated from the rate constant at the storage temperature k_1 using $t_{0.9} = 0.105/k_1$.
- Nonisothermal stability testing methods may be used to further reduce the time taken to conduct stability studies; in these methods the temperature is usually increased in accordance with a predetermined temperature-time programme.

3.5.3 Protocol for stability testing

A stability-testing requirement for a Registration Application agreed within the three areas of the E.C., Japan and the USA exemplifies the core stability data package required for new drug substances and associated drug products.[37] Under this agreement, information on stability generated in any one of these three areas that meets the appropriate requirements of this guideline is mutually acceptable in both of the other two areas. The following summarises some of the main points of the guideline as it affects the stability testing of both drug substances and drug products; the original document should of course be consulted if a more detailed account is required.

Drug substances

Stability information from accelerated and long-term testing is required to be provided on at least three batches manufactured to a minimum of pilot plant scale by the same synthetic route and using a method of manufacture and procedure that simulates the final process to be used on a manufacturing scale. In this context, 'pilot plant scale' is taken to mean a minimum scale of one-tenth that of the full production process. The containers to be used in the long-term evaluation should be the same as, or simulate, the actual packaging used for storage and distribution. The overall quality of the batches of drug substance subjected to stability testing should be representative of both the quality of the material used in pre-clinical and clinical studies and the quality of material to be made on a manufacturing scale.

The testing should be designed to cover those features susceptible to change during storage and likely to influence quality, safety and/or efficacy, including, as necessary, the physical, chemical and microbiological characteristics. The length of the studies and the storage conditions should be sufficient to cover storage, shipment and subsequent use. The specifications for the long-term testing are a temperature of $25 \pm 2°C$ and $60\% \pm 5\%$ relative humidity (RH) for a period of 12 months. For accelerated testing the temperature is specified as $40 \pm 2°C$ and $75\% \pm 5\%$ RH for a period of 6 months. Other storage conditions are allowable if justified; in particular, temperature-sensitive drugs should be stored at a lower temperature, which then becomes the designated long-term testing temperature.

The 6-month accelerated testing should then be carried out at a temperature at least 15°C above this designated temperature together with the relative humidity appropriate to that temperature. Where 'significant change' occurs during the 6 months accelerated storage testing, additional testing at an intermediate temperature (such as $30 \pm 2°C/60\% \pm 5\%$ RH) should be conducted for drug substances to be used in the manufacture of dosage forms tested for long-term stability at 25°C/60% RH. 'Significant change' at 40°C/75% RH or 30°C/60% RH is defined as failure to meet the specification.

The long-term testing is required to be continued for a sufficient period of time beyond 12 months to cover all appropriate re-test periods. The frequency of testing should be sufficient to establish the stability characteristics of the drug substance; under the long-term conditions this will normally be every 3 months over the first year, every 6 months over the second year, and then annually.

Drug product

The design of the stability programme for the finished product is based on the knowledge of the behaviour and properties of the drug substance and the experience gained from clinical formulation studies and from stability studies on the drug substance. Stability information from long term and accelerated testing is required to be presented on three batches of the same formulation and dosage form in the containers and closure proposed for marketing. Two of the three batches should be at least pilot-scale; the third batch may be smaller, for example 25 000–50 000 tablets or capsules for solid dosage forms. Data on laboratory-scale batches are not acceptable as primary stability information. It is stipulated that the manufacturing process to be used should meaningfully simulate that which would be applied to large-scale batches for marketing and should provide product of the same quality intended for marketing, and meeting the same quality specification as to be applied for release of material. Where possible, batches of the finished product should be manufactured using identifiably different batches of drug substance.

As with the stability testing of drug substance, the testing of the product should cover those features susceptible to change during storage and likely to influence quality, safety and/or efficacy. The range of testing should cover not only chemical and biological stability but also loss of preservative, physical

properties and characteristics, organoleptic properties and, where required, microbiological attributes. The conditions and time periods for long-term and accelerated storage testing are the same as those outlined above for drug substances but with special considerations arising from the nature of the drug product. If it is necessary to store the product at a lower temperature because of its heat sensitivity, then consideration should be given to any physical or chemical change in the product that might occur at this temperature; for example, suspensions or emulsions may sediment or cream, while oils and semi-solid preparations may show an increased viscosity. Storage under conditions of high relative humidity applies particularly to solid dosage forms. For products such as solutions and suspensions contained in packs designed to provide a permanent barrier to water loss, specific storage under conditions of high RH is not necessary, but the same range of temperatures should be applied. It is recognised that low RH (10–20%) can adversely affect products packed in semipermeable containers such as solutions in plastic bags and nose drops in small plastic containers, and consideration should be given to appropriate testing under such conditions.

In the case of drug products, 'significant change' at the accelerated condition is defined as

- A 5% potency loss from the initial assay value of a batch
- Any specified degradant exceeding its specification limit
- The product exceeding its pH limits
- Dissolution exceeding the specification limits for 12 capsules or tablets
- Failure to meet specifications for appearance and physical properties, e.g. colour, phase separation, resuspendability, delivery per actuation, caking and hardness

If significant change occurs at 40°C/75% RH then it is necessary to submit a minimum of 6 months' data from an ongoing one-year study at 30°C/60% RH using the same criteria for 'significant change'.

Summary

In this chapter we have examined the various ways in which drugs can chemically breakdown in both liquid and solid dosage forms and discussed possible means of preventing or minimising this loss of activity. The most common cause of degradation of drugs in aqueous solution is the hydrolysis of groups such as esters, amides, lactones, lactams, imides or carbamates. The stability of solutions of drugs containing these groups can be improved by formulation at the pH of maximum stability. Care must be taken, however, in the choice of buffer used because hydrolysis is catalysed not only by hydrogen or hydroxyl ions (specific acid–base hydrolysis) but also by the components of buffer solutions (general acid–base catalysis). Drugs possessing carbon–carbon double bonds such as the steroids, polyunsaturated fatty acids and polyene antibiotics are susceptible to oxidative degradation; liquid formulations of these drugs may be stabilised by replacing the oxygen in the system with inert gases such as nitrogen; by avoiding contact with metals such as iron, cobalt and nickel; and by adding antioxidants or reducing agents to the solution. Some oxidative reactions are pH-dependent, in which case the product can be stabilised by buffering the system. Other less common types of drug decomposition include photochemical breakdown (necessitating storage in amber containers), epimerisation and polymerisation.

We have seen how reactions may follow zero-, first- and second-order kinetics and examined how to determine the rate constant, and in some cases the half-life, of the decomposition process. With this information we are able to make a prediction of the shelf-life of the product, which is usually the time taken for the drug to be reduced to 95% of its original potency. Although the breakdown of most drugs in solution follows first-order or pseudo first-order kinetics, the decomposition process may be complicated by more complex breakdown schemes involving parallel, reversible or consecutive reactions.

Assessment of the optimum pH for formulation of liquid dosage forms is greatly speeded up by measuring the hydrolysis rate at a series of elevated temperatures and extrapolating to room temperature using the Arrhenius equation. A protocol for stability testing that has been agreed in the EC, Japan and the USA has been described.

The kinetics of drug decomposition in solid dosage forms is less well understood. Decomposition of drugs susceptible to hydrolysis can occur if moisture is allowed to adsorb onto the surface of the dosage form

and the packaging should be selected to minimise this effect. Excipients of the solid dosage form can affect the drug breakdown by increasing the moisture content of the dosage form. Film coating of tablets can markedly reduce moisture ingress, as discussed in Chapter 7.

References

1. LePree JM, Connors KA. Hydrolysis of drugs. In: Swarbrick J, ed. *Encyclopedia of Pharmaceutical Technology*. 3rd edn. New York: Informa Healthcare; 2006: 2040–2047.
2. Wells PR. Linear free energy relationships. *Chem Rev* 1963;63:171–219.
3. Cartensen JT *et al.* Use of Hammett graphs in stability programs. *J Pharm Sci* 1964;53:1547–1548.
4. Hovorka SW, Schöneich C. Oxidative degradation of pharmaceuticals: theory, mechanisms and inhibition. *J Pharm Sci* 2001;90:253–269.
5. Johnson DM, Taylor WF. Degradation of fenprostalene in polyethylene glycol 400 solution. *J Pharm Sci* 1984;73:1414–1417.
6. Halbaut L *et al.* Oxidative stability of semi-solid excipient mixtures with corn oil and its implication in the degradation of vitamin A. *Int J Pharm* 1997;147:31–40.
7. Smith GB *et al.* Autooxidation of simvastatin. *Tetrahedron* 1993;49:4447–4462.
8. Lamy-Freund MT *et al.* Effect of aggregation on the kinetics of autoxidation of the polyene antibiotic amphotericin B. *J Pharm Sci* 1993;82:162–166.
9. Tønnesen HH. Formulation and stability testing of photolabile drugs. *Int J Pharm* 2001;225:1–14.
10. Greenhill JV, McLelland MA. Photodecomposition of drugs. *Prog Med Chem* 1990;27:51–121.
11. Huang CL, Sands FL. Effect of ultraviolet irradiation on chlorpromazine. II. Anaerobic condition. *J Pharm Sci* 1967;56:259–264.
12. Matsuda Y *et al.* Stabilization of sulfisomidine tablets by use of film coating containing UV absorber: Protection of coloration and photolytic degradation from exaggerated light. *J Pharm Sci* 1978;67:196–201.
13. Bundgaard H. Polymerization of penicillins: kinetics and mechanism of di- and polymerization of ampicillin in aqueous solution. *Acta Pharm Suec* 1976;13:9–26.
14. Carstensen JT. Stability of solids and solid dosage forms. *J Pharm Sci* 1974;63:1–14.
15. Carstensen JT. *Drug Stability. Principles and Practices.* 2nd edn. New York: Marcel Dekker; 1995.
16. Andersin R, Tammilehto S. Photochemical decomposition of midazolam. IV. Study of pH-dependent stability by high-performance liquid chromatography. *Int J Pharm* 1995;123:229–235.
17. Torniainen K *et al.* The effect of pH, buffer type and drug concentration on the photodegradation of ciprofloxacin. *Int J Pharm* 1996;132:53–61.

18. Ong JTH, Kostenbauder HB. Effect of self-association on rate of penicillin G degradation in concentrated aqueous solutions. *J Pharm Sci* 1975;64:1378–1380.

19. Allen AE, Das Gupta V. Stability of hydrocortisone in polyethylene glycol ointment base. *J Pharm Sci* 1974; 63:107–109.

20. Das Gupta V. Effect of vehicles and other active ingredients on stability of hydrocortisone. *J Pharm Sci* 1978; 67:299–302.

21. Busse MJ. Dangers of dilution of topical steroids. *Pharm J* 1978;22025.

22. Ullmann E *et al.* The stability of sodium penicillin G in the presence of ionic surfactants, organic gel formers, and preservatives. *Pharm Acta Helv* 1963;38:577–586.

23. Testa B, Etter JC. Hydrolysis of pilocarpine in Carbopol hydrogels. *Can J Pharm Sci* 1975;10:16–20.

24. Poust RI, Colaizzi JC. Copper-catalyzed oxidation of ascorbic acid in gels and aqueous solutions of polysorbate 80. *J Pharm Sci* 1968;57:2119–2125.

25. Tingstad J, Dudzinski J. Preformulation studies. II. Stability of drug substances in solid pharmaceutical systems. *J Pharm Sci* 1973;62:1856–1860.

26. Jun HW *et al.* Decomposition of aspirin in polyethylene glycols. *J Pharm Sci* 1972;61:1160–1152.

27. Whitworth CW *et al.* Stability of aspirin in liquid and semisolid bases. II. Effect of fatty additives on stability in a polyethylene glycol base. *J Pharm Sci* 1973;62:1372–1374.

28. Ekman R *et al.* Formation of indomethacin esters in polyethylene glycol suppositories. *Acta Pharm Suec* 1982;19:241–246.

29. Amirjahed AK. Simplified method to study stability of pharmaceutical preparations. *J Pharm Sci* 1977;66:785.

30. Rogers AR. An accelerated storage test with programmed temperature rise. *J Pharm Pharmacol* 1963; 15:101T.

31. Maudling HV, Zoglio MA. Flexible nonisothermal stability studies. *J Pharm Sci* 1970;59:333–337.

32. Madsen BW *et al.* Integral approach to nonisothermal estimation of activation energies. *J Pharm Sci* 1974; 63:777–781.

33. Kay AI, Simon TH. Use of an analog computer to simulate and interpret data obtained from linear nonisothermal stability studies. *J Pharm Sci* 1971;60: 205–208.

34. Zoglio MA *et al.* Nonisothermal kinetic studies III: rapid nonisothermal–isothermal method for stability prediction. *J Pharm Sci* 1975;641381.

35. ICH Harmonised Tripartite Guideline. Q1B: Photostability Testing of New Drug Substances and Products. Federal Register, 62, 27115.(1997).

36. Lachman L. Physical and chemical stability testing of tablet dosage forms. *J Pharm Sci* 1965;54:1519–1526.

37. *Stability Testing of new drug substances and products (ICH).* MCA EuroDirect Publication No. 3335/92.

4

The solubility of drugs

There are many reasons why it is vital to understand the way in which drugs dissolve in solution and the factors that maintain solubility or cause drugs to come out of solution, that is, to precipitate. These include the facts that:

- Many drugs are formulated as solutions or are added in powder or solution form to the liquids, such as infusion fluids, in which they must remain in solution for a given period.
- In whatever way drugs are presented to the body, they must usually be in a molecularly dispersed form (that is in solution) before they can be absorbed across biological membranes*.
- The solution process will precede absorption unless the drug is administered as a solution, but even solutions may precipitate in the stomach contents or in blood, and the precipitated drug will then have to re-dissolve before being absorbed.
- Drugs of low aqueous solubility (e.g. Taxol) frequently present problems in relation to their formulation and bioavailability.

In this chapter we will consider the factors controlling the solubility of drugs in solution, in particular the nature of the drug molecule and the crystalline form in which it exists, its hydrophobicity, its shape, its surface area, its state of ionisation, the influence of pH of the medium and the importance of the pK_a of the drug. The equation linking solubility to solution pH and drug pK_a (equation 4.11) is possibly one of the most important in this book. Experimental methods of measurement of solubility are essential in drug development, as is the ability to predict the solubility of a drug from a knowledge of its chemical structure,

*In section 9.2.1 we discuss the special circumstances under which microparticulate materials can be taken up by specialised cells in the gut and, by way of the lymphatic circulation, reach the liver and blood and other organs. It may be that very insoluble colloidal drug suspensions are absorbed by this route also.

recognising hydrophilic and hydrophobic groups and their influence on solubility. How additives such as salts, co-solvents, surfactants and other agents can affect the solubility of a drug should to an extent be predictable from the theory, bearing in mind the complexity of many formulations.

Pharmaceutical solutions might appear to be extremely simple systems, but it is in the solution state that degradation takes place most rapidly, and the solubilisation of poorly soluble compounds is often very difficult. It is ideal if a drug can be formulated as a simple stable aqueous solution when required for injection, but resort to additives such as water-miscible solvents and surfactants, hydrotropes and cyclo-dextrins to increase the water solubility of the drug complicates the formulation. Here we deal with simple solutions. Some of the special problems related to peptide and protein solubility are discussed in Chapter 12.

Aqueous solvents are the most common in pharmaceutical and, of course, in biological systems, so this chapter is concerned mainly with solutions of aqueous and mixed aqueous solvents, such as alcohol–water mixtures. The solution of drugs in nonaqueous media (such as oils) is also considered because of the many pharmaceutical applications of nonaqueous solutions and formulations such as oil-in-water emul-sions, and because of the need to understand the process of the transport of drugs across biological and artificial membranes, which are effectively structured nonaqueous phases. A primary factor in passive membrane transport is the relative solubility of the drug in an aqueous medium and in the lipid cell membrane, the relative affinities being quantified in the partition coefficient of the compound, a topic discussed at the end of this chapter.

4.1 Definitions

A *solution* can be defined as a system in which mole-cules of a solute (such as a drug or protein) are dis-solved in a solvent vehicle. When a solution contains a solute at the limit of its solubility at any given temper-ature and pressure, it is said to be *saturated*. If the solubility limit is exceeded, solid particles of solute may be present and the solution phase will be in equi-librium with the solid, although under certain circum-stances *supersaturated* solutions may be prepared, where the drug exists in solution above its normal solubility limit.

The maximum *equilibrium solubility* of a drug in a given medium is of practical pharmaceutical interest because it dictates the *rate of solution* (*dissolution*) of the drug (the rate at which the drug dissolves from the solid state). The higher the solubility, the more rapid is the rate of solution when no chemical reaction is involved.

4.1.1 Expressions of solubility

The solubility of a solute in a solvent can be expressed quantitatively in several ways (see Chapter 2, section 2.1). The British Pharmacopoeia and other chemical and pharmaceutical compendia frequently use less-specific forms of noting solubility such as parts per parts of solvent (for example, parts per million, ppm) and also the expressions 'insoluble', 'very highly soluble' and 'soluble'. These are imprecise and often not very helpful. For quantitative work, specific concentration terms must be used.

Most substances have at least some degree of sol-ubility in water and while they may appear to be 'insoluble' by a qualitative test, their solubility can be measured and quoted precisely. In aqueous media at pH 10, chlorpromazine base has a solubility of $8 \times 10^{-6} \, \text{mol dm}^{-3}$, that is it is very slightly soluble, but it might be considered to be 'insoluble' if judged visually by the lack of disappearance of solid placed in a test-tube of water.

4.2 Factors influencing solubility

Progress has been made in ways of predicting the sol-ubility of solutes in aqueous media, both from esti-mates of their molecular surface area and from the nature of the key chemical groups in the parent

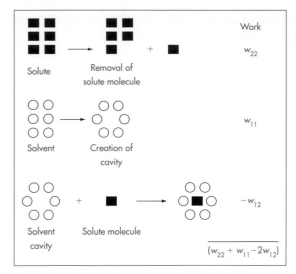

Figure 4.1 Diagrammatic representation of the three processes involved in the dissolution of a crystalline solute: the expression for the work involved is $w_{22} + w_{11} - 2w_{12}$ (solute–solvent interaction in the last stage is $-2w_{12}$ as bonds are made with one solute and two solvent molecules).

structure. The importance of the surface area becomes clear if we think of the processes involved in the dissolution of a crystal (Fig. 4.1). The process can be considered in three stages:

1 A solute (drug) molecule is 'removed' from its crystal.
2 A cavity for the molecule is created in the solvent.
3 The solute molecule is inserted into this cavity.

Placing the solute molecule in the solvent cavity requires a number of solute–solvent contacts; the larger the solute molecule, the more contacts are created. If the surface area of the solute molecule is A, the solute–solvent interface increases by $\sigma_{12}A$, where σ_{12} is the interfacial tension between the solvent (subscript 1) and the solute (subscript 2). σ is a parameter not readily obtained for solid interfaces on the molecular scale, but reasonable estimates can be made from knowledge of the interfacial tensions of molecules at normal interfaces.[1–5]

The number of solvent molecules that can pack around the solute molecule is considered in calculations of the thermodynamic properties of the solution. The molecular surface area of the solute is therefore the key parameter and good correlations can be obtained between aqueous solubility and this parameter.[1,5]

Of course, most drugs are not simple nonpolar hydrocarbons and we have to consider polar molecules and weak organic electrolytes. The term w_{12} in Fig. 4.1, a measure of solute–solvent interactions, has to be further divided to take into account the interactions involving the nonpolar part and the polar portion of the solute. The molecular surface area of each portion can be considered separately: the greater the area of the hydrophilic portion relative to the hydrophobic portion, the greater is the aqueous solubility. For a hydrophobic molecule of area A, the free energy change in placing the solute in the solvent cavity is $-\sigma_{12}A$. Indeed, it can be shown that the reversible work of solution is $(w_{11} + w_{22} - 2w_{12})A$.

Implicit in this derivation is the assumption that the solution formed is dilute, so that solute–solute interactions are unimportant. The success of the molecular area approach is evidenced by the fact that equations can be written to relate solubility to surface area. For example, equation (4.1) has been shown to hold for a range of 55 compounds (some of which are listed in Table 4.1):

$$\ln S = -4.3A + 11.78 \tag{4.1}$$

where S is the molal (not molar) solubility, and A is the total surface area in nm^2.

The compounds in Table 4.1 are liquids, so the process of dissolution is simpler than that outlined in Fig. 4.1.

4.2.1 Structural features and aqueous solubility

Shape

Interactions between nonpolar groups and water were discussed above, where the importance of both size and shape was indicated. Chain branching of hydrophobic groups influences aqueous solubility, as shown by the solubilities of a series of straight and branched-chain alcohols in Table 4.2.

What other predictors of solubility might there be? The boiling point of liquids and the melting point of solids are useful in that both reflect the strengths of interactions between the molecules in the pure liquid or the solid state. Boiling point correlates with total surface area, and in a large enough range of compounds we can detect the trend of decreasing aqueous solubility with increasing boiling point (see data in Table 4.2).

Table 4.1 Experimental aqueous solubilities, boiling points, surface areas and predicted aqueous solubilities[a]

Compound	Solubility (mol kg^{-1})	Surface area (nm^2)	Boiling point (°C)	Predicted solubilities (mol kg^{-1})
1-Butanol	1.006	2.721	117.7	0.821
1-Pentanol	2.5×10^{-1}	3.039	137.8	2.09×10^{-1}
1-Hexanol	6.1×10^{-2}	3.357	157	5.32×10^{-2}
1-Heptanol	1.55×10^{-2}	3.675	176.3	1.36×10^{-2}
Cyclohexanol	3.83×10^{-1}	2.905	161	4.3×10^{-1}
1-Nonanol	1×10^{-3}	4.312	213.1	0.88×10^{-3}

[a] Reproduced from reference 1.

Table 4.2 Solubilities of pentanol isomers in water[a]

Compound	Solubility (molality, m)	Surface area (nm^2)	Boiling point (°C)	Structure
1-Pentanol	2.6×10^{-1}	3.039	137.8	
3-Methyl-1-butanol	3.11×10^{-1}	2.914	131.2	
2-Methyl-1-butanol	3.47×10^{-1}	2.894	128.7	
2-Pentanol	5.3×10^{-1}	2.959	119.0	
3-Pentanol	6.15×10^{-1}	2.935	115.3	
3-Methyl-2-butanol	6.67×10^{-1}	2.843	111.5	
2-Methyl-2-butanol	1.403	2.825	102.0	

[a] Reproduced from reference 1.

As boiling points of liquids and melting points of solids are indicators of molecular cohesion, these can be useful indicators of trends in a series of similar compounds. There are other empirical correlations that are useful. Melting points, even of compounds that form nonideal solutions, can be used as a guide to the order of solubility in a closely related series of compounds, as can be seen in the properties of sulfonamide derivatives listed in Table 4.3. Such correlations depend on the relatively greater importance of w_{22} in the solution process in these compounds.

Substituents

The influence of substituents on the solubility of molecules in water can be due to their effect on the properties of the solid or liquid (for example, on its molecular cohesion) or to the effect of the substituent on its interaction with water molecules. It is not easy to predict what effect a particular substituent will have on crystal properties, but as a guide to the solvent interactions, substituents can be classified as either hydrophobic or hydrophilic, depending on their polarity (see Table 4.4). The position of the substituent on the molecule can influence its effect, however. This can be seen in the aqueous solubilities of o-, m- and p-dihydroxybenzenes; as expected, all are much greater than that of benzene, but they are not the same, being 4, 9 and 0.6 mol dm^{-3}, respectively. The relatively low solubility of the *para* compound is due to its greater stability. The melting points of the derivatives indicate that is so, as they are 105°C, 111°C and 170°C, respectively. In the case of the *ortho* derivative, the possibility of intramolecular hydrogen bonding in aqueous solution, decreasing the ability of the OH group to interact with water, may explain why its solubility is lower than that of its *meta* analogue.

One can best illustrate the use of the information in Table 4.4 by considering the solubility of a series of substituted acetanilides, data for which are provided in Table 4.5. The strong hydrophilic characteristics of polar groups capable of hydrogen bonding with water molecules are evident. The presence of hydroxyl groups can therefore markedly change the solubility characteristics of a compound; phenol, for example, is 100 times more soluble in water than is benzene. In the case of phenol, where there is considerable hydrogen-bonding capability, the solute–solvent interaction (w_{12}) outweighs other factors (such as w_{22} or w_{11}) in the solution process. But, as we have discovered, the position of any substituent on the parent molecule will affect its contribution to solubility.

Table 4.3 Correlation between melting points of sulfonamide derivatives and aqueous solubility

Compound	Melting point (°C)	Solubility
Sulfadiazine	253	1 g in 13 dm^3 (0.077 g dm^{-3})
Sulfamerazine	236	1 g in 5 dm^3 (0.20 g dm^{-3})
Sulfapyridine	192	1 g in 3.5 dm^3 (0.29 g dm^{-3})
Sulfathiazole	174	1 g in 1.7 dm^3 (0.59 g dm^{-3})

Table 4.4 Substituent group classification

Substituent	Classification
$-CH_3$	Hydrophobic
$-CH_2-$	Hydrophobic
$-Cl, -Br, -F$	Hydrophobic
$-N(CH_3)_2$	Hydrophobic
$-SCH_3$	Hydrophobic
$-OCH_2CH_3$	Hydrophobic
$-OCH_3$	Slightly hydrophilic
$-NO_2$	Slightly hydrophilic
$-CHO$	Hydrophilic
$-COOH$	Slightly hydrophilic
$-COO^-$	Very hydrophilic
$-NH_2$	Hydrophilic
$-NH_3^+$	Very hydrophilic
$-OH$	Very hydrophilic

Steroid solubility

The steroids as a group tend to be poorly soluble in water. Their complex structure makes prediction of

Table 4.5 The effect of substituents on solubility of acetanilide derivatives in water

Derivative	X	Solubility (mg dm^{-3})
NHCOCH$_3$ structure with X	H	6.38
	Methyl	1.05
	Ethoxyl	0.93
	Hydroxyl	13.9
	Nitro	15.98
	Aceto	9.87

solubility somewhat difficult, but one can generally rationalise, *post hoc*, the solubility values of related steroids. Table 4.6 gives solubility data for 14 steroids. As examples, the substitution of an ethinyl group has conferred increased solubility on the estradiol molecule, as would be expected. Estradiol benzoate with its

3-OH substituent is much less soluble than the parent estradiol because of the loss of the hydroxyl and its substitution with a hydrophobic group. The same relationships are seen in testosterone and testosterone propionate. As both estradiol benzoate and testosterone propionate are oil soluble, they are used as solutions in castor oil and sesame oil for intramuscular and subcutaneous injection (see Chapter 10).

Methyltestosterone might be expected to be less soluble in water than is testosterone, but in fact it is not; this demonstrates again the importance of crystal properties in determining solubility. The methyl compound is more soluble because of the smaller heat of fusion of this derivative, hence the solid state more readily 'disintegrates' in the solvent.

Dexamethasone and betamethasone are isomeric fluorinated derivatives of methylprednisolone, but their solubilities are not identical, which might be a crystal property or a solution property. A simpler example of differences in isomeric solubility is that of the *o*-, *m*- and *p*-dihydroxybenzenes referred to above. A steric argument may be applied to the case of dexamethasone,

Table 4.6 The effect of substituents on solubility of acetanilide derivatives in water[a]

Structure	Compound	Solubility (μg cm^{-3})
(I)	Estradiol (I)	5
(II)	Ethinylestradiol (II)	10
(III)	Estradiol benzoate (III)	0.4

(continued overleaf)

Table 4.6 *(continued)*

Structure	Compound	Solubility ($\mu g\ cm^{-3}$)
(IV)	Testosterone (**IV**) Testosterone propionate	24 0.4
(V)	Methyltestosterone (**V**)	32
(VI)	Prednisolone (**VI**)	215
(VII)	Prednisone (**VII**) Prednisone acetate	115 23
(VIII)	Cortisone (**VIII**)	230

(continued overleaf)

Table 4.6 *(continued)*

Structure	Compound	Solubility ($\mu g\,cm^{-3}$)
(IX)	Dexamethasone (**IX**)	84
(X)	Betamethasone (**X**)	58
(XI)	Progesterone (**XI**)	9
(XII)	Hydrocortisone (**XII**)	285

[a] Reproduced from reference 6.

water molecules being less able to move close to the 17-OH group than in the case of betamethasone.

4.2.2 Hydration and solvation

The way in which solute molecules interact with the water molecules of the solvent is crucial to determining their affinity for the solvent. Ionic groups and electrolytes interact avidly with the polar water molecules, but nonelectrolytes also do not leave the structure of water unchanged, nor even do nonpolar groups and molecules such as the hydrocarbons.

Hydration of nonelectrolytes

Solvation is the general term used to describe the process of binding of solvent to solute molecules. If the solvent is water, the process is hydration. In a solution of sucrose (**XIII**), six water molecules are bound to each sucrose molecule with such avidity that the water and sucrose move as a unit in solution, and the extent of hydration can therefore be measured by hydrodynamic techniques.

Structure XIII Sucrose

Chemically very similar molecules such as mannitol (**XIV**), sorbitol (**XV**) and inositol have very different affinities for water. The solubility of sorbitol in water is about 3.5 times that of mannitol.

Structure XIV Mannitol

Structure XV Sorbitol

Most favourable hydration occurs when there is an equatorial –OH group on pyranose sugars.[7] This is thought to be due to the compatibility of the equatorial OH with the organised structure of water in bulk. Axial hydroxyl groups cannot bond onto the water 'lattice' without causing it to distort considerably. This may be one explanation of the difference, although differences in the lattice energies of the crystals may also contribute.

Hydration of ionic species: water structure breakers and structure makers

The study of ionic solvation is complicated but is relevant in pharmaceutics because of the effect ions have on the solubility of other species. The forces between cations and water molecules are so strong that the cations may retain a layer of water molecules in their crystals. The effect of ions on water structure is complex and variable. All ions in water possess a layer of tightly bound water – the water molecules being directionally orientated. Four water molecules are in the bound layer of most monovalent, monatomic ions. The firmly held layer can be regarded as being in a 'frozen' condition around a positive ion. The water molecules could be oriented with all the hydrogen atoms of the water molecules pointing outwards (see Fig. 4.2). Because of this and because their orientation depends on the ion size, they cannot all participate in the normal tetrahedral arrangements of bulk water (see section 5.3.1). For this to be feasible, two of the water molecules must be orientated with the hydrogens of the water molecules pointing in towards the ion. Inevitably, then, with cations and many small anions there tends to be a layer of water around the bound layer which is *less ordered* than bulk water (Fig. 4.2). Such ions, which include all the alkali and halide ions except Li^+ and F^-, are called *structure breakers*. The size of the ion is important, as the surface area of the ion determines the constraints on the polarised water molecules. Many polyvalent ions, for example Al^{3+}, increase the structured nature of water beyond the immediate hydration layer, and are therefore *structure makers*.

Hydration numbers

Hydration numbers (the number of water molecules in the primary hydration layer) can be determined by various physical techniques (for example, compressibility) and the values obtained tend to differ depending on the method used. The overall total action of the ion on water may be replaced conceptually by a strong binding between the ion and some effective number (solvation number) of solvent molecules; this effective number may well be almost zero in the case of large ions such as iodide, caesium and tetraalkylammonium ions. The solvation numbers decrease with increase of ionic radius because the ionic force field diminishes with increasing radius, and consequently water molecules are less inclined to be abstracted from their position in bulk water.

Hydrophobic hydration

Water is associated in a dynamic manner with nonpolar groups, but only in rare cases (where crystalline

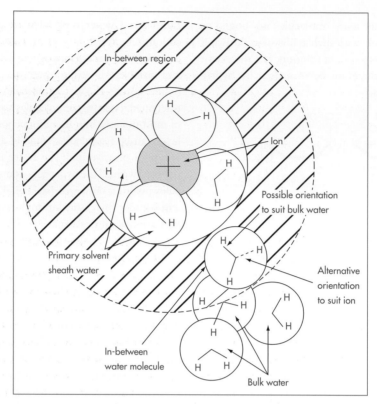

Figure 4.2 Schematic diagram to indicate that, in the (hatched) region between the primary solvated ion and bulk water, the orientation of the 'in-between' water molecules must be a compromise between that which suits the ion (oxygen-facing ion) and that which suits the bulk water (hydrogen-facing ion).

Reproduced with permission from Bockris JO'M, Reddy AKN, *Modern Electrochemistry*, Vol. 1, London: MacDonald, 1970.

clathrates can be formed) is this water able to be isolated along with the hydrophobic groups. The phrase 'hydrophobic hydration' is used to describe this layer of water. The motion of water molecules is slowed down in the vicinity of nonpolar groups. Hydrophobic groups induce structure formation in water, hence the negative entropy $(-\Delta S)$ of their dissolution in water and the positive entropy $(+\Delta S)$ gained on their removal. In the discussion of hydrophobic bonding (section 5.3.1) and nonpolar interactions, this special relationship between water and hydrocarbon chains is elaborated.

The solubility of inorganic materials in water

While a minority of therapeutic agents are inorganic electrolytes, it is nevertheless pertinent to consider the manner of their interaction with water. Electrolytes are, of necessity, components of replacement fluids, injections and eye drops and many other formulations. An increasing number of metal-containing compounds

are used in diagnosis and therapy, some of which have interesting solution behaviour.

First consider the simpler salts. What determines the solubility of a salt such as sodium chloride and its solubility in relation to, say, silver chloride? The solubility of NaCl is in excess of $5 \, \text{mol dm}^{-3}$ while the solubility of AgCl is 500 000 times less. The heats of solution $(\Delta H_{\text{solution}})$ are $62.8 \, \text{kJ mol}^{-1}$ for silver chloride and $4.2 \, \text{kJ mol}^{-1}$ for sodium chloride, suggesting a substantial difference either in the crystal properties or in the interaction of the ions with water. In fact the very great strength of the silver chloride crystal is due to the high polarisability of the silver ion. The heat of solution of an ionic solute can be written as

$$\Delta H_{\text{solution}} = \Delta H_{\text{sublimation}} - \Delta H_{\text{hydration}} \quad (4.2)$$

Conceptually, the solid salt (sodium chloride, for instance) is converted to the gaseous (g) state, $Na^+(g) + Cl^-(g)$, and each unit is then hydrated to form the species $Na^+(aq)$ and $Cl^-(aq)$. If the heat of hydration is sufficient to provide the energy needed to overcome the lattice forces, the salt will be freely soluble at a given temperature and the ions will readily dislodge from the crystal lattice. If the partial molal enthalpy of solution of the substance is positive, the solubility will increase with increasing temperature; if it is negative the solubility will decrease, in agreement with Le Chatelier's principle.

4.2.3 The effect of simple additives on solubility

Solubility products

For poorly soluble materials such as silver chloride and barium sulfate the concept of the solubility product can be used. The following equilibrium exists in solution between crystalline silver chloride $AgCl_c$ and ions in solution:

$$AgCl_c \rightleftharpoons Ag^+ + Cl^- \qquad (4.3)$$

An equilibrium constant K can be defined as

$$K = \frac{[Ag^+][Cl^-]}{[AgCl_c]} \qquad (4.4)$$

Strictly, K should be written in terms of thermodynamic activities and not concentrations, but activities can be replaced by concentrations (denoted by square brackets) because of the low solubilities involved (see section 2.3.1). At saturation the concentration of the crystalline silver chloride $[AgCl_c]$ is essentially constant and the solubility product, K_{sp}, may therefore be written

$$K_{sp} = [Ag^+][Cl^-] \qquad (4.5)$$

The sparingly soluble compound silver chloride is an example of a 1:1 salt, i.e. each molecule ionises to give one ion of Ag^+ and one of Cl^-. When a compound has more than one ion of each type, for example the poorly soluble salt calcium hydroxide $Ca(OH)_2$, then the solubility product is defined as the product of each ion raised to the appropriate power. Calcium hydroxide ionises to give one ion of Ca^{2+} and two OH^- ions and the solubility product becomes

$$K_{sp} = [Ca^{2+}][OH^-]^2$$

Some values of solubility products are quoted in Table 4.7.

Common ion effect

The solubility product is useful for evaluating the influence of other species on the solubility of salts of low aqueous solubility. One of the most important influences on the solubility of poorly soluble salts occurs on addition of another compound that has an identical ion to one of those of the salt. For example, if sodium chloride is added to a saturated solution of silver chloride, the concentration of Cl^- ions in solution will be increased as therefore will the product $[Ag^+][Cl^-]$. Consequently, to maintain K_{sp} constant the concentration of Ag^+ in solution will decrease, i.e. solid AgCl will be precipitated. This effect whereby the solubility of a sparingly soluble salt is decreased by the addition of another compound having an ion in common is referred to as the *common ion effect*. Several examples of the influence of the common ion effect on drug solubilities *in vivo* are discussed in section 4.7.2.

Salting in and salting out

In general, additives may either increase or decrease the solubility of a solute in a given solvent. The effect that they have will depend on several factors:

- The effect the additive has on the structure of water
- The interaction of the additive with the solute
- The interaction of the additive with the solvent

The effect of a solute additive on the solubility of another solute may be quantified by the Setschenow equation:

$$\log \frac{S}{S_a} = kc_a \qquad (4.6)$$

where S_a is the solubility in the presence of an additive, S is the solubility in its absence, c_a is the concentration of additive, and k is the salting coefficient. The sign of k is positive when the activity coefficient is increased; it is negative if the activity coefficient is decreased by

Table 4.7 Solubility products of some inorganic salts	
Compound	K_{sp} **(mol^2 dm^{-6})**
AgCl	1.25×10^{-10}
Al(OH)$_3$	7.7×10^{-13}
BaSO$_4$	1.0×10^{-10}

the additive. The Setschenow equation frequently holds up to additive concentrations of $1 \, \mathrm{mol \, dm^{-3}}$, a measure of the sensitivity of the activity coefficient of the solute towards the salt.

Salts that increase solubility are said to *salt in* the solute and those that decrease solubility *salt out* the solute. Salting out may result from the removal of water molecules that can act as solvent because of competing hydration of the added ion. The opposite effect, salting in, can occur when salts with large anions or cations that are themselves very soluble in water are added to the solutions of nonelectrolytes. Sodium benzoate and sodium *p*-toluenesulfonate are good examples of such agents and are referred to as *hydrotropic salts*; the increase in the solubility of other solutes is known as *hydrotropy*. Values of k (in $(\mathrm{mol \, dm^{-3}})^{-1}$) for three salts added to benzoic acid in aqueous solution are 0.17 for NaCl; 0.14 for KCl; and -0.22 for sodium benzoate. That is, NaCl and KCl decrease the solubility of benzoic acid, and sodium benzoate increases it.

4.2.4 The effect of pH on the solubility of ionisable drugs

pH is one of the primary influences on the solubility of most drugs that contain ionisable groups. As the great majority of drugs are organic electrolytes, there are four parameters that determine their solubility:

- Their degree of ionisation
- Their molecular size
- Interactions of substituent groups with solvent
- Their crystal properties

In this section consideration is given to the solubility of weak electrolytes and the influence of pH on aqueous solubility, important in both formulation and dissolution of drugs *in vivo*, and ultimately and importantly their biological activity.

Acidic drugs

Acidic drugs such as the nonsteroidal anti-inflammatory agents, are less soluble in acidic solutions than in alkaline solutions because the predominant undissociated species cannot interact with water molecules to the same extent as the ionised form, which is readily hydrated. Equation (4.11), which is a form of the

Henderson–Hasselbalch equation relating drug solubility to the pH of the solution and to the pK_a of the drug, is derived in Box 4.1

$$pH - pK_a = \log\left(\frac{S - S_0}{S_0}\right)$$

where S is the total saturation solubility of the drug and S_0 is the solubility of the undissociated species.

Box 4.1 Derivation of an equation for the solubility of an acidic drug as a function of pH

If we represent the drug as HA and the total saturation solubility of the drug as S, and if S_0 is the solubility of the undissociated drug, it is clear that the total solubility is the sum of the solubility of the un-ionised and ionised species, that is

$$S = S_0 + (\text{concentration of ionised species})$$

The dissociation of the acid in water can be written

$$HA + H_2O \rightleftharpoons H_3O^+ + A^- \qquad (4.7)$$

and the dissociation constant K_a is given by

$$K_a = \frac{[H_3O^+][A^-]}{[HA]} \qquad (4.8)$$

Rearranging and substituting S_0 for [HA] gives

$$\frac{K_a}{[H_3O^+]} = \frac{[A^-]}{S_0} \qquad (4.9)$$

but as $[A^-] = S - S_0$,

$$\frac{K_a}{[H_3O^+]} = \frac{S - S_0}{S_0} \qquad (4.10)$$

Taking logarithms,

$$pH - pK_a = \log\left(\frac{S - S_0}{S_0}\right) \qquad (4.11)$$

Hence the solubility of the drug at any pH can be calculated provided pK_a and S_0 are known.

Examples of the use of equation (4.11) to calculate the effect of pH on the solubility of acidic drugs are given below.

Example 4.1 Calculation of the effect of pH on the solubility of an acidic drug

What is the pH below which sulfadiazine ($pK_a = 6.48$) will begin to precipitate in an infusion fluid, when the initial molar concentration of sulfadiazine sodium is $4 \times 10^{-2}\,\mathrm{mol\,dm^{-3}}$ and the solubility of sulfadiazine is $3.07 \times 10^{-4}\,\mathrm{mol\,dm^{-3}}$?

Answer

The pH below which the drug will precipitate is calculated using equation (4.11):

$$pH = 6.48 + \log\frac{(4.00 \times 10^{-2}) - (3.07 \times 10^{-4})}{3.07 \times 10^{-4}}$$
$$= 8.60$$

Example 4.2 Calculation of the effect of pH on the solubility of an acidic drug

What is the solubility of benzylpenicillin G at a pH sufficiently low to allow only the nondissociated form of the drug to be present?

The pK_a of benzylpenicillin G is 2.76 and the solubility of the drug at pH 8.0 is 0.174 mol dm^{-3}. (From Notari RE, *Biopharmaceutics and Pharmacokinetics*, 2nd edn, New York: Marcel Dekker, 1978.)

Answer

If only the undissociated form is present at low pH then we need to find S_0. This can be obtained from the information given using equation (4.11):

$$pH - pK_a = \log\left(\frac{S - S_0}{S_0}\right)$$

Therefore,

$$8.0 - 2.76 = \log\left(\frac{0.174 - S_0}{S_0}\right)$$

i.e.,

$$5.24 = \log\left(\frac{0.174 - S_0}{S_0}\right)$$

Therefore, $S_0 = 1 \times 10^{-6}\,\mathrm{mol\,dm^{-3}}$.

Basic drugs

Basic drugs such as ranitidine are more soluble in acidic solutions, where the ionised form of the drug is predominant. If S_0 is the solubility of an undissociated base, RNH_2, the Henderson–Hasselbalch expression for the solubility (S) as a function of pH (see derivation in Box 4.2) is

$$pH - pK_a = \log\left(\frac{S_0}{S - S_0}\right)$$

Solubility–pH profiles of a basic drug (chlorpromazine) and an acidic drug (indometacin) and values for the more complex profile of the amphoteric drug oxytetracycline are plotted in Fig. 4.3.

In general, this approach is valid in dilute ideal solutions for which the solubility of the ionised species is much greater than that of the uncharged species. Despite its widespread use to predict the pH dependence of drug solubility, a study of the accuracy of equation (4.15) in predicting the solubility of a series of cationic drugs as a function of pH in divalent buffer systems mimicking the intestinal fluid highlighted some limitations of this equation and the authors cautioned against its uncritical use.[8]

Box 4.2 Derivation of equations for solubility of basic drugs as a function of pH

The dissociation of the base in water can be written:

$$RNH_2 + H_2O \rightleftharpoons RNH_3^+ + OH^- \qquad (4.12)$$

Therefore,

$$K_b = \frac{[RNH_3^+][OH^-]}{[RNH_2]} \qquad (4.13)$$

That is

$$\frac{K_b}{[OH^-]} = \frac{[H^+]}{K_a} = \frac{S - S_0}{S_0} \qquad (4.14)$$

Taking logarithms,

$$pK_a - pH = \log\left(\frac{S - S_0}{S_0}\right) \qquad (4.15)$$

or

$$pH - pK_a = \log\left(\frac{S_0}{S - S_0}\right) \qquad (4.16)$$

Figure 4.3 Solubility of (a) indometacin, (b) chlorpromazine and (c) oxytetracycline as a function of pH, plotted as logarithm of the solubility.

Example 4.3 Calculation of the effect of pH on the solubility of a basic drug

A drug is found to have the following saturation solubilities at room temperature:

pH	S (μmol dm^{-3})
7.4	205.0
9.0	10.0
10.0	5.5
12.0	5.0

What type of compound is it likely to be and what is its pK_a?

Answer

As the solubility decreases with increasing pH, the compound is a base. At pH 12 the solubility quoted is likely to be the solubility of the unprotonated species, that is, S_0. Using the figures given, we can apply equation (4.15) at each of the other pH values:

$$pK_a = pH + \log\left(\frac{S - S_0}{S_0}\right)$$

$$= 7.4 + \log\frac{200}{5}$$

$$= 7.4 + \log 40 = 7.4 + 1.602 = 9.0$$

$$pK_a = 9.0 + \log\frac{10 - 5}{5} = 9.0 + \log 1 = 9.0$$

$$pK_a = 10.0 + \log\frac{5.5 - 5}{5} = 10.0 + \log 0.1 = 9.0$$

The drug has a pK_a value of 9.0 and is thus likely to be an amine.

Amphoteric drugs

Several drugs and amino acids, peptides and proteins are amphoteric, displaying both basic and acidic characteristics. Frequently encountered drugs in this category are the sulfonamides and the tetracyclines. If, for simplicity, we were to use a generalised structure for an amphoteric compound

$$R - X - COOH$$
$$|$$
$$NH_2$$

and if the solution equilibrium between the species were written down, we would obtain the following equations relating solubility to pH (see Box 4.3).

$$pH - pK_a = \log\left(\frac{S_0}{S - S_0}\right)$$

at pH values below the isoelectric point, and

$$pH - pK_a = \log\left(\frac{S - S_0}{S_0}\right)$$

at pH values above the isoelectric point.

Table 4.8 gives solubility data for oxytetracycline (**XVI**) as a function of pH. Oxytetracycline has three pK_a values: $pK_{a1} = 3.27$, $pK_{a2} = 7.32$, and $pK_{a3} = 9.11$, corresponding to the regions 1, 2 and 3 in the structure shown.

Structure XVI Oxytetracycline

The equations for the solubilities of acidic, basic and zwitterionic drugs (equations 4.11, 4.16, 4.23 and 4.24) can all be used to calculate the pH at which a drug will precipitate from solution of a given concentration (or the concentration at which a drug will reach its maximum solubility at a given pH). This is especially important in determining the maximum allowable levels of a drug in infusion fluids or formulations. Some idea of the range of pH values encountered in common infusion fluids is given in Table 4.9. The variation in pH between preparations and within batches of the same infusion fluid (the monograph for Dextrose Infusion BP allows a pH ranging from 3.5 to 5.5) means that the fluids vary considerably in their solvent capacity for weak electrolytes.

Box 4.3 Derivation of equations for solubility of amphoteric drugs as a function of pH

The equilibria between the species can be written as

More simply,

The two dissociation constants can be defined in the normal way as

$$K_{a_1} = \frac{[HA^\pm][H^+]}{[HAH^+]} \tag{4.17}$$

and

$$K_{a_2} = \frac{[A^-][H^+]}{[HA^\pm]} \tag{4.18}$$

That is

$$\frac{K_{a_1}}{[H^+]} = \frac{[HA^\pm]}{[HAH^+]} \tag{4.19}$$

and (4.20)

$$\frac{K_{a_2}}{[H^+]} = \frac{[A^-]}{[HA^\pm]} \tag{4.20}$$

It is observed that the zwitterion has the lowest solubility (see Fig. 4.3 and Table 4.8), which we take to be S_0.

$$\frac{K_{a_1}}{[H^+]} = \frac{S_0}{S - S_0} \tag{4.21}$$

and

$$\frac{K_{a_2}}{[H^+]} = \frac{S - S_0}{S_0} \tag{4.22}$$

Therefore,

$$pH - pK_a = \log\left(\frac{S_0}{S - S_0}\right) \tag{4.23}$$

at pH values below the isoelectric point, and

$$pH - pK_a = \log\left(\frac{S - S_0}{S_0}\right) \tag{4.24}$$

at pH values above the isoelectric point.

Table 4.8 Oxytetracycline: pH dependence of solubility at 20°C[a]

pH	Solubility (g dm^{-3})
1.2	31.4
2	4.6
3	1.4
4	0.85
5	0.5
6	0.7
7	1.1
8	28.0
9	38.6

[a] Data from the *United States Dispensatory*, 25th edn.

Table 4.9 pH of some parenteral solutions[a]

Solution	pH
5% Dextrose in water (5% D/W)	4.40, 4.70
5% D/W (1 dm^3 containing 2 cm^3 of vitamins)	4.30, 4.38
5% D/W (1 dm^3 containing 100 mg thiamine hydrochloride)	3.90, 3.96
5% D/W (1 dm^3 containing 300 mg thiamine hydrochloride)	3.82, 4.00
5% D/W (1 dm^3 containing 2 cm^3 of vitamins, 200 mg thiamine hydrochloride)	4.15
5% D/W (1 dm^3 containing 4 cm^3 of vitamins, 300 mg thiamine hydrochloride)	4.28
Normal saline	5.35, 5.40
Lactated Ringer's solution (Ringer)	7.01
Ringer (1 dm^3 containing 2 cm^3 of vitamins)	5.50
Ringer (1 dm^3 containing 2 cm^3 of vitamins, 100 mg thiamine hydrochloride)	5.38
Ringer (1 dm^3 containing 2 cm^3 of vitamins, 200 mg thiamine hydrochloride)	5.16

[a] Reproduced from Tse RL, Lee MW, *J Am Med Assoc*, 1971; 215: 642.

Not only is it important to consider the pH of the formulation when deciding on the concentration of drug that can be incorporated, it is equally important to bear in mind possible changes in pH that might occur following administration of the formulation as these might be responsible for drug precipitation from formulations in which the drug concentration is close to the solubility limit. Several examples of the precipitation of drugs *in vivo* resulting from alteration of pH are considered in Chapter 11 and we will consider here only one example,

that of precipitation from eye drop formulations containing amphoteric fluoroquinolone drugs.

Rule of thumb

From equations (4.11), (4.16), (4.23) and (4.24) it is seen that, as a rough guide, the solubility of drugs with un-ionised species of low solubility varies by a factor of 10 for each pH unit change. A compilation of the dissociation constants of drugs is given in Chapter 2 (Table 2.6).

 Clinical point

Eye drops containing norfloxacin (Chibroxin), ciprofloxacin (Ciloxan) and ofloxacin (Ocuflox) are used for the treatment of external ocular infection and corneal ulcer. Although these products are all formulated as sterile, isotonic, aqueous solutions, preserved with benzalkonium chloride and all contain 0.3% of the respective fluoroquinolone drug, there have been observations of crystallised corneal deposits only following the clinical use of Ciloxan. The reason for the precipitation of this drug is seen from a consideration of differences in the pH of the formulations (Chibroxin 5.2, Ciloxan 4.5 and Ocuflox 6.4) and also the solubilities of the three fluoroquinolones. As we have seen above, solubility of this class of drug generally exhibits a minimum near physiological pH corresponding to the zwitterionic form of the drug; ciprofloxacin is the least soluble of the commercially available fluoroquinolones, with particularly low solubility near the pH of tears. Figure 4.4 shows the solubility–pH plots for the three drugs up to pH 7.5 (the solubility would, of course, increase at higher pH values as the compounds are amphoteric) and provides an explanation for the precipitation of ciprofloxacin. The pH of the tear film immediately following instillation of the eyedrops is determined by the pH of the formulation but returns to the physiological value (pH 6.8) within 15 minutes due to tear turnover and drainage.

Superimposed on the solubility profile of each drug in Fig. 4.4 are the total drug concentration and the concentration of drug dissolved in the tear fluid. The decrease of total drug concentration with time is a result of tear turnover and drainage. Following dosing of ofloxacin and norfloxacin (Fig. 4.4a,b), the soluble drug concentration is identical to the total drug concentration at all time points and the tear solution remains clear and particulate-free. Following ciprofloxacin dosing (Fig. 4.4c), however, the soluble drug concentration falls significantly below the total drug concentration at approximately 8 minutes after drug addition (tear pH 6.1). At this pH the drug concentration exceeds the solubility limit, a supersaturated solution is formed and precipitation of ciprofloxacin occurs, producing a milky white tear solution. At approximately 12 minutes post dose (tear pH 6.6), the soluble ciprofloxacin concentration is reduced to almost half (54%) of the total drug concentration due to continued precipitation.

Figure 4.4 Relationship between drug concentration in a tear turnover model (solid lines) and drug solubility (dashed lines) for (a), ofloxacin (Ocuflox) (b), norfloxacin (Chibroxin) and (c), ciprofloxacin (Ciloxan).

Reproduced with permission from Firestone BA *et al., Int J Pharm*, 1998; 164: 119.

Example 4.4 Calculation of the solubility of an amphoteric drug

Tryptophan has two pK_a values: 2.4 and 9.4, and an isoelectric point of 5.9. Calculate the solubility of tryptophan at pH 2 and at pH 10, given that the solubility of the compound in neutral solutions, S_0, is $2 \times 10^{-2}\,mol\,dm^{-3}$.

Answer

At pH 2.0: This pH is below the isoelectric point so we must use equation (4.23):

$$pH - pK_a = \log\left(\frac{S_0}{S - S_0}\right)$$

$$2 - 2.4 = \log\left(\frac{2 \times 10^{-2}}{S - (2 \times 10^{-2})}\right)$$

Rearranging,

$$\log\left(\frac{S - (2 \times 10^{-2})}{2 \times 10^{-2}}\right) = 0.4$$

That is,

$$\frac{S - (2 \times 10^{-2})}{2 \times 10^{-2}} = 2.5118$$

Therefore, $S = (5.02 \times 10^{-2}) + (2 \times 10^{-2}) = 7.02 \times 10^{-2}\,mol\,dm^{-3}$.

At pH 10 (using equation 4.24):

$$10 - 9.4 = \log\left(\frac{S - (2 \times 10^{-2})}{2 \times 10^{-2}}\right)$$

That is,

$$\frac{S - (2 \times 10^{-2})}{2 \times 10^{-2}} = 3.981$$

Therefore, $S = (7.96 \times 10^{-2}) + (2 \times 10^{-2}) = 9.96 \times 10^{-2}\,mol\,dm^{-3}$.

Example 4.5 Calculation of the effect of pH on solubility

Calculate the pH at which the following drugs will precipitate from solution given the information supplied.

Drug	pK_a	Solubility of un-ionised species	Concentration of solution
(a) Thioridazine HCl (mol wt 407 Da)	9.5	1.5×10^{-6} mol dm^{-3}	0.407% w/v
(b) Oxytetracycline HCl	3.3, 7.3 and 9.1	0.5 g dm^{-3}	1.4 mg cm^{-3}

Answer

(a) We use equation (4.15) or (4.16) to calculate the pH above which thioridazine will precipitate:

$$pH = pK_a + \log\left(\frac{S_0}{S - S_0}\right)$$

The concentration of solution is the saturation solubility at the point of precipitation. 0.407% w/v = 1×10^{-2} mol dm^{-3} = S. $S_0 = 1.5 \times 10^{-6}$ mol dm^{-3}.

$$pH = 9.5 + \log\left(\frac{1.5 \times 10^{-6}}{(1 \times 10^{-2}) - (1.5 \times 10^{-6})}\right)$$

$$= 9.5 + \log\left(\frac{1.5 \times 10^{-6}}{1.0 \times 10^{-2}}\right)$$

$$= 9.5 - 3.284$$

$$= 5.68$$

(b) The concentration of solution is 1.4 mg cm^{-3}, which is 1.4 g dm^{-3}. $S_0 = 0.5$ g dm^{-3}. At pH values below 7, the pH at which S is the maximum solubility is given by

$$pH = pK_a + \log\left(\frac{S_0}{S - S_0}\right)$$

$$= 3.3 + \log(0.556)$$

$$= 3.3 - 0.255$$

$$= 3.05$$

At pH values above 7, the pH at which S is the maximum value is given by

$$pH = pK_a + \log\left(\frac{S - S_0}{S_0}\right)$$

$$= 7.3 + \log(1.8)$$

$$= 7.3 + 0.255$$

$$= 7.56$$

Thus at pH values between 3.05 and 7.56 the solution containing 1.4 mg cm^{-3} will precipitate.

4.3 Measurement of solubility

In the traditional method of determining drug solubility, often referred to as the 'shake flask' method, the drug is added to a standard buffer solution until saturation occurs, indicated by undissolved excess drug. The pH is remeasured and, if necessary, readjusted with dilute acid or alkali. The flasks are then shaken for a minimum of 24 hours and the amount of dissolved drug is determined by a suitable assay of the supernatant solution after filtration. This method is, however, manually intensive and time-consuming, and several alternative procedures have been proposed.

A simple turbidimetric method for the determination of the solubility of acids and bases in buffers of different pH can be used.[9] Solutions of the hydrochloride (or other salt) of a basic drug, or the soluble salt of an acidic compound, are prepared in water over a range of concentrations. Portions of each solution are added to buffers of known pH and the turbidity of the solutions is determined in the visible region. Typical results are shown in Fig. 4.5. Below the solubility limit there is no turbidity. As the solubility limit is progressively exceeded, the turbidity rises. The solubility can be determined by extrapolation as shown in Fig. 4.5. Table 4.10 shows results obtained by this method for some phenothiazines and tricyclic antidepressant compounds. Determination of the solubility of weak electrolytes at several pH values provides one method of obtaining the dissociation constant of the drug substance. For basic drugs, equation (4.16) is rearranged to give

$$pH = pK_a + \log\left(\frac{S_0}{S - S_0}\right)$$

S_0, the solubility of the undissociated species (base), is determined at high pH, and S is determined at several different lower pH values. A plot of $\log[S_0/(S - S_0)]$ versus pH will have the pK_a as the intercept on the pH axis.

Alternatively, S may be plotted against [H$^+$] as in Fig. 4.5b. Equation (4.14) can be written in the form

$$[H^+] = \left(\frac{K_a S}{S_0}\right) - K_a \tag{4.25}$$

Plotting data as in Fig. 4.5b yields S_0 when the line crosses the x-axis as [H$^+$] = 0 (and $S = S_0$). The intercept

Figure 4.5 (a) Plot of extinction against concentration of amitriptyline hydrochloride at pH 9.78 (O) and pH 9.20 (●). (b) Relationship between hydrogen ion concentration and solubility of pecazine (●) and amitriptyline (O).

Reproduced from reference 9.

Table 4.10 Water solubilities and pK_a values of aminoalkylphenothiazines and related compounds[a]

Structure	Trivial or approved name	pK_a, solubility method	pK_a, Chatten–Harris[b]	Solubility ($\mu mol\ dm^{-3}$)	Calculated relative solubility at pH 7.4
R=H; R'=CH$_2$CH(Me)·NMe$_2$	Promethazine	9.1	9.1	55	4.5
R=H; R'=[CH$_2$]$_3$·NMe$_2$	Promazine	9.4	–	50	8.0
R=Cl; R'=[CH$_2$]$_3$·NMe$_2$	Chlorpromazine	9.3	9.2	8	1.0
R=CF$_3$; R'=[CH$_2$]$_3$·NMe$_2$	Triflupromazine	9.2	9.4	5	0.4
R = H; R'= CH$_2$— (piperidine, N–Me)	Pecazine	9.7	–	18	5.0
R = SMe; R'= [CH$_2$]$_2$— (piperidine, N–Me)	Thioridazine	9.5	9.2	1.5	0.3

[a] Reproduced from reference 9.

[b] Data from Chatten LG, Harris LE, *Anal Chem*, 1962; 34: 1495.

on the y-axis gives $-K_a$ and the slope of the line is K_a/S_0.

4.4 The solubility parameter

Regular solution theory characterises nonpolar solvents in terms of solubility parameter, δ_1, which is defined as

$$\delta_1 = \left(\frac{\Delta U}{V}\right)^{1/2} = \left(\frac{\Delta H - RT}{V}\right)^{1/2} \qquad (4.26)$$

where ΔU is the molar energy and ΔH is the molar heat of vaporisation of the solvent. ΔH is determined by calorimetry at temperatures below the boiling point at constant volume. V is the molar volume of the solvent. The solubility parameter is thus a measure of the intermolecular forces within the solvent and gives us information on the ability of the liquid to act as a solvent. Table 4.11 gives the solubility parameters of some common solvents calculated using equation (4.26).

$\Delta U/V$ is the liquid's *cohesive energy density*, a measure of the attraction of a molecule from its own liquid, which is the energy required to remove it from the liquid and is equal to the energy of vaporisation per unit volume. Because cavities have to be formed in a solvent, by separating other solvent molecules, to accommodate solute molecules (as discussed earlier) the solubility parameter δ_1 enables predictions of solubility to be made in a semiquantitative manner, especially in relation to the solubility parameter of the solute, δ_2.

By itself the solubility parameter can explain the behaviour of only a relatively small group of solvents – those with little or no polarity and those unable to participate in hydrogen-bonding interactions. The difference between the solubility parameters expressed as $(\delta_1 - \delta_2)$ will give an indication of solubility relationships.

For solid solutes a hypothetical value of δ_2 can be calculated from $(U/V)^{1/2}$, where U is in this case the lattice energy of the crystal. In a study of the solubility of ion pairs in organic solvents it has been found that the logarithm of the solubility ($\log S$) correlates well with $(\delta_1 - \delta_2)^2$.

Table 4.11 Solubility parameters of common solvents

Solvent	δ_1 (cal$^{1/2}$ cm$^{-3/2}$)*
Methanol	14.50
Ethanol	12.74
1-Propanol	11.94
2-Propanol	11.56
1-Butanol	11.40
1-Octanol	10.24
Ethyl acetate	8.58
Isoamyl acetate	8.07
Hexane	7.30
Hexadecane	8
Carbon disulfide	10
Membrane (erythrocytes)	10.3 ± 0.40
Cyclohexane	8.2
Benzene	9.2

* The solubility parameter is commonly expressed in hildebrand units: 1 hildebrand unit = 1 (cal cm^{-3})$^{1/2}$.
1 cal = 4.18 J.

4.4.1 Solubility parameters and biological processes

The solubility of small molecules in biological membranes is of importance from pharmacological, physiological and toxicological viewpoints. Biological membranes are not simple solvents – the bilayer has an interior core of hydrocarbon chains about 2.5–3.5 nm thick – and therefore one would not expect simple solution theory to hold. Regular solution theory has been applied to biomembranes to obtain a value of

δ_1 for a membrane.[10] From experimental solubility data for anaesthetic gases in erythrocyte ghosts, mean empirical solubility parameters of 10.3 ± 0.40 for the whole membrane and 8.7 ± 1.03 for membrane lipid were calculated. The values compare with solubility parameters of 7.3 for hexane and 8.0 for hexadecane. The value for the whole membrane (10.3) is very close to the solubility parameter of 1-octanol (10.2), a solvent that is used widely in partition coefficient work to simulate biological lipid phases.

Solubility parameters of drugs (δ_2) have also been correlated with membrane absorption rates in model systems. A reasonable relationship was obtained between δ_2 and a logarithmic absorption term, thus providing one predictive index of absorption. Scott[11] has said of solubility parameters and equations employing them that 'the theory offers a useful initial approach to a very wide area of solutions. Like a small-scale map for a very broad long-distance view of a sub-continent they are unlikely to prove highly accurate when a small area is examined carefully, but they are equally unlikely to prove completely absurd.'

4.5 Solubility in mixed solvents

The device of using mixed solvents (co-solvents) is resorted to when drug solubility in one solvent is limited or perhaps when the stability characteristics of soluble salts forbid the use of single solvents. Many pharmaceutical preparations are complex systems. Common water-miscible solvents used in pharmaceutical formulations include glycerol, propylene glycol, ethyl alcohol and polyoxyethylene glycols. As can be imagined, the addition of another component complicates any system and explanations of the often complex solubility patterns are not easy. Only relatively recently has there been any attempt to predict solubility in mixed solvents theoretically, although the solubility parameters of the mixed solvent systems have been used for this purpose for some time. Toxicity considerations are, of course, a constraint on the choice of solvent for products for administration by any route.

Figure 4.6 shows the solubility of phenobarbital in glycerol–water, ethanol–water and ethanol–glycerol mixtures. Phenobarbital dissolves up to 0.12% w/v

Figure 4.6 The solubility of phenobarbital in glycerol–water, ethanol–water and absolute ethanol–glycerol mixtures as a function of the percentage composition of the mixtures. Abscissa indicates percentage of: A, glycerol in water; B, ethanol in water; C, absolute ethanol in glycerol.

Reproduced from Krause GM, Cross JM, *J Am Pharm Assoc*, 1951; 40; 137.

in water at 25°C. Glycerol, even in high concentrations, does not significantly increase the solubility of the drug. Ethanol is a much more efficient co-solvent than glycerol as it is less polar. Solubility is at a maximum at 90% ethanol in ethanol–water mixtures, and at 80% ethanol in ethanol–glycerol mixtures. It is naive to assume that the drug dissolves in 'pockets' of the cosolvent (for example, ethanol in ethanol–water mixtures), although obviously the affinity of cosolvent for the solute is of importance.

Additives will influence solute–solvent interfacial energies or dissociation of electrolytes through changes in dielectric constant. A reduction in ionisation through a decrease in dielectric constant will favour decreased solubility, but this effect may be counterbalanced by the greater affinity of the undissociated species in the presence of the cosolvent.

Clinical point

A potential problem associated with the administration of mixed solvent formulations of poorly water-soluble drugs is drug precipitation when these preparations are added to an aqueous solution such as blood plasma. For example, precipitation of the relatively water-insoluble diazepam has been reported when formulations of this drug in a mixed solvent solution containing propylene glycol (40%) and alcohol (10%) are administered by injection using an intravenous infusion set, rather than directly into the vein of the patient as instructed by the supplier. Precipitation occurs because of changes in the proportions of the solvents on dilution with plasma in the infusion set; we discuss this problem in more detail in Chapter 11 (section 11.2).

Precipitation of a poorly water-soluble drug during IV injection may also be a consequence of a rapid infusion rate or abnormally slow venous flow rate, both of which result in unfavourable changes in solvent composition. The critical parameters that determine whether a drug will precipitate during IV injection are its solubility in plasma, the drug dose and the plasma flow rate in the vein. The maximum infusion rate ($mg\ min^{-1}$) is the product of the plasma solubility ($mg\ cm^{-3}$) and the venous flow rate (normally between 40 and 60 cm^3 min^{-1}). Example 4.6 shows the calculation of minimum injection times for a poorly water-soluble drug and illustrates the influence of the rate of venous flow on the time required to prevent precipitation of drug in the plasma. Note that in this calculation it is assumed that the injected solution mixes instantaneously with the plasma; in practice longer injection times should be used to ensure safety.

 Example 4.6 Calculation of minimum injection times for poorly water-soluble drugs

What is the minimum time required for the IV injection of a 20 mg dose of a poorly water-soluble drug (solubility in plasma = 0.60 mg cm^{-3}) to ensure that precipitation does not occur? Assume a venous flow rate of (a) 60 cm^3 min^{-1} and (b) 40 cm^3 min^{-1}

Answer

(a) Maximum infusion rate = plasma solubility × venous flow rate:

$$= 0.60 \times 60 = 36.0\ mg\ min^{-1}$$

Therefore, a 20 mg dose should be injected over a period of at least 33 seconds to avoid drug precipitation.

(b) Maximum infusion rate = $0.60 \times 40 = 24.0\ mg\ min^{-1}$.

Therefore, at least 50 seconds should be allowed for injection at this venous flow rate.

4.6 Cyclodextrins as solubilising agents

Solubilisation by surface-active agents is discussed in Chapter 5. Alternatives to micellar solubilisation (or solubilisation in vesicles) include the use of the cyclodextrin family. When the first edition of this book was published in 1981 (and a diagram of a cyclodextrin–drug complex was used to adorn the cover), the use of cyclodextrins was in its infancy. Attention was then focused around α-, β- and γ-cyclodextrins, but a veritable industry has grown up with an array of derivatives that can lend useful new properties to the complexes they form. There is now Encapsin HPB (hydroxypropyl-β-cyclodextrin), which is available commercially for pharmaceutical use. Ten per cent of this cyclodextrin can enhance the aqueous solubility of betamethasone 118 times, of diazepam 21 times and of ibuprofen 55 times.

Table 4.12 Properties of α, β and γ cyclodextrins[a]

Property	Alpha (α)	Beta (β)	Gamma (γ)
Molecular weight	973	1135	1297
Glucose monomers	6	7	8
Internal cavity diameters (nm)	0.5	0.6	0.8
Water solubility (g/100 cm³; 25°C)	14.2	1.85	23.2
Surface tension (mN m⁻¹)	71	71	71
Melting range (°C)	255–260	255–260	240–245
Water of crystallisation (no. of molecules)	10.2	13–15	8–18
Water in cavity (no. of molecules)	6	11	17

[a] Reproduced from Brewster ME *et al.*, *J Parenter Sci Technol*, 1989; 43: 262.

$n = 1$ α-CD	
$n = 2$ β-CD	
$n = 3$ γ-CD	

Cyclodextrin structure

Cavity volume:

0.174 nm³   0.262 nm³   0.427 nm³

α-CD   β-CD   γ-CD

In one mole:
104 cm³   157 cm³   256 cm³

In one gram:
0.10 cm³   0.14 cm³   0.20 cm³

Figure 4.7 Structures of the α-, β- and γ-cyclodextrins.
Reproduced from Szejtli J, *Pharm Tech Int*, 1991; 3(2); 15.

Cyclodextrins (CDs) are enzymatically modified starches. Their glucopyranose units form a ring: α-CD a ring of 6 units; β-CD a ring of 7 units; and γ-CD a ring of 8 units (Table 4.12; Fig. 4.7). The 'ring' is cylindrical, the outer surface being hydrophilic and the internal surface of the cavity being nonpolar. Appropriately sized lipophilic molecules can be accommodated wholly or partially in the complex, in which the host–guest ratio is usually 1 : 1 (Fig. 4.8), although other stoichiometries are possible, one, two or three CD molecules complexing with one or more drug molecules. The dissolution–dissociation–crystallisation process that can occur on dissolution is illustrated in Fig. 4.9.

Not all cyclodextrins are free of adverse effects; di-*O*-methyl β-CD, for example, has a strong affinity for cholesterol and is haemolytic. It is also one of the best solubilisers technically.

The cyclodextrins have obvious uses in parenteral formulations, including use as components of vehicles for peptides and other biologicals (ovine growth hormone, IL-2 and insulin)

Calixarenes

Research continues into other agents, apart from surfactants (which are discussed in Chapter 5), that can enhance the solubility of drugs. The calixarenes are another type of host, existing in a 'cup-shape' in a rigid conformation. The 4-sulfonic calix[*n*]arenes can form

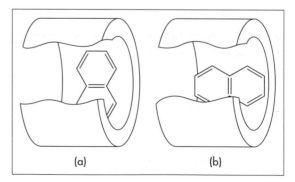

(a)   (b)

Figure 4.8 Two models of a complex of cyclodextrin with a lipophilic guest compound: (a) equatorial inclusion, (b) axial inclusion.
Reproduced from Harata K, Uedaira H, *Bull Chem Soc Jpn*, 1975; 48: 375.

Figure 4.9 Schematic representation of the dissolution–dissociation–recrystallisation process of a cyclodextrin complex with a poorly soluble guest. The complex rapidly dissolves, and a metastable oversaturated solution is obtained. The anomalously high level of dissolved guest drops back but remains higher than the level that can be obtained with non-complexed drug. Solid curve = complexed drug; broken curve = non-complexed drug.

Redrawn after Szejtli J, *Pharm Tech Int*, 1991; 3(2); 15.

host–guest type interactions with drugs such as nifedipine, a poorly water soluble agent,[12] seen in Fig. 4.10.

4.7 Solubility problems in formulation

4.7.1 Mixtures of acidic and basic compounds

Sometimes a combination formulation requires the admixture of acidic and basic drugs. One example (Septrin infusion) is discussed here.

Because sulfamethoxazole (**XVII**) is a weakly acidic substance and trimethoprim (**XVIII**) is a weakly basic one, for optimal solubility basic and acidic solutions, respectively, are required. In consequence, in an ordinary aqueous solution sulfamethoxazole and trimethoprim demonstrate a high degree of incompatibility and mutual precipitation occurs on mixing. To optimise mutual dissolution, an aqueous solution that includes 40% propylene glycol is used in the formulation of the infusion. This solution, which has a pH between 9.5 and 11.0, allows adequate amounts of both substances to coexist in solution to give the correct ratio of concentration for antibacterial action. On dilution, the infusion becomes less stable and at the recommended 1 in 25 dilution stability is about 7 hours. Owing to incompatibility of the two constituents, their degrees of solubility are sensitive to changes in ionic composition, pH and any drug additives. If there is imbalance in pH or ionic composition, then precipitation of one or other of the components may well occur.

Structure XVII Sulfamethoxazole, $pK_a = 6.03$

Structure XVIII Trimethoprim, $pK_a = 7.05$

4.7.2 Choice of drug salt to optimise solubility

The choice of a particular salt of a drug for use in formulations may depend on several factors. The solubility of the drug in aqueous media may be markedly dependent on the salt form. The chemical stability rather than the solubility may be a criterion and in many cases this is dependent on the choice of salt, sometimes through a pH effect. Deliberate choice of an insoluble form for use in suspensions is an obvious ploy; the formation of water-soluble entities from poorly soluble acids or bases by the use of hydrophilic

Figure 4.10 Molecular structures of (a) nifedipine and (b) 4-sulfonic calix[n]arenes. As n increases (4, 6, 8) the cavity size (see (c)) increases from 0.3 nm, through 0.76 nm to 1.16 nm. The solubility increase for nifedipine is greatest with calix[8]arene, being nearly 250% at a concentration of $0.008 \, mol \, dm^{-3}$ and pH of 5.

Reproduced from Yang W, de Villiers MM, *Eur J Pharm Biopharm*, 2004; 58: 629–636.

counterions is frequently attempted to produce injectable solutions of a drug. Table 4.13 gives some indication of the range of solubilities that can be obtained through the use of different salt forms, in this case of an experimental antimalarial drug (**XIX**).

Structure XIX   Compound used in Table 4.13

The large hydrophobic compound **XIX**, even as its hydrochloride salt, is poorly soluble and this is presumably the reason for its poor oral bioavailability. Similar conclusions were drawn several years ago for novobiocin. The acid salt administered to dogs at $12.5 \, mg \, kg^{-1}$ was not absorbed, but the monosodium salt, which is about 300 times as soluble in water, produced plasma levels of $22 \, \mu g \, cm^{-3}$ after 3 hours. Unfortunately, the sodium salt is unstable in solution. An amorphous form of the acid produced even higher levels of drug than the sodium salt, illustrating the fact that choice of salt and crystalline form of a drug substance may be of critical importance.

Some of the solubility differences obviously arise from differences in the pH of the salt solutions, which in the case of compound **XIX** ranged from 2.4 to 5.8 pH units. This is not atypical. The pH of solutions of salts of a 3-oxyl-1,4-benzodiazepine derivative at $5 \, mg \, cm^{-3}$ ranged from 2.3 for its dihydrochloride, to 4.3 for the maleate, and to 4.8 for the methanesulfonate.

Table 4.13 Solubilities of salts of an antimalarial drug (XIX)[a]

Salt	Melting point (°C)[b]	Solubility (mg cm^{-3})	Saturated solution pH
Free base	215	7–8	–
Hydrochloride	331	32–15	5.8
dl-Lactate	172 (dec)	1800	3.8
l-Lactate	193 (dec)	900	–
2-Hydroxy-1-sulfonate	250 (dec)	620	2.4
Methanesulfonate	290 (dec)	300	5.1
Sulfate	270 (dec)	20	–

[a] Reproduced from Agharkar S *et al.*, *J Pharm Sci*, 1976; 65: 747.
[b] (dec) = with decomposition.

Further examples of the solubility range in drug salts and derivatives are shown in Table 4.14. The increase in the solubility on the formation of the hydrochloride is readily attributable in the case of tetracycline to a lowering of the solution pH by the hydrochloride. The common ion effect (see section 4.2.3) can, however, produce an unexpected trend in the solubilities and dissolution rates (since these are proportional to the solubility in the diffusion layer at the surface of the solid) of bases in the presence of high concentrations of hydrochloric acid.[13] Increase in Cl⁻ concentrations will cause the equilibrium between solid (s) and solution (aq) forms

$$BH^+Cl^-_s \overset{K_{sp}}{\rightleftharpoons} (BH^+)_{aq} + (Cl^-)_{aq}$$

to be pushed to the left-hand side, with a resultant decrease in solubility. The solubility of **XIX** as the hydrochloride decreases from 24×10^{-5} mol dm^{-3} in 1.3 mmol dm^{-3} chloride ion, to 3×10^{-5} mol dm^{-3} in 40 mmol dm^{-3} chloride ion concentration. It should be noted that the stomach contents are rich in chloride ions. The common ion effect will be apparent in many infusion fluids to which drugs may be added, and therefore the effect of pH as well as electrolyte concentrations must be considered.

Consideration of Table 4.14 suggests that the hydrochloride salts of tetracyclines are always more readily dissolved than the base. The situation is more complex than at first appears, however. In dilute HCl at pH 1.2, the free base dissolves more than the hydrochloride, probably owing to the differences in crystallinity. The amount of compound derived from the base in solution decreases with time as the drug is converted to the hydrochloride. At pH 1.6 the rate of solution of the two forms is identical, and at pH 2.1 the hydrochloride has a higher solubility owing to its effect on local pH around the dissolving particles.

Erythromycin (**XX**) is labile at pH values below pH 4, and hence is unstable in the stomach contents. Erythromycin stearate (the salt of the tertiary aliphatic amine and stearic acid), being less soluble, is not as susceptible to degradation. The salt dissociates in the intestine to yield the free base, which is absorbed. There are differences in the absorption behaviour of the erythromycin salts and differences in toxicity, which may be related to their aqueous solubilities. Erythromycin ethylsuccinate was originally developed for paediatric use because its low water solubility and relative tastelessness was suited to paediatric formulations. The soluble lactobionate is used in intravenous infusions.

Structure XX Erythromycin

Table 4.14 Aqueous solubilities of tetracycline, erythromycin and chlorhexidine salts

Compound	Solubility in water (mg cm^{-3})
Tetracycline	1.7
Tetracycline hydrochloride	10.9
Tetracycline phosphate	15.9
Erythromycin	2.1
Erythromycin estolate[a]	0.16
Erythromycin stearate	0.33
Erythromycin lactobionate	20
Chlorhexidine	0.08
Chlorhexidine dihydrochloride	0.60
Chlorhexidine digluconate	>700

[a] Lauryl sulfate ester of erythromycin propionate

4.7.3 Drug solubility and biological activity

There should be a broad correlation between aqueous solubility and indices of biological activity. On the one hand, as drug solubility in aqueous media is inversely related to the solubility of the agent in biological lipid phases, there will be some relationship between pharmacodynamic activity and drug solubility. On the other, we should expect that drug or drug salt solubility might influence the absorption phase; drugs of very low aqueous solubility will dissolve slowly in the gastrointestinal tract, and in many cases the rate of dissolution is the rate-controlling step in absorption.

With drugs of low aqueous solubility such as digoxin, chlorpropamide, indometacin, griseofulvin and many steroids, the physical properties of the drug can influence biological properties. At early stages in a drug's development, pharmacological and toxicological tests are frequently carried out on extemporaneously prepared suspensions whose physical characteristics are not always well defined. This is not good practice as the toxicity of some drugs given by gavage to rats is dependent on the drug species used[14] (Table 4.15). This has been shown to be true with polymorphic forms of the same drug, but in the cases discussed in Table 4.15 different salts of the drugs were used.

There are other examples in which aqueous solubility acts as a rough and ready guide to absorption characteristics. The least soluble of the cardiotonic glycosides (digitoxin, digoxin and ouabain), being the most lipid soluble, are best absorbed. But because of the lipophilicity of digitoxin and digoxin, the rate-limiting step is the rate of solution, which is influenced directly by the solubility of the compounds.

High-molecular-weight quaternary salts such as bephenium hydroxynaphthoate (**XXI**) and pyrvinium embonate (**XXII**), being quaternary, have low lipid solubility but also have low aqueous solubility. They are virtually unabsorbed from the gut and indeed are used in the treatment of worm infestation of the lower bowel.

Table 4.15 The effect of solubility in water on the toxicity of drugs given by gavage to albino rats[a]

Drug	Salt	Solubility	$LD_{50} \pm SEM$
Benzylpenicillin	Ammonium	$<20\ mg\ cm^{-3}$	8.4 ± 0.13
Benzylpenicillin	Potassium	$>20\ mg\ cm^{-3}$	6.7 ± 0.1
Iron	Free metal	Insoluble	98.6 ± 26.7
Iron	Ferrous sulfate	Soluble	0.78
Spiramycin	Free base	Poorly soluble	9.4 ± 0.8
Spiramycin	Adipate	Soluble	4.9 ± 0.2

[a] Modified from reference 14.

Structure XXI Bephenium hydroxynaphthoate

Structure XXII Pyrvinium embonate

Key points

- As predicted from a simple model of the processes involved in the dissolution of a solute, there is often a good correlation between the molecular surface area and the aqueous solubility; the solubility of simple nonpolar hydrocarbons decreases with increase of surface area. With polar molecules and weak organic electrolytes, it is, however, necessary to consider the surface area of each portion of the molecule separately in predicting the overall effect; the greater the surface area of the hydrophilic portion relative to the hydrophobic portion, the greater will be the solubility.

- There is a trend for a decrease of solubility with increasing boiling point of liquids and increasing melting points of closely related series of solids.

- The influence of substituents on solubility can be due to their effect on the molecular cohesion of solids or liquids and/or their interaction with water molecules. Substituents can be classified as either hydrophobic or hydrophilic, depending on their polarity.

- The way in which solute molecules interact with water determines their affinity for the solvent; ionic substituents readily interact with the polar water molecules and confer solubility on the solute.

- Additives may either increase or decrease the solubility of a solute depending on the effect of the additive on water structure, and the interaction of the additive with the solute and the solvent. Addition of another compound with an identical ion to that of a poorly soluble salt will cause precipitation of the salt; this is known as the common ion effect. Additives that increase solubility are said to 'salt in' the solute, those that decrease the solubility 'salt out' the solute. Very soluble salts such as sodium benzoate with large anions or cations can salt in other solutes and are known as hydrotropic salts; the increase in solubility caused by their addition is referred to as hydrotropy. The effect of an additive on solubility is given by the Setschenow equation.

- pH has a major influence on solubility of solutes with ionisable substituents: acidic drugs are less soluble in acidic solutions, whereas basic drugs are less soluble in alkaline solutions. Amphoteric drugs are least soluble at their isoelectric point where they exist as zwitterions. The solubility of each type of drug may be calculated at any given pH from a knowledge of the pK_a of the drug and its solubility in the un-ionised form.

- Solubility of acids and bases in buffers of different pH may be measured by 'shake flask' or turbidimetric methods.

- Drug solubility may be increased by the use of mixed solvents, for example glycerol–water, ethanol–water and ethanol–glycerol mixtures, or by choice of drug salt. Cyclodextrins may be used to encapsulate the water-insoluble drug.

4.8 Partitioning

Here we discuss the topic of partitioning of a drug or solute between two immiscible phases. One phase might be blood or water and the other a biomembrane, or an oil or a plastic. As many processes (not least the absorption process) depend on the movement of molecules from one phase to another, it is vital that this topic is mastered. Here we will learn of the simple concepts of the partitioning of drugs and the calculation of partition coefficient (P) of the un-ionised form of the solute (and its logarithm, log P), as well as the use of the log P concept in determining the relative activities or toxicities of drugs from a knowledge of log P between an oil, most commonly octanol, and water. Where P cannot be measured, calculations of log P can be accomplished.[15,16] An outline of the methods available is given here.

Whether in formulations containing more than one phase or in the body, drugs move from one liquid phase to another in ways that depend on their relative concentrations (or chemical potentials) and their affinities for each phase. So a drug will move from the blood into extravascular tissues if it has the appropriate affinity for the cell membrane and the non-blood phase.

The movement of molecules from one phase to another is called *partitioning*. Examples of the process include:

- Drugs partitioning between aqueous phases and lipid biophases
- Preservative molecules in emulsions partitioning between the aqueous and oil phases
- Antibiotics partitioning into microorganisms
- Drugs and preservative molecules partitioning into the plastic of containers or giving sets

Plasticisers will sometimes partition from plastic containers into formulations. It is, therefore, important that the process can be quantified and understood.

4.8.1 The partition coefficient

If two immiscible phases are placed in contact, one containing a solute soluble to some extent in both phases, the solute will distribute itself so that when equilibrium is attained no further net transfer of solute takes place, as then the chemical potential of the solute in one phase is equal to its chemical potential in the other phase. If we think of an aqueous (w) and an organic (o) phase, we can write, according to equations (2.49) and (2.52),

$$\mu_w^\ominus + RT \ln a_w = \mu_o^\ominus + RT \ln a_o \qquad (4.27)$$

Rearranging equation (4.27) we obtain

$$\frac{\mu_o^\ominus - \mu_w^\ominus}{RT} = \ln \frac{a_w}{a_o} \qquad (4.28)$$

The term on the left-hand side of equation (4.28) is constant at a given temperature and pressure, so it follows that $a_w/a_o =$ constant and, of course $a_o/a_w =$ constant. These constants are the *partition coefficients* or *distribution coefficients*, P. If the solute forms an ideal solution in both solvents, activities can be replaced by concentration, so that

$$P = \frac{C_o}{C_w} \qquad (4.29)$$

P is therefore a measure of the relative affinities of the solute for an aqueous and a nonaqueous or lipid phase. Unless otherwise stated, P is calculated according to the convention in equation (4.29), where the concentration in the nonaqueous (oily) phase is divided by the concentration in the aqueous phase. The higher the value of P, the greater is the lipid solubility of the solute.

It has been shown for several systems that the partition coefficient can be approximated by the solubility of the agent in the organic phase divided by its solubility in the aqueous phase, a useful starting point for estimating relative affinities.

As early as 1891, Nernst stressed the fact that the partition coefficient as a function of concentration would be constant only if a single molecular species were involved. In some systems the association of the solute in one of the solvents complicates the calculation of partition coefficient; a simple example of the treatment of the partitioning of a dimerising compound is given in Box 4.4.

Being weak electrolytes, many drugs will ionise in at least one phase, usually the aqueous phase. The partitioning of the drug between the organic and water phases depends on the ionic state of the drug and, as we have seen in section 2.5, this is determined by its pK_a and the pH of the aqueous phase. The partition coefficient refers to the distribution of one species, in this case the un-ionised drug, whereas the assay method will usually determine both the ionised and un-ionised drug in the aqueous phase. Because ionised species cannot, in general, partition into organic hydrophobic solvents, the ratio of drug concentrations in organic and aqueous phases determined from assay data will yield an *apparent partition coefficient*, P_{app}, which will vary with pH, rather than the true partition coefficient P. The relationship between the true thermodynamic P and P_{app} is given by the following equations, which have been derived in Box 4.4 (equations (4.30) to (4.40)):

For acids:

$$\log P = \log P_{app} - \log \left(\frac{1}{1 + 10^{pH - pK_a}} \right)$$

For bases:

$$\log P = \log P_{app} - \log \left(\frac{1}{1 + 10^{pK_a - pH}} \right)$$

4.8.2 Free energies of transfer

The standard free energy of transfer of a solute between two phases is given by

$$\Delta G^{\ominus}_{trans} = \mu^{\ominus}_w - \mu^{\ominus}_o = RT \ln P \qquad (4.41)$$

In a homologous series, P can be measured and the increase in its value observed for each substituent group (for example, $-CH_2-$). As the chain length of nonpolar aliphatic compounds increases, it has been found that P increases by a factor of 2–4 per methylene group. The substituent contributions to P are additive, so a *substituent constant*, π_X, may be defined as

$$\pi_X = \log P_X - \log P_H \qquad (4.42)$$

where P_X is the partition coefficient of the derivative of the parent compound whose partition coefficient is P_H and π_X is the logarithm of the partition coefficient of the function X. For example, π_{Cl} can be obtained by subtracting $\log P_{benzene}$ from $\log P_{chlorobenzene}$.

4.8.3 Octanol as a nonaqueous phase

Octanol is often used as the nonaqueous phase in experiments to measure the partition coefficient of drugs. Its polarity means that water is solubilised to some extent in the octanol phase and thus partitioning is more complex than with an anhydrous solvent, but perhaps its usefulness stems from the fact that biological membranes are also not simple anhydrous lipid phases. While octanol is favoured, other alcohols have also been used. For example, isobutanol has been used to show that the binding of many drugs to serum protein is determined by the hydrophobicity or lipophilicity of the drug, following the relationship

$$\log K = 0.9 \log P_{isobutanol} + \text{constant} \qquad (4.43)$$

where K is an equilibrium constant measuring the binding of solute to protein. Transfer of a hydrophobic drug from an aqueous phase to a protein is, of course, a type of partitioning.

The correlation of lipophilicity and biological activity usually involves equations of the type

$$\log \frac{1}{C} = A \log P + \text{constant} \qquad (4.44)$$

where C is the concentration required to produce a given pharmacological response.

4.9 Biological activity and partition coefficients: thermodynamic activity and Ferguson's principle

As the site of action of many biologically active species is in lipid components such as membranes, correlations between partition coefficients and biological activity were found early on by investigators of structure–action relationships. For example, a wide range of simple organic compounds can exert qualitatively identical depressant actions (narcosis) on many simple organisms. Lack of any chemical specificity in the compounds tested led to the suggestion that physical, rather than chemical, properties governed the activity of the compounds. Early work by Meyer and Overton

Box 4.4 Partitioning of aggregating and ionising species

Aggregating species

If the solute forms aggregates or otherwise self-associates, the simple expression for partition coefficient given in equation (4.29) no longer applies. For example, the following equilibrium between the two phases 1 and 2 occurs when dimerisation occurs in phase 2:

$$\underset{\text{phase 1}}{2A} \; \rightleftharpoons \; \underset{\text{phase 2}}{A \cdot A}$$

$$K = \frac{[A]_{\text{phase2}}}{[A]_{\text{phase1}}^2}$$

Hence

$$K' = \frac{\sqrt{C_2}}{C_1} \tag{4.30}$$

K' is a constant combining the partition coefficient and the association constant. Table 4.16 illustrates the use of equations (4.29) and (4.30).

Ionisable species

We will consider the distribution of *weakly acidic drugs* between organic and aqueous phases. If we express the dissociation of a weak acid as

$$HA \rightleftharpoons H^+ + A^-$$

the dissociation constant in the aqueous phase, K_a will be given by

$$K_a = \frac{[H^+][A^-]}{[HA]} \tag{4.31}$$

The true partition coefficient is the ratio of the concentrations of the un-ionised species in organic and aqueous phases, i.e.

$$P = \frac{[HA]_o}{[HA]_w} \tag{4.32}$$

whereas the apparent partition coefficient is the ratio of the concentration of the un-ionised species in organic phase to the sum of the un-ionised and ionised species in the aqueous phase, i.e.

$$P_{\text{app}} = \frac{[HA]_o}{[HA]_w + [A^-]_w} \tag{4.33}$$

Substituting for $[A^-]_w$ from equation (4.31) and rearranging using the expression for P from equation (4.32) gives

$$P_{\text{app}} = \frac{[H^+][HA]_o}{[HA]_w \{[H^+] + K_a\}} = \frac{P[H^+]}{[H^+] + K_a} \tag{4.34}$$

Therefore,

$$\frac{P}{P_{\text{app}}} = 1 + \frac{K_a}{[H^+]} \tag{4.35}$$

Taking logarithms and rearranging gives

$$\log P = \log P_{\text{app}} - \log \left[\frac{1}{1 + \frac{K_a}{[H^+]}} \right] \tag{4.36}$$

Substituting from equation (4.31),

$$\log P = \log P_{\mathrm{app}} - \log \left[\frac{1}{1 + \frac{[A^-]}{[HA]}} \right] \qquad (4.37)$$

Since, from equation (2.70),

$$pH - pK_a = \log \frac{[A^-]}{[HA]}$$

and therefore,

$$\frac{[A^-]}{[HA]} = 10^{pH - pK_a} \qquad (4.38)$$

Substituting into equation (4.37) gives

$$\log P = \log P_{\mathrm{app}} - \log \left(\frac{1}{1 + 10^{pH - pK_a}} \right) \qquad (4.39)$$

The equivalent expression for the relationship between true and apparent partition coefficients for weakly basic drugs, which may be derived in a similar manner, is

$$\log P = \log P_{\mathrm{app}} - \log \left(\frac{1}{1 + 10^{pK_a - pH}} \right) \qquad (4.40)$$

Table 4.16 Distribution of two acids between immiscible phases at 25°C[a]

C_1 (mol dm^{-3})[b]	C_2 (mol dm^{-3})[c]	C_2/C_1	$\sqrt{C_2}/C_1$
Succinic acid			
0.191	0.0248	0.130	
0.370	0.0488	0.132	
0.547	0.0736	0.135	
0.749	0.1010	0.135	
Benzoic acid			
4.88×10^{-3}	3.64×10^{-2}	7.46	39.06
8.00×10^{-3}	8.59×10^{-2}	10.75	36.63
16.00×10^{-3}	33.8×10^{-2}	21.13	36.36
23.7×10^{-3}	75.3×10^{-2}	31.77	36.63

[a] Reproduced from Glasstone S, Lewis D, *Elements of Physical Chemistry*, 2nd edn, London: Macmillan; 1964.
[b] Aqueous phase concentration.
[c] Nonaqueous phase concentration (succinic acid in ether; benzoic acid in benzene).

related narcotic potency to the oil/water partition coefficient of the compounds concerned, and in a later re-interpretation of the data it was concluded that narcosis commences when any chemically nonspecific substance has attained a certain molar concentration in the lipids of the cells.

In 1939 Ferguson placed the Overton–Meyer theory on a more quantitative basis by applying thermodynamics to the problem of narcotic action. By expressing compound potency in terms of thermodynamic activity, rather than concentration, he avoided the problem of there being various distribution coefficients between the numerous different phases within the cell, any of which might be the phase in which the drug exerted its pharmacological effects (the biophase). The fact that the narcotic action of a drug remains at a constant level while a critical concentration of drug is applied, decreasing rapidly when administration of the drug is stopped, indicates that an equilibrium exists between some external phase and the biophase.

According to equation (2.49) the chemical potentials in two phases at equilibrium are equal. Thus, from equation (2.52),

$$\mu_A^\ominus + RT \ln a_A = \mu_B^\ominus + RT \ln a_B \qquad (4.45)$$

If the standard states are identical, the activities will consequently be equal in the two phases. The activity of a substance in the biophase at equilibrium is thus identical to the readily determined value in an external phase.

For narcotic agents applied as a vapour, the standard state can be taken to be the saturated vapour, and thus activity $a = p_t/p_s$ where p_t is the partial pressure of the vapour and p_s is the saturated vapour pressure at the same temperature. When the narcotic agent was applied in solution and was also of limited solubility, activity was equated with the ratio S_t/S_0 where S_t is the molar concentration of the narcotic solution and S_0 its limiting solubility; the ratio S_t/S_0 therefore represents proportional saturation. This is in contrast to the normal procedure of taking the standard state as an infinitely dilute solution.

From recalculations of published data and also from measurements of the potency of many different compounds, Ferguson concluded that, within reasonable limits, substances present at approximately the same proportional saturation (that is with the same thermodynamic activity) in a given medium have the same biological potency. For example, Table 4.17 shows that while the bactericidal concentrations against *Bacillus typhosus* vary widely (0.0022–3.89 mol dm^{-3}), the thermodynamic activities vary within a relatively restricted range (0.11–0.76).

As with most physicochemical theories there may be problems in applying the equations to real life. If an attempt is made to correlate hydrophobicity with the rate of inhibition of local anaesthetic activity, the answers are complex, i.e. there is not necessarily a clear correlation because (1) molecular size as well as hydrophobicity is a factor in kinetics, (2) membranes are nonhomogeneous and if adsorption occurs at phospholipid head groups there is no way to mimic this with octanol and water; and (3) there is the problem of using equilibrium measurements for kinetic predictions.

4.10 Using log *P*

As we have seen, the value of log *P* is a measure of lipophilicity and, as so many pharmaceutical and

Table 4.17 Bactericidal concentrations and activities of organic substances in solution[a]

Substance	Bactericidal concentration (mol dm^{-3}) (S_1)	Solubility at 25°C (mol dm^{-3}) (S_0)	Activity or S_1/S_0
Phenol	0.097	0.90	0.11
o-Cresol	0.039	0.23	0.17
Propionaldehyde	1.08	2.88	0.37
Thymol	0.0022	0.0057	0.38
Acetone	3.89	∞	0.40
Methyl ethyl ketone	1.25	3.13	0.40
Aniline	0.17	0.40	0.44
Cyclohexanol	0.18	0.38	0.47
Resorcinol	3.09	6.08	0.54
Methyl propyl ketone	0.39	0.70	0.56
Butyraldehyde	0.39	0.51	0.76

[a] Reproduced from Meyer KH, Hemmi H, *Biochem Z*, 1935; 277; 39.

Table 4.18 Log P values for representative drugs[a]

Drug	log P
Acetylsalicylic acid (aspirin)	1.19
Amiodarone	6.7
Benzocaine	1.89
Bupivacaine	3.4
Bromocriptine	6.6
Caffeine	0.01
Chlorpromazine	5.3
Cisapride	3.7
Ciprofloxacin	−1.12
Desipramine	4.0
β-Estradiol	2.69
Glutethimide	1.9
Haloperidol	1.53
Hydrocortisone	4.3
Hyoscine	1.90
Indometacin	3.1
Lidocaine	2.26
Methadone	3.9
Misoprostil	2.9
Nicotinamide	−0.37
Norfloxacin	1.55
Ondansetron	3.2
Oxytetracycline	−1.12
Pergolide	3.8
Phenytoin	2.5
Physostigmine	2.2
Prednisone	1.46
Sulfadiazine	0.12
Sulfadimethoxine	1.56
Sulfafurazole	1.01
Sulfaguanidine	−1.22
Sulfamerazine	0.13
Sulfanilamide	−1.05
Sulfapyridine	0.90
Sulfathiazole	0.35
Tetracaine	3.56
Thiopental	2.8
Xamoterol	0.5
Zimeldine	2.7

[a] Data from Herbert BJ, Dorsey JG, *Anal Chem*, 1995; 67: 744; Butterworth JF, Strichartz GR, *Anaesthesiology*, 1990; 72: 711; Jack DB, *Handbook of Clinical Pharmacokinetic Data*, London: Macmillan; 1992.

biological events are dependent on lipophilic characteristics, the examples where correlations can be found between $\log P$ and biological indices are legion. A selection of applications of the $\log P$ concept is discussed here. Table 4.18 provides a sample of $\log P$ data for a range of pharmaceuticals. The relatively simple *in vitro* measurement of P can give an accurate prediction of activity in a complex biological system, provided that the obvious limitations of the simple system are recognised and that the biological activity of the drug depends on its lipophilic nature. Applications of P or $\log P$ come into their own particularly in homologous series or series of closely related compounds, where the influence of substituent groups can be accurately examined.

4.10.1 The relationship between lipophilicity and behaviour of tetracyclines

The lipid solubility of four tetracyclines (minocycline, doxycycline, tetracycline and oxytetracycline) correlates inversely with the mean concentration of antibiotic in plasma and with renal uptake and excretion. Only the more lipophilic minocycline and doxycycline pass across the blood–brain and blood–ocular barriers in detectable concentrations. Table 4.19 gives some of these characteristics of the tetracyclines. These analogues of tetracycline, while active *in vitro* against meningococci, are not of equal value in clinical use; oxytetracycline and doxycycline fail to change the state of 'carriers' of the disease, whereas minocycline has a significant effect. It is thought that the ability to enter the saliva and tears influences the clinical activity, for although saliva does not usually wet the nasopharynx, tears pass into the nasopharynx as the normal route of drainage from the conjunctival sac.

The pH dependence of partition coefficients of tetracyclines is more complex than for most drugs, as the tetracyclines are amphoteric.

For slightly simpler amphoteric compounds, such as p-aminobenzoic acid and sulfonamides, the apparent partition coefficient is maximal at the isoelectric point. Figure 4.11 illustrates the variation with pH of $\log P_{app}$ for p-aminobenzoic acid and for two sulfonamides.

The participation of the zwitterionic species in the partitioning can be excluded because of its low concentration, thus $K_t \rightarrow 0$ in Scheme 4.1. From this we obtain P and P_{app} as follows:

$$P = \frac{[I]_o}{[I]_w} \tag{4.46}$$

and

$$P_{app} + \frac{[I]_o}{[II]_w + [I]_w + [IV]_w + [III]_w}$$

$$= P \left[\frac{1}{\dfrac{[H^+]}{K_a} + \dfrac{K_c}{[H^+]} + K_t + 1} \right] \tag{4.47}$$

If $K_t \rightarrow 0$,

$$P_{app} = P \left[\frac{1}{\dfrac{[H^+]}{K_A} + \dfrac{K_c}{[H^+]} + 1} \right] \tag{4.48}$$

Passive diffusion of sulfonamides into human red cells is determined by plasma drug binding and lipid solubility. Apparent partition coefficients between chloroform and water at pH 7.4 show an almost linear relation with penetration constant for sulfonamides and a number of other acids. Penetration rates of sulfonamides into the aqueous humour and cerebrospinal fluid also correlate with partition coefficients (Fig. 4.12); moreover, as can be seen from the data in Fig. 4.13, the antibacterial effects of fatty acids and esters towards *B. subtilis* correlate with octanol/water partition coefficients.

Scheme 4.1 Partitioning of p-aminobenzoic acid. K_a, K_b, K_c and K_d are microdissociation constants for each equilibrium and the relation between them is

$$K_1 = K_a + K_b$$
$$\frac{1}{K_2} = \frac{1}{K_c} + \frac{1}{K_d}$$
$$K_t = \frac{[\text{zwitterion}]}{[\text{neutral form}]} = \frac{K_b}{K_a} = \frac{K_c}{K_d}$$

where K_1 and K_2 are composite or macroscopic acid dissociation constants and K_t is the tautomeric constant between the zwitterionic and neutral forms.

Reproduced from Terada H, Chem Pharm Bull, 1972; 20: 765.

There are many quantitative relationships between physiological action and $\log P$ or $\log P_{app}$. A few examples are given in Box 4.5.

Local anaesthetic action on peripheral nerves is also proportional to P since the un-ionised form must diffuse across the continuous cell layer of the perineurium. Once across the perineurium, the molecules

Absorption of acidic drugs from the colon may be quantified according to P and pK_a by the equation

$$\log (\text{percentage absorption}) = 0.156(pK_a - 6.8) - 0.366 \log P + 0.755 \quad (4.49)$$

Absorption of bases from the small intestine has been similarly treated:

$$\log (\text{percentage absorbed}) = -0.131(\log P)^2 + 0.362 \log P \quad (4.50)$$

4.10.2 Sorption

Figure 4.15 summarises the physicochemical problems in the use of preservative molecules in formulations. Solubility and partition coefficients of ionised species are determined, as we have seen, by the pH and ionic strength of the system. In this example, partitioning may occur from the aqueous phase to the oily phase of an emulsion, to the micellar phase of a surfactant, or to a closure. Adsorption may also occur onto container closures and suspended solid particles.

Permeation of antimicrobial agents into rubber stoppers and other closures is another example of partitioning. Although rubber is an amorphous solid, partitioning between the aqueous phase and rubber depends, as in liquid systems, on the relative affinities of the solute for each phase.

Glyceryl trinitrate, a volatile drug with a chloroform/water partition coefficient of 109, diffuses from simple tablet bases into the walls of plastic bottles and into plastic liners used in packaging tablets. This partitioning can be prevented if there is included in the tablet formulation an agent (such as polyoxyethylene glycol) that complexes with the drug substance, thereby increasing its affinity for the 'tablet phase' – in other words, reducing its escaping tendency or 'fugacity'. Significant losses of glyceryl trinitrate have been detected when the drug was given as an infusion

ionise and they combine with the receptors in the nerve membrane in their ionised form.

The toxicity of some agents such as X-ray contrast media and penicillins has also been related to lipophilicity. Rates of entry into the brain of X-ray contrast agents used in cerebral angiography are proportional to P, and P correlates with clinical neurotoxicity. Figure 4.14 shows the positive relationship between toxicity of the penicillins and partition coefficient.

Table 4.19 Some characteristics of four tetracyclines

Compound	P_{app} (chloroform/water)[a]	P_{app} (octanol/water)[b]	Serum protein binding (%)
Minocycline	30	1.1	76–83
Doxycycline	0.48	0.60	25–93
Tetracycline	0.09	0.036	20–67
Oxytetracycline	0.007	0.025	10–40

[a] pH 7.4.
[b] pH 7.5.

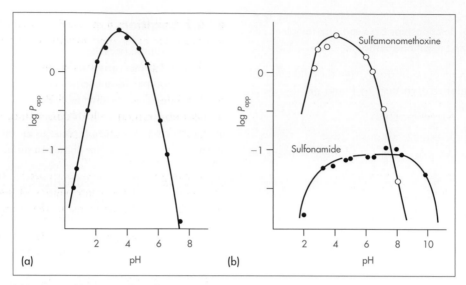

Figure 4.11 (a) Variation of $\log P_{app}$ with pH for *p*-aminobenzoic acid. (b) Variation of $\log P_{app}$ with pH for sulfamonomethoxine and sulfonamide.

Reproduced from Terada H, *Chem Pharm Bull*, 1972; 20: 765.

through plastic giving sets from a plastic reservoir, the absorption (of as much as 50% of the drug) resulting in the necessity to use unusually high doses of the drug.

Some relation has been found between the rate of sorption by poly(vinyl chloride) (PVC) bags of a series of drugs and their hexane/water partition coefficients.[17] Table 4.20 shows the data for sorption of $100\,cm^3$ PVC infusion bags (equivalent to $11\,g$ of PVC). In the table, P_{app} values have been calculated from

$$P_{app} = \left(\frac{1 - F_\infty}{F_\infty}\right) \frac{W_s}{W_p} \qquad (4.51)$$

where W_s is the weight of solution in contact with a given weight W_p of plastic and F_∞ is the equilibrium fraction of drug remaining in solution. Only the un-ionised form of the drug is sorbed; the kinetics of the process can be accounted for by considering the diffusion of the molecules in the plastic matrix.

There are concerns over phthalates in medical devices, including diethylhexylphthalate (DEHP), used in medical products made of PVC such as IV bags, blood bags and tubing. DEHP can 'leach' out of PVC

into liquids such as intravenous fluids, especially in the presence of formulations containing additives such as surfactants, as with Cremophor EL in Taxol. Figure 4.16 illustrates some of the problems that can occur in giving sets.

4.10.3 A chromatographic model for the biophase

Octanol/water partition coefficients, as we have seen, have been useful predictors of biological activity. In spite of this it has been suggested that bulk liquid phases may not be the most appropriate models for a structured biophase such as a biological membrane, and chromatographic stationary phases have been proposed as an alternative because of the structuring of the 'membranous' hydrophobic chains.

4.10.4 Calculating $\log P$ from molecular structures

The large number of methods used to calculate $\log P$ values have been elegantly reviewed by Leo.[16] The

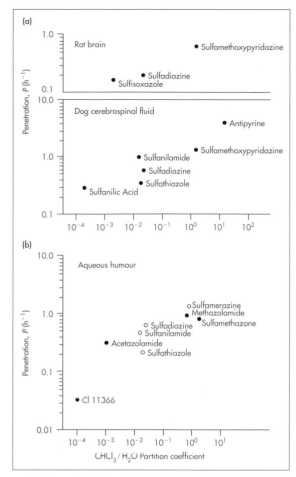

Figure 4.12 (a) Penetration rates of sulfonamides from plasma into rat brain and into canine cerebrospinal fluid. (b) Penetration rates of sulfonamides from plasma into aqueous humour for the rabbit (O) and for the rat (●) against partition coefficients (chloroform/water).

(a) Dog cerebrospinal fluid data from Rall DP, *J Pharm Exp Ther*, 1959; 125; 185. (b) Data from Wistrand PJ, *Acta Pharmacol Toxicol*, 1960; 17: 337 and Sorsby A, *Br J Ophthalmol*, 1949; 33: 347.

method proposed in 1964 by Fujita, Iwasa and Hansch[18] used values for the 'parent' molecule and values for substituents gathered by analysis of thousands of values of $\log P$ for homologous and other series. In this method of 'substituents', $\log P$ is considered to be an additive-constitutive free-energy-related property, where one can define Π for substituent X as

the difference between the $\log P$ values for the parent solute and the compound with the substituent:

$$\Pi_{(X)} = \log P_{(R-X)} - \log P_{(R-H)} \tag{4.52}$$

By definition $\Pi_{(H)} = 0$. For example,

$$\log P_{NO_2-C_6H_4CH_3} = \log P_{C_6H_6} + \Pi_{NO_2} + \Pi_{CH_3}$$
$$\log P = 2.13 - 0.28 + 0.56 = 2.41$$

against a measured value of 2.45.

The fragmental method developed by Rekker and Mannhold[19] uses the contributions of simple fragments. This may be illustrated by the example:

$$\log P_{C_6H_5OCH_2COOH} = f_{C_6H_5} \pm f_O + f_{CH_2} + f_{COOH} + PE1$$

where PE1 is a 'proximity effect,' an adjusting fraction for polar fragments in nonpolar surroundings. So

$$\log P_{C_6H_5OCH_2COOH} = 1.866 - 0.433 + 0.53 - 0.954 + 0.861 = 1.87$$

compared with a measured value of 1.34.

A method based on the surface areas of molecules has also been proposed to obtain measures of $\log P$ in a manner analogous to the calculation of solubility.[20] Computer programs for calculation of $\log P$ are also in use and are described in detail in Leo's 1993 review.[16]

4.10.5 Drug distribution into human milk

The distribution of drugs into the milk of breastfeeding mothers is of obvious importance. Nearly all drugs find their way into milk and it is, therefore, useful to be able to predict which of them will achieve high concentrations in milk in relation to their plasma level, defined in one model[21] described below as the milk: plasma (*M/P*) ratio (see Table 4.21). Three key parameters are the pK_a of the drug, plasma protein binding and the octanol/water partition coefficients of the drugs. Protein binding is the most important single predictor, an increase in M/P ratios generally being found as protein binding decreases. The equations used to calculate milk : plasma ratios are shown in Box 4.6.

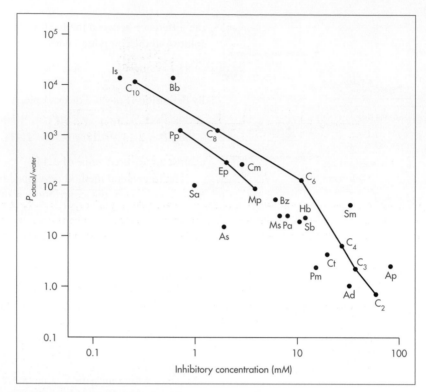

Figure 4.13 Relationship between the partition coefficient (*P*) and growth inhibitory concentration of a wider range of compounds. The octanol/water partition coefficient of the undissociated compounds is plotted against the concentrations of compounds needed to inhibit growth of *B. subtilis* by 50%.

Reproduced from Sheu GW *et al., Antimicrob Agents Chemother*, 1975; 7: 349.

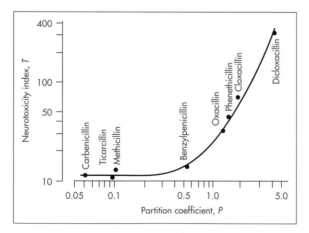

Figure 4.14 Relation of neurotoxicity to the hydrophobic character of various penicillins: the hydrophobic character is measured by the partition coefficient *P* and toxicity by a neurotoxicity index *T*.

Reproduced from Weihrauch TR *et al., Arch Pharmacol (NS)*, 1975; 289: 55.

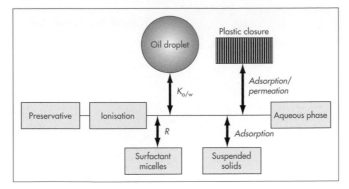

Figure 4.15 The potential fate of preservative molecules in pharmaceutical products. Much depends on the state of ionisation of the molecules. Partitioning into oil droplets or surfactant micelles can occur, as well as adsorption onto suspended solids. Adsorption, sorption or permeation of plastic closures can occur, leaving the less active form in the aqueous phase.

Table 4.20 Sorption into PVC and partitioning of drugs[a]				
Compound	Initial rate of sorption ($10^{-2}\,h^{-1}$)	Extent of sorption at equilibrium (%)	log P_{app}	log P (hexane/water)
Medazepam	51	85	1.7	2.9
Diazepam	27	90	1.9	0.9
Warfarin (pH 2–4)	22	90	1.9	0.2
Glyceryl trinitrate	20	83	1.6	0.2
Thiopental (pH 4)	6	73	1.4	0.1
Oxazepam	4.6	46	0.9	−0.1
Nitrazepam	4.1	47	0.9	−0.1
Hydrocortisone acetate	0	0		−1.2
Pentobarbital (pH 4)	0	0	–	−1.3

[a] Reproduced from reference 17.

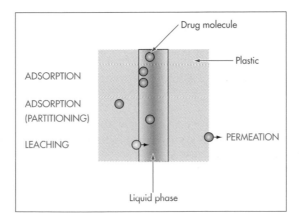

Figure 4.16 Diagram showing opportunities in plastic systems for adsorption of drug molecules, partitioning into and eventually permeation through the plastic. Leaching of molecules from the plastic also may occur.

Table 4.21 Distribution of drugs into milk: the M/P ratio[a,b]

Drug	M/P
Acidic drugs	
Carbenicillin	0.02
Ethosuximide	0.78
Ibuprofen	0
Paracetamol	0.76
Valproic acid	0.05
Basic drugs	
Amitriptyline	0.83
Atenolol	0.32
Cimetidine	1.7
Clonazepam	0.33
Codeine	2.16
Lamotrigine	0.4–0.45
Morphine	2.46
Verapamil	0.6
Vigabatrin	0.01–0.05
Neutral drugs	
Alcohol	0.89
Digoxin	0.55
Medroxyprogesterone	0.72
Norethisterone	0.19
Prednisolone	0.13

[a] Reproduced from reference 21.
[b] M/P = Milk : plasma drug concentration ratio.

Box 4.6 The calculation of milk : plasma ratios

The two key equations, each with three independent variables, are as follows:

For basic drugs:

$$\ln\left(\frac{M}{P}\right) = 0.025 + 2.28 \ln\left(\frac{M_u}{P_u}\right) + 0.89 \ln f_{u,p} + 0.51 \ln K \tag{4.53}$$

For acidic drugs:

$$\ln\left(\frac{M}{P}\right) = -0.405 + 9.36 \ln\left(\frac{M_u}{P_u}\right) - 0.69 \ln f_{u,p} - 1.54 \ln K \tag{4.54}$$

where

M_u/P_u = milk : plasma unbound drug concentration ratio
$f_{u,p}$ = fraction of drug unbound in plasma
$f_{u,m}$ = fraction of drug unbound in milk
$K = (0.955/f_{u,m}) + [0.045 P_{app}(\text{milk/lipid})]$
P_{app} = apparent partition coefficient at pH 7.2

Few measurements of $f_{u,m}$ and P_{app}(milk/lipid) have been made, but these parameters can be predicted from $f_{u,p}$ and $\log P$.[22]

It is clear from equations (4.53) and (4.54) that there is a degree of empiricism about these equations, which arises in their derivation from the fitting of data sets based on the independent variables. The ratio M_u/P_u can be obtained from the modified Henderson–Hasselbalch equation.

For basic drugs,

$$\frac{M_u}{P_u} = \frac{1 + 10^{(pK_a - pH_m)}}{1 + 10^{(pK_a - pH_p)}} \tag{4.55}$$

and for acidic drugs,

$$\frac{M_u}{P_u} = \frac{1 + 10^{(pH_m - pK_a)}}{1 + 10^{(pH_p - pK_a)}} \tag{4.56}$$

where pH_m and pH_p are the pH values of milk and plasma, respectively. Milk has a mean pH of 7.2, slightly lower than that of plasma at 7.4.

For neutral drugs the predicted M_u/P_u ratio would be unity, since the distribution of unbound un-ionised drugs would not be expected to be altered by pH gradients.

Key points

- The partitioning of a drug or solute between two immiscible phases is quantified by the partition coefficient P (and its logarithm $\log P$). P is the ratio of concentration in the organic (or lipid) phase to that in the aqueous phase; the greater the value of P the higher the lipid solubility.
- In the calculation of partition coefficient, consideration must be given to any aggregation or self-association of the drug in either of the solvents, and to changes of the ionisation of the drug with pH. In the case of ionisable drugs, the *true* partition coefficient refers to the distribution of the un-ionised form of the drug and this may be determined from measurements of the *apparent* partition coefficient as a function of pH.
- Ferguson's principle correlates the partition coefficient of a drug with its biological activity; it states that substances present at approximately the same proportional saturation (i.e. with the same thermodynamic activity) in a given medium have the same biological potency.
- $\log P$, usually measured using octanol as the nonaqueous solvent, is an indicator of the lipophilicity of a drug and can give a reasonably accurate prediction of *in vivo* activity if the biological activity of the drug depends on its lipophilic nature.
- Several methods are available for calculating $\log P$ from molecular structure.

Summary

Definitions of solubility, modes of expression of solubility and means of estimating solubility from the surface area of molecules were some of the key subjects discussed in this chapter. Molecular shape factors and substituents on molecules affect solubility, one of the key parameters of a drug substance. Effects such as solvation (or hydration in aqueous media) and the effects of additives on solubility are also dealt with, but perhaps the most important effect of all is that of pH on the solubility of ionisable drugs. This is treated in detail, and equations for acids, bases and zwitterions are considered. An understanding of pH–solubility relationships is vital to predicting the behaviour of ionic drugs in pharmaceutical formulations and in the body.

When additives, such as surfactants and cyclodextrins, do not achieve appropriate levels of practical solubility, we can resort to the use of co-solvents. The relative advantages and disadvantages of these different approaches to formulating a solution have to be considered, but in the last analysis other factors such as stability may determine which is the best approach to achieve a satisfactory solution formulation.

References

1. Amidon GL *et al.* Solubility of nonelectrolytes in polar solvents. II. Solubility of aliphatic alcohols in water. *J Pharm Sci* 1974;63:1858–1866.
2. Amidon GL. Theoretical calculation of heats of complexation in carbon tetrachloride. *J Pharm Sci* 1974;63: 1520–1523.
3. Amidon GL *et al.* Solubility of nonelectrolytes in polar solvents. V. Estimation of the solubility of aliphatic monofunctional compounds in water using a molecular surface area approach. *J Phys Chem* 1975;79: 2239–2246.
4. Hermann RB. Theory of hydrophobic bonding. II. Correlation of hydrocarbon solubility in water with solvent cavity surface area. *J Phys Chem* 1972;76: 2754–2759.
5. Hermann RB. Theory of hydrophobic bonding. I. Solubility of hydrocarbons in water, within the context of the significant structure theory of liquids. *J Phys Chem* 1971;75:363–368.
6. Kabasakalian P *et al.* Solubility of some steroids in water. *J Pharm Sci* 1966;55:642.
7. Franks F. In: Duckworth RD, ed. *Water Relations of Foods.* London: Academic Press; 1975.
8. Bergstrom CAS *et al.* Accuracy of calculated pH-dependent aqueous drug solubilities. *Eur J Pharm Sci* 2004;22:387–398.
9. Green AL. Ionisation constants and water solubilities of some aminoalkyl phenothiazine tranquillizers and related compounds. *J Pharm Pharmacol* 1967;19:10–16.

10. Bennett LJ, Miller KW. Application of regular solution theory to biomembranes. *J Med Chem* 1974; 17:1124–1125.

11. Scott RS. Solutions of nonelectrolytes. *Annu Rev Phys Chem* 1956;7:43–66.

12. Yang W, deVilliers MM. The solubilization of the poorly water soluble drug nifedipine by water soluble 4-sulphonic calix[n]arenes. *Eur J Pharm Biopharm* 2004; 58:629–36.

13. Serajuddin ATM. Salt formation to improve drug solubility. *Adv Drug Del Rev* 2007;59:603–616.

14. Boyd E. *Predictive Toxicometrics*. Bristol: Scientechnica; 1972.

15. Leo AJ *et al*. Partition coefficients and their uses. *Chem Rev* 1971;71:525–616.

16. Leo AJ *et al*. Calculating log P_{oct} from structures. *Chem Rev* 1993;93:1281–306.

17. Illum L, Bundgaard H. Sorption of drugs by plastic infusion bags. *Int J Pharm* 1982;10:339–351.

18. Fujita T *et al*. A new substituent constant, π, derived from partition coefficients. *J Am Chem Soc* 1964; 86:5175–5180.

19. Rekker R, Mannhold R. *Calculations of Drug Lipophilicity*. Weinheim: VCH; 1992.

20. Broto P, Moreau G, Vandycke C *et al*. Molecular structures: perception, autocorrelation descriptor and SAR studies. Perception of molecules: topological structure and 3-dimensional structure. *Eur J Med Chem* 1984; 19:61–65.

21. Atkinson HC, Begg EJ. Prediction of drug distribution into human milk from physicochemical characteristics. *Clin. Pharmacokinet* 1990;18:151–167.

22. Begg EJ *et al*. Prospective evaluation of a model for the prediction of milk: plasma drug concentrations from physicochemical characteristics. *Br J Clin Pharmacol* 1992;33:501–505.

5

Surfactants

Certain compounds, because of their chemical structure, have a tendency to accumulate at the boundary between two phases. Such compounds are termed *amphiphiles*, *surface-active agents*, or *surfactants*. Their adsorption at the various interfaces between solids, liquids and gases results in changes in the nature of the interface that are of considerable importance in pharmacy. For example, the lowering of the interfacial tension between oil and water phases facilitates emulsion formation; the adsorption of surfactants on insoluble particles enables these particles to be dispersed in the form of a suspension; and the incorporation of insoluble compounds within micelles of the surfactant can lead to the production of clear solutions.

In this chapter we will see how the surface activity of a molecule is related to its molecular structure and look at the properties of some surfactants which are commonly used in pharmacy. We will examine the nature and properties of films formed when water-soluble surfactants accumulate spontaneously at liquid–air interfaces and when insoluble surfactants are spread over the surface of a liquid to form a monolayer. We will look at some of the factors that influence adsorption onto solid surfaces and how experimental data from adsorption experiments may be analysed to gain information on the process of adsorption. An interesting and useful property of surfactants is that they may form aggregates or *micelles* in aqueous solutions when their concentration exceeds a critical concentration. We will examine why this should be so and some of the factors that influence micelle formation. The ability of micelles to solubilise water-insoluble drugs has obvious pharmaceutical importance and the process of solubilisation and its applications will be examined in some detail.

5.1 Amphipathic compounds

Surface-active compounds are characterised by having two distinct regions in their chemical structure, termed *hydrophilic* ('water-liking') and *hydrophobic* ('water-hating') regions. The existence of two such moieties in a molecule is referred to as *amphipathy* and the molecules are consequently often referred to as *amphipathic* molecules.

The hydrophobic portions are usually saturated or unsaturated hydrocarbon chains or, less commonly, heterocyclic or aromatic ring systems. The hydrophilic regions can be anionic, cationic, zwitterionic, or nonionic. Surfactants are generally classified according to the nature of the hydrophilic group. Typical examples are given in Box 5.1.

The most commonly encountered *anionic* surfactants have carboxylate, sulfate, sulfonate, and phosphate polar groups in combination with counterions such as sodium and potassium (for water solubility) or calcium and magnesium (for oil solubility). In the most common *cationic* surfactants the charge is carried on a

nitrogen atom as, for example, with amine and quaternary ammonium surfactants. The quaternary ammonium compounds retain this charge over the whole pH range, whereas the amine-based compounds only function as surfactants in the protonated state and therefore cannot be used at high pH. By far the most common *nonionic* surfactants are those with a poly(oxyethylene) chain as the hydrophilic group. In principle, it is possible to ethoxylate any material containing an active hydrogen, but the most commonly used starting materials are fatty alcohols, alkylphenols, fatty acids and fatty amines. *Zwitterionic* and *amphoteric* surfactants possess polar head groups which on ionisation may impart both positive and negative charges. The positive charge is almost always carried by an ammonium group and the negative charge is often a carboxylate. If the ammonium group is quaternary the molecule will exist as a zwitterion over a wide pH range since the quaternary ammonium group will be permanently charged. If not, the molecule will behave as a true amphoteric surfactant, that is, the molecule will change from net cationic to zwitterionic and finally to net anionic as the pH is

Box 5.1 Classification of surfactants[a]

Anionic

Alkyl sulfate

Alkylbenzene sulfonate

Cationic

Alkyltrimethylammonium bromide

Alkylpyridinium chloride

Zwitterionic

Alkyl betaine

Alkyldimethylamine oxide

Nonionic

Alcohol ethoxylate

Polyoxyethylene–polyoxypropylene–polyoxyethylene block copolymer

[a] Hydrophobic areas of the molecules are shaded.

increased; such surfactants will only therefore be zwitterionic over a certain range of pH that depends on the pK_a values of each charge group. At the isoelectric point both charged groups will be fully ionised and the molecule will have properties similar to those of nonionic surfactants. As the pH shifts away from the isoelectric point, the molecule will gradually assume the properties of either a cationic or anionic surfactant. Common examples are N-alkyl derivatives of simple amino acids such as glycine (NH_2CH_2COOH), aminopropionic acid ($NH_2CH_2CH_2COOH$) and the alkyl betaines shown in Box 5.1.

The dual structure of amphipathic molecules is the unique feature that is responsible for the characteristic behaviour of compounds of this type. Thus their surface activity arises from adsorption at the solution–air interface – the means by which the hydrophobic region of the molecule 'escapes' from the hostile aqueous environment by protruding into the vapour phase above. Similarly, adsorption at the interface between nonaqueous solutions occurs in such a way that the hydrophobic group is in the solution in the nonaqueous phase, leaving the hydrophilic group in contact with the aqueous solution. Adsorption on hydrophobic particles such as carbon again represents a means of reduction of the contact between the hydrophobic groups and water and allows the consequent attainment of a minimum energy state. Perhaps the most striking consequence of the dual structure is micellisation – the formation in solution of aggregates in which the component molecules arc usually arranged in a spheroidal structure with the hydrophobic cores shielded from the water by a mantle of hydrophilic groups.

In the following sections we will examine in more detail the various characteristic properties of surfactants which arise as a consequence of their amphipathic nature.

5.2 Surface and interfacial properties of surfactants

5.2.1 Effects of amphiphiles on surface and interfacial tension

The molecules at the surface of a liquid are not completely surrounded by other molecules as they are in the bulk of the liquid. As a result there is a net inward force of attraction exerted on a molecule at the surface from the molecules in the bulk solution, which results in a tendency for the surface to contract.

The contraction of the surface is spontaneous; that is, it is accompanied by a decrease in free energy. The contracted surface thus represents a minimum free energy state and any attempt to expand the surface must involve an increase in the free energy. The surface free energy of a liquid is defined as the work, w, required to increase the surface area A by $1\,m^2$:

$$w = \gamma \Delta A \qquad (5.1)$$

where ΔA is the increase in surface area. γ is also referred to as *surface tension* and in this context is defined as the force acting at right angles to a line 1 m in length along the surface. Surface free energy and surface tension have SI units of $J\,m^{-2}$ and $N\,m^{-1}$ respectively (the units are, of course, identical since $1\,J = 1\,N\,m$). It is usual to quote values of surface tension in $mN\,m^{-1}$ (which is numerically equivalent to the cgs unit, dyne cm^{-1}).

A similar imbalance of attractive forces exists at the interface between two immiscible liquids. Table 5.1 lists surface tensions of various liquids and also

Table 5.1 Surface tensions of pure liquids and interfacial tensions against water at 20°C

Substance	Surface tension ($mN\,m^{-1}$)	Interfacial tension ($mN\,m^{-1}$)
Water	72	–
Glycerol	63	–
Oleic acid	33	16
Benzene	29	35
Chloroform	27	33
n-Octanol	27	8.5
Carbon tetrachloride	27	45
Castor oil	39	–
Olive oil	36	33
Cottonseed oil	35	–
n-Octane	22	51
Ethyl ether	17	11

interfacial tensions at the liquid–water interface. The value of the interfacial tension is generally between those of the surface tensions of the two liquids involved except where there is interaction between them. Table 5.1 includes several such examples. The interfacial tension at the octanol–water interface is considerably lower than the surface tension of octanol due to hydrogen bonding between these two liquids.

Amphiphilic molecules in aqueous solution have a tendency to seek out the surface and to orientate themselves in such a way as to remove the hydrophobic group from the aqueous environment and hence achieve a minimum free energy state (see Fig. 5.1). A consequence of the intrusion of surfactant molecules into the surface or interfacial layer is that some of the water molecules are effectively replaced by hydrocarbon or other nonpolar groups. Since the forces of intermolecular attraction between water molecules and nonpolar groups are less than those existing between two water molecules, the contracting power of the surface is reduced and so therefore is the surface tension. In some cases the interfacial tension between two liquids may be reduced to such a low level $(10^{-3}\,\mathrm{mN\,m^{-1}})$ that spontaneous emulsification of the two immiscible liquids is observed. These very low interfacial tensions are of relevance in understanding the formation and stabilisation of emulsions and are dealt with in more detail in Chapter 6.

5.2.2 Change of surface tension with surfactant concentration – the critical micelle concentration

Figure 5.2 shows a typical plot of surface tension against the logarithm of concentration for a surfactant

solution. Appreciable lowering of surface tension is evident even at low concentrations. As the surfactant concentration is increased, the surface tension continues to decrease as the concentration of surfactant molecules at the surface increases. A concentration is reached, however, when the surface layer becomes saturated with surfactant molecules and no further decrease in surface tension is possible. An alternative means of shielding the hydrophobic portion of the amphiphile from the aqueous environment now occurs as the surfactant molecules form small spherical aggregates or *micelles* in the bulk of the solution. The hydrophobic groups of the surfactants form the core of these aggregates and are protected from contact with water by their hydrophilic groups, which form a shell around them. The concentration of surfactant molecules in the surface layer remains approximately constant in the presence of micelles and hence the γ–log(concentration) plot becomes almost horizontal. The concentration at which the micelles first form in solution is called the *critical micelle concentration* (cmc) and corresponds to the concentration at which there is an abrupt change of slope of the plot. We will consider the formation and properties of micelles in more detail in section 5.3. At the moment we will concentrate on the region of the γ–log(concentration) plot below the cmc and see how it is possible to calculate the area occupied by a surfactant molecule at the surface using the Gibbs equation.

5.2.3 Gibbs adsorption equation

It is important to remember that an equilibrium is established between the surfactant molecules at the surface or interface and those remaining in the bulk

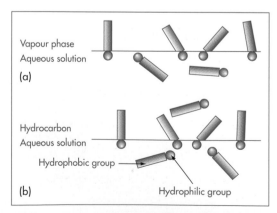

Figure 5.1 Orientation of amphiphiles at (a) solution–vapour interface, and (b) hydrocarbon–solution interface.

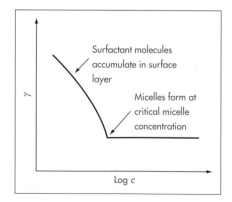

Figure 5.2 Typical plot of the surface tension, γ, against logarithm of surfactant concentration, c.

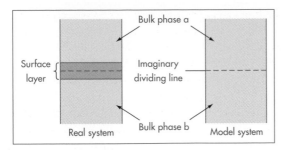

Figure 5.3 Diagrammatic representation of an interface between two bulk phases in the presence of an adsorbed layer.

of the solution. This equilibrium is expressed in terms of the Gibbs equation. In developing this expression it is necessary to imagine a definite boundary between the bulk of the solution and the interfacial layer (see Fig. 5.3). The real system containing the interfacial layer is then compared with this reference system, in which it is assumed that the properties of the two bulk phases remain unchanged up to the dividing surface. A thermodynamic derivation of the Gibbs equation is provided in Box 5.2, equations (5.2) to (5.11).

The form of the Gibbs equation applicable to dilute solutions is

$$\Gamma_2 = -\frac{1}{RT}\frac{d\gamma}{d\ln c} = -\frac{c}{RT}\frac{d\gamma}{dc} \qquad (5.12)$$

where activity in equation (5.11) has been replaced by concentration, c. Equation (5.12) is the form of the Gibbs equation applicable to the adsorption of nonionic surfactants at the surface of the solution. For ionic surfactants the derivation becomes more complex since consideration must be taken of the adsorption of both surfactant ion and counterion. The general form of the Gibbs equation is then written

$$\Gamma_2 = -\frac{1}{xRT}\frac{d\gamma}{d\ln c}$$
$$= -\frac{1}{xRT}\frac{d\gamma}{2.303\,d\log c} \qquad (5.13)$$

where x has a numerical value varying from 1 (for ionic surfactants in dilute solution or in the presence of excess electrolyte) to 2 (in concentrated solution).

Application of the Gibbs equation to surfactant solutions

The slope of the plot of surface tension against log (concentration) reaches a limiting value at concentrations just below the cmc (Fig. 5.2). The surfactant molecules are closely packed in the surface over this narrow concentration range and we can calculate the area A that each molecule occupies at the surface from

$$A = \frac{1}{N_A\Gamma_2} \qquad (5.14)$$

where Γ_2 is the value of surface excess concentration calculated from the Gibbs equation using the limiting $d\gamma/(d\ln c)$ value and N_A is the Avogadro constant. The calculation is shown in Example 5.1 using surface tension data for the surface-active drug, diphenhydramine.

Example 5.1 Calculation of area per molecule using the Gibbs equation

The limiting slope of a plot of γ against $\log c$ just below the cmc for the antihistamine diphenhydramine hydrochloride (see Box 5.3) is $-0.0115\,\mathrm{N\,m^{-1}}$ at 30°C. Calculate the area per molecule of this drug at the air–solution interface.

Answer

The surface excess concentration, Γ_2, may be calculated from equation (5.13), assuming a value of $x = 1$:

$$\Gamma_2 = \frac{0.0115}{8.314 \times 303 \times 2.303}$$
$$= 1.982 \times 10^{-6}\,\mathrm{mol\,m^{-2}}$$

Substituting in equation (5.14),

$$A = 1/(6.023 \times 10^{23} \times 1.982 \times 10^{-6})$$
$$= 83.8 \times 10^{-20}\,\mathrm{m^2\,molecule}$$

The area per molecule of diphenhydramine = $0.84\,\mathrm{nm^2}$.

Box 5.2 The Gibbs equation

We can treat the thermodynamics of the surface layer in a similar way to the bulk of the solution. The energy change, dU, accompanying an infinitesimal, reversible change in the system is given by

$$dU = dq_{rev} - dw$$

or

$$dU = T\,dS - dw \tag{5.2}$$

where dq_{rev} and dw are, respectively, the heat absorbed and the work done during the reversible change (see section 2.2.1).

For an open system (one in which there is a transfer of material between phases) equation (5.2) must be written

$$dU = T\,dS - dw + \Sigma\mu_i\,dn_i \tag{5.3}$$

where μ_i and n_i are the chemical potential and number of moles of the ith component, respectively.

When applying equation (5.3) to the surface layer, the work is that required to increase the area of the surface by an infinitesimal amount, dA, at constant T, P and n. This work is done against the surface tension and is given by equation (5.1) as $dw = \gamma\,dA$.

Thus, equation (5.3) becomes

$$dU^s = T\,dS^s + \gamma\,dA + \Sigma\mu_i\,dn_i^s \tag{5.4}$$

where the superscript, s, denotes the surface layer.

If the energy, entropy and number of moles of component are allowed to increase from zero to some finite value, equation (5.4) becomes

$$U^s = TS^s + \gamma A + \Sigma\mu_i n_i^s \tag{5.5}$$

General differentiation of equation (5.5) gives

$$dU^s = T\,dS^s + S^s\,dT + \gamma\,dA$$
$$+ A\,d\gamma + \Sigma\mu_i\,dn_i^s + \Sigma n_i^s\,d\mu_i \tag{5.6}$$

Comparison with equation (5.4) gives

$$0 = S^s\,dT + \Sigma n_i^s\,d\mu_i + A\,d\gamma \tag{5.7}$$

At constant temperature, equation (5.7) becomes

$$d\gamma = -\Sigma\Gamma_i\,d\mu_i \tag{5.8}$$

where $\Gamma_i = n_i^s/A$ and is termed the *surface excess concentration*. Γ_i is the amount of the ith component in the surface phase s, in excess of that which there would have been had the bulk phases a and b extended to the dividing surface without change in composition.

For a two-component system at constant temperature, equation (5.8) reduces to

$$d\gamma = -\Gamma_1\,d\mu_i - \Gamma_2\,d\mu_2 \tag{5.9}$$

where subscripts 1 and 2 denote solvent and solute, respectively. The surface excess concentrations are defined relative to an arbitrarily chosen dividing surface. A convenient choice of location of this surface is that at which the surface excess concentration of the solvent, Γ_1, is zero. Indeed, this is the most realistic position since we are now considering the surface layer of adsorbed solute. Equation (5.9) then becomes

$$d\gamma = -\Gamma_2 \, d\mu_2 \tag{5.10}$$

The chemical potential of the solute is given by equation (2.52) as

$$\mu_2 = \mu_2^\ominus + RT \ln a_2$$
$$d\mu_2 = RT \, d(\ln a_2)$$

Substituting in equation (5.10) gives the Gibbs equation:

$$\Gamma_2 = -\frac{1}{RT}\frac{d\gamma}{d(\ln a_2)} = -\frac{a_2}{RT}\frac{d\gamma}{da_2} \tag{5.11}$$

Box 5.3 Structures of some surface-active drugs[a]

Antidepressants

Chlorpromazine

Amitriptyline

Antihistamines

Diphenhydramine

Brompheniramine

Anticholinergic drugs

Orphenadrine

Local anaesthetics

Tetracaine

[a] Hydrophobic areas of the molecules are shaded.

An interesting effect arises when the surfactant is contaminated with surface-active impurities. A pronounced minimum in the surface tension–$\log c$ plot is observed at the cmc, which would seem to be an apparent violation of the Gibbs equation, suggesting a desorption (positive $d\gamma/d[\log c]$ value) in the vicinity of the cmc. The minimum in fact arises because of the release below the cmc of the surface-active impurities on the breakup of the surfactant micelles in which they were solubilised.

5.2.4 The influence of the surfactant structure on surface activity

The surface activity of a particular surfactant depends on the balance between its hydrophilic and hydrophobic properties. For the simplest case of a homologous series of surfactants, an increase in the length of the hydrocarbon chain as the series is ascended results in increased surface activity. Conversely, an increase in the hydrophilicity, which for polyoxyethylated nonionic surfactants may be effected by increasing the length of the ethylene oxide chain, results in a decreased surface activity. This latter effect is demonstrated by Fig. 5.4, from which it is noted that lengthening the hydrophilic chain results in an increase in both the surface tension (decrease of surface activity) and the cmc.

The relationship between hydrocarbon chain length and surface activity is expressed by *Traube's rule*, which states that 'in dilute aqueous solutions of surfactants belonging to any one homologous series, the molar concentrations required to produce equal lowering of the surface tension of water decreases threefold for each additional CH_2 group in the hydrocarbon chain of the solute'. Traube's rule also applies to the interfacial tension at oil–water interfaces.

Example 5.2 Use of Traube's rule

The surface tension lowering of an anionic surfactant (mol wt $= 328$ Da) with a hydrocarbon chain length of 16 carbon atoms, is $15\ \text{mN m}^{-1}$ at a concentration of 0.0276% w/v. For a surfactant with an identical hydrophilic group and a hydrocarbon chain length of 14 carbon atoms, estimate the percentage concentration that is required to produce an equal lowering of surface tension, assuming that both concentrations are below the cmc.

Answer

The molar concentration of the first surfactant $= 8.415 \times 10^{-4}\ \text{mol dm}^{-3}$. Since the second surfactant has two CH_2 groups fewer than the first, the concentration required to produce an equal lowering of surface tension is, according to Traube's rule,

$$8.415 \times 10^{-4} \times 3 \times 3 = 75.74 \times 10^{-4}\ \text{mol dm}^{-3}$$

The molecular weight of the second surfactant $= 328 - 28 = 300$ Da. Thus, the concentration required $= 0.227\%$ w/v.

5.2.5 Surface activity of drugs

The surface activity at the air–solution interface has been reported for a wide variety of drugs.[1,2] This surface activity is a consequence of the amphiphilic nature of the drugs. The hydrophobic portions of the drug molecules are in general more complex than those of typical surfactants, often being composed of aromatic or heterocyclic ring systems. Examples of the types of drug that exhibit surface activity are illustrated in Box 5.3. They include the phenothiazine tranquillisers such as promazine, chlorpromazine, promethazine, and the antidepressants, such as imipramine, amitriptyline and nortriptyline, which have tricyclic hydrophobic moieties; the antihistamines (for example, chlorcyclizine and diphenhydramine) and the antiacetylcholine drugs such as orphenadrine, which are based on a diphenylmethane hydrophobic group; the local anaesthetics (tetracaine, for example); and several antihistamines, such as brompheniramine and mepyramine, which have a hydrophobic group consisting of a single phenyl ring. Many peptides also

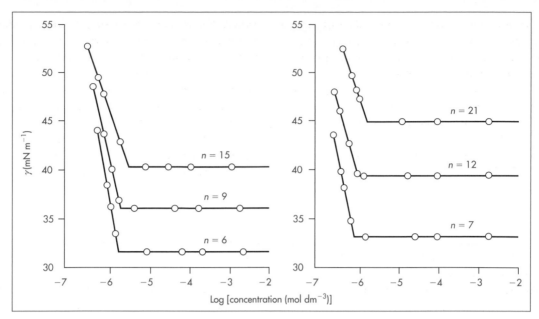

Figure 5.4 Surface tension versus log concentration plots for nonionic surfactants with the general formula $CH_3(CH_2)_{15}(OCH_2CH_2)_nOH$ for a series of ethylene oxide chain lengths, n.

Reproduced with permission from Elworthy PH, Macfarlane CB, *J Pharm Pharmacol*, 1962; 14; 100T.

have amphiphilic structures and adsorb at the air–water interface.

As with typical surfactants, the surface activity depends on the nature of the hydrophobic and hydrophilic portions of the drug molecule. The presence of any substituents on the aromatic ring systems can have an appreciable effect on hydrophobicity. Figure 5.5 shows the decrease of cmc and increased surface activity that is associated with the Br substituent on the phenyl ring of an antihistaminic drug. Similarly, substitution on the phenothiazine ring systems increases surface activity in the order $CF_3 \gg Cl > H$.

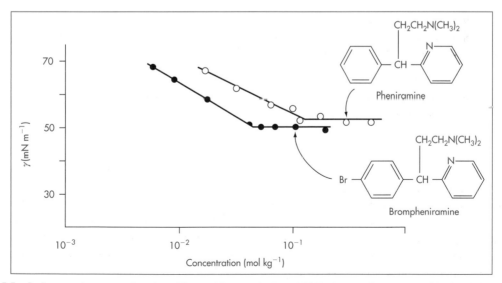

Figure 5.5 Surface tension, γ, as a function of log molal concentration at 30 °C showing the increase of hydrophobicity associated with a Br substituent on the phenyl ring of an antihistamine.

Reproduced with permission from Attwood D, Udeala OK, *J Pharm Pharmacol*, 1975; 27; 754.

The surface activity of drugs may have biological consequences because of their propensity to bind hydrophobically to proteins and to other biological macromolecules and to associate with other amphipathic substances such as bile salts and of course with receptors.[1] The surface activity of drug solutions, whether caused by an excipient such as benzylkonium chloride or the drug itself, e.g. salbutamol sulfate, can have a direct effect on the spray pattern from nebulisers[3] (see Chapter 10).

Key points

- Surface and interfacial tensions arise because of an imbalance of attractive forces on the molecules of a liquid at these interfaces such that the surface or interface has a tendency to contract.
- Surfactant molecules are amphiphilic, i.e. they have both hydrophilic and hydrophobic regions. They are classified according to the nature of the hydrophilic group as anionic, cationic, nonionic and zwitterionic surfactants. As a consequence of their amphiphilic nature they adsorb at interfaces in such a way that their hydrophobic regions are removed from the aqueous environment. The forces of attraction between surfactant and water molecules in the interface are weaker than those between two water molecules and hence the surface tension is reduced as a result of adsorption.
- The extent of adsorption at the interface can be calculated using the Gibbs equation. The lowering of surface tension increases with increase of surfactant concentration until the critical micelle concentration is reached, i.e. until the surfactant forms micelles; at higher concentrations the surface tension remains effectively constant.
- The surface activity of a surfactant depends on the balance between its hydrophilic and hydrophobic properties. An increase in the overall hydrophobicity of the surfactant molecule, by for example increasing the length of the hydrocarbon chain, results in increased surface activity. Conversely, an increase in the hydrophilicity of the molecule, by for example increasing the length of the ethylene oxide chain of a polyoxyethylated nonionic surfactant, results in a decreased surface activity.

5.2.6 Insoluble monolayers

In section 5.2.4 we examined the case in which the surface of a solution containing an amphiphile became covered with a monomolecular film as a result of spontaneous adsorption from solution. The molecules in such films are in equilibrium with those in the bulk of the solution, i.e. there is a continuous movement of molecules between the surface and the solution below it. If, however, a surfactant has a very long hydrocarbon chain it will be insufficiently water-soluble for a film to be formed in this way. In such cases we can spread a film on the surface of the solution by dissolving the surfactant in a suitable volatile solvent and carefully injecting the solution on to the surface. The *insoluble monolayer*

formed by this process contains all of the molecules injected on the surface; there is no equilibrium with the bulk solution because of the low water solubility of the surfactant. Consequently, the number of molecules per unit area of surface is generally known directly.

Although the films are called insoluble films, this is not meant to imply that any insoluble substance will form a stable monolayer; in fact, only two classes of materials will do so. The simpler and larger of the two classes includes the water-insoluble amphiphiles discussed above. Such structures orientate themselves at the water surface in the manner of typical surfactants, with the polar group acting as an anchor and the hydrocarbon chain protruding into the vapour phase.

The other class of film-forming compounds includes a range of amphipathic polymeric materials such as proteins and synthetic polymers. With these compounds a high degree of water insolubility is not so essential and stable films will form, providing there is a favourable free energy of adsorption from the bulk solution.

Experimental study of insoluble films

One of the earliest studies of insoluble films was conducted by Benjamin Franklin in 1765 on a pond in Clapham Common in London. Surprisingly Franklin's experiment was sufficiently controlled to establish that olive oil formed a film of monolayer thickness (quoted as one ten millionth of an inch: approximately 2.5 nm). Figure 5.6 illustrates an apparatus – the Langmuir trough – commonly used to study monolayers on a laboratory scale.

In its simplest form the apparatus consists of a shallow trough with waxed or Teflon sides (nonwetting), along which a nonwetting barrier may be mechanically moved. In use, the trough is filled completely so as to build up a meniscus above the level of the sides. The surface is swept clean with the moveable barrier and any surface impurities are sucked away using a water pump. The film-forming material

is dissolved in a suitable volatile solvent and an accurately measured amount, usually about $0.01\,\mathrm{cm}^3$, of this solution is carefully distributed on to the surface. The solvent evaporates and leaves a uniformly spread film entirely contained in the well-defined surface area between the two barriers. The film is compressed by moving the moveable barrier towards the fixed barrier in a series of steps. At each position of the two barriers the surface tension of the film-covered surface is measured directly using a Wilhelmy plate partially immersed in the subphase and attached to a sensitive electrobalance. The surface pressure, π, of the film is then calculated from the difference between the surface tension of the clean surface γ_0 and that of the film-covered surface, γ_m:

$$\pi = \gamma_0 - \gamma_m \qquad (5.15)$$

There have been steady improvements in the design of Langmuir troughs over recent years and, in modern instruments, operation and data collection are under computer control.

The results are generally presented as graphs of π against the surface area per molecule, A, which is readily calculated from the number of molecules added to the surface and the area enclosed between the two barriers as shown by Example 5.3.

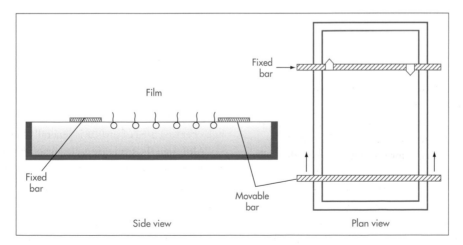

Figure 5.6 Langmuir trough for monolayer studies (not to scale). A Wilhelmy plate or other device is used to measure surface tension as the surface is compressed or expanded.

Example 5.3 Calculation of the area per molecule in an insoluble monolayer

When 1 cm^3 of a solution containing 8.5 mg per 100 cm^3 of stearic acid (mol wt $= 284.3$ Da) dissolved in a volatile organic solvent is placed on the surface of water in a Langmuir trough, the solvent evaporates off, leaving the stearic acid spread over the surface as an insoluble monomolecular film. If the surface area occupied by the film is 400 cm^2, calculate the area occupied by each molecule of stearic acid in the film.

Answer

1 cm^3 of the solution contains $8.5 \times 10^{-5} \text{ g}$ of stearic acid $= 2.99 \times 10^{-7} \text{ mol}$.

Since 1 mol contains 6×10^{23} (Avogadro constant) molecules, the solution contains

$$2.99 \times 10^{-7} \times 6 \times 10^{23}$$
$$= 1.79 \times 10^{17} \text{ molecules}$$

Therefore, the area per molecule of stearic acid in the film is

$$\frac{400 \times 10^{-4}}{1.79 \times 10^{17}} = 2.23 \times 10^{-19} \text{ m}^2$$
$$= 0.22 \text{ nm}^2$$

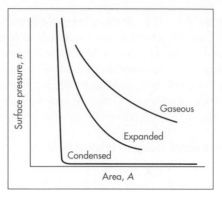

Figure 5.7 Surface pressure, π, versus area per molecule, A, for the three main types of monolayer.

Monolayer states

The surface film acts as a two-dimensional analogue to normal matter in that it may exist in different physical states, which in some ways resemble solids, liquids and gases. In this section we shall consider the three different states of monolayers of simple amphiphiles, referred to as solid (or condensed), liquid (or expanded), and gaseous monolayers (see Fig. 5.7).

Solid or condensed monolayers

Figure 5.8 shows the π–A curve for cholesterol, which produces a typical condensed film on an aqueous substrate. The film pressure remains very low at high film areas and rises abruptly when the molecules become tightly packed on compression. Simultaneous electron microscopy of the film-covered surface has shown cholesterol clusters or islands which gradually pack more tightly at greater pressures. The film becomes continuous as the pressure is further increased and at such high pressures the molecules are in contact and orientated as depicted in Fig. 5.8. The extrapolated limiting surface area of 0.39 nm^2 is very close to the cross-sectional area of a cholesterol ring system calculated from molecular models, confirming a vertical orientation.

Similar films are formed by long-chain fatty acids such as stearic and palmitic acid, for which a limiting surface area of about 0.20 nm^2 is found. This value is very close to the cross-sectional area of the compounds in the bulk crystal as determined by X-ray diffraction techniques.

Gaseous monolayers

These films represent the opposite extreme in behaviour to the condensed film. They resemble the gaseous state of three-dimensional matter in that the molecules move around in the film, remaining a sufficiently large distance apart so as to exert very little force on each other. Upon compression, there is a gradual change in the surface pressure, in marked contrast to the behaviour of solid films. It is thought that the molecules in these types of monolayer lie along the surface and this is certainly so with those dibasic esters with terminal polar groups that anchor the molecules flat on the surface. Those steroids in which the polar groups are distributed about the molecule tend to form gaseous films for similar reasons.

Expanded monolayers

Variously named liquid-expanded, expanded or liquid, these monolayers represent intermediate states between gaseous and condensed films. The π–A plots are quite steeply curved and extrapolation to a limiting

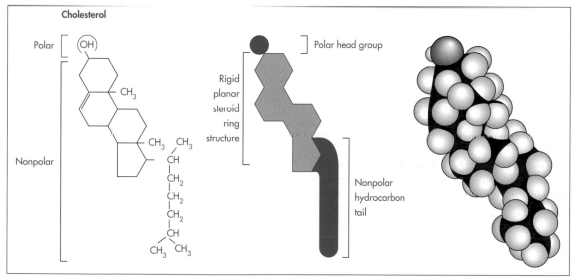

Figure 5.8 Surface pressure, π, versus area per molecule, A, for cholesterol, which shows a typical condensed monolayer, and schematic drawings of the oriented molecule including a space-filling model.

Reproduced with permission from Reiss HE *et al.*, *J Colloid Interface Sci*, 1976; 57: 396.

Figure 5.9 Surface pressure, π, versus area per molecule, A, for oleyl alcohol, which forms a typical expanded monolayer.

Reproduced with permission from Crisp DJ, in; Danielli JF *et al.*, eds, *Surface Phenomena in Chemistry and Biology*, Oxford: Pergamon Press; 1958: 23.

surface area yields a value that is usually several times greater than the cross-sectional area from molecular models. Films of this type tend to be formed by molecules in which close packing into condensed films is prohibited by bulky side-chains or, as in the case of oleyl alcohol (Fig. 5.9), by a *cis* configuration of the molecule.

Factors influencing monolayer state

Many factors, including both external factors such as temperature and also modifications to the molecular structure, influence the type of monolayer formed. Many simple molecules, rather than exhibiting behaviour exclusively characteristic of one monolayer state, show transitions between one state and another as the film is compressed. Estradiol diacetate, for example (Fig. 5.10), shows typical gaseous behaviour at a large area per molecule, and in this state the molecules are thought to be lying along the surface, as might be expected from the location of the hydrophilic groups on the molecule. As compression is applied, the molecules are gradually pressed closer together until at a molecular surface area of approximately $0.96\,\text{nm}^2$ the molecules begin to stand upright. The film now undergoes a gradual transition to a condensed film as the proportion of upright molecules increases with further compression, until at approximately $0.38\,\text{nm}^2$ the film is wholly in the condensed form.

In some compounds, notably myristic acid, the extent of the gaseous, expanded and condensed regions varies with temperature (Fig. 5.11). There is an analogy between the π–A curves of such

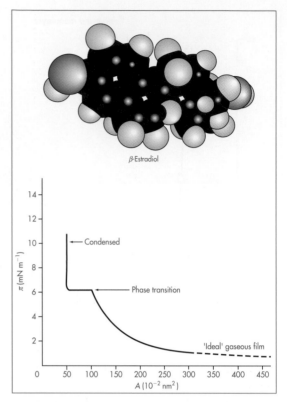

Figure 5.10 Surface pressure, π, versus area per molecule, A, for β-estradiol diacetate showing a transition from a gaseous to a condensed film on compression.

Reproduced from Cadenhead DA, Philips MC, *J Colloid Interface Sci*, 1967; 24: 491.

Figure 5.11 Surface pressure, π, versus area per molecule for myristic acid spread on $0.01\,\text{mol}\,\text{dm}^{-3}$ HCl at different temperatures, showing a transition from condensed to an expanded film with temperature increase.

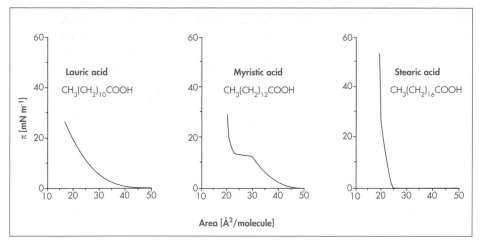

Figure 5.12   Surface pressure, π, versus area per molecule, A, for lauric acid, myristic acid and stearic acid spread on 0.001 mol dm^{-3} HCl aqueous subphase at 20 °C, showing changes in the nature of the isotherm caused by increasing the length of the hydrophobic chain.

Reprinted from Dynarowicztka P *et al.*, *Modern Physicochemical Research on Langmuir Monolayers*, Advances in Colloid and Interface Science 91, New York: Elsevier; 2001: 221–293 with permission from Elsevier.

compounds and the *PV* isotherms of three-dimensional gases.

Figure 5.12 shows changes in monolayer type as the length of the alkyl chain is increased from lauric acid (*n*-dodecanoic acid) to stearic acid (*n*-octadecanoic acid). Lauric acid represents the minimum alkyl chain length for the formation of monolayers; shorter chain length compounds have sufficient aqueous solubility to cause loss of molecules from monolayer and resultant decrease of monolayer area. Lauric acid forms slightly soluble, gaseous monolayers; the addition of two more carbon atoms causes myristic acid (*n*-tetradecanoic acid) to exhibit a condensed gaseous phase region as well as an expanded phase, and further increase in the hydrocarbon chain length results in the additional formation of the solid phase. Replacement of the hydrogen atoms of the alkyl chain with a halogen such as fluorine also affects the type of monolayer. Monolayers containing fluorocarbon chains are more stable than those formed from their hydrocarbon counterparts and, because the fluorocarbon chain is more hydrophobic than a hydrocarbon chain, compounds with shorter chains are able to form insoluble monolayers. Similarly, changes in the polarity, size and shape of the head group can influence the arrangements of the hydrocarbon chains and hence the monolayer

structure, as illustrated by early studies with alcohols, esters, amides, amines and nitriles.

Visualisation of monolayer structures

There has been considerable interest in probing the structure of films transferred from the water surface onto solid substrates, the *Langmuir–Blodgett (LB) films*. The usual method of depositing a LB monolayer on to a hydrophilic substrate is to slowly raise the substrate upward through the monolayer-covered surface. A wide range of imaging techniques, including X-ray diffraction, neutron reflection, infrared and Raman spectroscopy, fluorescence microscopy and atomic force microscopy, have recently been used to study the structures formed in monolayers both *in situ* on the water surface and after deposition on to solid surfaces as LB films (see reviews by Peng *et al.*[4] and Dynarowicz-Łatka *et al.*[5]). Flanders and co-workers[6] used atomic force microscopy (AFM) to visualise the disorder induced in a monolayer of palmitic acid (PA) when increasing amounts of a peptide (the 25-peptide amino terminus of lung surfactant protein B, SP-B$_{1-25}$) were added. Elliptically shaped liquid expanded (LE) domains roughly 10 μm in diameter were shown to coexist with liquid condensed (LC) phase in monolayers containing 5 wt% peptide. When the peptide content was increased to 10 wt% the LE phase existed as a sheet-like region that covered more than one-third of the area of the image and contained clover-shaped LC domains roughly 5 μm in dimension. AFM images at peptide contents of 15 and 20 wt% showed the existence of a broad, sheet-like region of LE phase containing circular (approximately 20 μm diameter) LC regions with uniformly smooth boundaries.

Polymer monolayers

Monolayers of polymers and proteins lack the characteristic features described in the previous section. Most produce smooth curves, typical of those for gaseous monolayers of amphiphiles.

Lung surfactant monolayers

Lung surfactant is a lipid–protein complex secreted as vesicles or other aggregates by type II pneumocytes into the thin aqueous layer that covers the alveoli; it spontaneously adsorbs from the aggregates to form a film at the air–water interface, which acts to control surface tension during breathing.[7] Lung surfactant is a complex mixture of lipids and proteins consisting of 78–90% phospholipid, 5–10% protein and 4–10% neutral lipid. Phosphatidylcholine is by far the most abundant component of lung surfactant accounting for 70–80% of total lipid. About 50–70% of the phosphatidylcholine is dipalmitoylphosphatidylcholine (DPPC) but other saturated and unsaturated phosphatidylcholines are present as well as other phospholipid classes. The neutral lipids are mainly accounted for by cholesterol. There are four specific surfactant-associated proteins, SP-A, SP-B, SP-C and SP-D, which are closely associated with the membrane and play varied roles in modifying its physical properties.

The different components of lung surfactant interact to determine the overall behaviour of the surfactant film. Maintenance of a stable surface film requires efficient transfer of phospholipids between the extracellular large aggregate surfactant pool and the air–liquid interface. This process involves rapid insertion of phospholipids into the expanding film during inhalation followed by tight phospholipid packing and partial exclusion from the compressed film during exhalation. Rigid monolayers formed by DPPC alone can provide the necessary low surface tension (less than 5 mN m^{-1}) on compression of the alveolar interface that accompanies exhalation. However, pure DPPC is not able to spread rapidly

enough to cover the greatly enlarged interface that is formed when the lungs expand during inhalation. The re-spreading of the film is greatly enhanced by the presence of the neutral lipids and the surfactant proteins. In particular, the presence of SP-B has been correlated to the high compressibility and reversible re-spreading properties required for proper functioning of the membrane. SP-B is a relatively small (mol wt ~8700 Da), very hydrophobic amphipathic protein which is found in mammalian lung surfactant as a disulfide-linked dimer consisting of alpha-helices. Studies on model lung surfactant systems have led to the view that SP-B readily penetrates and fluidises the lipid membrane so that the liquid-expanded phase survives at higher degrees of compression. The effect of synthetic SP-B derived peptides on the surface pressure–area plots of monolayers formed from mixtures of DPPC and palmitoyloleoylphosphatidylglycerol (POPG) is shown in Fig. 5.13; increasing amounts of the SP-B peptides result in a more liquid-expanded film.[8]

 Clinical point

The lung surfactant membrane comprises a complex mixture of lipids and proteins that act to lower the surface tension of the alveolar air–water interface, thus facilitating the large surface area changes that occur during the successive compression–expansion cycles that accompany the breathing process. When formation of this membrane is incomplete, as may occur for example in prematurely born infants suffering from respiratory distress syndrome, breathing is laboured and there is insufficient transport of oxygen into the bloodstream.

5.2.7 Pharmaceutical applications of surface film studies

Study of polymers used as packaging materials and film coatings

Packaging materials must protect the drug without altering in any way the composition of the product.

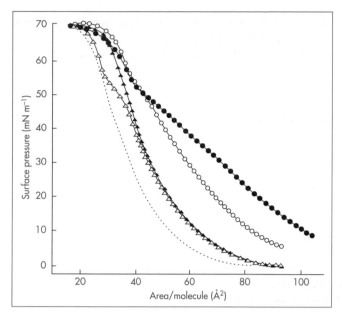

Figure 5.13 Effect of SP-B-derived peptide (N-term helix 1,2) on the surface pressure versus area per molecule plots of monolayers of 7:3 dipalmitoylphosphatidylcholine–palmitoyloleoylphosphatidylglycerol showing a more expanded monolayer with increasing amount of added peptide. Key: ···, 0; ▲, 1.3; △, 6.5; ○, 13; ●, 26% peptide. Note: 1 Å^2 = 0.01 nm^2.

Redrawn from Serrano AG *et al.*, Critical structure-function determinants within the N-terminal region of pulmonary surfactant protein SP-B, *Biophys J*, 2006; 90: 238–249 with permission of Elsevier.

One problem is that of adsorption of constituents, for example preservatives, from the drug product (see section 5.2.8). The permeability of the packing material to gases or liquids should also be considered, since this may result in deterioration of the product due to oxidation, hydrolysis or loss of volatile ingredients. Monolayers are useful models by which the properties of polymers used as packaging materials can be investigated.

Several methods have been employed in the determination of the resistance of monolayers to evaporation. The evaporation rate may be determined from the increase in mass of a desiccant suspended over the monolayer, or from the loss of weight of a Petri dish containing solution and spread monolayer, under carefully controlled conditions. Such experiments are useful in determining the effect on permeability of incorporation of a plasticiser into the polymer structure.[9]

Polymer monolayers have been used as models to assess the suitability of new polymers and of polymer mixtures as potential enteric and film coatings for solid dosage forms. The effects of substrate pH on the properties of three esters of cellulose, namely, cellulose acetate phthalate (Cellacefate), cellulose acetate butyrate, and cellulose acetate stearate have been examined. Monolayers of the butyrate and stearate esters were virtually unaffected by changes of pH of the substrate from 3 to 6.5. Condensed films were formed at both pH values, indicating that disintegration in either the stomach or small intestine would be prevented. Neither of these cellulose esters would therefore be of use as enteric coatings. The phthalate ester, on the other hand, formed a much more condensed monolayer at pH 3 than at pH 6.5 (Fig. 5.14). The conformational changes of this ester suggested its suitability as an enteric coating: the more tightly packed film at low pH would restrict dissolution in the stomach, whereas the more expanded film at higher pH would allow penetration of water and tablet disintegration in the small intestine where the environmental pH is approximately 6.

Cell membrane models

Phospholipid monolayers provide useful models for studying drug–lipid interactions as we can see from the following recent example[10], which explores the interaction of the phenothiazine drugs trifluoperazine (TFP) and chlorpromazine (CPZ) with the anionic

Figure 5.14 Surface pressure, π, versus area per molecule, A, for cellulose acetate phthalate (CAP) spread on an aqueous substrate, showing a more condensed monolayer at a substrate pH of 3 than at pH 6.5.

Reproduced with permission from Zatz JL, Knowles B, *J Pharm Sci*, 1970; 57: 1188.

glycerophospholipid dipalmitoylphosphatidylglycerol (DPPG). The surface pressure isotherms of Fig. 5.15 show interesting differences in the interaction of the two drugs with this phospholipid. Incorporation of CPZ expands the monolayer and an additional phase transition appears at higher drug concentrations; at high surface pressures there is little increase in area, suggesting that this drug is being excluded from the interface. TFP also expands the monolayer, although there is no appearance of an additional phase transition; the increase of area per molecule is noted even at high surface pressures, indicating that this drug remains in the monolayer. The considerable expansion of the monolayer observed even at relatively low drug/phospholipid ratios for both systems suggests that phospholipid molecules not in immediate contact with the drug are affected by incorporation of the drug into the monolayer. This 'cooperative effect', which is thought to be a consequence of either a significant reorientation and different packing of the DPPG

molecules or a change in their hydration state, may explain why drugs such as these with relatively nonspecific effects on the membrane are highly effective at very low concentrations.

Cholesterol monolayers are also used to model drug–membrane interactions. Figure 5.16 shows the surface pressure–area isotherms for equimolar mixtures of valinomycin (a cyclic peptide), which orientates horizontally at the air–solution interface to give an expanded film, and cholesterol, which orientates vertically giving a solid film. The shape of the mixed isotherm at low and intermediate pressures is similar to that of valinomycin, while the behaviour at high surface pressures is similar to that of cholesterol, suggesting that the valinomycin has been squeezed out of the mixed film. The position of the mixed curve to the left of the calculated average curve suggests some form of interaction between the components that condenses the mixed film.

Figure 5.15 Surface pressure isotherms for mixed monolayers of dipalmitoylphosphatidylglycerol (DPPG) and (a) trifluoperazine (TFP) and (b) chlorpromazine (CPZ) for a range of drug/phospholipid molar ratios.

Reproduced with permission from Hidalgo AA *et al., Biophys Chem*, 2004, 109: 85.

5.2.8 Adsorption at the solid–liquid interface

The term *adsorption* is used to describe the process of accumulation at an interface. Adsorption is essentially a surface effect and should be distinguished from *absorption*, which implies the penetration of one component throughout the bulk of a second. The distinction between the two processes is not always clear-cut, however, and in such cases the noncommittal word *sorption* is sometimes used.

There are two general types of adsorption: physical adsorption, in which the adsorbate is bound to the surface through weak van der Waals forces, and chemical adsorption or *chemisorption*, which involves the stronger valence forces. Of the two processes, chemisorption is the more specific, and usually involves an

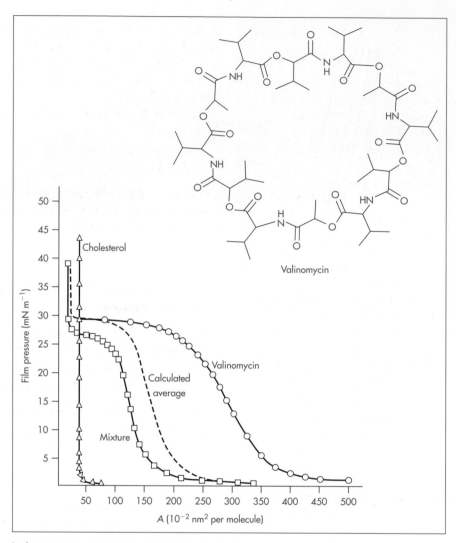

Figure 5.16 Surface pressure–area isotherms for cholesterol, valinomycin and an equimolar mixture of the two.

Reproduced with permission from Reiss HE, Swift HS, *J Colloid Interface Sci*, 1978; 64: 111.

ion-exchange process. Frequently both physical and chemical adsorption may be involved in a particular adsorption process. This is the case with the adsorption of toxins in the stomach by attapulgite and kaolin: there is both chemisorption involving cation exchange with the basic groups of the toxins and physical adsorption of the remainder of the molecule.

Adsorption isotherms

The study of adsorption from solution is experimentally straightforward. A known mass of the adsorbent material is shaken with a solution of known concentration at a fixed temperature. The concentration of the supernatant solution is determined by either physical or chemical means and the experiment is continued until no further change in the concentration of the supernatant is observed, that is, until equilibrium conditions have been established. Equations originally derived for the adsorption of gases on solids are generally used in the interpretation of the data, the Langmuir and Freundlich equations being the most commonly used.

Key points

- Insoluble amphiphilic compounds may form films when injected on to water surfaces using volatile solvents. An important difference between these insoluble monolayers and the films produced when surfactant molecules accumulate spontaneously at the surface of surfactant solutions is that the molecules of the insoluble monolayers remain in the surface film and are not in equilibrium with surfactant molecules in the bulk of the solution as they are in surfactant solutions.

- Insoluble films may be tightly packed, as in solid (or condensed) films, or more loosely packed, as in liquid (or expanded) and gaseous films. The three types of film are identified from plots of surface pressure against area per molecule derived from measurements using a Langmuir trough. Many factors, including external factors such as temperature and also modifications to the molecular structure, influence the type of monolayer formed.

- Films formed by lung surfactants at the alveolar air–water interface facilitate the large surface area changes that occur during the successive compression–expansion cycles that accompany the breathing process.

- Surface film studies are useful when selecting polymers for use as packaging materials and as film coatings, and in the study of models of the cell membrane.

Langmuir equation

When applied to adsorption from solution, the Langmuir equation becomes

$$\frac{x}{m} = \frac{abc}{1 + bc} \tag{5.16}$$

where x is the amount of solute adsorbed by a weight, m, of adsorbent, c is the concentration of solution at

equilibrium, b is a constant related to the enthalpy of adsorption, and a is related to the surface area of the solid. Figure 5.17 shows a typical Langmuir isotherm for the adsorption of the antidepressant drug amitriptyline on carbon black.

Equation (5.16) can be arranged into the linear form

$$\frac{c}{x/m} = \frac{1}{ab} + \frac{c}{a} \tag{5.17}$$

Values of a and b may be determined from the intercept and slope of plots of $c/(x/m)$ against concentration as shown in Example 5.4.

Example 5.4 Use of the Langmuir equation

Calculate the Langmuir constants for the adsorption of amitriptyline on carbon black using the following data (taken from Fig. 5.17)

$10^3\,x/m$ (mol g^{-1})	0.75	0.95	1.10	1.25	1.40	1.55	1.65
$10^4\,c$ (mol dm^{-3})	0.25	0.40	0.60	0.70	1.10	1.35	1.95
$10^2\,c/(x/m)$ (g dm^{-3})	3.33	4.21	5.45	5.60	7.86	8.71	11.82

Answer

The gradient of the plot of $c/(x/m)$ against c (see Fig. 5.18) $= 4.88 \times 10^2\,\text{g mol}^{-1} = 1/a$. Therefore,

$$a = 1/\text{gradient} = 2.05 \times 10^{-3}\,\text{mol g}^{-1}$$

Intercept $= 2.35 \times 10^{-2} = 1/ab$. Therefore,

$$b = 1/(2.35 \times 10^{-2} \times 2.05 \times 10^{-3})$$
$$= 2.07 \times 10^4\,\text{dm}^3\,\text{mol}^{-1}$$

The value of a is a measure of the adsorptive capacity of the adsorbent for the particular adsorbate under examination. Table 5.2 gives the adsorptive capacity of carbon black for a series of antidepressant and phenothiazine drugs, arranged in order of decreasing degree of adsorption.

Figure 5.17 Langmuir adsorption isotherm of amitriptyline on carbon black from aqueous solution at 30 °C.

Reproduced with permission from Nambu N *et al.*, *Chem Pharm Bull*, 1975; 23: 1404.

Deviations from the typical Langmuir plot can occur at high concentrations and are then usually attributed to the formation of multilayers.

Freundlich equation

The Freundlich equation is generally written in the form:

$$\frac{x}{m} = ac^{1/n} \qquad (5.18)$$

where a and n are constants, the form $1/n$ being used to emphasise that c is raised to a power less than unity. $1/n$ is a dimensionless parameter and is related to the intensity of drug adsorption. Equation (5.18) can be written in a linear form by taking logarithms of both sides, giving

$$\log(x/m) = \log a + (1/n)\log c \qquad (5.19)$$

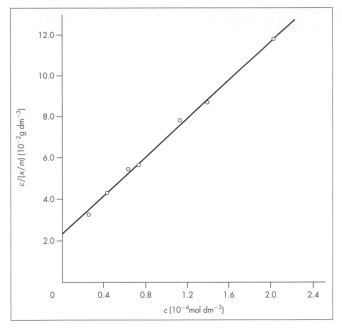

Figure 5.18 Adsorption of amitriptyline by carbon black plotted according to equation (6.17) using the data from Fig. 5.17.

A plot of $\log(x/m)$ against $\log c$ should be linear, with an intercept of $\log a$ and gradient of $1/n$; it is generally assumed that, for systems that obey this equation, adsorption results in the formation of multi-layers rather than a single monolayer. Figure 5.19 shows Freundlich isotherms for the adsorption of local anaesthetics on activated carbon; the method of calculating the constants a and $1/n$ from these plots is given in Example 5.5.

Example 5.5 Use of the Freundlich equation

The following data refer to the adsorption of tetracaine from aqueous solution at 25°C on to a sample of activated charcoal:

Equilibrium conc. ($mg\,dm^{-3}$)	0.155	0.468	1.259	2.510	5.370
Amount adsorbed ($mg\,g^{-1}$)	202.8	217.8	232.0	243.2	254.7

Show that these data can be represented by the Freundlich isotherm and calculate the constants a and $1/n$.

Answer

Plot a graph of $\log(x/m)$ against $\log c$, noting that the data for the amount adsorbed are given per gram of carbon (x/m). This graph is linear, showing that the data can be represented by the Freundlich equation.

At $\log c = 0$, the value of $\log(x/m)$ interpolated from this graph is 2.359. Therefore,

$$a = 229\,mg\,g^{-1}$$

The gradient of this plot $= 0.065$. Therefore,

$$1/n = 0.065$$

Table 5.2 Langmuir constants *a* and *b* in the adsorption of antidepressants and phenothiazines by carbon black[a]

Drug	*a* ($10^3 \, mol \, kg^{-1}$)	*b* ($10^{-4} \, dm^3 \, mol^{-1}$)
Antidepressants		
Amitriptyline	2.05	2.07
Imipramine	1.80	1.48
Opipramol	1.51	1.77
Desipramine	1.36	4.70
Phenothiazines		
Promazine	1.70	3.36
Chlorpromazine	1.70	4.37
Isothipendyl	1.30	2.23
Chlorpromazine sulfoxide	1.13	3.18

[a] Reproduced from Nambu N et al., *Chem Pharm Bull*, 1975; 23: 1404.

Factors affecting adsorption

Solubility of the adsorbate

Solubility is an important factor affecting adsorption. In general, the extent of adsorption of a solute is inversely proportional to its solubility in the solvent from which adsorption occurs. This empirical rule is termed *Lundelius's rule*. There are numerous examples of the applicability of this rule; for example, in Lundelius's original work it was noted that the adsorption of iodine onto carbon from CCl_4, $CHCl_3$ and CS_2 was $1 : 2 : 4.5$, respectively. These ratios are close to the inverse ratios for the solubilities of iodine in the respective solvents. The effect of solubility on adsorption might be expected since, in order for adsorption to occur, solute–solvent bonds must first be broken. The greater the solubility, the stronger are these bonds and hence the smaller the extent of adsorption.

For homologous series, adsorption from solution increases as the series is ascended and the molecules become more hydrophobic. There is, for example, a good correlation between the Freundlich adsorption constant, $1/n$ (related to the extent of adsorption) and the molecular weight of the local anaesthetics discussed above (Figure 5.20). The data for phenobarbital deviated from this linear relationship possibly as a result of the difficulty of adhesion of the phenobarbital molecules to the carbon surface because the barbiturate ring and benzene ring are not aligned in the same plane.

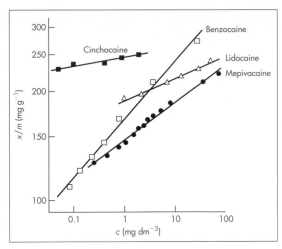

Figure 5.19 Freundlich adsorption isotherms of local anaesthetics on activated carbon at pH 7.0 and 25 °C.

Reproduced with permission from Abe I et al., *J Pharm Sci*, 1990; 79: 354.

pH

pH affects adsorption for a variety of reasons, the most important from a pharmaceutical viewpoint being its effect on the ionisation and solubility of the adsorbate drug molecule. In general, for simple molecules adsorption increases as the ionisation of the drug is suppressed, the extent of adsorption reaching a

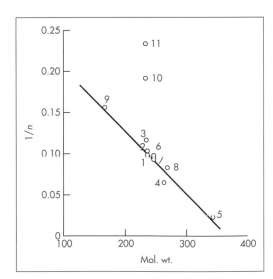

Figure 5.20 Relationship between the Freundlich adsorption constant, $1/n$, and the molecular weight for (1) procaine, pH 7; (2) procaine, pH 11; (3) lidocaine, pH 7; (4) tetracaine, pH 7; (5) cinchocaine, pH 7; (6) mepivacaine, pH 6.6; (7) mepivacaine, pH 8.6; (8) chloroprocaine, pH 7; (9) benzocaine, pH 7; (10) phenobarbital, pH 7; (11) phenobarbital, pH 9.

Reproduced with permission from Abe I et al., *J Pharm Sci*, 1990; 79: 354.

Figure 5.21 pH profile for the sorption of benzocaine by nylon 6 powder from buffered solutions at 30 °C and ionic strength 0.5 mol dm^{-3} (○) and the corresponding drug dissociation curve (●).

Reproduced with permission from Richards NE, Meakin BJ *J Pharm Pharmacol*, 1974; 26: 166.

maximum when the drug is completely un-ionised. Figure 5.21 shows that the pH profile for the sorption (this is not a true adsorption process) of benzocaine by nylon 6 powder is indeed almost super-imposable on the drug dissociation curve. For amphoteric compounds, adsorption is at a maximum at the isoelectric point, that is, when the compound bears a net charge of zero. In general, pH and solubility effects act in concert, since the un-ionised form of most drugs in aqueous solution has low solubility. Of the two effects, the solubility effect is usually the stronger. Thus, in the adsorption of hyoscine and atropine on magnesium trisilicate it was noted[11] that hyoscine, although in its completely un-ionised form, was less strongly adsorbed than atropine, which at the pH of the experiment was 50% ionised. The reason for this apparently anomalous result is clear when the solubilities of the two bases are considered. Hyoscine base is freely soluble (1 in 9.5 parts of water at 15°C) compared with atropine base (1 in 400 at 20°C). Even when 50% ionised, atropine is less soluble than hyoscine and consequently more strongly adsorbed.

Nature of the adsorbent

The physicochemical nature of the adsorbent can have profound effects on the rate and capacity for adsorption. The most important property affecting adsorption is the surface area of the adsorbent; the extent of adsorption is proportional to the specific surface area. Thus the more finely divided or the more porous the solid, the greater will be its adsorption capacity. Indeed, adsorption studies are frequently used to calculate the surface area of a solid.

Adsorbent–adsorbate interactions are of a complex nature and beyond the scope of this book. Particular adsorbents have affinities for particular adsorbates for a wide variety of reasons. The surfaces of adsorbent clays such as bentonite, attapulgite and kaolin carry cation-exchange sites, and such clays have strong affinities for protonated compounds, which they adsorb by an ion-exchange process. In many cases, different parts of the surface of the same adsorbent have different affinities for different types of adsorbents. There is evidence, for example, that anionic materials are adsorbed on the cationic edge of kaolin particles, while cationics are adsorbed on the cleavage surface of the particles, which are negatively charged. An example of the differing affinities of a series of adsorbents used an antacids is shown in Fig. 5.22. The adsorptive capacity of a particular

adsorbent often depends on the source from which it was prepared and also on its pretreatment.

Temperature

Since adsorption is generally an exothermic process, an increase in temperature normally leads to a decrease in the amount adsorbed. The changes in enthalpy of adsorption are usually of the order of those for condensation or crystallisation. Thus small variations in temperature tend not to alter the adsorption process to a significant extent.

Some medical and pharmaceutical applications and consequences of adsorption

Adsorption at the solid–liquid interface plays a crucial role in preparative and analytical chromatography, and in heterogeneous catalysis, water purification and solvent recovery. These applications are, however, outside the scope of this book and we will be concerned with examples of the involvement of adsorption in more medical and pharmaceutical situations.

 Clinical point

The 'universal antidote' for use in reducing the effects of poisoning by the oral route is composed of activated charcoal, magnesium oxide and tannic acid. A more recent use of adsorbents has been in dialysis to reduce toxic concentrations of drugs by passing blood through a haemodialysis membrane over charcoal and other adsorbents. Several drugs are adsorbed effectively by activated charcoal. These include chlorphenamine, dextropropoxyphene hydrochloride, colchicine, diphenylhydantoin and aspirin. Some of these are easily recognisable as surface-active molecules (chlorphenamine, dextropropoxyphene) and will be expected to adsorb onto solids. Highly ionised substances of low molecular weight are not well adsorbed, neither are drugs such as tolbutamide that are poorly soluble in acidic media. The formation of a monolayer of drug molecules covering the surface of the charcoal particles through nonpolar interactions is indicated.

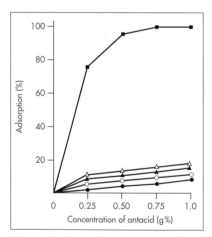

Figure 5.22 Adsorption of digoxin by some antacids at $37 \pm 0.1\,^{\circ}C$. (■) Magnesium trisilicate; (△) aluminium hydroxide gel BP (Aludrox was used in the concentration range 2.5–10%v/v); (▲) light magnesium oxide; (○) light magnesium carbonate; (●) calcium carbonate. Initial concentration of the glycoside: 0.25 mg%.

Reproduced with permission from Khalil SAH, *J Pharm Pharmacol*, 1974; 26: 961.

Adsorption of poisons/toxins

The direct application of *in vitro* data for estimating doses of activated charcoal for antidotal purposes may lead to use of inadequate amounts of adsorbent.[12] In an animal study, charcoal:drug ratios of 1:1, 2:1, 4:1 and 8:1 reduced absorption of drugs as follows: pentobarbital sodium, 7%, 38%, 62% and 89%; chloroquine phosphate 20%, 30%, 70% and 96%; isoniazid 1.2%, 7.2%, 35% and 80%. Activated charcoal, of course, is not effective in binding all poisons. Biological factors such as gastrointestinal motility, secretions and pH may influence charcoal adsorption. While 5 g of activated charcoal has been said to be capable of binding 8 g of aspirin *in vitro*[13], 30 g of charcoal *in vivo* was reported to inhibit the gastrointestinal absorption of 3 g of aspirin by only 50%.[14] The surface area of the charcoal is a factor in its effectiveness; charcoal tablets have been found to be approximately half as effective as powdered material.

Taste masking

The intentional adsorption of drugs such as diazepam onto solid substrates should be mentioned, the object being to minimise taste problems. Desorption of the drug *in vivo* is essential but should not occur during the shelf-life of the preparation. Desorption may be a rate-limiting step in absorption. Diazepam adsorbed onto an inorganic colloidal magnesium aluminium silicate (Veegum) had the same potency in experimental animals as a solution of the drug, but when adsorbed onto microcrystalline cellulose (Avicel) its efficacy was much reduced. Flocculation of the cellulose in the acidic environment of the stomach probably retards the desorption process.

Haemoperfusion

Carbon haemoperfusion is an extracorporeal method of treating cases of severe drug overdoses, and originally involved perfusion of the blood directly over charcoal granules. Although activated charcoal granules were very effective in adsorbing many toxic materials, they were found to give off embolising particles and also to lead to removal of blood platelets. Microencapsulation of activated charcoal granules by coating with biocompatible membranes such as acrylic hydrogels was found to be a successful means of eliminating charcoal embolism and to lead to a much reduced effect on platelet count. *In vitro* tests showed that the coated granules had a reduced adsorption rate although the adsorptive capacity was unchanged.[15] A large proportion of drug overdoses in Great Britain at one time involved barbiturates, and the applicability of carbon haemoperfusion in the treatment of such cases was demonstrated.[16] Many other drugs taken as overdoses are also present in the plasma at sufficiently high concentration to allow removal by this technique.

Adsorption in drug formulation

Examples of the adsorption of drugs and excipients on to solid surfaces are found in many aspects of drug formulation, some of which, for example the adsorption of surfactants and polymers in the stabilisation of suspensions, are considered elsewhere in this book (see section 6.4). An interesting approach to the improvement of the dissolution rate of poorly water-soluble drugs is to adsorb very small amounts of surfactant onto the drug surface. For example, the adsorption of Pluronic F127 onto the surface of the hydrophobic drug phenylbutazone significantly increased its dissolution rate when compared with untreated material.[17]

In addition to the beneficial use of surfactants in the preparation of formulations, we should also be aware of problems that can arise as a result of inadvertent adsorption occurring both in the manufacture and storage of the product and in its subsequent usage. Problems arising from the adsorption of medicaments by adsorbents such as antacids which may be taken simultaneously by the patient, or which may be present in the same formulation, are discussed in section 11.7. Problems also arise from the adsorption of medicaments onto the container walls. Containers for medicaments, whether glass or plastic, may adsorb a significant quantity of the drug or bacteriostatic or fungistatic agents present in the formulation and thereby affect the potency and possibly the stability of the product. The problem is particularly significant where the drug is highly surface active and present in low concentration. With plastic containers the process is often referred to as sorption rather than adsorption since it often involves significant penetration of the drug into the polymer matrix. Plastics are a large and varied group of materials and their properties are often modified by various additives, such as plasticisers, fillers and stabilisers (see Chapter 7). Such additives may have a pronounced effect on the sorption characteristics of the plastics. The sorption of the fungistatic agent sorbic acid from aqueous solution by plastic cellulose acetate and cellulose triacetate shows an appreciable pH dependence; the sorption declining to zero in the vicinity of the point of maximum ionisation of the sorbic acid. The sorption of local anaesthetics by polyamide and polyethylene depends on the kind of plastic, the reaction conditions and the chemical structure of the drugs. As with sorbic acid, significant sorption was observed only when the drugs were in their un-ionised forms.

Key points

- Adsorption of solutes on to solid surfaces from solution can occur by physical adsorption, involving weak van der Waals forces, or by a chemical process. Adsorption data can be analysed using the Langmuir equation or, if multilayer adsorption occurs, by the Freundlich equation.
- The extent of adsorption is influenced by pH mainly through its effect on ionisation of the solute; adsorption increases as the ionisation of the solute decreases and is at a maximum for an un-ionised compound. The greater the solubility of a solute in a particular solvent, the lower is the extent of its adsorption. The extent of adsorption is proportional to the surface area of the adsorbent; the more finely divided or the more porous the solid, the greater will be its adsorption capacity. An increase of temperature normally leads to a decrease in the amount adsorbed.
- The adsorption processes can be used advantageously, as in the removal of toxic drugs in the case of overdosing, or can cause problems, as in the unintentional adsorption of drugs by antacids from the gastrointestinal tract, or the adsorption of drugs on to the walls of the container.

5.3 Micellisation

As the concentration of aqueous solutions of many amphiphilic substances increases, there is a pronounced change in the physical properties of the solution. For example, we have seen in section 5.2.2 that an inflection appears in surface tension plots of

surfactant solutions at a critical concentration (the *critical micelle concentration*, cmc) which is attributable to the self-association of the amphiphile into small aggregates called *micelles*. Similar inflection points are observed when other physical properties such as solubility, conductivity, osmotic pressure and light scattering intensity are plotted as a function of concentration (see Fig. 5.23).

The idea that molecules should come together at a critical concentration to form aggregates in solution was quite controversial when first proposed by McBain in 1913, but the concept of micellisation has long gained universal acceptance. The micelles are in dynamic equilibrium with free molecules (monomers) in solution; that is, the micelles are continuously breaking down and reforming. It is this fact that distinguishes micellar solutions from other types of colloidal solution and this difference is emphasised by referring to micelle-forming compounds as *association colloids*.

The primary reason for micelle formation is the attainment of a state of minimum free energy. At low concentration, amphiphiles can achieve an adequate decrease in the overall free energy of the system by accumulation at the surface or interface, in such a way as to remove the hydrophobic group from the aqueous environment. As the concentration is increased, this method of free energy reduction becomes inadequate and the monomers form into

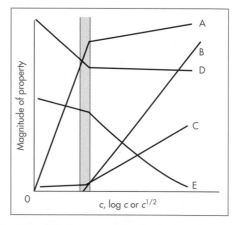

Figure 5.23 Solution properties of an ionic surfactant as a function of concentration, c. A, Osmotic pressure (against c); B, solubility of a water-insoluble solubilisate (against c); C, intensity of light scattered by the solution (against c); D, surface tension (against $\log c$); E, molar conductivity (against $c^{1/2}$).

micelles. The hydrophobic groups form the core of the micelle and so are shielded from the water.

The free energy change of a system is dependent on changes in both the entropy and the enthalpy; that is, $\Delta G = \Delta H - T\Delta S$. For a micellar system at normal temperatures the entropy term is by far the most important in determining the free energy changes ($T\Delta S$ constitutes approximately 90–95% of the ΔG value). Micelle formation entails the transfer of a hydrocarbon chain from an aqueous to a nonaqueous environment (the interior of the micelle). To understand the changes in enthalpy and entropy that accompany this process, we must first consider the structure of water itself.

5.3.1 Water structure and hydrophobic bonding

Water possesses many unique features that distinguish it from other liquids. These arise from the unusual structure of the molecule in which the O and H atoms are arranged at the apices of a triangle (see Fig. 5.24).

Each of the covalent bonds between a hydrogen atom and the oxygen atom of the water molecule involves the pairing of the electron of the hydrogen atom with an electron in the oxygen atom's outer shell of six electrons. This pairing leaves two lone pairs of electrons in the outer-shell, the orbitals of which point to the vertices of an approximately regular tetrahedron formed by the lone pairs and the OH bonds. The resulting tetrahedral structure has two positively charged sites at one side and two negatively charged sites at the other. It will readily attach itself by hydrogen bonds to four neighbouring molecules, two at the negatively charged sites and two at the positively charged sites. In its usual form, ice demonstrates an almost perfect tetrahedral arrangement of bonds with

a distance of about 0.276 nm between neighbouring oxygen atoms. There is much unfilled space in the crystal, which accounts for the low density of ice.

When ice melts, a high degree of hydrogen bonding persists in the resulting liquid. In spite of extensive investigation by a variety of techniques such as X-ray diffraction, thermochemical determination, infrared and Raman spectroscopy, the structural nature of liquid water is still to be completely resolved. There are, broadly speaking, two distinct types of model: those that involve distortion but not breaking of hydrogen bonds, and a second type in which unbonded detached water molecules exist in addition to the hydrogen-bonded structures. Of the former type, the model that is considered to be the most acceptable is one in which all the water molecules continue to be hydrogen-bonded to their four neighbours, but the intermolecular links are bent or stretched to give an irregular framework. Such distorted networks are known to exist in some of the denser forms of ice.

Many proposed structures for water involve mixtures of structured material and free water molecules. One of the most highly developed theories encompasses the so-called 'flickering cluster' concept of water structure. The model is based on the cooperative nature of hydrogen bonding. The formation of one hydrogen bond on a water molecule leaves the molecule more susceptible to further hydrogen bonding, and similarly when one bond breaks there is a tendency for large groups of bonds to break. As a result, clusters of ice-like hydrogen-bonded material are imagined to be suspended in a fluid of unbonded water (Fig. 5.25). Because of the continual formation and

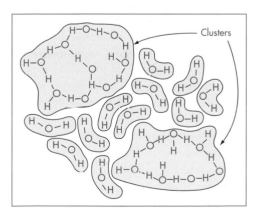

Figure 5.25 Water clusters with unassociated water molecules around them.

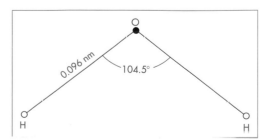

Figure 5.24 Diagram of the water molecule showing bond angle and length.

rupture of hydrogen bonds throughout the liquid, these clusters have only a temporary existence, and are aptly described by the term 'flickering'.

Most of the models proposed for the structure of water, only two of which have been considered here, can account for some, but not all of the physical and thermodynamic anomalies that have been observed with water.

The flickering cluster model can be used to describe possible structural changes that occur when nonpolar and polar solutes are dissolved in water. A nonpolar molecule or portion of a molecule tends to seek out the more ice-like regions within the water. Such regions, as we have seen, contain open structures into which the nonpolar molecules may fit without breaking hydrogen bonds or otherwise disturbing the surrounding ice-like material. In solution, therefore, hydrophobic molecules tend always to be surrounded by structured water. This concept is important in discussing interactions between nonpolar molecules in aqueous solution, such as those that occur in micelle formation. The interaction of hydrocarbons in aqueous solution was first thought to arise simply as consequence of the van der Waals forces between the hydrocarbon molecules. It was later realised, however, that changes in the water structure around the nonpolar groups must play an important role in the formation of bonds between the nonpolar molecules – the so-called *hydrophobic bonds*. In fact the contribution from the van der Waals forces is only about 45% of the total free energy of formation of a hydrophobic bond. When the nonpolar groups approach each other until they are in contact, there will be a decrease in the total number of water molecules in contact with the nonpolar groups. The formation of the hydrophobic bond in this way is thus equivalent to the partial removal of hydrocarbon from an aqueous environment and a consequent loss of the ice-like structuring that always surrounds the hydrophobic molecules. The increase in entropy and decrease in free energy that accompany the loss of structuring make the formation of the hydrophobic bond an energetically favourable process.

There is much experimental evidence to support this explanation for the decrease in ΔG. Thus the enthalpy of micelle formation becomes more negative as the temperature is increased, a fact which was attributed to a reduction in water structure as temperature is increased. Nuclear magnetic resonance (NMR) measurements indicate an increase in the mobility of water protons at the onset of micellisation. The addition of urea, a water-structure-breaking compound, to surfactant solutions leads to an increase of cmc, again indicating the role of water structure in the micellisation process. An alternative explanation of the free energy decrease emphasises the increase in internal freedom of the hydrocarbon chains that occurs when these chains are transferred from the aqueous environment, where their motion is restrained by the hydrogen-bonded water molecules, to the interior of the micelle. It has been suggested that the increased mobility of the hydrocarbon chains, and of course their mutual attraction, constitute the principal hydrophobic factor in micellisation.

5.3.2 Theories of micelle formation

Two general approaches have been employed in attempting to describe the process of micellisation. In one of these, the phase separation model, the cmc is assumed to represent the saturation concentration of the unassociated molecules and the micelles are regarded as a distinct phase that separates out at the cmc. In the alternative approach, the micelle and associated monomers are assumed to be in an association–dissociation equilibrium to which the law of mass action may be applied. Neither of these models is rigorously correct, although the mass action approach seems to give a more realistic description of micellisation, and thus will be considered in more detail.

The aggregation process may in its simplest form be described by

$$ND^+ + (N-p)X^- \rightleftharpoons M^{p+} \qquad (5.20)$$

Equation (5.20) represents the formation of a cationic micelle M^{p+} from N surfactant ions D^+ and $(N-p)$ firmly held counterions X^-. Whenever the thermodynamics of a process is under consideration, it is important to define the standard states of the species. In this example, the standard states are such that the mole fractions of the ionic species are unity and the solution properties are those of the infinitely dilute solutions. The equilibrium constant K_m may be written in the usual way,

$$K_m = \frac{[M^{p+}]}{[D^+]^N[X^-]^{N-p}} \tag{5.21}$$

where activity coefficients have been neglected. The analogous equation for nonionic micelles is of a simpler form since counterion terms and charges need not be considered.

$$K_m = \frac{[M]}{[D]^N} \tag{5.22}$$

Equations (5.21) and (5.22) are important in that they can be used to predict the variation of both monomers and micelles with total solution concentration.

Figure 5.26 shows the result of such a calculation for a model system. It illustrates several important points about the micellisation process. According to the mass action treatment, the monomer concentration decreases very slightly above the cmc: this is a very small effect (although it can be detected experimentally from very precise surface-tension measurements) and for most purposes it is reasonable to assume that the monomer concentration remains constant at the cmc value. A second point of interest illustrated by the mass action treatment concerns the predicted sharpness of the cmc. It is readily shown by calculations that combinations of low values of N and K_m lead to gradual changes of slope of the cmc region, while larger values for both of these parameters give sharp inflections. The cmc, rather than being an exact concentration, is often a range of concentration over which the

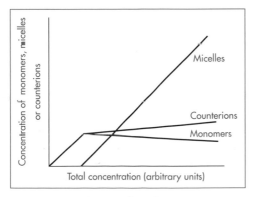

Figure 5.26 Concentration of micelles, monomers and counterions against total concentration (arbitrary units) calculated from equation (6.21) for an aggregation number (N) of 100, micellar equilibrium constant (K_m) of 1, and with 85% of the counterions bound to the micelle.

solution properties exhibit a gradual change and hence is often difficult to locate exactly.

5.3.3 Micellar structure

Critical packing parameter

The shape of the micelle formed by a particular surfactant is influenced to a large extent by the geometry of the surfactant molecule, as can be seen if we consider the packing of space-filling models of the surfactants. The dimensionless parameter of use in these considerations is called the *critical packing parameter* (CPP) and is defined as

$$CPP = \frac{v}{l_c a}$$

where v is the volume of one chain, a is the cross-sectional area of the surfactant head group and l_c is the extended length of the surfactant alkyl chain (see Fig. 5.27). This parameter provides a simple geometric characterisation of the surfactant molecule, which is useful when we consider the structure of the aggregate that will be formed in solution. Consideration of the packing of molecules into spheres shows that when CPP $\leq 1/3$, which is the case for surfactants having a single hydrophobic chain and a simple ionic or large nonionic head group, a spherical micelle will be formed. Most surfactants of pharmaceutical interest fall into this category. It is easily seen that if we double v by adding a second alkyl chain then the value of CPP will exceed 1/3 and nonspherical structures such as bilayers (CPP ≈ 1) will form in solution, from which vesicles are formed (see section 5.4.2). One important factor not considered in this simple geometrical model is the interaction between the head groups in the aggregate. The 'effective' cross-sectional area of the surfactant molecule is strongly influenced by the interaction forces between adjacent head groups in the micelle surface. These forces are decreased by addition of electrolyte, leading to a decrease of a, an increase of the CPP, and a change of shape of the aggregate, as discussed below.

In nonaqueous media, reverse (or inverted) micelles may form, in which the hydrophilic charge groups form the micellar core shielded from the nonaqueous environment by the hydrophobic chains; such structures are generally formed when CPP > 1 (see Fig. 5.27).

(a) Micelles when CPP $\leq 1/3$

(b) Bilayers when CPP ≈ 1

(c) Reverse micelles when CPP > 1

Figure 5.27 Influence of the critical packing parameter, CPP ($v/l_c a$), on the type of aggregate formed by surfactants in solution.

Ionic micelles

As we have seen from consideration of the simple geometrical packing model, charged micelles of low aggregation number have a CPP $< 1/3$ and consequently adopt a spherical or near-spherical shape at concentrations not too far removed from the cmc. The hydrophobic part of the amphiphile is located in the core or the micelle. Around this core is a concentric shell of hydrophilic head groups with $(1 - \alpha)N$ counterions, where α is the degree of ionisation. This compact region is termed the *Stern layer* (see Fig. 5.28). For most ionic micelles the degree of ionisation α is between 0.2 and 0.3; that is, 70–80% of the counterions may be considered to be bound to the micelles.

The outer surface of the Stern layer is the shear surface of the micelle. The core and the Stern layer together constitute what is termed the *kinetic micelle*. Surrounding the Stern layer is a diffuse layer called the *Gouy–Chapman electrical double layer*, which contains the αN counterions required to neutralise the charge on the kinetic micelle. The thickness of the double layer is dependent on the ionic strength of the solution and is greatly compressed in the presence of electrolyte.

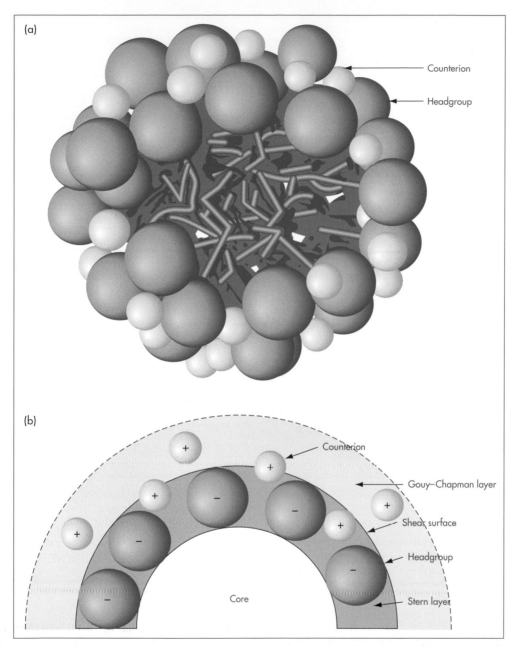

Figure 5.28 (a) Diagrammatic representation of a spherical ionic micelle and (b) partial cross-section of an anionic micelle showing charged layers.

In highly concentrated solution, a gradual change in micellar shape is thought to occur with many ionic systems, the micelles elongating to form cylindrical structures (see Fig. 5.29).

Nonionic micelles

In general, nonionic surfactants form larger micelles than their ionic counterparts. The reason for this is clearly attributable to the removal of electrical work that must be done when a monomer of an ionic surfactant is added to an existing charged micelle. As a consequence of the larger size, the nonionic micelles are frequently asymmetric. The micelles of Cetomacrogol 1000 ($C_{16}H_{33}(OCH_2CH_2)_{21}OH$, abbreviated to $C_{16}E_{21}$), for example, are thought to be ellipsoidal with an axial ratio not exceeding $2:1$.

Figure 5.29 Elongation of a spherical micelle to form a cylindrical micelle at high concentration.

Nonionic micelles have a hydrophobic core surrounded by a shell of oxyethylene chains, which is often termed the *palisade layer* (Fig. 5.30). This layer is capable of mechanically entrapping a considerable number of water molecules, as well as those that are hydrogen-bonded to the oxyethylene chains. Micelles of nonionic surfactants tend, as a consequence, to be highly hydrated. The outer surface of the palisade layer forms the shear surface; that is, the hydrating molecules form part of the kinetic micelle.

5.3.4 Factors affecting the critical micelle concentration and micellar size

Structure of the hydrophobic group

The hydrophobic group plays an important role in determining the type of association of the amphiphile. Compounds with rigid aromatic or heteroaromatic ring structures (many dyes, purines and pyrimidines, for example) associate by a nonmicellar process involving the face-to-face stacking of molecules one on top of the other, rather than by

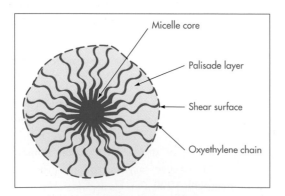

Figure 5.30 Diagrammatic representation of the cross-section of a nonionic micelle.

micellisation. Such systems do not exhibit cmcs. Association usually commences at very low concentrations and growth of aggregates may occur by the stepwise addition of monomers. Consequently, the aggregates continuously increase in size rather than attain an equilibrium size as in micellisation. Some drugs are thought to associate in this manner[1,2].

Micellar amphiphiles of the most common type have hydrophobic groups constructed from hydrocarbon chains. Increase in length of this chain results in a decrease in cmc, and for compounds with identical polar head groups this relationship is expressed by the linear equation

$$\log[\text{cmc}] = A - Bm \tag{5.23}$$

where m is the number of carbon atoms in the chain and A and B are constants for a homologous series. A corresponding increase in micellar size with increase in hydrocarbon chain length is also noted.

Many drugs are surface active and form small micelles in aqueous solution. For these and other amphiphiles with more complex hydrophobic regions, the effect of substituents on hydrophobicity can be roughly estimated from Table 4.4 (section 4.2.1). In the series of micellar diphenylmethane drugs shown in Table 5.3 there is an increased hydrophobicity (as evidenced by a decrease in cmc and increase in aggregation number) following the introduction of $-CH_3$, $-Br$ and $-Cl$ substituents to the hydrophobic ring systems.

Nature of the hydrophilic group

The most important point to be noted here is the pronounced difference in properties between amphiphiles with ionic hydrophilic groups and those in which this group is uncharged. In general, nonionic surfactants

Table 5.3 Effect of substituents on the micellar properties of some diphenylmethane drugs[a]

Drug	R[1]	R[2]	R[3]	Critical micellar concentration $(mol\,kg^{-1})$	Micellar aggregation number
Diphenhydramine	H	H	H	0.132	3
Orphenadrine	H	CH_3	H	0.096	7
Bromodiphenhydramine	Br	H	H	0.053	11
Chlorphenoxamine	Cl	H	CH_3	0.045	13

[a] Reproduced from Attwood D, *J Pharm Pharmacol*, 1972; 24: 751; 1976; 28: 407.

have very much lower cmc values and higher aggregation numbers than their ionic counterparts with similar hydrocarbon chains, mainly because the micellisation process for such compounds does not involve any electrical work.

The properties of the polyoxyethylated nonionic surfactants show a pronounced dependence on the length of the polyoxyethylene chain. An increase in the chain length confers a greater hydrophilicity to the molecule and the cmc increases, as shown in Table 5.4.

Nature of the counterion

The counterion associated with the charged group of ionic surfactants has a significant effect on the micellar properties. There is an increase in micellar size for a particular cationic surfactant as the counterion is changed according to the series $Cl^- < Br^- < I^-$, and for a particular anionic surfactant according to $Na^+ < K^+ < Cs^+$. Generally, the more weakly hydrated a counterion, the larger the micelles formed by the surfactant. This is because the weakly hydrated ions can be adsorbed more readily in the micellar surface and so decrease the charge repulsion between the polar groups. A greater depression of cmc and a greater increase in micellar size is noted with organic counterions such as maleates, than with inorganic ions.

Addition of electrolytes

Addition of electrolytes to ionic surfactants decreases the cmc and increases the micellar size. The effect is simply explained in terms of a reduction in the magnitude of the forces of repulsion between the charged

Table 5.4 Values of cmc and micellar weights of hexadecyl polyoxyethylene ethers $CH_3(CH_3)_{15}(CH_2CH_2)_nOH$[a]

Property	n =					
	6	7	9	12	15	21
10^6 cmc $(mol\,kg^{-1})$	1.7	1.7	2.1	2.3	3.1	3.9
10^{-5} Micellar weight	12.3	3.27	1.4	1.17	–	0.82
Aggregation number	2430	590	220	150	–	70

[a] Reproduced from Elworthy PH, Macfarlane CB, *J Chem Soc*, 1963: 907; 1962: 537.

Table 5.5 Effect of electrolyte on the micellar properties of dodecyltrimethylammonium bromide $CH_3(CH_2)_{11}N^+(CH_3)_3Br^-$ [a]

NaCl concentration (mol dm^{-3})	Critical micellar concentration (mol dm^{-3})	Aggregation number
0.00	0.014 6	61
0.10	0.004 28	74
0.50	0.001 71	90

[a] Reproduced from Anacker EW, in: Jungermann E, ed., *Cationic Surfactants*, New York: Marcel Dekker; 1970.

head groups in the micelle and a consequent decrease in the electrical work of micellisation. At sufficiently high electrolyte concentration the reduction of head group interaction is sufficient to increase CPP to such an extent that spherical micelles can no longer form. Table 5.5 shows the effect of sodium chloride addition on the micellar properties of the cationic surfactant dodecyltrimethylammonium bromide. The micellar properties of nonionic surfactants, in contrast, are little affected by electrolyte addition.

Effect of temperature

If aqueous solutions of many nonionic surfactants are heated, they become turbid at a characteristic temperature called the *cloud point* (see Fig. 5.33 in section 5.4). Other nonionic surfactants have cloud points above 100°C. The process is reversible; that is, cooling the solution restores clarity. The turbidity at the cloud point is due to separation of the solution into two phases. At temperatures up to the cloud point, an increase in micellar size and a corresponding decrease in cmc is noted for many nonionic surfactants (Fig. 5.31). The cloud point is very sensitive to additives in the system, which can increase or decrease the clouding temperature.

Temperature has a comparatively small effect on the micellar properties of ionic surfactants. The temperature dependence of the cmc of sodium lauryl (dodecyl) sulfate shown in Fig. 5.31 is typical of the effect observed.

  Key points

- Micelles form at the critical micelle concentration, which has a characteristic value for a particular surfactant under a given set of conditions. Micelles are in dynamic equilibrium with free molecules of surfactant in solution, that is, they are continuously breaking down and reforming. The main driving force for the formation of micelles is the increase of entropy that occurs when the hydrophobic regions of the surfactant are removed from water and the ordered structure of the water molecules around this region of the molecule is lost.
- An increase in hydrophobic chain length causes a decrease in the cmc and increase of size of ionic and nonionic micelles; an increase of polyoxyethylene chain length has the opposite effect on these properties in nonionic micelles. Electrolyte addition to micellar solutions of ionic surfactants reduces the cmc and increases the micellar size, sometimes causing a change of shape from sphere to ellipsoids. Solutions of some nonionic surfactants become cloudy on heating and separate reversibly into two phases at the cloud point.
- The core of the micelle contains the hydrophobic region of the surfactant. The core of ionic micelles is surrounded by a concentric shell (the Stern layer) that encloses the charged head groups and about 70–80% of the counterions. Surrounding the Stern layer is a diffuse layer (the Gouy–Chapman layer) that contains the remaining counterions. The core of nonionic micelles is surrounded by a shell of oxyethylene chains (the palisade layer), which contains entrapped water.

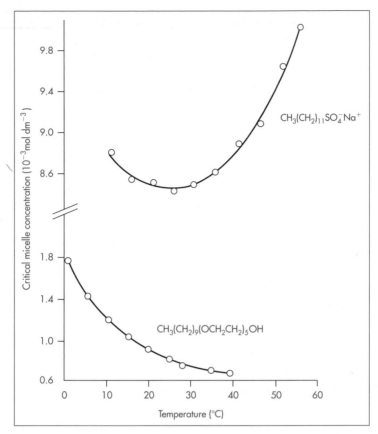

Figure 5.31 Variation of cmc with temperature for sodium dodecyl sulfate ($CH_3(CH_2)_{11}SO_4^-$ Na^+) and pentaoxyethylene glycol monodecyl ether ($CH_3(CH_2)_9(OCH_2CH_2)_5OH$).

Modified with permission from Goddard ED, Benson GC, *Can J Chem*, 1957; 35: 986.

5.4 Liquid crystals and surfactant vesicles

5.4.1 Liquid crystals

Lyotropic liquid crystals

Surfactant solutions at concentrations close to the cmc are clear and isotropic; that is, the magnitudes of such physical properties as viscosity and refractive index do not depend on the direction in which these properties are measured. As the concentration is increased, there is frequently a transition from the typical spherical micellar structure to a more elongated or rod-like micelle. Further increase in concentration may cause the orientation and close packing of the elongated micelles into hexagonal arrays. A new phase containing these ordered arrays separates out from the remainder of the solution, which

contains randomly orientated rods, but remains in equilibrium with it. This new phase is a liquid crystalline state termed the *middle phase* or *hexagonal phase*. With some surfactants, further increase of concentration results in the separation of a second liquid crystalline state, the *neat phase* or *lamellar phase*. In some surfactant systems another liquid crystalline state, the *cubic phase*, occurs between the middle and neat phases. The most common type of cubic phase is the micellar cubic phase formed by the close packing of spherical micelles; a more complex cubic phase, the bicontinuous cubic phase, occurs with some amphiphilic lipids such as glyceryl monooleate (see section 5.4.2). Finally, in all systems, surfactant separates out of solution. The liquid crystalline phases that occur on increasing the concentration of surfactant solutions are referred to as *lyotropic* liquid crystals; their structure is shown diagrammatically in Fig. 5.32. The phase diagram in Fig. 5.33 shows the transition from micellar solution to liquid crystalline phase and finally to pure amphiphile for the polyoxyethylated nonionic surfactant $C_{12}E_6$ [$CH_3(CH_2)_{11}(OCH_2CH_2)_6OH$].

Liquid crystals are anisotropic; that is, their physical properties vary with direction of measurement. The middle phase, for example, will flow only in a direction parallel to the long axis of the arrays. It is rigid in the other two directions. On the other hand, the neat phase is more fluid and behaves as a solid only in the direction perpendicular to that of the layers. Similarly, plane-polarised light is rotated when travelling along any axis except the long axis in the middle phase and a direction perpendicular to the layers in the neat phase. Because of this ability to rotate polarised light, the liquid crystals are visible when placed between crossed polarisers, and this provides a useful means of detecting the liquid crystalline state.

Thermotropic liquid crystals

A second category of liquid crystals is the type produced when certain substances, notably the esters of cholesterol, are heated. These systems are referred to as *thermotropic* liquid crystals and, although not formed by surfactants, their properties will be described here for purposes of comparison. The formation of a cloudy liquid when cholesteryl benzoate is heated to temperatures between 145 and 179°C was first noted in 1888 by the Austrian botanist, Reinitzer. The name 'liquid crystal' was applied to this cloudy intermediate phase because of the presence of areas with crystal-like molecular structure within this solution.

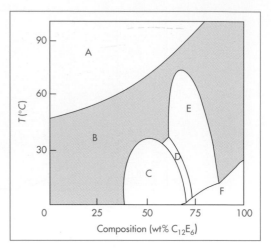

Figure 5.33 Phase diagram of the $CH_3(CH_2)_{11}(OCH_2CH_2)_6OH$ ($C_{12}E_6$)–H_2O system: A, two isotropic liquid phases; B, micellar solution; C, middle or hexagonal phase; D, cubic phase; E, neat or lamellar phase; F, solid phase. The boundary between phases A and B is the cloud point.

Modified from Clunie JS *et al.*, *Trans Farad Soc*, 1969; 65: 287.

Although the compounds that form thermotropic liquid crystalline phases are of a variety of chemical types such as azo compounds, azoxy compounds or esters, the molecular geometries of the molecule have some characteristic features in that they are generally elongated, flat and rigid along their axes. The presence of easily polarisable groups often enhances liquid crystal formation.

The arrangement of the elongated molecules in thermotropic liquid crystals is generally recognisable as one of three principal types: namely, *smectic* (soap-like), *nematic* (thread-like) and *cholesteric*. The molecular arrays are illustrated diagrammatically in Fig. 5.34.

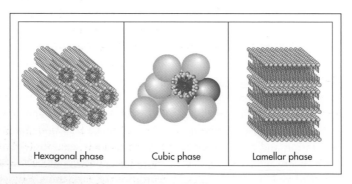

| Hexagonal phase | Cubic phase | Lamellar phase |

Figure 5.32 Diagrammatic representation of forms of lyotropic liquid crystals.

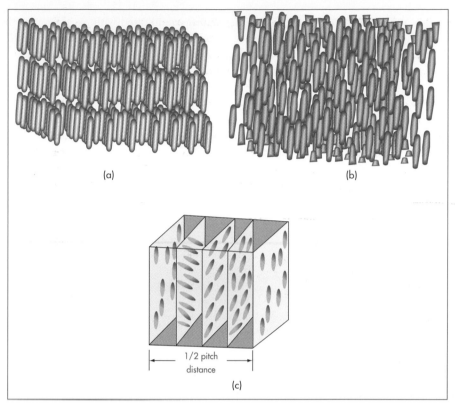

Figure 5.34 Diagrammatic representation of forms of thermotropic liquid crystals: (a) smectic, (b) nematic, and (c) a stylised diagram of cholesteric liquid crystals.

In the nematic liquid crystalline state, groups of molecules orientate spontaneously with their long axes parallel, but they are not ordered into layers. Because the molecules have freedom of rotation about their long axis, the nematic liquid crystals are quite mobile and are readily orientated by electric or magnetic fields. Nematic liquid crystals are formed, for example, when p-azoxyanisole is heated.

The molecules in smectic liquid crystals are more ordered than the nematic since not only are they arranged with their long axes parallel but they are also arranged into distinct layers. As a result of this two-dimensional order, the smectic liquid crystals are viscous and are not orientated by magnetic fields. Examples of compounds forming smectic liquid crystals are octyl p-azoxycinnamate and ethyl p-azoxybenzoate.

If a nematic liquid crystal is made of chiral molecules, i.e. the molecules differ from their mirror image, a cholesteric (or chiral nematic) liquid crystal is obtained. The cholesteric phase is formed by several cholesteryl esters and can be visualised as a stack of very thin two-dimensional nematic-like layers in which the elongated molecules lie parallel to each other in the plane of the layer. The orientation of the long axes in each layer is displaced from that in the adjacent layer and this displacement is cumulative through successive layers so that the overall displacement traces out a helical path through the layers. The helical path causes very pronounced rotation of polarised light, which can be as much as 50 rotations per millimetre. The pitch of the helix (the distance required for one complete rotation) is very sensitive to small changes in temperature and pressure and dramatic colour changes can result from variations in these properties. When nonpolarised light is passed through the cholesteric material, the light is separated into two components, one with the electric vector rotating clockwise and the other with the electric vector rotating anticlockwise. One of these components is transmitted and the other reflected, depending on the material involved. This process is called *circular dichroism* and it gives the cholesteric phase a characteristic iridescent appearance when illuminated by white light.

5.4.2 Liposomes, niosomes and surfactant vesicles

Phospholipids and other surfactants having two hydrophobic chains have CPP values of approximately 1 (see section 5.3.3) and tend to form lamellar phases.

When equilibrated with excess water, these lamellar phases may form vesicles that can entrap drug and these have potential use as drug carriers. In this section we will consider several types of vesicular structures; Box 5.4 shows some of the amphiphiles that form such structures.

Liposomes

Liposomes are formed by naturally occurring phospholipids such as lecithin (phosphatidylcholine). When first formed in solution they are usually composed of several bimolecular lipid lamellae

---

Box 5.4 Some vesicle-forming amphiphiles

Dioctadecyldimethylammonium chloride

Glyceryl monooleate

Lecithin

separated by aqueous layers (*multilamellar liposomes*). Figure 5.35 shows a diagrammatic representation of a multilamellar liposome with three phospholipid bilayers. Sonication of these units can give rise to *unilamellar liposomes*. The net charge of the liposome can be varied by incorporation of, for example, a long-chain amine such as stearylamine (to give positively charged vesicles) or dicetyl phosphate (to give negatively charged species). Positively charged vesicles are being used experimentally as carriers for DNA: the anionic DNA condenses around the cationic vesicles to provide compact units for cell delivery. Water-soluble drugs can be entrapped in liposomes by intercalation in the aqueous layers, while lipid-soluble drugs can be solubilised within the hydrocarbon interiors of the lipid bilayers (see Fig. 5.35). The use of liposomes as drug carriers has been reviewed.[18] Since liposomes can encapsulate drugs, proteins and enzymes, the systems can be administered intravenously, orally or intramuscularly in order to decrease toxicity, to increase specificity of uptake of drug and in some cases to control release. Liposomes have several disadvantages as carriers for delivery of drugs, however; for example, phospholipids are liable to oxidative degradation and must be stored and handled in a nitrogen atmosphere.

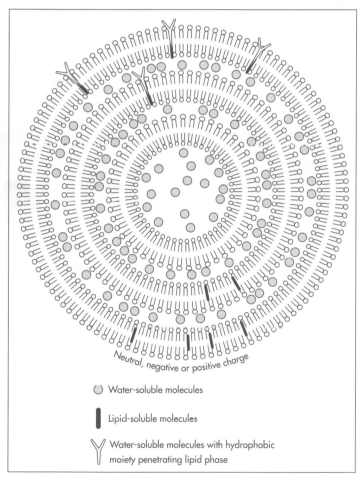

Neutral, negative or positive charge

- Water-soluble molecules
- Lipid-soluble molecules
- Water-soluble molecules with hydrophobic moiety penetrating lipid phase

Figure 5.35 Diagrammatic representation of a liposome in which three bilayers of polar phospholipids alternate with aqueous compartments; water-soluble and lipid-soluble substances may be accommodated in the aqueous and lipid phases, respectively. Certain macromolecules can insert their hydrophobic regions into the lipid bilayers with the hydrophilic portions extending into water.

Surfactant vesicles and niosomes

Surfactants having two alkyl chains can pack in a similar manner to the phospholipids (see Box 5.4 for examples). Vesicle formation by the dialkyldimethylammonium cationic surfactants has been studied extensively. As with liposomes, sonication of the turbid solution formed when the surfactant is dispersed in water leads ultimately to the formation of optically transparent solutions that may contain single-compartment vesicles. For example, sonication of dioctadecyldimethylammonium chloride for 30 seconds gives a turbid solution containing bilayer vesicles of 250–450 nm diameter, while sonication for 15 minutes produces a clear solution containing monolayer vesicles of diameter 100–150 nm. The main use of such systems has been as membrane models rather than as drug delivery vehicles because of the toxicity of ionic surfactants.

Some dialkyl polyoxyethylene ether nonionic surfactants also form vesicles, as do mixtures of cholesterol and a single alkyl-chain nonionic surfactant with a glyceryl head group. The resultant vesicles have been termed *niosomes*. These vesicles behave *in vivo* like liposomes, prolonging the circulation of entrapped drug and altering its organ distribution and metabolic stability. As with liposomes, the properties of niosomes depend both on the composition of the bilayer and on the method of production; Fig. 5.36 shows a freeze-fracture electron micrograph of a multilamellar niosome. Being nonionic, niosomes are likely to be less toxic than vesicles produced from ionic surfactants and represent promising vehicles for drug delivery.[19,20]

Figure 5.36 Freeze-fracture electron micrograph of a multilamellar niosome.

Monoolein vesicles

Polar amphiphilic lipids such as glyceryl monooleate (monoolein) also form bilayers, the nature of which depends on the temperature and concentration. An interesting phase formed at monoolein concentrations of 60–80% w/w is the bicontinuous cubic phase. The structure of this phase is unique and consists of a curved bicontinuous lipid bilayer extending in three dimensions, separating two networks of water channels with pores of about 5 nm diameter (see Fig. 5.37). On dilution, these structures coexist with excess water and there is the formation of dispersed cubic phase vesicles or *cubosomes*. Cubic phases have been shown to incorporate and deliver small-molecule drugs and large proteins by oral and parenteral routes, in addition to local delivery in vaginal and periodontal cavities.[21]

Key points

- There are two main categories of liquid crystal: lyotropic liquid crystals, which are observed in highly concentrated surfactant solutions; and thermotropic liquid crystals, which are produced when certain substances, notably cholesterol esters, are heated.

- Phase diagrams of surfactants may show transitions from micellar solutions to hexagonal (or middle), cubic, and lamellar (or neat) liquid crystalline phases as the surfactant concentration is increased.

- There are three main types of thermotropic liquid crystals: nematic, in which the groups of molecules are ordered with their long axes parallel; smectic, which are similar to nematic but are also arranged into distinct layers; and cholesteric, which are stacks of nematic-like layers in which the orientation of the long axes traces out a helical path through the layers.

Figure 5.37 Structure of glyceryl monooleate–water cubic phase with inset showing the lipid bilayer.

Redrawn from Shah JC *et al.*, *Adv Drug Deliv Rev*, 2001; 47: 229.

5.5 Properties of some commonly used surfactants

5.5.1 Anionic surfactants

Sodium Lauryl Sulfate BP is a mixture of sodium alkyl sulfates, the chief of which is sodium dodecyl sulfate, $C_{12}H_{25}SO_4^-Na^+$. It is very soluble in water and is used pharmaceutically as a preoperative skin cleaner, having bacteriostatic action against Gram-positive bacteria, and also in medicated shampoos. It is a component of Emulsifying Wax BP.

Sodium dodecyl sulfate has been studied in depth. The cmc at 25°C is $8.2 \times 10^{-3}\,\mathrm{mol\,dm^{-3}}$ (0.23% w/v). The effect of temperature on the cmc is shown in Fig. 5.31.

5.5.2 Cationic surfactants

The quaternary ammonium and pyridinium cationic surfactants are important pharmaceutically because of their bactericidal activity against a wide range of Gram-positive and some Gram-negative organisms. They may be used on the skin especially in the cleaning of wounds. Aqueous solutions are used for cleaning contaminated utensils.

Cetrimide BP consists mainly of tetradecyltrimethylammonium bromide together with smaller amounts of dodecyl- and hexadecyltrimethylammonium bromides. The properties of the individual components have been studied in detail and are summarised in Table 5.6. Solutions containing 0.1–1% of cetrimide are used for cleaning the skin, wounds and burns, for cleaning contaminated vessels, polythene tubing and catheters, and for storage of sterilised surgical instruments. Solutions of cetrimide are also used in shampoos to remove scales in seborrhoea. In the form of Cetrimide Emulsifying Wax BP, it is used as an emulsifying agent for producing oil-in-water creams suitable for the incorporation of cationic and nonionic medicaments (anionic medicaments would, of course, be incompatible with this cationic surfactant).

Benzalkonium chloride is a mixture of alkylbenzyldimethylammonium chlorides of the general formula $[C_6H_5CH_2N(CH_3)_2R]Cl$, where R represents a mixture of the alkyls from C_8H_{17} to $C_{18}H_{37}$. In dilute solution (1 in 1000 to 1 in 2000) it may be used for the preoperative disinfection of skin and mucous membranes, for application to burns and wounds, and for

Table 5.6 Micellar properties of a commercial sample of cetrimide and its main constituents at 25°C[a]

Constituent	Percentage (calculated on dry weight basis)	Critical micellar concentration (mmol dm^{-3})	Micellar molecular weight ($\times 10^{-4}$)
Tetradecyltrimethylammonium bromide	68	3.3	2.7
Dodecyltrimethylammonium bromide	22	5.3	2.1
Hexadecyltrimethylammonium bromide	7	0.82	3.3
Cetrimide	–	2.9	2.5

[a] Data from Barry BW *et al.*, *J Colloid Interface Sc*, 1970; 33: 554; 1972; 40: 174.

cleaning polythene and nylon tubing and catheters. Benzalkonium chloride is also used as a preservative for eye-drops and as a permitted vehicle for the preparation of certain eye-drops.

5.5.3 Nonionic surfactants

The amphiphilic nature of nonionic surfactants is often expressed in terms of the balance between the hydrophobic and hydrophilic portions of the molecule. An empirical scale of HLB (hydrophile–lipophile balance) numbers has been devised (see Chapter 6, section 6.3.2). The lower the HLB number, the more lipophilic is the compound and vice versa. HLB values for a series of commercial nonionic surfactants are quoted in Tables 5.7 and 5.8. The choice of surfactant for medicinal use involves a consideration of the toxicity of the substance, which may be ingested in large amounts. The following surfactants are widely used in pharmaceutical formulations.

Sorbitan esters

The commercial products are mixtures of the partial esters of sorbitol and its mono- and dianhydrides with oleic acid. They are generally insoluble in water

and are used as water-in-oil emulsifiers and as wetting agents. The main sorbitan esters are listed in Table 5.7 together with a space-filling model of a representative component of sorbitan palmitate.

Polysorbates

Commercial products are complex mixtures of partial esters of sorbitol and its mono- and dianhydrides condensed with approximately 20 moles (usually) of ethylene oxide for each mole of sorbitol and its anhydride. The space-filling model of a representative component of polysorbate 20 is shown in Table 5.8. The polysorbates are miscible with water, as reflected in their higher HLB values (see Table 5.8), and are used as emulsifying agents for oil-in-water emulsions.

Cetomacrogol 1000 BP and other macrogol ethers

Cetomacrogol is a water-soluble substance with the general structure $CH_3(CH_2)_m(OCH_2CH_2)_nOH$, where m may be 15 or 17 and the number of oxyethylene groups, n, is between 20 and 24. It is used in the form of Cetomacrogol Emulsifying Wax BP in the preparation of oil-in-water emulsions and also as a solubilising agent for volatile oils. The cmc and

Table 5.7 HLB values of sorbitan esters

Chemical name	Commercial name	HLB
Sorbitan laurate	Span 20	8.6
Sorbitan palmitate	Span 40	6.7
Sorbitan stearate	Span 60	4.7
Sorbitan tristearate	Span 65	2.1
Sorbitan oleate	Span 80	4.3
Sorbitan trioleate	Span 85	1.8

Table 5.8 HLB and cmc values of polysorbates

Chemical name	Commercial name	HLB	cmc^a (g dm^{-3})
Polyoxyethylene (20) sorbitan laurate	Polysorbate (Tween) 20	16.7	0.060
Polyoxyethylene (20) sorbitan palmitate	Polysorbate (Tween) 40	15.6	0.031
Polyoxyethylene (20) sorbitan stearate	Polysorbate (Tween) 60	14.9	0.028
Polyoxyethylene (20) sorbitan tristearate	Polysorbate (Tween) 65	10.5	0.050
Polyoxyethylene (20) sorbitan oleate	Polysorbate (Tween) 80	15.0	0.014
Polyoxyethylene (20) sorbitan trioleate	Polysorbate (Tween) 85	11.0	0.023

^{a} Data from Wan LS, Lee PFS, *J Pharm Sci*, 1974; 63: 136.

micellar molecular weight in aqueous solution are 6×10^{-2} g dm^{-3} and 1.01×10^5 Da, respectively. Other macrogol ethers are commercially available as the Brij series – for example, Brij 30 [polyoxyethylene (4) lauryl ether, $C_{12}H_{35}(OCH_2CH_2)_4OH$], Brij 72 [polyoxyethylene (2) stearyl ether, $C_{18}H_{37}(OCH_2CH_2)_2OH$] and Brij 97 [polyoxyethylene (10) oleyl ether, $C_{18}H_{35}(OCH_2CH_2)_{10}OH$].

Cremophor EL is a polyoxyethylated castor oil containing approximately 40 oxyethylene groups to each triglyceride unit. It is used as a solubilising agent in the preparation of intravenous anaesthetics and other products, although care should be taken when Cremophor is used in injection formulations because

of the possibility of an anaphylactic response to this surfactant. However, other nonionic surfactants including polysorbate 80 also can cause adverse reactions in some patients.

Poloxamers

Poloxamers are synthetic block co-polymers of hydrophilic poly(oxyethylene) and hydrophobic poly(oxypropylene) with the general formula $E_mP_nE_m$, where E – oxyethylene (OCH_2CH_2) and P – oxypropylene (OCH_2CHCH_3) and the subscripts m and n denote chain lengths. Properties such as viscosity, HLB, and physical state (liquid, paste or solid) are dependent on the relative chain lengths of the hydrophilic and hydrophobic blocks. The convention for naming these compounds is to use a number, the first two digits of which, when multiplied by 100, correspond to the approximate average molecular weight of the poly-(oxypropylene) block and the third digit, when multiplied by 10, corresponds to the percentage by weight of the poly(oxyethylene) block. For example, the poly-(oxypropylene) block of poloxamer 188 has a molecular weight of approximately 1800 Da and about 80% by weight of the molecule is poly(oxypropylene). These co-polymers were introduced to the market in 1951 by the Wyandotte Chemical Corp. (now BASF-Wyandotte) under the trade name Pluronic. The nomenclature adopted by this company indicates the physical state by a letter (F, P or L, denoting solid, paste or liquid, respectively) followed by a two- or three-digit number. The last digit of this number is the same as that for the equivalent poloxamer and is approximately one-tenth of the weight percentage of poly(oxyethylene), the first digit (or two digits in a three-digit number) multiplied by 300 gives a rough estimate of the molecular weight of the hydrophobe. So, for example, Pluronic F68 is a solid, the molecular weight of the hydrophobe is approximately 1800 Da, and the poly(oxyethylene) content is approximately 80% of the molecule by weight. A grid was developed by BASF to interrelate the properties of the Pluronics

(see Fig. 5.38a). The BASF nomenclature has been adopted by the other major supplier of poloxamers, Uniqema, who market the co-polymers as the Synperonic series. The relationship between the Pluronic (and Synperonic) and poloxamer nomenclatures is shown in Table 5.9, which also gives the composition of each co-polymer.

Included in Table 5.9 are examples of block co-polymers of poly(oxyethylene) and poly(oxypropylene) with the general formula $P_nE_mP_n$ (meroxapols). The nomenclature for these 'reverse' block co-polymers uses three digits, the first two (approximately one-hundredth of the molecular weight of the poly(oxypropylene) block) separated from the third (approximately one-tenth of the weight percentage of poly(oxyethylene) in the molecule) by the letter R. For example, 25R4 contains 40% by weight of poly(oxyethylene), and the total molecular weight of the poly(oxypropylene) blocks is approximately 2500 Da. The properties of the members of the Pluronic R series are interrelated using the grid shown in Fig. 5.38b.

The poloxamers are water-soluble and, as might be expected from their amphiphilic structure, are also surface active. Many of the series form micelles, the properties of which have been reviewed by several authors.[22,23]

Poloxamers are used as emulsifying agents for intravenous fat emulsions, as solubilising agents to

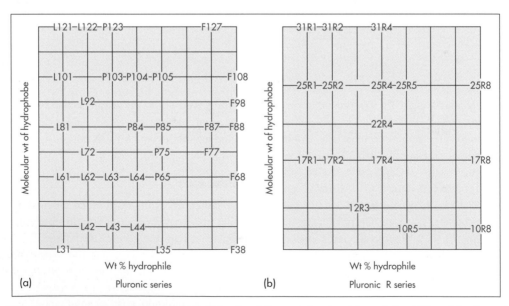

Figure 5.38 The Pluronic grid for (a) the poly(oxyethylene)–poly(oxypropylene)–poly(oxyethylene) [Pluronic] series and (b) the poly(oxypropylene)–poly(oxyethylene)–poly(oxypropylene) [Pluronic R] series of block co-polymers.

Table 5.9 Nomenclature of $E_mP_nE_m$ and $P_nE_mP_n$(*) block copolymers[a]

Poloxamer	Pluronic	Mol. wt. of P block	Chain length, n	Weight % of E block	Chain length, m	Mol. wt. of copolymer
188	F68	1 750	30	80	80	8 750
217	F77	2 050	35	70	54	6 835
237	F87	2 250	39	70	60	7 500
238	F88	2 250	39	80	102	11 250
288	F98	2 750	47	80	125	13 750
338	F108	3 250	56	80	148	16 250
407	F127	4 000	69	70	106	13 335
105	L35	5 950	103	50	68	11 900
123	L43	1 200	21	30	6	1 715
124	L44	1 200	21	40	9	2 000
181	L61	1 750	30	10	2	1 945
182	L62	1 750	30	20	5	2 190
183	L63	1 750	30	30	9	2 500
184	L64	1 750	30	40	13	2 915
212	L72	2 050	35	20	6	2 565
231	L81	2 250	39	10	3	2 500
282	L92	2 750	47	20	8	3 440
331	L101	3 250	56	10	4	3 610
401	L121	4 000	69	10	5	4 445
402	L122	4 000	69	20	11	5 000
185	P65	1 750	30	50	20	3 500
333	P103	3 250	56	30	16	4 645
334	P104	3 250	56	40	25	5 415
335	P105	3 250	56	50	37	6 500
403	P123	4 000	69	30	19	5 715
171*	17R1	1 410	–	10	–	1 565
252*	25R2	2 100	–	20	–	2 625
258*	25R8	2 100	–	80	–	10 500
311*	31R1	2 450	–	10	–	2 720

[a] Modified from Edens MW, in: Nace VM, ed., *Nonionic Surfactants. Polyoxyalkylene Block Copolymers*, Surfactant Science Series 60, New York: Marcel Dekker; 1996: 185–210.

maintain clarity in elixirs and syrups, and as wetting agents for antibacterials. They may also be used in ointment or suppository bases and as tablet binders or coaters.

5.6 Solubilisation

As we have seen in section 5.3, the micellar core is essentially a paraffin-like region and as such is capable of dissolving oil-soluble molecules. This process, whereby water-insoluble substances are brought into solution by incorporation into micelles, is termed *solubilisation* and the incorporated substance is referred to as the *solubilisate*. The subject of solubilisation has been reviewed extensively[1,24] and it is only possible in this book to give an outline of this phenomenon.

5.6.1 Determination of maximum additive concentration

The maximum amount of solubilisate that can be incorporated into a given system at a fixed concentration is termed the *maximum additive concentration*

(MAC). The simplest method of determining the MAC is to prepare a series of vials containing surfactant solution of known concentration. Increasing concentrations of solubilisate are added and the vials are then sealed and agitated until equilibrium conditions are established. The maximum concentration of solubilisate forming a clear solution can be determined by visual inspection or from extinction or turbidity measurement on the solutions.

Solubility data are expressed as solubility–concentration curves or as phase diagrams. The latter are preferable since a three-component phase diagram completely describes the effect of varying all three components of the system – namely, the solubilisate, the solubiliser and the solvent. The axes of the phase diagram form an equilateral triangle (see Fig. 5.39), each side of which is divided into 100 parts to correspond to percentage composition.

A typical phase diagram of a solubilised system is shown in Fig. 5.40. In solutions of high water content the oil is solubilised in the micelles of the nonionic surfactant Brij 97 ($C_{18}H_{35}(OCH_2CH_2)_{10}OH$), forming an isotropic micellar solution (often referred to as the L_1 region). When the concentration of the oil is

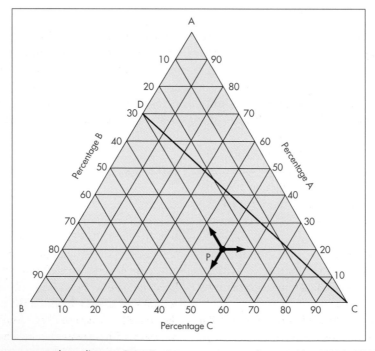

Figure 5.39 Three-component phase diagram. Point P represents a system of composition 20% A, 30% B and 50% C. Line CD represents the dilution of a mixture, originally containing 70% A and 30% B, with component C.

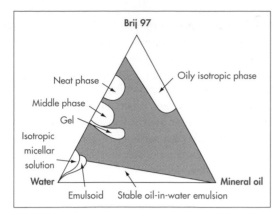

Figure 5.40 Partial phase diagram for the Brij 97 $(C_{18}H_{35}(OCH_2CH_2)_{10}OH)$–water–mineral oil solubilised system.

Redrawn from Lachampt R, Vila RM, *Am Perfum Cosmet*, 1967; 82: 29.

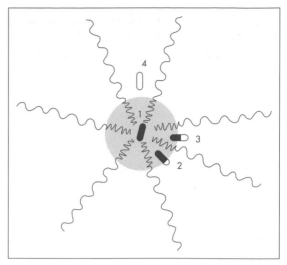

Figure 5.41 Schematic representation of sites of solubilisation depending on the hydrophobicity of the solubilisate. Completely water-insoluble hydrophobic molecules are incorporated in the micelle core (case 1); water-soluble molecules may be solubilised in the polyoxyethylene shell of a nonionic micelle (case 4); solubilisates with intermediate hydrophobicities (cases 2 and 3) are incorporated in the micelle with the hydrophobic region (black) in the core and the hydrophilic region (white) at the micelle–water interface.

Redrawn from Torchilin V, *J Control Release*, 2001; 73: 137.

increased, stable oil-in-water emulsions may be formed, while an increase in the surfactant concentration results in the formation of the liquid-crystalline regions, labelled middle and neat phases (see section 5.4). It is important in formulation to avoid boundary regions, as otherwise there is a danger of unwanted phase transitions.

5.6.2 Location of the solubilisate

The site of solubilisation within the micelle is closely related to the chemical nature of the solubilisate (see Fig. 5.41). It is generally accepted that nonpolar solubilisates (aliphatic hydrocarbons, for example) are dissolved in the hydrocarbon core of ionic and nonionic micelles. Water-insoluble compounds containing polar groups are orientated with the polar group at the core–surface interface of the micelle and the hydrophobic group buried inside the hydrocarbon core of the micelle. In addition, solubilisation in nonionic polyoxyethylated surfactants can occur in the polyoxyethylene shell (palisade layer) that surrounds the core. *p*-Hydroxybenzoic acid, for example, is solubilised entirely within this region of the cetomacrogol micelle, while esters of *p*-hydroxybenzoic acid are located at the palisade–core junction, with the ester group just within the core.

Solubilisates that are located within the micellar core increase the size of the micelles in two ways. Micelles become larger not only because their core is enlarged by the solubilisate but also because the number of surfactant molecules per micelle (the aggregation number) increases in an attempt to cover the swollen core. Solubilisation within the palisade layer, on the other hand, tends not to alter the aggregation number, the increase in micellar size resulting solely from the incorporation of solubilisate molecules.

5.6.3 Factors affecting solubilisation

Nature of the surfactant

Chain length of hydrophobe

It is difficult to generalise about the way in which the structural characteristics of a surfactant affect its solubilising capacity because this is influenced by the solubilisation site within the micelle. In cases where the solubilisate is located within the core or deep within the micelle structure, the solubilisation capacity increases with increase in alkyl chain length as might be expected. Table 5.10 clearly shows an increase of solubilising capacity of a series of polysorbates for

Table 5.10 Solubilising capacity of polysorbates for the barbiturates at 30°C[a]

Drug	Surfactant	Solubility (mg drug per g surfactant)
Phenobarbital	Polysorbate 20	55
	Polysorbate 40	61
	Polysorbate 60	63
	Polysorbate 80	66
Amobarbital	Polysorbate 20	32
	Polysorbate 40	38
	Polysorbate 80	40
Secobarbital	Polysorbate 20	111
	Polysorbate 80	144

[a] Reproduced from Ismail AA *et al.*, *J Pharm Sci*, 1970; 59: 220.

selected barbiturates as the alkyl chain length is increased from C_{12} (polysorbate 20) to C_{18} (polysorbate 80). Similar effects have been noted for the solubilisation of barbiturates in polyoxyethylene surfactants with the general structure $CH_3(CH_2)_m(OCH_2CH_2)_nOH$ with increasing alkyl chain length, m. There is a limit, however, to the improvement of solubilising capacity caused by increase of alkyl chain length in this way: an increase of m from 16 to 22, although producing larger micelles, does not result in a corresponding increase of solubilisation.[25]

Ethylene oxide chain length

The effect of an increase in the ethylene oxide chain length of a polyoxyethylated nonionic surfactant on its solubilising capacity is again dependent on the location of the solubilisate within the micelle and is complicated by corresponding changes in the micellar size. Table 5.11 shows the solubilisation capacity of a series of polyoxyethylated nonionic surfactants with a hydrocarbon chain length of 16 (C_{16}) and an increasing number of ethylene oxide units (E) in the polyoxyethylene chain. As seen from this table, the aggregation number decreases with increase in the hydrophilic chain length so, although the number of

steroid molecules solubilised per micelle also decreases, the total amount solubilised per mole of surfactant (number of steroid molecules per micelle × number of micelles per mole) actually increases because of the increasing number of micelles.

Similar results were observed in a study of the solubilisation of the poorly water-soluble mydriatic drug tropicamide by a series of poloxamers.[26] Figure 5.42 shows an increase of solubilisation (expressed as moles of tropicamide per mole of poloxamer) with increase of the oxyethylene content of the poloxamer. When the data were expressed as the moles of drug solubilised per ethylene oxide unit of the poloxamer, however, the solubilisation capacity decreased with increasing ethylene oxide chain length. Again, the reason for this decrease is that the micellar size per ethylene oxide equivalent decreases with increasing length of the ethylene oxide chain.

Nature of the solubilisate

Although many possible relationships between the amount solubilised and various physical properties of the solubilisate molecule (for example, molar volume, polarity, polarisability and chain length) have been explored, it has not been possible to establish simple correlations between them. In general, a decrease in solubility in a surfactant solution occurs when the alkyl chain length of a homologous series is increased. Unsaturated compounds are generally more soluble than their saturated counterparts. Branching of the hydrocarbon chain of the solubilisate has little effect, but increased solubilisation is often noted following cyclisation. Unfortunately, these generalisations apply only to very simple solubilisates.

More specific rules can be formulated for particular series of solubilisates. For example, it is clear from studies of the effect of steroid structure on solubilisation by a series of surfactants that the more hydrophilic is the substituent in position 17 of the ring structure the lower the quantity of surfactant required to effect solubilisation of the hormone. Thus the extent of solubilisation of hormones in sodium lauryl sulfate follows the series progesterone < testosterone < deoxycorticosterone, the C_{17} substituents being $COCH_3$, OH and $COCH_2OH$, respectively (Box 5.5).

A relationship between the lipophilicity of the solubilisate, expressed by the partition coefficient between octanol and water, $P_{octanol}$ (see Chapter 4),

Table 5.11 Micellar solubilisation parameters for steroids in *n*-alkyl polyoxyethylene surfactants C_nE_m (where *n* = alkyl (C) chain length and *m* = polyoxyethylene (E) chain length) at 25°C[a]

Surfactant	Aggregation number	Micelles per mole ($\times 10^{-21}$)	Steroid molecules per micelle			
			Hydrocortisone	Dexamethasone	Testosterone	Progesterone
$C_{16}E_{17}$	99	6.1	9.1	6.7	6.0	5.6
$C_{16}E_{32}$	56	10.8	7.6	5.3	4.6	4.3
$C_{16}E_{44}$	39	15.4	5.8	4.2	3.6	3.3
$C_{16}E_{63}$	25	24.1	4.0	3.3	2.4	2.3

[a] Reproduced from Barry BW, El Eini DID, *J Pharm Pharmacol*, 1976; 28: 210.

and its extent of solubilisation has been noted for the solubilisation of substituted barbituric acids by polyoxyethylene stearates, of substituted benzoic acids by polysorbate 20, and of several steroids by polyoxyethylene nonionic surfactants. An exhaustive survey of data for the solubilisation of some 64 drugs by bile salt micelles revealed linear relationships between $\log P_m$ and $\log P_{octanol}$ for each of seven bile salts examined.[27]

Effect of temperature

In most systems the amount solubilised increases as temperature increases. The effect is particularly pronounced with some nonionic surfactants where it is a

Figure 5.42 Moles of tropicamide solubilised per mole of Pluronic plotted against the oxyethylene content of the poloxamer (see Table 5.9 for details of the Pluronics).

Reproduced with permission from Saettone MF *et al.*, *Int J Pharm*, 1988; 43: 67.

Box 5.5 Structures of some steroid solubilisates

Progesterone   R = — COCH$_3$
Testosterone   R = — OH
Deoxycorticosterone   R = — COCH$_2$OH

consequence of an increase in the micellar size with temperature increase. Table 5.12 shows an increased solubilisation of two drugs by aqueous micellar solutions of bile salts as temperature is increased over the range 27–45°C.

A complicating factor when considering the effect of temperature on the amount solubilised is the change in the aqueous solubility of the solubilisate with temperature increase. In some cases, although the amount of drug that can be taken up by a surfactant solution increases with temperature increase, this may simply reflect an increase in the amount of drug dissolved in the aqueous phase rather than an increased solubilisation by the micelles. This point is illustrated by a

study of the solubilisation of benzoic acid by a series of polyoxyethylated nonionic surfactants, details of which are given in Table 5.13. Although the extent of solubilisation of benzoic acid increases with temperature, the data when plotted reveal a minimum micelle/water distribution coefficient, P_m, at about 27°C. The decrease in P_m (and therefore the amount of drug solubilised in the micelles) with temperature increase up to this temperature is possibly due to the increase in aqueous solubility of benzoic acid; the subsequent increase of P_m at higher temperatures is due to a rapid increase of micellar size as the cloud point is approached and a consequent ability of the micelles to incorporate more solubilisate.

Methods of preparation of solubilised systems

The method of preparation of the solubilised system can have a significant influence on the solubilisation capacity.[28] The simplest and most commonly used method of incorporation of the drug is the so-called 'shake flask' method in which excess solid drug is equilibrated with the micellar solution and unsolubilised drug is subsequently removed by filtration or centrifugation. Larger amounts of drug can often be solubilised by co-mixing the drug and copolymer at elevated temperature (typically about 60°C) and adding the resultant intimate mixture to water or buffer to

Table 5.12 The effect of temperature on the maximum additive concentrations (MAC) of griseofulvin and hexestrol in bile salts[a]

Solubilisate	Bile salt	10^3 MAC (moles solubilisate/mole surfactant)		
		27°C	37°C	45°C
Griseofulvin	Sodium cholate	5.36	6.18	6.80
	Sodium deoxycholate	4.68	6.18	7.54
	Sodium taurocholate	3.77	4.90	6.15
	Sodium glycocholate	3.85	5.13	5.29
Hexestrol	Sodium cholate	187	195	197
	Sodium deoxycholate	164	167	179
	Sodium taurocholate	220	225	223
	Sodium glycocholate	221	231	251

[a] Reproduced from Wiedmann TS, Kamel L, *J Pharm Sci*, 2002; 91: 1743.

Table 5.13 Micelle/water distribution coefficients, P_m, for the solubilisation of benzoic acid by *n*-alkyl polyoxyethylene surfactants C_nE_m (where n = alkyl (C) chain length and m = polyoxyethylene (E) chain length) as a function of temperature[a]

Surfactant formula	18°C	25°C	31°C	37°C	45°C
$C_{16}E_{16}$	59.51	50.07	43.75	44.11	_[b]
$C_{16}E_{30}$	47.80	45.55	35.42	38.23	38.66
$C_{16}E_{40}$	37.07	32.72	28.76	29.90	37.06
$C_{16}E_{96}$	31.22	27.43	25.13	27.46	32.35

[a] Reproduced from Humphries KJ, Rhodes CT, *J Pharm Sci*, 1968; 57: 79.

[b] No P_m value determined at this temperature for $C_{16}E_{16}$ because the cloud point temperature was exceeded.

form the solubilised micellar solution; a method often referred to as 'melt loading'. Other methods, including dialysis, solvent evaporation and cosolvent evaporation methods, involve the use of nonaqueous solvents to dissolve the drug and copolymer. In the dialysis method drug and copolymer are dissolved in a water-miscible organic solvent followed by dialysis against water until the organic phase is replaced with water. In the solvent evaporation method, the drug and copolymer are dissolved in volatile organic solvents that are allowed to evaporate at room temperature; the resultant dried drug–copolymer film is then pulverised and dispersed in water. Alternatively, a micellar solution is formed by adding water slowly to a solution of drug and polymer in a water-miscible organic solvent (cosolvent) and removing the organic solvent by evaporation (cosolvent evaporation method). In a variation of this method, an oil-in-water emulsion is formed by mixing the organic solvent containing dissolved drug with an aqueous solution of the copolymer; the volatile solvent is then allowed to evaporate leaving the solubilised micellar solution.

5.6.4 Pharmaceutical applications of solubilisation

A wide range of insoluble drugs has been formulated using the principle of solubilisation. Only a few representative examples will be discussed in this section.

Phenolic compounds such as cresol, chlorocresol, chloroxylenol and thymol are frequently solubilised with soap to form clear solutions that are widely used for disinfection. Solution of Chloroxylenol BP, for example, contains 5% w/v chloroxylenol with terpineol in an alcoholic soap solution.

Nonionic surfactants are efficient solubilisers of iodine, and will incorporate up to 30% iodine by weight, of which three-quarters is released as available iodine on dilution. Such iodine–surfactant systems (referred to as *iodophors*) are more stable than iodine–iodide systems. They are preferable in instrument sterilisation since corrosion problems are reduced. Loss of iodine by sublimation from iodophor solutions is significantly less than from simple iodine solutions such as Iodine Solution NF. There is also evidence of an ability of the iodophor solution to penetrate hair follicles of the skin, so enhancing activity.

The low solubility of steroids in water presents a problem in their formulation for ophthalmic use. The requirements of optical clarity preclude the use of oily solutions or suspensions and there are many examples of the use of nonionic surfactants as a means of producing clear solutions that are stable to sterilisation. In most formulations, solubilisation has been achieved using polysorbates or polyoxyethylene sorbitan esters of fatty acids.

Essential oils are extensively solubilised by surfactants, polysorbates 60 and 80 being particularly well suited to this purpose.

The polysorbate nonionics have also been employed in the preparation of aqueous injections of the water-insoluble vitamins A, D, E and K. Table 5.14 shows the solubility of these vitamins in 10% polysorbate solutions, polysorbate 20 and 80 being the best two solubilisers.

Table 5.14 Solubilisation of vitamins by 10% polysorbate solutions[a]

Polysorbate	Vitamin D$_2$ (IU cm^{-3})	Vitamin E (mg cm^{-3})	Vitamin K$_3$ (mg cm^{-3})	Vitamin A alcohol (IU cm^{-3})
20	20 000	5.7	4.7	80 000
40	16 000	3.8	4.0	60 000
60	15 000	3.2	3.7	60 000
80	20 000	4.5	4.5	80 000

[a] Reproduced from Gstirner F, Tata PS, *Mitt dt Pharm Ges*, 1958; 28: 191.

One of the problems encountered with the use of nonionic surfactants as solubilisers is that they are prone to clouding on heating (see section 5.3.4). Moreover the presence of solubilisate can reduce the cloud point. For this reason, sucrose esters may be more suitable as alternative solubilisers for the vitamins, although they do have the disadvantage of a slightly higher haemolytic activity.

It has been possible to give only a brief description of the types of drugs that have been formulated using solubilisation. Many other drugs have been formulated in this way, including the analgesics, sedatives, sulfonamides and antibiotics. The reader is referred to reference 1 for a more complete survey of this topic and for a discussion of the effects of solubilisation on drug activity and absorption characteristics.

 Key points

- An important property of surfactant micelles is their ability to solubilise water-insoluble compounds. The location of solubilisates in the micelles is closely related to the chemical nature of the solubilisate.
- In general, nonpolar solubilisates are dissolved in the micelle core and water-insoluble compounds having polar groups are orientated with the polar group at the surface and the hydrophobic group in the core. Solubilisation in nonionic surfactants can also occur in the palisade layer.
- The extent of solubilisation is influenced by the volume of the micelle core, the ethylene oxide chain length of nonionic surfactants, the lipophilicity of the solubilisate, and the temperature.
- Some pharmaceutical applications of solubilisation have been discussed.

Summary

In this chapter we have seen that molecules having distinct hydrophilic and hydrophobic regions (so-called amphiphiles or surfactants) will accumulate at air–water and oil–water interfaces and in so doing will reduce respectively the surface and interfacial tension. This process is spontaneous and leads to the removal of the hydrophobic regions from solution by their protruding into the air or lipophilic phase. At concentrations above a critical value (the cmc), such molecules will form small spherical aggregates or micelles in solution, the cores of which are formed from the hydrophobic region of the surfactant and protected from the aqueous environment by a shell of polar groups or polyoxyethylene chains. Micelles are transient structures composed of typically 60–100 molecules that are in equilibrium with free surfactant molecules in solution, the concentration of which effectively remains at the cmc value as the solution concentration is increased. Micelles are useful in pharmaceutical formulation because of their ability to incorporate poorly water-soluble drugs. The balance between the hydrophobic and hydrophilic regions of the surfactant determines the degree of lowering of surface or interfacial tension, the critical micelle concentration and the micellar properties. The tendency for accumulation at surfaces also leads to the adsorption of amphiphilic molecules onto solid surfaces; this process can lead to removal of active ingredients from solution, which is advantageous when this material is a poison or toxin but problematic when the active ingredient is a drug or preservative.

As the surfactant concentration is increased there is frequently a transition from the typical spherical micellar structure to a more elongated or rod-like micelle. Further increase in concentration may lead to the formation of a liquid crystalline state termed the *middle phase* or *hexagonal phase* in which the elongated micelles are arranged into hexagonal arrays. With some surfactants, further increase of concentration results in the formation of a cubic phase and eventually at very high concentrations a further liquid crystalline state, the *neat phase* or *lamellar phase* may be observed.

Water-insoluble amphiphilic molecules will form films or monolayers when spread over the water surface. Depending on the molecular structure of the amphiphile, these may be tightly packed as in solid or condensed films, or more loosely packed as in liquid or expanded films and gaseous films. Lung surfactants form films at the alveolar air–water interface that facilitate the large surface area changes that occur during the successive compression–expansion cycles accompanying the breathing process.

References

1. Attwood D, Florence AT. *Surfactant Systems*. London: Chapman and Hall; 1983.
2. Attwood D. The mode of association of amphiphilic drugs in aqueous solution. *Adv Colloid Interface Sci* 1995;55:271–303.
3. Arzhavitina A, Steckel H. Surface active drugs significantly alter the drug output rate from medical nebulizers. *Int J Pharm* 2010;384:128–136.
4. Peng JB *et al*. The structures of Langmuir–Blodgett films of fatty acids and their salts. *Adv Colloid Interface Sci* 2001;91:163–219.
5. Dynarowicz-Łatka P *et al*. Modern physicochemical research on Langmuir monolayers. *Adv Colloid Interface Sci* 2001;91:221–293.
6. Flanders BN *et al*. Imaging of monolayers composed of palmitic acid and lung surfactant protein B. *J Microsc* 2001;202:379–385.
7. Notter RH. Lung surfactants. Basic science and clinical applications. In: C. Lenfant C, ed. *Lung Biology in Health and Disease, 149*. New York: Marcel Dekker; 2000: 1–444.
8. Serrano AG *et al*. Critical structure-function determinants within the N-terminal region of pulmonary surfactant protein SP-B. *Biophys J* 2006;90:238–249.
9. Zatz JL *et al*. Monomolecular film properties of protective and enteric film formers. II. Evaporation resistance and interactions with plasticizers of poly (methyl vinyl ether-maleic anhydride). *J Pharm Sci* 1969;58: 1493–1496.
10. Hidalgo AA *et al*. Oliveira. Interaction of two phenothiazine derivatives with phospholipid monolayers. *Biophys Chem* 2004;109:85–104.
11. El-Masry S, Khalil SAH. Adsorption of atropine and hyoscine on magnesium trisilicate. *J Pharm Pharmacol* 1974;26:243–248.
12. Chin L *et al*. Laird. Optimal antidotal dose of activated charcoal. *Toxicol Appl Pharmacol* 1973;26:103–108.
13. Decker WJ *et al*. Absorption of drugs and poisons by activated charcoal. *Toxicol Appl Pharmacol* 1968;13: 454–460.
14. Decker WJ *et al*. Inhibition of aspirin absorption by activated charcoal and apomorphine. *Clin Pharm Ther* 1969;10:710–713.
15. Kolthammer J. In vitro adsorption of drugs from horse serum onto carbon coated with an acrylic hydrogel. *J Pharm Pharmacol* 1975;27:801–805.
16. Vale JA *et al*. Use of charcoal haemoperfusion in the management of severely poisoned patients. *Br Med J* 1975;1:5–9.
17. Rouchotas C *et al*. Comparison of surface modification and solid dispersion techniques for drug dissolution. *Int J Pharm* 2000;195:1–6.
18. Crommelin DJA, Schreier H. In: Kreuter J, ed. *Colloidal Drug Delivery Systems*. New York: Marcel Dekker; 1994, Chap. 3.
19. Bouwstra JA, Hofland HEJ. In: Kreuter J, ed. *Colloidal Drug Delivery Systems*. New York: Marcel Dekker; 1994, Chap. 4.
20. Uchegbu IF, Florence AT. Nonionic surfactant vesicles (niosomes): physical and pharmaceutical chemistry. *Adv Colloid Interface Sci* 1995;58:1–55.
21. Shah JC *et al*. Cubic phase gels as drug delivery systems. *Adv Drug Del Rev* 2001;47:229–250.
22. Booth C, Attwood D. Effect of block copolymer architecture and composition on the association properties of poly(oxyalkylene) copolymers in aqueous solution. *Macromol Rapid Commun* 2000;21:501–527.
23. Nace VM. *Nonionic Surfactants. Polyoxyalkylene Block Copolymers*, Surfactant Science Series 60. New York: Marcel Dekker; 1996: 185–210.

24. Hurter PN *et al.* Solubilisation in amphiphilic copolymer solutions. In: Christian SD, Scamehorn JF, eds. *Solubilisation in Surfactant Aggregates.* Surfactant Science Series 55. New York: Marcel Dekker; 1995: 191–235.

25. Arnarson T, Elworthy PH. Effects of structural variations of nonionic surfactants on micellar properties and solubilisation: surfactants based on erucyl and behenyl (C_{22}) alcohols. *J Pharm Pharmacol* 1980;32:381–385.

26. Saettone MF *et al.* Solubilisation of tropicamide by poloxamers: physicochemical data and activity data in rabbits and humans. *Int J Pharm* 1988;43:67–76.

27. Wiedmann TS, Kamel L. Examination of the solubilisation of drugs by bile salt micelles. *J Pharm Sci* 2002;91:1743–1764.

28. Aliabadi HM, Lavasanifar A. Polymeric micelles for drug delivery. *Expert Opin Drug Deliv* 2006;3: 139–162.

rces – essentially short-range and repulsive
rces, which are dependent on the
y and conformation of molecules
arly macromolecules) at the particle

n forces due to changes in quantities of
d solvent on the very close approach of
uring particles

ent consideration of the electrostatic
d van der Waals forces of attraction by
d Landau and by Verwey and Overbeek
quantitative approach to the stability of
suspensions, known as the DLVO theory
bility.

Vaals forces between particles of the same
ays attractive. The multiplicity of interac-
n pairs of atoms or molecules on neigh-
icles must be taken into account in the
f attractive forces. Hamaker first deter-
ons for these forces on the basis of the
van der Waals energies between neigh-
ecules, assuming that the energies of
ried with the inverse 6th power of the
een them. At greater separations of the
power law changes to the inverse 7th
model considers two spherical particles
a distance H, R being $2a + H$ (Fig. 6.3).
calculated the energy of attraction, V_A,

$$\left(\frac{2a^2}{R^2 - 4a^2} + \frac{2a^2}{R^2} + \frac{R^2 - 4a^2}{R^2} \right)$$ (6.2)

ker constant, A, depends on the proper-
articles and of the medium in which

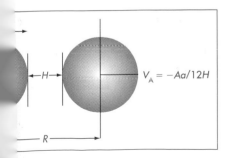

ram of the interaction between two spheres of
ance of separation H with a centre-to-centre
$H + 2a$) used in calculating energies of

they are dispersed. When H/a is small, that is when
the particles are large relative to the distance of
separation, equation (6.2) reduces to the simpler form:

$$V_A = -\frac{Aa}{12H}$$ (6.3)

The electrical charge on particles is due either to
ionisation of surface groups or to adsorption of ions
that confer their charge to the surface. A particle surface with a negative charge is shown in Fig. 6.4 along
with the layer of positive ions that are attracted to the
surface in the Stern layer, and the diffuse or electrical
double layer that accumulates and contains both
positive and negative ions.

Electrostatic forces arise from the interaction of
the electrical double layers surrounding particles in
suspension (see Fig. 6.4). This interaction leads to
repulsion if the particles have surface charges and surface potentials of the same sign and magnitude. When
the surface charge is produced by the adsorption of
potential-determining ions, the surface potential, ψ_0, is
determined by the activity of these ions and remains
constant during interaction with other particles, if the
extent of adsorption does not change. The interaction
therefore takes place at *constant surface potential*. In
emulsion systems where the adsorbed layers can
desorb, or in conditions of low availability of potential-determining ions, the interaction takes place not at
constant surface potential but at *constant surface
charge* (or at some intermediate state). The electrostatic repulsive force decays as an exponential function
of the distance and has a range of the order of the
thickness of the electrical double layer, equal to the
Debye–Hückel length, $1/\kappa$:

$$1/\kappa = \left(\frac{\varepsilon \varepsilon_0 RT}{F^2 \Sigma c_i z_i^2} \right)^{1/2}$$ (6.4)

where ε_0 is the permittivity of the vacuum, ε is the
dielectric constant (or relative permittivity) of the dispersion medium, R is the gas constant, T is temperature, F is the Faraday constant, and c_i and z_i are the
concentration and the charge number of the ions of
type i in the dispersion medium. For monovalent ions
in water, $c = 10^{-15}\kappa^2$ (with c in mol dm^{-3} and κ in
cm^{-1}). No simple equations can be given for the repulsive interactions. However, for small surface potentials and low values of κ (that is, when the double

6

Emulsions, suspensions and other disperse systems

Emulsions and suspensions are 'disperse' systems, that is they comprise respectively a liquid or solid phase
dispersed in an external liquid phase. Aerosols are either liquids or solids dispersed in a gas. While
emulsions have been formulated from oily drugs or nutrient oils, they also provide vehicles for drug
delivery with the drug dissolved in the oil or water phase. Suspensions, on the other hand, are usually
prepared from water-insoluble drugs for delivery orally or by injection, usually by the intramuscular route.
An increasing number of modern delivery systems are suspensions – of liposomes or of polymer or protein
microspheres, nanospheres or dendrimers – hence the need to understand the formulation and stabilisation
of these systems. Pharmaceutical emulsions and suspensions are in the colloidal state, that is where the
particles range from the nanometre size to visible or 'coarse' dispersions several micrometres in diameter.

After a general introduction to colloidal systems (disperse systems with particles below about 1 μm in
diameter) this chapter introduces the main types of emulsions, which are:

- Oil-in-water (o/w)
- Water-in-oil (w/o)
- Multiple emulsions (w/o/w; o/w/o)
- Microemulsions

The chapter will allow an appreciation of the factors leading to emulsion stability and physical
instability, including flocculation and coalescence. Approaches to the formulation of emulsions to provide vehicles for drug delivery and parenteral nutrition should be understood.

We then deal with aqueous and nonaqueous pharmaceutical suspensions and their formulation and
forms of instability, which are principally sedimentation, flocculation and caking. As concentrated
suspensions are used in a variety of pharmaceutical processes, e.g. granulation and spheronisation, we
will deal briefly with some of the physicochemical phenomena involved in wetting compacts.

6.1 Colloids and their classification

The word 'colloid' derives from the Greek *kolla* (glue) and was coined with the impression that colloidal substances were amorphous or glue-like rather than crystalline forms of matter. The colloidal state was recognised by Thomas Graham in 1861 and described poetically by Wolfgang Ostwald some fifty years later as the 'world of neglected dimensions', a reference both to the fact that colloid science had somehow remained a Cinderella topic, and to the special world of systems in which the particles are extremely small. Colloid chemistry is important in pharmacy because of the growing number of nanoparticles and other colloidal systems used in drug delivery and targeting.

Colloids can be broadly classified as those that are *lyophobic* (solvent-hating) or more specifically in aqueous systems, *hydrophobic* (water-hating) and those that are *lyophilic* or *hydrophilic*. Surfactant molecules, because of their dual affinity for water and oil and their consequent tendency to associate into micelles, form hydrophilic colloidal dispersions in water. Proteins and gums also form lyophilic colloidal systems. Water-insoluble drugs in fine dispersion or clays and oily phases will form lyophobic dispersions. While lyophilic dispersions (such as phospholipid vesicles and micelles) are inherently stable, lyophobic colloidal dispersions have a tendency to coalesce because they are thermodynamically unstable as a result of their high surface energy.

Pharmaceutical colloids such as emulsions and suspensions (Fig. 6.1) and aerosols are readily identified (Table 6.1). The *disperse phase* is the phase that is subdivided. The *continuous phase* is the phase in which the disperse phase is distributed. Many colloidal systems that exist in nature, including suspensions of microorganisms, blood, platelets and isolated cells in culture, are also in effect colloidal dispersions. Colloid science is interdisciplinary, for although it deals with complex systems it is nevertheless a unifying discipline as it bridges the physical and biological sciences. The concepts of the stability of colloidal systems derived for suspensions can be applied with little modification to our understanding of interactions between living cells, for example (see section 6.5).

It is because of the subdivision of matter in colloidal systems that they have special properties. The large

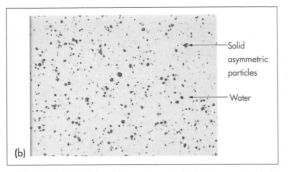

Figure 6.1 Photomicrographs of (a) an oil-in-water emulsion and (b) a suspension.

Table 6.1 Main types of colloidal systems

Type	Disperse phase	Continuous phase
o/w emulsion	Oil	Water
w/o emulsion	Water	Oil
Suspension	Solid	Water or oil
Aerosol	Solid or liquid	Air

surface-to-volume ratio of the particles dispersed in a liquid medium results in a tendency for particles to associate to reduce their surface area, so reducing their contact with the medium. Emulsions and aerosols are thermodynamically unstable two-phase systems that reach equilibrium only when the globules have coalesced to form one phase, for which the surface area is at a minimum. Many pharmaceutical problems revolve around the stabilisation of colloidal systems.

Some biological phenomena can be understood in terms of the association of cells with other cells or with inanimate or other substrates. This chapter describes various colloidal systems, deals with the theoretical approaches to colloid stability, and discusses the pharmaceutical problems encountered with colloidal dosage forms. At the close of the chapter some of the biological implications of the subject are indicated, which include the increasing use of particles in the nanometre (nm) size range (*nanoparticles*) and particles in the micrometer (µm) size range (*microparticles*) as carriers for drugs for targeting and for modifying the disposition of drug molecules contained within them. The dividing line between the colloidal and non-colloidal systems in terms of the nature of the dispersing medium and the dispersed material is not one that can be defined exactly.

6.2 Colloid stability

In dispersions of fine particles in a liquid or of particles in a gas, frequent encounters between the particles occur owing to

- Brownian movement
- Creaming or sedimentation
- Convection

Creaming of emulsions occurs when the oil droplets of an o/w emulsion migrate to the emulsion surface or the water droplets in a w/o emulsion move toward the bottom of the container. The rate of creaming depends on the difference in density between the dispersed particles and the dispersion medium, the particle radius, *a*, and the viscosity of the dispersion medium η. According to Stokes' law the rate of sedimentation (or creaming) of a spherical particle, *v*, in a fluid medium, is given by

$$v = \frac{2ga^2(\rho_1 - \rho_2)}{9\eta} \tag{6.1}$$

where ρ_1 is the density of the particles, ρ_2 is the density of the medium and *g* is the gravitational constant.

Creaming of an emulsion or sedimentation of a given suspension can be reduced in several ways:

- By forming smaller particles
- By increasing the viscosity of the continuous phase

- By decreasin
  two phases

Particles will
impact of the co
fate of particles
The encounters
particles or to co
allowed to cont
destroys itself t
and excessive c
particles; with e
to as the *cracki*
lisions result i
particles rebou
ance of the attr
tion between t
surface of the p

An additio
tendency for tl
expense of sm
Ostwald ripen
droplets to th
phase, with a
size, driven by
ically more fa

6.2.1 Forc
colloi

There are fi
particles:

- Electrost
- van der V
  attractio

Figure 6.2
a small particle
the molecules
smaller particl

- Born f
- Steric f
  geome
  (particl
  interfac
- Solvati
  adsorb
  neighb

Indepen
repulsion ar
Deryagin ar
produced a
hydrophobic
of colloid st

Van der
kind are alw
tions betwee
bouring par
calculation
mined equat
additivity of
bouring mo
attraction va
distance betv
particles, the
power. The
of radius *a* a

Hamaken
to be

$$V_A = -\frac{}{}$$

The Ham
ties of the p

Figure 6.3 Dia
radius *a* at a dis
distance of (*R* =
interaction.

6

Emulsions, suspensions and other disperse systems

Emulsions and suspensions are 'disperse' systems, that is they comprise respectively a liquid or solid phase dispersed in an external liquid phase. Aerosols are either liquids or solids dispersed in a gas. While emulsions have been formulated from oily drugs or nutrient oils, they also provide vehicles for drug delivery with the drug dissolved in the oil or water phase. Suspensions, on the other hand, are usually prepared from water-insoluble drugs for delivery orally or by injection, usually by the intramuscular route. An increasing number of modern delivery systems are suspensions – of liposomes or of polymer or protein microspheres, nanospheres or dendrimers – hence the need to understand the formulation and stabilisation of these systems. Pharmaceutical emulsions and suspensions are in the colloidal state, that is where the particles range from the nanometre size to visible or 'coarse' dispersions several micrometres in diameter.

After a general introduction to colloidal systems (disperse systems with particles below about 1 μm in diameter) this chapter introduces the main types of emulsions, which are:

- Oil-in-water (o/w)
- Water-in-oil (w/o)
- Multiple emulsions (w/o/w; o/w/o)
- Microemulsions

The chapter will allow an appreciation of the factors leading to emulsion stability and physical instability, including flocculation and coalescence. Approaches to the formulation of emulsions to provide vehicles for drug delivery and parenteral nutrition should be understood.

We then deal with aqueous and nonaqueous pharmaceutical suspensions and their formulation and forms of instability, which are principally sedimentation, flocculation and caking. As concentrated suspensions are used in a variety of pharmaceutical processes, e.g. granulation and spheronisation, we will deal briefly with some of the physicochemical phenomena involved in wetting compacts.

6.1 Colloids and their classification

The word 'colloid' derives from the Greek *kolla* (glue) and was coined with the impression that colloidal substances were amorphous or glue-like rather than crystalline forms of matter. The colloidal state was recognised by Thomas Graham in 1861 and described poetically by Wolfgang Ostwald some fifty years later as the 'world of neglected dimensions', a reference both to the fact that colloid science had somehow remained a Cinderella topic, and to the special world of systems in which the particles are extremely small. Colloid chemistry is important in pharmacy because of the growing number of nanoparticles and other colloidal systems used in drug delivery and targeting.

Colloids can be broadly classified as those that are *lyophobic* (solvent-hating) or more specifically in aqueous systems, *hydrophobic* (water-hating) and those that are *lyophilic* or *hydrophilic*. Surfactant molecules, because of their dual affinity for water and oil and their consequent tendency to associate into micelles, form hydrophilic colloidal dispersions in water. Proteins and gums also form lyophilic colloidal systems. Water-insoluble drugs in fine dispersion or clays and oily phases will form lyophobic dispersions. While lyophilic dispersions (such as phospholipid vesicles and micelles) are inherently stable, lyophobic colloidal dispersions have a tendency to coalesce because they are thermodynamically unstable as a result of their high surface energy.

Pharmaceutical colloids such as emulsions and suspensions (Fig. 6.1) and aerosols are readily identified (Table 6.1). The *disperse phase* is the phase that is subdivided. The *continuous phase* is the phase in which the disperse phase is distributed. Many colloidal systems that exist in nature, including suspensions of microorganisms, blood, platelets and isolated cells in culture, are also in effect colloidal dispersions. Colloid science is interdisciplinary, for although it deals with complex systems it is nevertheless a unifying discipline as it bridges the physical and biological sciences. The concepts of the stability of colloidal systems derived for suspensions can be applied with little modification to our understanding of interactions between living cells, for example (see section 6.5).

It is because of the subdivision of matter in colloidal systems that they have special properties. The large

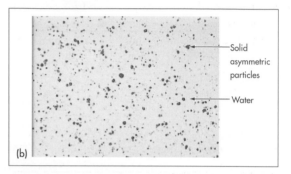

Figure 6.1 Photomicrographs of (a) an oil-in-water emulsion and (b) a suspension.

Table 6.1 Main types of colloidal systems

Type	Disperse phase	Continuous phase
o/w emulsion	Oil	Water
w/o emulsion	Water	Oil
Suspension	Solid	Water or oil
Aerosol	Solid or liquid	Air

surface-to-volume ratio of the particles dispersed in a liquid medium results in a tendency for particles to associate to reduce their surface area, so reducing their contact with the medium. Emulsions and aerosols are thermodynamically unstable two-phase systems that reach equilibrium only when the globules have coalesced to form one phase, for which the surface area is at a minimum. Many pharmaceutical problems revolve around the stabilisation of colloidal systems.

Some biological phenomena can be understood in terms of the association of cells with other cells or with inanimate or other substrates. This chapter describes various colloidal systems, deals with the theoretical approaches to colloid stability, and discusses the pharmaceutical problems encountered with colloidal dosage forms. At the close of the chapter some of the biological implications of the subject are indicated, which include the increasing use of particles in the nanometre (nm) size range (*nanoparticles*) and particles in the micrometer (μm) size range (*microparticles*) as carriers for drugs for targeting and for modifying the disposition of drug molecules contained within them. The dividing line between the colloidal and non-colloidal systems in terms of the nature of the dispersing medium and the dispersed material is not one that can be defined exactly.

6.2 Colloid stability

In dispersions of fine particles in a liquid or of particles in a gas, frequent encounters between the particles occur owing to

- Brownian movement
- Creaming or sedimentation
- Convection

Creaming of emulsions occurs when the oil droplets of an o/w emulsion migrate to the emulsion surface or the water droplets in a w/o emulsion move toward the bottom of the container. The rate of creaming depends on the difference in density between the dispersed particles and the dispersion medium, the particle radius, a, and the viscosity of the dispersion medium η. According to Stokes' law the rate of sedimentation (or creaming) of a spherical particle, v, in a fluid medium, is given by

$$v = \frac{2ga^2(\rho_1 - \rho_2)}{9\eta} \qquad (6.1)$$

where ρ_1 is the density of the particles, ρ_2 is the density of the medium and g is the gravitational constant.

Creaming of an emulsion or sedimentation of a given suspension can be reduced in several ways:

- By forming smaller particles
- By increasing the viscosity of the continuous phase
- By decreasing the density difference between the two phases

Particles will still collide, but the frequency or the impact of the collisions can be minimised. What is the fate of particles when they come into close contact? The encounters may lead to permanent contact of solid particles or to coalescence of liquid droplets. If they are allowed to continue unchecked, the colloidal system destroys itself through growth of the disperse phase and excessive creaming or sedimentation of the large particles; with emulsions this process is often referred to as the *cracking* of the emulsion. Whether these collisions result in permanent contact or whether the particles rebound and remain free depends on the balance of the attractive and repulsive forces of interaction between the particles and on the nature of the surface of the particles.

An additional cause of emulsion instability is the tendency for the growth of the larger droplets at the expense of smaller droplets in a process known as *Ostwald ripening*. Molecules diffuse from the smaller droplets to the larger ones through the continuous phase, with a resultant increase of the mean droplet size, driven by the fact that large particles are energetically more favoured than smaller ones (Fig. 6.2).

6.2.1 Forces of interaction between colloidal particles

There are five possible forces between colloidal particles:

- Electrostatic forces of repulsion
- van der Waals forces, or electromagnetic forces of attraction

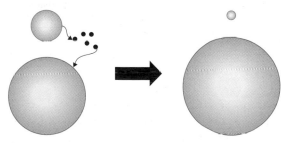

Figure 6.2 Representation of the process of Ostwald ripening: a small particle partially dissolves in the continuous phase and the molecules are taken up by the larger particle, until the smaller particle disappears completely.

- Born forces – essentially short-range and repulsive
- Steric forces, which are dependent on the geometry and conformation of molecules (particularly macromolecules) at the particle interface
- Solvation forces due to changes in quantities of adsorbed solvent on the very close approach of neighbouring particles

Independent consideration of the electrostatic repulsion and van der Waals forces of attraction by Deryagin and Landau and by Verwey and Overbeek produced a quantitative approach to the stability of hydrophobic suspensions, known as the DLVO theory of colloid stability.

Van der Waals forces between particles of the same kind are always attractive. The multiplicity of interactions between pairs of atoms or molecules on neighbouring particles must be taken into account in the calculation of attractive forces. Hamaker first determined equations for these forces on the basis of the additivity of van der Waals energies between neighbouring molecules, assuming that the energies of attraction varied with the inverse 6th power of the distance between them. At greater separations of the particles, the power law changes to the inverse 7th power. The model considers two spherical particles of radius a at a distance H, R being $2a + H$ (Fig. 6.3).

Hamaker calculated the energy of attraction, V_A, to be

$$V_A = -\frac{A}{6}\left(\frac{2a^2}{R^2 - 4a^2} + \frac{2a^2}{R^2} + \frac{R^2 - 4a^2}{R^2}\right) \quad (6.2)$$

The Hamaker constant, A, depends on the properties of the particles and of the medium in which they are dispersed. When H/a is small, that is when the particles are large relative to the distance of separation, equation (6.2) reduces to the simpler form:

$$V_A = -\frac{Aa}{12H} \quad (6.3)$$

The electrical charge on particles is due either to ionisation of surface groups or to adsorption of ions that confer their charge to the surface. A particle surface with a negative charge is shown in Fig. 6.4 along with the layer of positive ions that are attracted to the surface in the Stern layer, and the diffuse or electrical double layer that accumulates and contains both positive and negative ions.

Electrostatic forces arise from the interaction of the electrical double layers surrounding particles in suspension (see Fig. 6.4). This interaction leads to repulsion if the particles have surface charges and surface potentials of the same sign and magnitude. When the surface charge is produced by the adsorption of potential-determining ions, the surface potential, ψ_0, is determined by the activity of these ions and remains constant during interaction with other particles, if the extent of adsorption does not change. The interaction therefore takes place at *constant surface potential*. In emulsion systems where the adsorbed layers can desorb, or in conditions of low availability of potential-determining ions, the interaction takes place not at constant surface potential but at *constant surface charge* (or at some intermediate state). The electrostatic repulsive force decays as an exponential function of the distance and has a range of the order of the thickness of the electrical double layer, equal to the Debye–Hückel length, $1/\kappa$:

$$1/\kappa = \left(\frac{\varepsilon\varepsilon_0 RT}{F^2 \Sigma c_i z_i^2}\right)^{1/2} \quad (6.4)$$

where ε_0 is the permittivity of the vacuum, ε is the dielectric constant (or relative permittivity) of the dispersion medium, R is the gas constant, T is temperature, F is the Faraday constant, and c_i and z_i are the concentration and the charge number of the ions of type i in the dispersion medium. For monovalent ions in water, $c = 10^{-15}\kappa^2$ (with c in $mol\,dm^{-3}$ and κ in cm^{-1}). No simple equations can be given for the repulsive interactions. However, for small surface potentials and low values of κ (that is, when the double

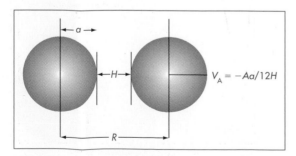

Figure 6.3 Diagram of the interaction between two spheres of radius a at a distance of separation H with a centre-to-centre distance of $(R = H + 2a)$ used in calculating energies of interaction.

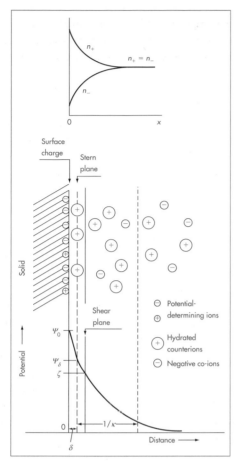

Figure 6.4 Representation of the conditions at a negative surface, with a layer of adsorbed positive ions in the Stern plane. The number of negative ions increases and the number of positive ions decreases (see upper diagram) as one moves away from the surface, the electrical potential becoming zero when the concentrations are equal. The surface potential, ψ_0, and the potential at the Stern plane, ψ_δ, are shown. As the particle moves, the effective surface is defined as the surface of shear, which is a little further out from the Stern plane, and would be dependent on surface roughness, adsorbed macromolecules, etc. It is at the surface of shear that the zeta potential, ζ, is located. The thickness of double layer is given by $1/\kappa$.

layer extends beyond the particle radius) and at constant ψ_0, the repulsive energy is

$$V_R = 2\pi\varepsilon\varepsilon_0 a\psi_\delta^2 \frac{\exp(-\kappa H)}{1 + H/2a} \qquad (6.5)$$

For small values of ψ_δ and $\exp(-\kappa H)$ this simplifies to

$$V_R = 2\pi\varepsilon\varepsilon_0 a\psi_\delta^2 \exp(-\kappa H) \qquad (6.6)$$

The equations do not take into account the finite size of the ions; the potential to be used is ψ_δ, the potential at the Stern plane (the plane of closest approach of ions to the surface), which is difficult to measure. The nearest experimental approximation to ψ_δ is often the zeta potential (ζ) measured by electrophoresis.

In the DLVO theory the combination of the electrostatic repulsive energy V_R with the attractive potential energy V_A gives the total potential energy of interaction: $V_{total} = V_A + V_R$.

V_{total} plotted against the distance of separation H gives a potential energy curve showing certain characteristic features, illustrated in Fig. 6.5. The maximum and minimum energy states are shown. If the maximum is too small, two interacting particles may reach the primary minimum and in this state of close approach the depth of the energy minimum can mean that escape is improbable. Subsequent irreversible changes in the system may then occur, such as sintering and recrystallisation in suspensions or coalescence in emulsions forming irreversible structures. When the

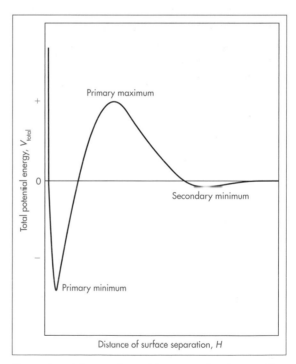

Figure 6.5 Schematic form of the curve of total potential energy (V_{total}) against distance of surface separation (H) for interaction between two particles, with $V_{total} = V_A + V_R$.

maximum in V_{total} is sufficiently high, the two particles do not reach the stage of being in close contact. The depth of the secondary minimum is important in determining events in a hydrophobic dispersion. If the secondary minimum is smaller than the thermal energy, kT (where k is the Boltzmann constant), the particles will always repel each other, but when the particles are large enough the secondary minimum can trap particles for some time as there is no energy barrier to overcome. At intermediate distances the energy of repulsion may be the larger of the two.

Effect of electrolytes on stability

Pharmaceutical colloids are rarely simple systems. Suspensions, except for some nanosuspensions rarely comprise only particles of a single size; they usually also contain additives. The influence of these, including electrolytes, has to be considered. Electrolyte concentration and valence (z) are accounted for in the term ($\Sigma c_i z_i^2$) in equation (6.4) and thus in equations (6.5) and (6.6). Figure 6.6 gives an

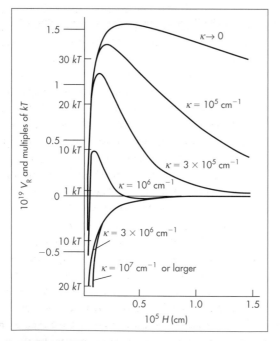

Figure 6.6 The energy of interaction of two spherical particles as a function of the distance, H, between the surfaces. For monovalent ions c (mol dm^{-3}) $= 10^{-15}\kappa^2$ (cm^{-1}). In this example, $a = 10^{-5}$ cm, $A = 10^{-19}$ J and $\psi_0 = RT/F = 26.5$ mV.

Reproduced from Overbeek J Th, *J Colloid Interface Sci* 1977; 58: 408.

example of the influence of electrolyte concentration on the electrostatic repulsive force. As the electrolyte concentration is increased, κ increases due to compression of the double layer with consequent decrease in $1/\kappa$.

At low electrolyte concentrations (low κ) the double layer is diffuse and V_R extends to large distances around the particles. Summation of V_R and V_A gives a total energy curve having a high primary maximum but no secondary minimum. The decrease of the double layer when more electrolyte is added produces a more rapid decay in V_R and the resultant total energy curve now has a small primary maximum but, more importantly, a secondary minimum. This concentration of electrolyte would produce a stable suspension, since flocculation could occur in the secondary minimum and the small primary maximum would be sufficient to prevent coagulation in the primary minimum. At high concentrations of added electrolyte, the range of V_R would be so small that the van der Waals attractive forces would dictate the shape of the total energy curve. As a consequence, this curve has no primary maximum, so the dispersion would be unstable with no energy barrier to prevent coagulation of the particles in the primary minimum. The practical importance of this can be seen when nanoparticles are dispersed in cell culture media with high levels of electrolyte and flocculate as a result.

We can see from equation (6.4) that the magnitude of the effect of an electrolyte of a given concentration on V_R also depends on the valence of the ion of opposite charge to that of the particles (the counterion): the greater the valence of the added counterion, the greater its effect on V_R. These generalisations are known as the Schulze–Hardy rule. Note that it does not matter which particular counterion of a given valence is added.

Effect of surface potential on stability

A second parameter that influences the shape of the total energy curve is the surface potential of the particles. We can see from equation (6.5) that V_R will increase with an increase in ψ_0; the changes that occur in the total curve are seen in Fig. 6.7. There is a decrease in the primary maximum as the surface potential decreases and you should note the appearance of a secondary minimum at the intermediate value of ψ_0 (see curve C).

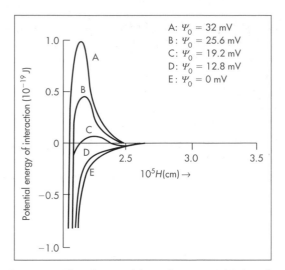

Figure 6.7 The influence of the surface potential (ψ_0) on the total potential energy of interaction of two spherical particles.

6.2.2 Repulsion between surfaces with macromolecular stabilisers

The increasing use of nonionic macromolecules as stabilisers, which has occurred since the development of the DLVO theory, has led to the awareness of other stabilising forces. The approach of particles with hydrated macromolecules adsorbed to their surfaces leads, on the interaction of these layers, to repulsion (Fig. 6.8), because of the consequent positive enthalpy

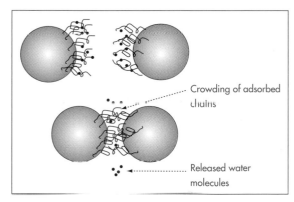

Figure 6.8 Enthalpic stabilisation: representation of enthalpic stabilisation of particles with adsorbed hydrophilic chains. The hydrated chains of the polyoxyethylene molecules —$(OCH_2CH_2)_nOH$ protrude into the aqueous dispersing medium. On close approach of the particles to within 2δ (twice the length of the stabilising chains), hydrating water is released, resulting in a positive enthalpy change which is energetically unfavourable.

change ($+\Delta H$) that ensues. In more general terms, the approach of two particles with adsorbed stabilising chains leads to a steric interaction when the chains interact. The repulsive forces may not always be enthalpic in origin. Loss of conformational freedom leads to a negative entropy change ($-\Delta S$). Each chain loses some of its conformational freedom and its contribution to the free energy of the system is increased, leading to repulsion. This volume restriction is compounded by an 'osmotic effect' that arises as the macromolecular chains on neighbouring particles crowd into each other's space, increasing the concentration of chains in the overlap region. The repulsion that arises is due to the osmotic pressure of the solvent attempting to dilute out the concentrated region: this can only be achieved by the particles moving apart.

Quantitative assessments of the steric effect depends on three parameters:

- The hydrophilic polymer chain length, δ
- The interaction of the solvent with the chains
- The number of chains per unit area of interacting surface

The steric effect does not come into play until $H = 2\delta$, so the interaction increases suddenly with decreasing distance. There are many problems in applying such equations in practice, the main ones being the lack of an accurate knowledge of δ, and the difficulty in taking account of desorption and changes in chain conformation or solvation during interaction. When the steric contribution is combined with the electrostatic and van der Waals interactions, a minimum in the energy at large separations still obtains, but repulsion is generally evident at all shorter distances, provided that the adsorbed macromolecules or surfactants do not desorb into the continuous phase or otherwise move away from the points of interaction (Fig. 6.9).

For particles with a hydrated stabilising layer of thickness δ, the volume of the overlapping region (V_v) is as derived as described in Fig. 6.10:

$$V_{ov} = \frac{2\pi}{3}\left(\delta - \frac{H}{2}\right)^2\left(3a + 2\delta + \frac{H}{2}\right) \qquad (6.7)$$

The difference between chemical potential in the overlap volume and the potential when the particles are at an infinite distance apart is a measure of the repulsive force, an osmotic force, caused by the

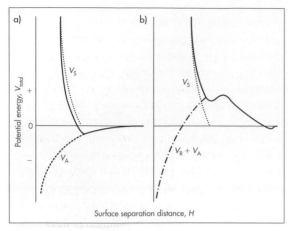

Figure 6.9 Entropic (steric) stabilisation: the potential energy–distance plots for (a) particles with no electrostatic repulsion, $V_{total} = V_S + V_A$ and (b) with electrostatic repulsion, $V_{total} = V_S + V_A + V_R$.

increased concentration of the polymer chains in the region of overlap. This can be written in terms of free energy as

$$\Delta G_m = 2\pi_E \frac{2\pi}{3} \left(\delta - \frac{H}{2}\right)^2 \left(3a + 2\delta + \frac{H}{2}\right) \quad (6.8)$$

Substituting for π_E (where $\pi_E = RTBc^2$) and using $R = kN_A$, where k is the Boltzmann constant and B the second virial coefficient, we obtain

$$\frac{\Delta G_m}{kT} = \frac{4\pi}{3} BN_A c^2 \left(\delta - \frac{H}{2}\right)^2 \left(3a + 2\delta + \frac{H}{2}\right) \quad (6.9)$$

where c is the concentration of surfactant in the interfacial layer and N_A is the Avogadro constant. This equation probably appears more complex than it is. Apart from telling us the effect of increasing or decreasing δ, for example by using different polymers of different length (δ), we can find out the effect of temperature and additives, as B is proportional to $(1 - \theta/T)$, where θ is the temperature (the theta temperature) at which the polymer and solvent have no affinity for each other. Thus when $T = \theta$, B tends to zero, and the stabilising influence of the hydrated layer disappears, as hydration is lost. Heating reduces ΔG_m in this case. Additives that salt out the macromolecules from solution will have the same effect.

The requirement for the strict applicability of the equations is that the particles are monosized, which is rarely the case with pharmaceutical emulsions and suspensions. Where particles of two radii, a_1 and a_2, interact, equation (6.3) is modified to:

$$V_A = - \frac{A a_1 a_2}{6(a_1 + a_2)H} \quad (6.10)$$

Similarly, V_R is expressed by an analogue of equation (6.5), namely,

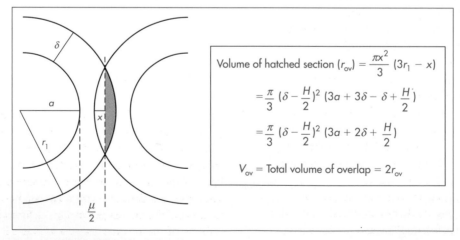

Figure 6.10 The model used in the derivation of equation (6.7): particles of radius a with adsorbed layer of thickness δ approach to a distance H between the particle surfaces; $r_1 = (a + \delta)$ and x is the distance between the surface and the line bisecting the volume of overlap.

$$V_R = \frac{\varepsilon}{4} \frac{a_1 a_2}{(a_1 + a_2)} (\psi_1 + \psi_2)^2 \ln[1 + \exp(-kH)]$$
$$+ (\psi_1 - \psi_2)^2 \ln[1 - \exp(-kH)]$$

(6.11)

where ψ_1 and ψ_2 are the surface potentials of particles 1 and 2.

These equations have been applied not only to the study of suspensions but to the reversible interaction of microbial cells with a solid substrate such as glass before permanent adhesion occurs due to the formation of polymeric bridges between cell and glass.

Key points

- Colloids can be broadly classified as
  - *Lyophobic* (solvent hating) (= *hydrophobic* in aqueous systems) or
  - *Lyophilic* (= *hydrophilic* in aqueous systems).
- Emulsions and suspensions are 'disperse' systems: a liquid or solid phase dispersed in an external liquid phase.
  - The *disperse phase* is the phase that is subdivided.
  - The *continuous phase* is the phase in which the disperse phase is distributed
- Emulsions and suspensions are intrinsically unstable systems. Creaming of an emulsion or sedimentation of a suspension can be minimised by reducing particle size, increasing the viscosity of the continuous phase, or decreasing the density difference between the continuous and disperse phases. If growth of the dispersed particles is unchecked, the colloidal system will be destroyed, for example an emulsion will separate into two phases (i.e. crack).
- Colloidal particles can interact by electrostatic forces of repulsion, van der Waals forces of attraction, short-range repulsive Born forces, steric forces and solvation forces. In the DLVO theory, the electrostatic repulsive energy, V_R, is combined with the attractive potential energy, V_A, to give the total potential energy of interaction, V_{total}. DLVO plots show the variation of V_{total} with distance of separation of the particles.

- Electrolyte addition affects the width of the double layer around the dispersed particles and hence the value of V_R. At low electrolyte concentration, DLVO plots have a high primary maximum but no secondary minimum; addition of more electrolyte compresses the double layer, producing plots with a small primary maximum but, more importantly, a secondary minimum (conditions for a stable suspension); at high electrolyte concentrations there is no primary maximum and the dispersion is unstable.
- Colloids can be stabilised by the repulsive forces that arise from adsorption of macromolecules and surfactants to their surfaces. Stabilisation arises because of loss of freedom of movement of the chains of the adsorbed molecules (negative entropy change), an osmotic effect, and release of hydrating water (positive enthalpy change).

6.3 Emulsions

Emulsions – liquid dispersions usually of an oil/lipid phase and an aqueous phase – are a traditional pharmaceutical dosage form. Oil-in-water systems have enjoyed a renaissance as vehicles for the delivery of lipid-soluble drugs (as with the anaesthetic propofol). Their use as a delivery system necessitates an understanding of the factors governing the formulation and stability of oil-in-water (o/w) and water-in-oil (w/o) emulsions, multiple emulsions (w/o/w or o/w/o) and microemulsions, which occupy a position between swollen micelles and 'emulsions with very small

Figure 6.11 Photomicrograph of emulsions: (a) an oil-in-water (o/w) emulsion, (b) a water-in-oil (w/o) system, (c) a water-in-oil-in-water emulsion in which the internal water droplets can be seen in the larger oil droplets.

globule sizes. Photomicrographs of o/w, w/o systems and multiple emulsions are shown in Fig. 6.11. It is also possible to formulate emulsions without water. Nonaqueous or anhydrous emulsions can also be formulated as o_1/o_2 systems or as oil in a polar solvent emulsions as well as multiple oil-in-oil-in-oil systems or variants.

6.3.1 Stability of o/w and w/o emulsions

Adsorption of a surfactant at the oil–water interface, by lowering interfacial tension during manufacture, aids the dispersal of the oil into droplets of a small size and maintains the particles in a dispersed state (Fig. 6.12). Unless the interfacial tension is zero, there is a natural tendency for the oil droplets to coalesce to reduce the area of oil–water contact, but the presence of the surfactant monolayer at the surface of the droplet reduces the possibility of collisions leading to coalescence. Charged surfactants will lead to an increase in negative or positive zeta potential and will thus help to maintain stability by increasing V_R. Nonionic surfactants such as the alkyl or aryl polyoxyethylene ethers, sorbitan polyoxyethylene derivatives, sorbitan esters and polyoxyethylene–polyoxypropylene–polyoxyethylene ABA block copolymers are widely used in pharmaceutical emulsions because of their lack of

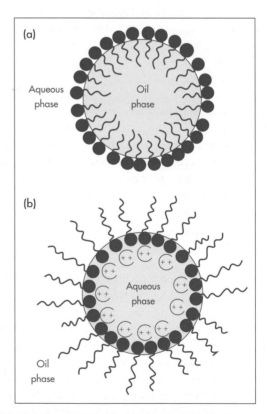

Figure 6.12 Surfactant films at the water–oil interface in o/w and w/o emulsions: (a) formation of a monomolecular film at the oil–water interface for the stabilisation of o/w emulsions; (b) stabilisation of w/o emulsions by the oriented adsorption of divalent soap salts (not to scale).

toxicity and their relatively low sensitivity to additives. These nonionic stabilisers adsorb onto the emulsion droplets and, although they generally reduce zeta potentials, they maintain stability by creating a hydrated layer on the hydrophobic particle in o/w emulsions. They effectively convert a hydrophobic colloidal dispersion into a hydrophilic dispersion.

In w/o emulsions the hydrocarbon chains of the adsorbed molecules protrude into the oily continuous phase. Stabilisation arises from steric and enthalpic forces as described in section 6.2.2; there is also a barrier to coalescence that is due to the presence of surfactant or polymer molecules and their effect on the elasticity of the interface. Emulsions are more complex than suspensions, because of the possibility (a) of movement of the surfactant into either the continuous or disperse phase, (b) of micelle formation in both phases, and (c) of formation of liquid crystalline phases between the disperse droplets.

It is usually observed that mixtures of surfactants form more stable emulsions than do single surfactants. This may be because complex formation at the interface results in a more 'rigid' stabilising film. Certainly where complex films can be formed, such as between sodium lauryl sulfate and cetyl alcohol, the stability of emulsions prepared with such mixtures is high. Theory has not developed to an extent that it can readily cope with mixtures of stabiliser molecules. Complex formation between surfactant and cosurfactants in the bulk phase of emulsion systems is dealt with in section 6.3.5, as this frequently leads to semisolid systems of high intrinsic stability.

6.3.2 HLB system

In spite of many advances in the theory of stability of lyophobic colloids, resort has still to be made to an empirical and practical approach to the choice of an optimal emulsifier, that devised in 1949 by Griffin. In this system a hydrophile–lipophile balance (HLB) can be calculated for each surfactant. This number is a measure of the relative contributions of the hydrophilic and lipophilic regions of the molecule. The method allows the effective HLB of surfactant mixtures to be calculated.

The HLB number of a surfactant is calculated according to an empirical formula. For nonionic surfactants the values range from 0 to 20 on an arbitrary scale (see Fig. 6.13). At the higher end of the scale the surfactants are hydrophilic and act as solubilising agents, detergents and o/w emulsifiers. To maintain stability, an excess of surfactant is required in the continuous phase; hence, in general, water-soluble surfactants stabilise o/w emulsions and water-insoluble (oil-soluble) surfactants stabilise w/o emulsions. In the stabilisation of oil globules it is essential that there is a degree of surfactant hydrophilicity to confer an enthalpic stabilising force and a degree of hydrophobicity to secure adsorption at the o/w interface. The balance between the two will depend on the nature of the oil and the mixture of surfactants; hence the need to apply the HLB system.

The HLB of polyhydric alcohol fatty acid esters such as glyceryl monostearate may be obtained from

$$HLB = 20\left(1 - \frac{S}{A}\right) \tag{6.12}$$

where S is the saponification number of the ester and A is the acid number of the fatty acid. The HLB of polysorbate 20 (Tween 20) calculated using this formula is 16.7, with $S = 45.5$ and $A = 276$.

Typically, the polysorbate (Tween) surfactants have HLB values in the range 9.6–16.7; the sorbitan ester (Span) surfactants have HLBs in the lower range of 1.8–8.6.

For those materials for which it is not possible to obtain saponification numbers, for example beeswax and lanolin derivatives, the HLB is calculated from

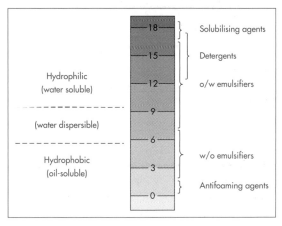

Figure 6.13 The HLB scale and the approximate ranges into which solubilising agents, detergents, emulsifiers and antifoaming agents fall.

$$HLB = (E + P)/5 \qquad (6.13)$$

where E is the percentage by weight of oxyethylene chains, and P is the percentage by weight of polyhydric alcohol groups (glycerol or sorbitol) in the molecule.

Calculation of HLB of a polysorbate

Polysorbate 20 has a molecular weight of approximately 1300 Da and contains 20 oxyethylene groups and two sorbitan rings. Thus,

$$E = \frac{20 \times 44 \times 100}{1300} = 68$$
$$P = \frac{182 \times 100}{1300} = 14$$

Hence,

$$HLB = 82/5 = 16.4$$

If the hydrophile consists only of oxyethylene groups ($[-CH_2CH_2O-]$, mol wt $= 44$ Da), a simpler version of the equation is

$$HLB = E/5 \qquad (6.14)$$

giving the upper end of the scale (20) for the polyoxyethylene glycol molecule itself. Some HLB values of typical surfactants used in pharmacy are given in Table 6.2. A more detailed list is given in Tables 5.7 and 5.8.

Group contribution

The HLB system has been put on a more quantitative basis by Davies, who calculated group contributions (group numbers) to the HLB number such that the HLB was obtained from

$$HLB = \Sigma(\text{hydrophilic group numbers}) \\ - \Sigma(\text{lipophilic group numbers}) + 7 \qquad (6.15)$$

Some group numbers are given in Table 6.3.

Choice of emulsifier or emulsifier mixture

Regardless of any theories, the appropriate choice of emulsifier or emulsifier mixture is usually made by preparing a series of emulsions with a range of surfactants of varying HLB values. It is assumed that the HLB of a mixture of two surfactants containing fraction f of A and $(1 - f)$ of B is the algebraic mean of the two HLB numbers:

$$HLB_{mixture} = f HLB_A + (1 - f) HLB_B \qquad (6.16)$$

For reasons not explained by the HLB system, mixtures of high HLB and low HLB give more stable emulsions than do single surfactants. Apart from the possibility of complex formation at the interface, the solubility of surfactant components in both the

Table 6.2 Typical HLB numbers of some surfactants

Compound	HLB
Glyceryl monostearate	3.8
Sorbitan monooleate (Span 80)	4.3
Sorbitan monolaurate (Span 20)	8.6
Triethanolamine oleate	12.0
Polyoxyethylene sorbitan monooleate (Tween 80)	15.0
Polyoxyethylene sorbitan monolaurate (Tween 20)	16.7
Sodium oleate	18.0
Sodium lauryl sulfate[a]	40.0

[a] Although applied mainly to nonionic surfactants it is possible to obtain numbers for ionic surfactants.

Table 6.3 Group contributions to HLB numbers

Group	Group number
Hydrophilic groups	
COO^-Na^+	19.1
Ester	2.4
Hydroxyl	1.9
Hydroxyl (sorbitan)	0.5
Lipophilic groups	
$-CH-$	0.475
$-CH_2-$	0.475
$-CH_3$	0.475
$=CH-$	0.475

disperse and the continuous phase maintains the stability of the surfactant film at the interface. Creaming of emulsions, (a function of particle size) is observed and is taken as an index of stability. The system with the minimum creaming or separation of phases is deemed to have an optimal HLB. It is therefore possible to determine optimum HLB numbers required to produce stable emulsions of a variety of oils. Table 6.4 shows the required HLB of surfactants to achieve stability of five oils. A more sensitive method would be to determine the mean globule size in emulsions using techniques such as laser diffraction methods to produce data such as those in Fig. 6.14. For a mineral oil-in-water emulsion stabilised by a mixture of two nonionic surfactants, an optimal HLB of between 7.5 and 8 is identified.

At the optimum HLB the mean particle size of the emulsion is at a minimum (Fig. 6.13) and this factor would explain to a large extent the stability of the system (see equations 6.1 and 6.2, for example).

Although the optimum HLB values for forming o/w emulsions are obtained in this way, it is possible to formulate stable systems with mixtures of surfactants well below the optimum. This is sometimes because of the formation of a viscous network of surfactant in the continuous phase. The high viscosity of the medium surrounding the droplets prevents their collision and this overrides the influence of the interfacial layer and barrier forces due to the presence of the adsorbed layer.

The HLB system has several drawbacks. The calculated HLB, of course, cannot take account of the effect of temperature or that of additives. The presence in emulsions of agents that salt-in or salt-out surfactants will respectively increase and decrease the

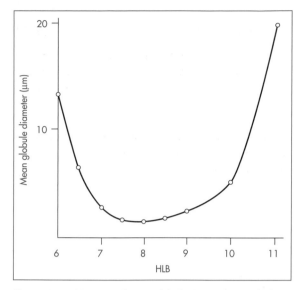

Figure 6.14 Variation of mean globule size in a mineral oil-in-water emulsion as a function of the HLB of the surfactant mixtures present at a level of 2.5%. Surfactants: Brij 92–Brij 96 mixtures.

Source: P. Depraetre, M. Seiller, A. T. Florence and F. Puisieux (unpublished material).

effective (as opposed to the calculated) HLB values. Salting-out the surfactant (for example, with NaCl) will make the molecules less hydrophilic and one can thus expect a higher optimal calculated HLB value for the stabilising surfactant for o/w emulsions containing sodium chloride. Examples are shown in Fig. 6.15 in which the effects of NaCl and NaI are compared.

6.3.3 Multiple emulsions

Multiple emulsions are emulsions whose disperse phase contains droplets of another phase (Fig. 6.11). Water-in-oil-in-water (w/o/w) or o/w/o emulsions may be prepared, both forms being of interest as drug delivery systems. Water-in-oil emulsions, in which a water-soluble drug is dissolved in the aqueous phase, may be injected by the subcutaneous or intramuscular routes to produce a delayed-action preparation. To escape, the drug has to diffuse through the oil to reach the tissue fluids. The main disadvantage of a w/o emulsion is generally its high viscosity, brought about through the influence of the oil on the bulk viscosity. Emulsifying a w/o emulsion using surfactants that stabilise an oily disperse phase can produce w/o/w

Table 6.4 Required HLB for different oils for o/w emulsion formation	
Oil	**HLB**
Cottonseed oil	7.5
Vaseline oil	8.5
Dodecane	9–9.5
Mineral oil	10–12
Cyclohexane	12

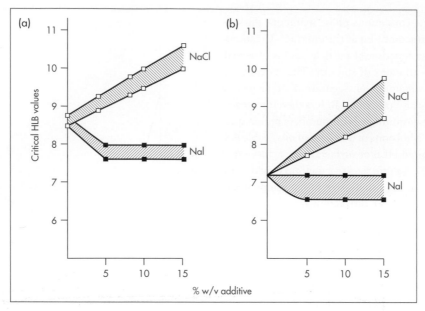

Figure 6.15 The change in critical HLB values as a function of added salt concentration, where the salt is either NaCl or NaI. Results were obtained from measurements of particle size, stability, viscosity and emulsion type as a function of HLB for liquid paraffin-in-water emulsions stabilised by Brij 92–Brij 96 mixtures. Data from different experiments showed different critical values; hence, on each diagram hatching represents the critical regions while data points actually recorded are shown. Results in (a) show particle size and stability data; those in (b) show the HLB at transition from pseudoplastic to Newtonian flow properties (see section 6.3.10) and emulsion type (o/w → w/o transitions).

Reproduced from Florence AT *et al.*, *J Pharm Pharmacol*, 1975; 27: 385.

emulsions with an external aqueous phase and lower viscosity than the primary emulsion. On injection, into muscle for example, the external aqueous phase dissipates rapidly, leaving behind the w/o emulsion. Nevertheless, biopharmaceutical differences have been observed between w/o and multiple emulsion systems (Fig. 6.16).

Physical degradation of w/o/w emulsions can arise by several routes: (Fig. 6.17a):

- Coalescence of the internal water droplets
- Coalescence of the oil droplets
- Rupture of the oil film separating the internal and external aqueous phases
- Osmotic flux of water to and from the internal droplets, possibly associated with inverse micellar species in the oil phase

The external oil particles may coalesce with others (which may or may not contain internal aqueous droplets), as in route (a); the internal aqueous droplets may be expelled individually (routes b, c, d, e) or more than one may be expelled (route f), or less frequently they may be expelled in one step (route g); the internal droplets may coalesce before being expelled (routes h, i, j, k); or water may pass by diffusion through the oil phase, gradually resulting in shrinkage of the internal droplets (routes l, m, n). Figure 6.17 is of course oversimplified; in practice the number of possible combinations is large. Several factors will determine the breakdown mechanisms in a particular system, but one of the main driving forces behind each step will be the reduction in the free energy of the system brought about by the reduction in the interfacial area.

Mechanisms of drug release from multiple emulsion systems include diffusion of the drug molecules from the internal droplets (1), from the medium of the 'external' droplets (2), or by mass transfer due to the coalescence of the internal droplets (3), as shown in Fig. 6.17b.

Nonaqueous emulsions

Relatively few studies have been carried out on non-aqueous emulsions, but these can be useful as topical vehicles or reservoirs for the delivery of hydrolytically

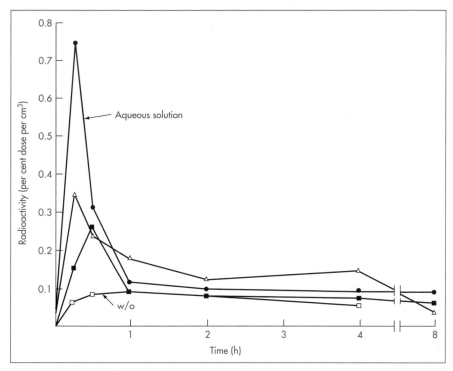

Figure 6.16 Blood levels of 5-fluoro(^{3}H)uracil (5-FU) following intramuscular injection of (●) an aqueous solution, (□) a w/o emulsion prepared with hexadecane, and a w/o/w emulsion prepared with (△) isopropyl myristate or (■) hexadecane as the oil phase.

unstable drugs.[1] Systems such as castor oil or propylene glycol in silicone oil can be formulated using silicone surfactants; the HLB number clearly does not help in formulation in these cases, especially if the continuous phase has low polarity. For hydrocarbon–formamide emulsions, surfactants that stabilise aqueous systems can be used, taking into account the change in effective HLB number of the replacement for the aqueous phase. The key to stabilisation lies in the sufficient solubility of the emulsifier in the continuous phase.

6.3.4 Microemulsions

Microemulsions consist of apparently homogeneous transparent systems of low viscosity that contain high concentrations (15–25%) of emulsifier mixture. They were first described by Schulman as disperse systems with spherical or cylindrical droplets in the size range 8–80 nm. They are essentially swollen micellar systems, but obviously the distinction between a swollen micelle and small emulsion droplet is difficult to assess.

Microemulsions form spontaneously when the components are mixed in the appropriate ratios and are thermodynamically stable. In their simplest form, microemulsions are small droplets (diameter 5–140 nm) of one liquid dispersed throughout another by virtue of the presence of a fairly large concentration of a suitable combination of surfactants. They can be dispersions of oil droplets in water (o/w) or water droplets in oil (w/o). An essential requirement for their formation and stability is the attainment of a very low interfacial tension, γ. Since microemulsions have a very large interface between oil and water (because of the small droplet size), they can only be thermodynamically stable if the interfacial tension is so low that the positive interfacial energy (given by γA, where A is the interfacial area) can be compensated by the negative free energy of mixing ΔG_m. We can calculate a rough measure of the limiting value required as follows: ΔG_m is given by $-T \Delta S_m$ (where T is the temperature), and the entropy of mixing (ΔS_m) is of the order of the Boltzmann constant. Hence $k_B T = 4\pi r^2 \gamma$. Hence, for a droplet radius r of about 10 nm, an

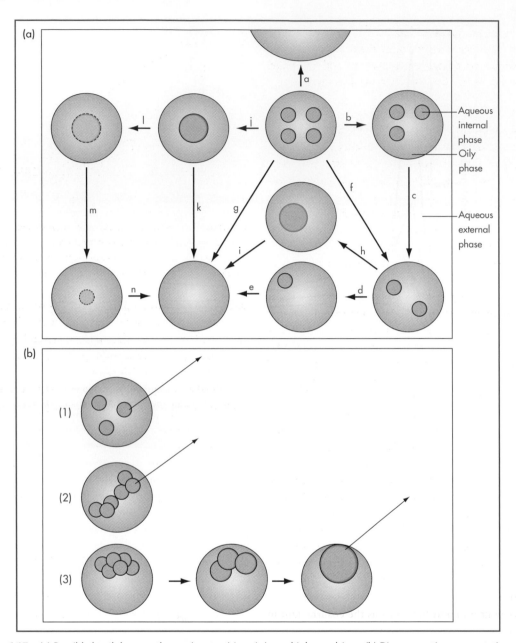

Figure 6.17 (a) Possible breakdown pathways (see text) in w/o/w multiple emulsions. (b) Diagrammatic representation of mechanisms of drug release. See text for explanation.

(a) From Whitehill D, Florence AT, *J Colloid Interface Sci*, 1981; 79: 243–256.
(b) After Davis SS, *J Clin Pharm* 1976; 1: 11.

interfacial tension of 0.03 mN m^{-1} would be required. The role of the surfactants in the system is thus to reduce the interfacial tension between oil and water (typically about 50 mN m^{-1}) to this low level.

Cosurfactants

With the possible exception of double alkyl chain surfactants and a few nonionic surfactants, it is generally not possible to achieve the required interfacial area with the use of a single surfactant. If, however, a second amphiphile (cosurfactant) is added to the system, the effects of the two surfactants can be additive provided that the adsorption of one does not adversely affect that of the other and that mixed micelle formation does not reduce the available concentration of surfactant molecules.

The importance of the cosurfactant is illustrated in the following example. The interfacial tension between cyclohexane and water is approximately 42 mN m^{-1} in the absence of any added surfactant. The addition of the ionic surfactant sodium dodecyl sulfate (SDS) in increasing amounts causes a gradual reduction of γ to a value of about 2 mN m^{-1} at an SDS concentration of 10^{-4} g cm^{-3}. Addition of 20% pentanol to the cyclohexane–water system in the absence of SDS reduces the interfacial tension to 10 mN m^{-1}. It is then theoretically possible by the addition of SDS to achieve a negative interfacial tension at SDS concentrations below the level at which it forms micelles (the critical micelle concentration, cmc). The changes in interfacial tension occurring in this system are illustrated in Fig. 6.18. Although pentanol is not generally regarded as a surfactant, it has the ability to reduce interfacial tension by virtue of its amphiphilic nature (a short hydrophobic chain and a terminal hydrophilic hydroxyl group) and functions as the cosurfactant in this system. Its presence means that in order to produce a microemulsion, the SDS is now required to produce a much smaller lowering of the interfacial tension (10 mN m^{-1} rather than 42 mN m^{1} in its absence).

The simplest representation of the structure of microemulsions is the droplet model in which microemulsion droplets are surrounded by an interfacial film consisting of both surfactant and cosurfactant molecules, as illustrated in Fig. 6.19. The orientation of the amphiphiles at the interface will, of course, differ in o/w and w/o microemulsions. As shown

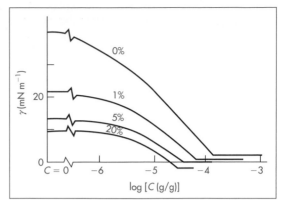

Figure 6.18 Interfacial tension, δ, between solutions of sodium dodecyl sulfate (SDS) of concentration C in aqueous 0.30 mol dm^{-3} NaCl and solutions of 1-pentanol in cyclohexane with the percentage concentrations indicated.

in Fig. 6.19, the hydrophobic portions of these molecules will be in the dispersed oil droplets of o/w systems, with the hydrophilic groups protruding in the continuous phase, while the opposite situation will be true of w/o microemulsions.

Whether the systems form o/w or w/o microemulsions is determined to a large extent by the nature of

Figure 6.19 Diagrammatic representation of microemulsion structures: (a) a water-in-oil microemulsion droplet; (b) an oil-in-water microemulsion droplet; and (c) an irregular bicontinuous structure.

the surfactant. The geometry of the surfactant molecule is important. If the volume of the surfactant molecule is v, the cross-sectional area of its head group is a, and its length is l, then when the *critical packing parameter* v/al (see section 6.3.3) has values between 0 and 1, o/w systems are likely to form; but when v/al is greater than 1, w/o microemulsions are favoured. Values of the critical packing parameter close to unity can result in the formation of a bicontinuous structure in which areas of water can be imagined to be separated by a connected amphiphile-rich interfacial layer as depicted in Fig. 6.19(c). Values of the parameters v, a and l can readily be estimated, but it should be noted that the critical packing parameter is based purely on geometric considerations. Penetration of oil and cosurfactant into the surfactant interface and hydration of the surfactant head groups will also influence the packing of the molecules in the interfacial film around the droplets. In many systems, inversion from w/o to o/w microemulsions can occur as a result of changing the composition or the temperature. In general, o/w microemulsions are favoured when small amounts of oil are present and w/o systems form in the presence of small amounts of water. Under such conditions the droplet model is a reasonable representation of the system. The structure of microemulsions containing almost equal amounts of oil and water is best represented by a bicontinuous structure.

Clinical point **A microemulsion formulation**

A formulation of ciclosporin (Sandimmun Neoral, Novartis) incorporates the drug in a preconcentrate that forms a microemulsion on dilution in aqueous fluids.[2,3] This formulation offers an alternative to the oil formulation of ciclosporin (Sandimmun), which *in vivo* would be emulsified by bile salts and pancreatic enzymes. The residence time of ciclosporin in the gastrointestinal tract is shorter and the rate of absorption is faster with the microemulsion formulation. Some data can be found in Fig. 6.20. Reviews of parenteral microemulsions as drug delivery systems have been published.[4,5]

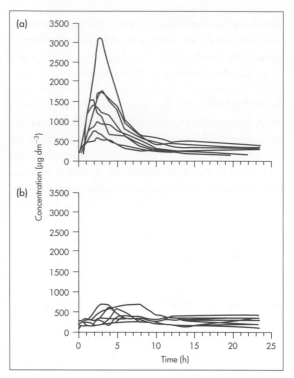

Figure 6.20 Blood ciclosporin concentration–time curves obtained following single oral doses (10 mg kg^{-1}) of (a) microemulsion and (b) conventional formulations in eight liver transplant recipients with external biliary diversion.

Reproduced with permission from Trull AK *et al.*, *Br J Clin Pharmacol*, 1995; 39: 627.

6.3.5 Structured (semisolid) emulsions

So far we have considered only relatively simple dilute emulsions. Many pharmaceutical preparations, lotions or creams are, in fact, complex semisolid or structured systems that contain excess emulsifier over that required to form a stabilising monolayer at the oil–water interface. The excess surfactant can interact with other components either at the droplet interface or in the bulk (continuous) phase to produce complex semisolid multiphase systems. Theories derived to explain the stability of dilute colloidal systems cannot be applied directly. In many cases the formation of stable interfacial films at the oil–water interface cannot be considered to play the dominant role in maintaining stability. Rather it is the structure of the bulk phase that maintains the disperse phase at a distance. Even very complex emulsions are often mobile at some point in their lifetime, e.g. during manufacture at elevated temperatures, or may become so during application of high shear rates in use. Under these conditions globules previously unable to interact become free to do so.

Stable o/w creams prepared with ionic or nonionic emulsifying waxes are composed of (at least) four phases (Fig. 6.21): (1) dispersed oil phase, (2) crystalline gel phase, (3) crystalline hydrate phase, and (4) bulk aqueous phase containing a dilute solution of surfactant. The interaction of the surfactant and fatty alcohol components of emulsifying mixtures to form these structures (body) is critical. It is also time-dependent, giving the name 'self-bodying' to these emulsions. The overall stability of a cream is dependent on the stability of the crystalline gel phase.

Emulsion stability is increased by the presence of liquid crystalline phases, as they form multilayers at the oil–water interface. These multilayers thus protect against coalescence by reducing the van der Waals forces of attraction and by retarding film thinning between approaching droplets, the viscosity of the liquid crystalline phases being at least 100 times that of the continuous phase in the absence of these structures. Guidelines have been devised for the formulation of self-bodied emulsions, the main ones of which are:[6]

- The *lipophilic component* should be an amphiphile that promotes the formation of w/o emulsions and is capable of complexing with the hydrophilic surfactant at the o/w interface.
- The *hydrophilic component* should be a surfactant that promotes the formation of o/w systems and is capable of complexing with the lipophilic component at the o/w interface.

The rigidity and strength of networks prepared with cetostearyl alcohol and alkyltrimethylammonium bromides (C_{12}–C_{18}) increase as the alkyl chain length increases. The rheological stability of ternary systems is markedly dependent on the alcohol chain length; networks prepared with ionic or nonionic surfactants and pure cetyl or pure stearyl alcohol are weaker than those prepared with cetostearyl alcohol.

6.3.6 Biopharmaceutical aspects of emulsions

Where traditionally emulsions have been used to deliver oils (castor oil, liquid paraffin) in a palatable form, a major use now is in intravenous nutrition. Lipid o/w

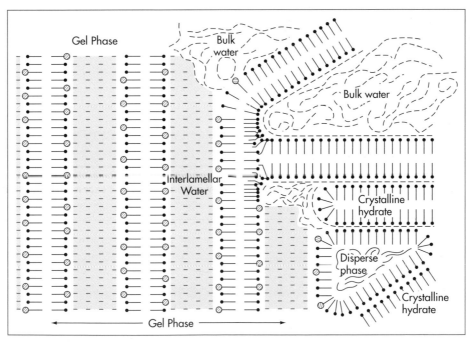

Figure 6.21 Schematic diagram of a typical semisolid cream prepared with cetostearyl alcohol and ionic surfactant. Note the four phases: (1) the dispersed oil phase; (2) the crystalline gel phase containing interlamellar fixed water; (3) phase composed of crystalline hydrates of cetostearyl alcohol; (4) bulk water phase.

Reproduced from Eccleston GM, *Pharm Int*, 1986; 7: 63.

emulsions are used as vehicles for lipophilic drugs (diazepam, propofol) for intravenous use. Griseofulvin, presented as an emulsion, exhibits enhanced oral absorption; an emulsion of indoxole has superior bioavailability over other oral forms. Medium-chain triglycerides and mono- and diglycerides promote the absorption of ceftriaxone and cefoxitin as well as ciclosporin.

In the case of griseofulvin, administration in a fatty medium enhances absorption. Fat is emulsified by the bile salts, and the administration of a pre-emulsified form increases the opportunity for solubilisation and hence transport across the microvilli by fat absorption pathways. The influence of the emulsifier on membrane permeability is one factor that must be considered. Knowledge that particles may be absorbed from the gut by the gut-associated lymphoid tissue suggests that we may have to revise our views on the nature of absorption of many drugs from the gastrointestinal tract.

Drug release from emulsions is related to the partition coefficient of the drug and the volume of the disperse phase, as well as to the concentration of surfactant that might solubilise the drug in the aqueous phase.

6.3.7 Preservative availability in emulsified systems

Microbial spoilage of emulsified products is avoided by the inclusion of appropriate amounts of a preservative in the formulation. Infected topical emulsions have been the cause of outbreaks of pseudomonal and other bacterial skin infections. The incorporation of preservatives into pharmaceutical emulsions is not without problems as most agents partition to the oily or micellar phases of complex systems; some are inactivated by surfactants.

The amount of preservative remaining in the aqueous phase (C_w) is related to the total amount (C) of preservative with a partition coefficient P in an emulsion with an oil/water phase ratio of Φ by equation (6.17):

$$C_w = \frac{C(\Phi + 1)}{R(P\Phi + 1)} \tag{6.17}$$

where R is the preservative/emulsifier ratio or interaction ratio. P and R need be determined experimentally.

The presence of surfactant micelles alters the native partition coefficient of the preservative molecule because the micellar phase offers an alternative site for preservative molecules. The partitioning then occurs between the oil globule and the aqueous micellar phases.

For preservatives that are less soluble in the oily phase ($P < 1$), the concentration in the oily, micellar or aqueous phases increases when the proportion of oil is increased. In contrast, for those preservatives that are more soluble in oil than in water ($P > 1$), the concentration in all phases decreases when the proportion of the oil phase is increased. This is the case with phenol and chlorocresol (see data given in Table 6.5).

Table 6.5 Percentage (W) of phenol and chlorocresol partitioned to various sites in arachis oil emulsions[a]

Arachis oil in water Φ (phase ratio)	Phenol				Chlorocresol			
	Oil W_o	Aqueous phase W_a	Micelles W_m	Water W_w	Oil W_o	Aqueous phase W_a	Micelles W_m	Water W_w
0.18	38	62	15.6	46.4	74.8	25.2	21.3	3.9
0.25	46.8	53.2	13.6	39.6	80.5	19.5	17	2.5
0.5	64	36	10.4	25.6	89.3	10.7	9.5	1.2
1.0	78.2	21.8	7.7	14.1	94.4	5.6	5.1	0.5
1.5	84.2	15.8	6.2	9.6	96.2	3.8	3.5	0.3

Note that $W_a = W_m + W_w$. Phenol and chlorocresol are present in 2.5% concentration.
Stabiliser: 1% polysorbate 80.
[a] Reproduced from Konning GK, *Can J Pharm Sci*, 1974; 9: 103.

In an emulsion containing 60% arachis oil ($\Phi = 1.5$) and 1% polysorbate, 9.6% of the phenol but only 0.3% of the more lipophilic chlorocresol is free in the water phase. As much as 93% of the phenol and 99.9% of chlorocresol are locked up in the oily phase or the micellar phases in emulsions containing 10% polysorbate 80.

The use of these equations can be criticised because of the simple manner in which R has been measured and defined, but they are useful to estimate effects of changing parameters. When the emulsified system is very complex, containing not one but at least two emulsifying agents (as most do), the determination of the parameters of the equation is a lengthy process, and a direct experimental approach to the determination of free aqueous concentration, such as a dialysis technique, may be the only approach.

6.3.8 Mass transport in oil-in-water emulsions

Not only preservative molecules partition from the phases in emulsions: drug molecules and flavouring and colouring agents also do. Interest in the extent and rate of flavour release on ingestion of a food emulsion has resulted in quantitative studies of the topic. The model used is equally applicable to drug release in the gastrointestinal tract as in the mouth, since dilution of the emulsion system occurs in both instances.

The concentration of the solute in the aqueous phase immediately after dilution C_w^0 and on re-establishing equilibrium C_w^e depends on the various properties of the solutes, such as the partition coefficient.

Usually, drugs dissolved in oils are absorbed mainly via the aqueous phase. Transport from one phase to the other and partitioning are therefore important. In the absorption of drugs from o/w emulsions when the drug partition coefficient is greater than 1, the *amount* of drug in the aqueous phase (rather than the concentration) is a critical factor for absorption. In the absorption of poorly oil-soluble drugs, drug absorption from emulsions is greater than from aqueous solution. In an emulsion of volume ratio, Φ, the drug concentration in the aqueous phase (C_w) is related to the overall concentration of the drug (C) by the expression:

$$C_w = C \frac{\Phi + 1}{P\Phi + 1} \tag{6.18}$$

where P is the oil/water partition coefficient of the drug or other agent.

6.3.9 Intravenous fat emulsions

Clinical point

Fat emulsions are used to supply a large amount of energy in a small volume of isotonic liquid; they supply the body with essential fatty acids and triglycerides. Fat emulsions for intravenous nutrition contain vegetable oil and phospholipid emulsifier. Several commercial fat emulsions are available, such as Intralipid, Lipiphysan, Lipofundin and Lipofundin S. They contain either cottonseed oil or soybean oil. In Intralipid, for example, purified egg-yolk phospholipids are used as the emulsifiers, and isotonicity is obtained by the addition of sorbitol, xylitol or glycerol. Intralipid has also been used as the basis of an intravenous drug carrier, for example for diazepam (Diazemuls) and propofol (Diprivan), as an alternative to solubilisation in nonionic micellar systems such as Cremophor EL.

To avoid adverse effects on injection it is important that the particle size of the emulsions is small and remains so on storage. After storage of Intralipid for two years at 4°C, more than 99% of the particles visible by light microscopy had a diameter of less than 1 μm; that is, there was practically no change in mean diameter.

Chylomicrons

Fat that finds its natural way into plasma occurs in three forms: as lipoprotein complexes, as free fatty acids bound to albumin, or as an emulsion of particles in the size range 0.4–3.0 μm. These natural emulsion globules are called *chylomicrons*. There are pronounced physical similarities between chylomicrons and the fat particles of the Intralipid emulsion.

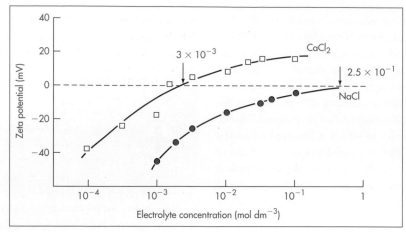

Figure 6.22 Zeta potential of Intralipid 20% diluted into varying concentrations (mol dm^{-3}) of ($\bullet$) NaCl, ($\square$) CaCl$_2$.
Reproduced from reference 7 with permission.

 Clinical point

The addition of electrolyte or drugs to intravenous fat emulsions is generally contraindicated because of the risk of destabilising the emulsion. Addition of cationic local anaesthetics reduces the electrophoretic mobility of the dispersed fat globules, and this contributes to instability.[7]

Minimum stability (and a minimum value of zeta potential) is caused by addition to Intralipid of 3×10^{-3} mol dm^{-3} CaCl$_2$ and 2.5×10^{-1} mol dm^{-3} NaCl, which are thus recommended as the maximum additive levels (see Fig. 6.22).

Prostaglandin E$_1$ (PGE$_1$) formulations

Lipid emulsion formulations of prostaglandin E$_1$ have been used in the treatment of vascular disorders. They exhibit a reduced incidence of side-effects at the site of injection, as does the diazepam lipid emulsion. A soybean emulsion stabilised by egg-yolk lecithin[8] releases the PGE$_1$ over a period of 4–16 hours depending on pH (Fig. 6.23). The partition coefficients of PGE$_1$ between soybean emulsion and aqueous buffers at 20°C are shown in Fig. 6.24, explaining why the release profiles have the pH dependency shown in Fig. 6.23. The release profile follows the expected pH trend, but a more detailed analysis shows that the majority of the drug is associated with the phospholipid.

6.3.10 Emulsion rheology

Most emulsions, unless very dilute, display both plastic and pseudoplastic flow behaviour rather than simple Newtonian flow. An attempt has been made[9] to calculate the shear conditions for simple pharmaceutical operations such as the spreading of an ointment or cream on the skin, ointment milling, and the flow of liquid through a hypodermic needle. The flow properties of fluid emulsions should have little influence on their biological behaviour, although the rheological characteristics of semisolid emulsions may affect their performance. The 'pourability', 'spreadability' and 'syringeability' of an emulsion will, however, be directly determined by its rheological properties. The

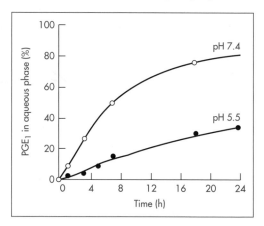

Figure 6.23 Release profiles of PGE$_1$ from particles in Lipo-PGE$_1$ diluted tenfold with buffer solutions at 5°C: ($\bullet$), pH 5.5; ($\circ$), pH 7.4.

Reproduced from reference 8.

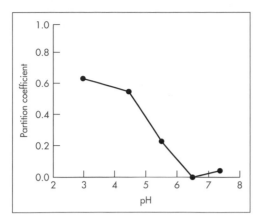

Figure 6.24 The pH–partition profiles of PGE_1 between soybean oil and water at 20°C, explaining why the release profiles have the pH dependency shown in Fig. 6.23.

Reproduced from reference 8.

high viscosity of w/o emulsions leads to problems with intramuscular administration of injectable formulations. Conversion to a multiple emulsion (w/o/w), in which the external oil phase is replaced by an aqueous phase, leads to a dramatic decrease in viscosity and consequent improved ease of injection.

The influence of phase volume on the flow properties of an emulsion is shown in Fig. 6.25. In this diagram the relative viscosity (η_{rel}) of the system increases with increasing ϕ, and at any given phase volume increases with decreasing mean particle size, D_m. These and other factors that affect emulsion viscosity are listed in Table 6.6.

As most emulsions are polydisperse, the influence of particle size and, in particular, of particle size distribution on viscosity is important. Figure 6.25 shows

the viscosity of w/o emulsions varying in mean particle size (D_m) stabilised with sorbitan trioleate.

Several equations for the viscosity of emulsion systems take the form

$$\eta_{rel} - 1 = \eta_{sp} = \frac{\alpha\phi}{1 - h\phi} \tag{6.19}$$

where $\alpha = 2.5$, and h is a measure of the fluid immobilised between the particles in concentrated emulsions and dispersions, which therefore reduces the total volume of liquid available for the particles to move around in. Immobilised liquid attached to solvated macromolecular stabilisers effectively increases the concentration of the particles and increases viscosity. In emulsions in which ϕ does not exceed 0.65, an equation of the form

$$\eta_{rel} = 1 + \frac{2.5\phi}{6(1 - h\phi)} \tag{6.20}$$

may be used, while for emulsions in which η_{rel} becomes infinite when $\phi \rightarrow 0.74$, the appropriate equation is

$$\eta_{rel} = 1 + \frac{2.5\phi}{2(1 - h\phi)} \tag{6.21}$$

where h has a value of 1.28–1.35.

Table 6.6 Factors that influence emulsion viscosity
Internal (disperse) phase
Volume fraction (ϕ)
Viscosity
Particle size and size distribution
Chemical nature
Continuous phase
Viscosity
Chemical constitution and polarity
Emulsifier
Chemical constitution and concentration
Solubility in the continuous and internal (disperse) phase
Physical properties of the interfacial film
Electroviscous effects
Presence of additional stabilisers, pigments, hydrocolloids, etc.

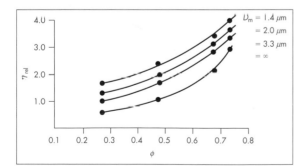

Figure 6.25 The relative viscosities of w/o emulsions stabilised with sorbitan trioleate; four emulsions have been studied with different mean particle diameters, D_m.

Reproduced from Sherman P, *J Pharm Pharmacol*, 1964; 16: 1.

When an emulsion is aged, its mean globule size increases. The ensuing changes in D_m and globule size distribution cause a fall in emulsion viscosity at high rates of shear. Provided no other changes have occurred in the system, the viscosity at any given time should be predictable from viscosity–D_m relationships derived from fresh emulsions of the same formulation. Viscosity changes at low rates of shear are more difficult to predict because of the complication of particle aggregation, which may change with time. Concentrated viscoelastic o/w emulsions stabilised by mixtures of nonionic emulsifiers and fatty alcohols are termed 'self-bodying' as the rheological characteristics change with time as a result of interactions between the components of the system.

Key points

- Emulsions can exist as oil-in-water (o/w) and water-in-oil (w/o) emulsions, multiple emulsions (w/o/w or o/w/o), microemulsions and semisolid emulsions.
- Adsorption of surfactant at the oil/water interface lowers the interfacial tension and aids the dispersal of the oil into droplets of a small size. Charged surfactants in the interfacial layer lead to an increase in zeta potential and will thus help to maintain stability by increasing V_R; nonionic surfactants maintain stability by creating a hydrated layer on the hydrophobic particle in o/w emulsions and by steric and enthalpic forces in w/o emulsions.
- Mixtures of surfactants usually form more stable emulsions than do single surfactants possibly because complex formation at the interface results in a more rigid stabilising film.
- Surfactants may be selected as emulsifiers on the basis of their HLB value (an empirical measure of the balance between hydrophobic and hydrophilic regions of the surfactant molecule). HLB values may be calculated from simple empirical equations or from summation of contributions from groups present in the molecule. Surfactants with a high HLB are water-soluble and are useful in the formation of o/w emulsions; those with low HLB are insoluble in water and are used in the formation of w/o emulsions. Mixtures of high- and low-HLB surfactants produce more stable emulsions than do single surfactants; the HLB of a mixture of two surfactants is the algebraic mean of the two HLB values. Optimum HLB values have been determined for a variety of oils used in o/w emulsions.
- Multiple emulsions are emulsions whose disperse phase contains droplets of another phase. They are made by emulsifying a w/o emulsion with a hydrophilic surfactant to produce a w/o/w system, or an o/w system with a low HLB surfactant to produce an o/w/o system. They are of interest in drug delivery as delayed-action formulations.
- Microemulsions are homogeneous transparent systems of low viscosity that form spontaneously when the components are mixed in the appropriate ratios and are thermodynamically stable. They can be dispersions of oil droplets in water (o/w) or water droplets in oil (w/o) with a mean droplet diameter of 5–140 nm. An essential requirement for their formation and stability is the attainment of a very low interfacial tension, which is achieved using a cosurfactant.
- Semisolid emulsions contain more emulsifier than is required to form a stabilising monolayer at the oil–water interface. Stable o/w creams prepared with ionic or nonionic emulsifying waxes are composed of (at least) four phases: a dispersed oil phase, a crystalline gel phase, a crystalline hydrate phase, and a bulk aqueous phase containing a dilute solution of surfactant. The overall stability of a cream is dependent on the stability of the crystalline gel phase.
- Emulsions are of interest as vehicles for drug delivery in which the drug is dissolved in the disperse phase. For example, lipid o/w emulsions are used as vehicles for lipophilic drugs (diazepam, propofol) for intravenous use. Intravenous fat emulsions such as Intralipid, Lipiphysan, Lipofundin and Lipofundin S are used to supply a large amount of energy in a small volume of isotonic liquid; they supply the body with essential fatty acids and triglycerides.

6.4 Suspensions

Suspensions are dispersions of an insoluble drug or other substance in an aqueous or nonaqueous continuous phase. Pharmaceutical suspensions tend to be coarse dispersions rather than true colloids, although there are many sub-micrometre polymer dispersions available as drug carriers. There are also suspensions of drug nanocrystals as discussed in Chapter 8. Drugs in suspension are prepared mainly for oral, intramuscular or subcutaneous use, but suspensions of drugs are also used as reservoirs in transdermal patch preparations and in conventional topical formulations. Many therapeutic aerosols are suspensions of drugs in a volatile propellant.

Problems can arise when a drug is dispersed in a liquid. Sedimentation, caking (leading to difficulty in resuspension), flocculation and particle growth (through dissolution and recrystallisation) all are possible. In practice we wish to avoid the problems of aggregation of particles in suspensions and in many lyophilised preparations and to ensure their efficient redispersion on reconstitution with water or other media. Adhesion of suspension particles to container walls has also been identified as a problem, particularly with low-dose drugs.

Formulation of pharmaceutical suspensions to minimise caking can be achieved by the production of flocculated systems. A flocculate, or floc, is a cluster of particles held together in a loose open structure; a suspension consisting of particles in this state is termed *flocculated* (Fig. 6.26). There are various states of flocculation and deflocculation. Unfortunately, flocculated systems clear rapidly and the preparation often appears unsightly, so a partially deflocculated formulation is the ideal pharmaceutical.

Suspensions of liposomes, microspheres and microcapsules, and nanospheres and nanocapsules formed from a variety of polymers or proteins form a relatively new class of pharmaceutical suspension in which physical stability is still paramount. It is important that on injection these carrier systems do not aggregate, as this will change the effective size and the fate of the particles. One exception to this would be the deliberate flocculation of latex particles administered to the eye, where aggregation leads to agglomerated particles that do not easily pass through the drainage ducts of the eye.

Figure 6.26 A flocculated suspension that has rapidly settled, clearly identifying the sedimentation layer, from which can be calculated the ratio R (equation 6.22) as $R = h_\infty/h_0$.

6.4.1 Stability of suspensions

In order to quantify the sedimentation of suspended particles, the ratio R of sedimentation layer volume (V_s) to total suspension volume (V_t) may be used. A measure of sedimentation may also be obtained from the height of the sedimented layer (h_∞) in relation to the initial height of the suspension (h_0).

$$R = \frac{V_s}{V_t} \approx \frac{h_\infty}{h_0} \tag{6.22}$$

In a completely deflocculated system the particles are not associated; pressure on the individual particles can lead in this layer to close packing of the particles to such an extent that the secondary energy barriers are overcome and the particles become irreversibly bound together. In flocculated systems (where the repulsive barriers have been reduced) particles settle as flocs and not as individual particles. The supernatant clears but, because of the random arrangement of the particles in the flocs, the sediment is not closely packed and caking does not readily occur.

In flocculated or concentrated suspensions, zone settling occurs (Fig. 6.27a). In the region A–B of Fig. 6.27b there is hindered settling of the particle interface at a constant rate; at B–C a transitional settling occurs; from C to D consolidation of the sediment occurs.

Suspension stability is governed by the same forces as in other disperse systems such as emulsions.

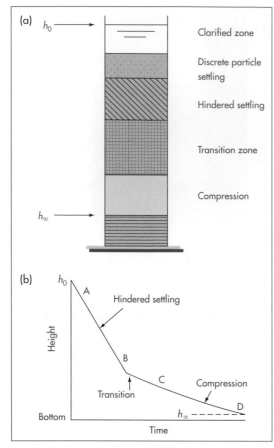

Figure 6.27 Zone sedimentation in a suspension. (a) The various zones are delineated, showing the clear layer at the top of the suspension and the sedimented layer at the bottom; immediately above this layer is a region in which the particles are crowded and begin to be compressed to form sediment. (b) The height of the interface between the clarified zone and the suspension as a function of time.

There are differences, however, as coalescence obviously cannot occur in suspensions; the adsorption of stabilising polymers and surfactants may also occur in a different fashion. Flocculation, unlike coalescence, can be a reversible process and partial or controlled flocculation is attempted in formulation, as discussed above.

Caking of the suspension, which arises on close packing of the sedimented particles, cannot be eliminated by reduction of particle size or by increasing the viscosity of the continuous phase. Fine particles in a viscous medium settle more slowly than coarse

particles but, after settling, they form a more closely packed sediment that may be difficult to re-disperse. Particles in a close-packed condition brought about by settling and by the pressure of particles above thus experience greater forces of attraction. Flocculating agents can prevent caking; deflocculating agents increase the tendency to cake. The addition of flocculating and deflocculating agents is often monitored by measurement of the zeta potential of the particles in a suspension.

Zeta potential and its relationship to stability

Most suspension particles dispersed in water have a charge acquired by specific adsorption of ions or by ionisation of ionisable surface groups, if present. If the charge arises from ionisation, the charge on the particle will depend on the pH of the environment. As with other colloidal particles, repulsive forces arise because of the interaction of the electrical double layers on adjacent particles. The magnitude of the charge can be determined by measurement of the electrophoretic mobility of the particles in an applied electric field. A microelectrophoresis apparatus in which this mobility may be measured is shown schematically in Fig. 6.28.

The velocity of migration of the particles (μ_E) under unit applied potential can be determined microscopically with a timing device and an eyepiece graticule. For nonconducting particles, the Henry equation is used to obtain ζ from μ_E. This equation can be written in the form

$$\mu_E = \frac{\zeta \varepsilon}{4\pi\eta} f(\kappa a) \tag{6.23}$$

where $f(\kappa a)$ varies between 1 for small κa and 1.5 for large κa; ε is the dielectric constant of the continuous phase and η its viscosity. In systems with low values of κa, the equation can be written in the form

$$\mu_\varepsilon = \frac{\zeta \varepsilon}{4\pi\eta} \tag{6.24}$$

The zeta potential (ζ) is not the surface potential (ψ_0) discussed earlier but is related to it. Therefore ζ can be used as a reliable guide to the magnitude of electric repulsive forces between particles. Changes in ζ on the addition of flocculating agents, surfactants and other

Figure 6.28 Schematic drawing of a microelectrophoresis apparatus showing the positioning of the anode and cathode and the capillary in which the velocity of particulates is monitored to allow calculation of zeta potential.

Figure 6.29 Caking diagram showing controlled flocculation of a bismuth subnitrate suspension employing dibasic potassium phosphate as the flocculating agent.

additives can then be used to predict the stability of the system.

The changes in a bismuth subnitrate suspension system on addition of dibasic potassium phosphate as flocculating agent are shown in Fig. 6.29. Bismuth subnitrate has a positive zeta potential; addition of phosphate reduces the charge and the zeta potential falls to a point where maximum flocculation is observed. In this zone there is no caking. Further addition of phosphate leads to a negative zeta potential and a propensity towards caking. Flocculation can therefore be controlled by the use of ionic species with a charge opposite to the charge of the particles dispersed in the medium.

The rapid clearance of the supernatant in a flocculated system is undesirable in a pharmaceutical suspension. The use of thickeners such as sodium carboxymethylcellulose hinders the movement of the particles by increasing the viscosity of the medium, slowing down sedimentation. The incompatibility of any anionic agents with cationic flocculating agents has to be considered. A technique to overcome the problem is the conversion of the particle surfaces into positive surfaces so that they require anions and not cations to flocculate them. Negatively charged or neutral particles can be converted into positively charged particles by addition of a surface-active amine. Such a suspension can then be treated with phosphate ions to induce flocculation.

It is perhaps not surprising that with some complex systems the interpretation of behaviour is open to debate. Consider the system shown in Fig. 6.30. One starts with a clumped suspension of sulfamerazine, a flocculated system that produces noncaking sediments. Addition of the surfactant sodium dioctyl sulfosuccinate (docusate sodium) confers a greater negative charge on the suspension particles and deflocculation results. Addition of aluminium chloride as a flocculating agent reduces the negative charge in a controlled way to produce the loose clusters illustrated in the diagram. These are the observable results of these procedures. The different interpretations of the effects are diagrammatically realised, the difference lying in the manner in which the aluminium ions adsorb onto the sulfamerazine particles; in one view they adsorb directly, and in the other view they interact with the surfactant ions on the surface.

Clinical point **Barium sulfate as an X-ray contrast medium**

The formulation of barium sulfate ($BaSO_4$) suspensions as a radiopaque material has to be carefully controlled for use. Flocculation of the suspended particles, which can be caused by the mucin in the gastrointestinal tract, causes artefacts to be seen in radiography. Such factors as particle size, zeta potential, pH-dependence of the properties of adjuvants and the whole suspension, and the film-forming characteristics of the formulation must be taken into account. The preparation must flow readily over the mucosal surface, penetrate into folds and coat the surface evenly with a thin radiopaque layer. A film 2 μm thick will absorb twice as much radiation as a layer 1 μm thick if the average $BaSO_4$ particle size and concentration are the same in both cases. The adhesion of wet films of barium sulfate suspensions to surfaces and their thickness have been assessed *in vitro* by a simple method in which a clean microscope slide is dipped into the suspension and allowed to drain for 30 seconds. The gross appearance displays evidence of irregular coating caused by foaming, bubble formation, or coagulation of particles. Commercially available suspensions preferred by radiologists are strongly negative at low pH, presumably resisting flocculation because of strong interparticle repulsion.

Polymers as flocculating agents

In many applications, such as water purification, suspended particles have to be removed by filtration. Flocculated particles are more readily removed than deflocculated particles. Polymers have been widely used as flocculating agents. Polymers used as flocculating or destabilising agents frequently act by adsorption and interparticle bridging. To be effective, the polymer must contain chemical groups that can interact with the surface of the colloidal particles. A particle–polymer complex is then formed, with polymer emerging into the

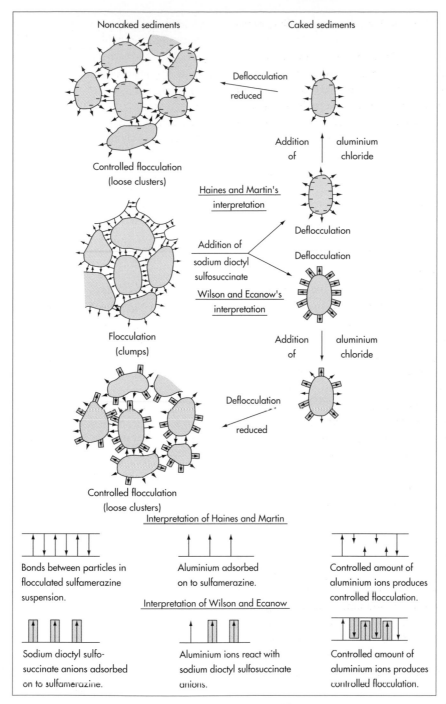

Figure 6.30 Diagrammatic drawing of flocculation and controlled flocculation in a sulfamerazine suspension: the effect of the addition of sodium dioctyl sulfosuccinate (docusate sodium) and aluminium chloride is shown and two interpretations of the results are outlined.

Reproduced from Woodford R, *Pharmacy Digest*, 1966; 29: 17.

aqueous phase. This free end will attach itself to another particle ('bridging') and thus promote flocculation. If there are no particles with which to interact, the polymer can coat the particle, leading to restabilisation. As can be seen in Fig. 6.31, however, the action of polymeric agents that can anchor at the particle surface is very concentration-dependent.

Polyacrylamide (30% hydrolysed) is an anionic polymer that can induce flocculation in kaolinite at very low concentrations. Restabilisation occurs by 'overdosing', probably by the mechanism outlined in Fig. 6.31. Dosages of polymer that are sufficiently large to saturate the colloidal surfaces produce a stable colloidal system, since no sites are available for the formation of interparticle bridges. Under certain conditions, physical agitation of the system can lead to breaking of polymer–suspension bonds and to a change in the state of the system.

 Key points

- Suspensions are coarse dispersions of an insoluble drug or other substance in an aqueous or nonaqueous continuous phase.
- They are inherently unstable due to sedimentation, caking (leading to difficulty in resuspension), flocculation and particle growth (through dissolution and recrystallisation).
- In a *deflocculated* system the particles settle separately and caking occurs because of close packing and irreversible binding of the sedimented particles. In *flocculated systems* particles settle as flocs, the sediment is not closely packed, and caking does not occur; clearance of the supernatant is, however, too rapid for an acceptable pharmaceutical formulation. The aim in the formulation of suspensions is, therefore, to achieve *partial or controlled flocculation* by the addition of flocculating agents, for example ions with opposite charge to that of the dispersed particles. Suspension stability may be assessed by measurement of the zeta potential of the particles and by the ratio of the height or volume of the sediment to that of the suspension.

6.4.2 Extemporaneous suspensions

Extemporaneous preparation of suspensions of drugs is still widely practised in hospital pharmacies, particularly to prepare dose forms for paediatric use when either a commercial product is unavailable or the dose has to be adjusted or the child cannot swallow tablets or capsules. Drugs such as acetazolamide, amiodarone and mercaptopurine are examples. In such formulations, alternatives to traditional suspending agents are required. The ideal suspending agent should:

- Be readily and uniformly incorporated in the formulation
- Be readily dissolved or dispersed in water without resort to special techniques
- Ensure the formation of a loosely packed system that does not cake
- Not influence the dissolution rate or absorption rate of the drug
- Be inert, nontoxic and free from incompatibilities

Among the alternative suspending agents are sodium carboxymethylcellulose, microcrystalline cellulose, aluminium magnesium silicate (Veegum), sodium alginate (Manucol) and sodium starch (Primojel). Pregelatinised starches, Primojel and Veegum, are promising alternatives to compound tragacanth powder. Paediatric formulations demand special care because of the potential toxicities of formulation additives. Some issues are discussed in the text *Paediatric Drug Handling*[10]

6.4.3 Suspension rheology

In deriving an equation for the viscosity of a suspension of spherical particles, Einstein considered particles that were far enough apart to be treated independently. The particle volume fraction is defined by

$$\phi = \frac{\text{volume occupied by the particles}}{\text{total volume of the suspension}} \quad (6.25)$$

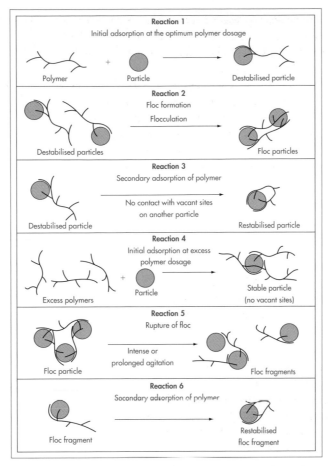

Figure 6.31 Schematic representation of the bridging model for the destabilisation of colloids by polymers: the concentration dependence of the process is illustrated.

Reproduced from Weber WJ, *Physicochemical Processes for Water Quality Control*, New York: Wiley; 1972.

The suspension could be assigned an effective viscosity, η_*, given by

$$\eta_* = \eta_0(1 + 2.5\phi) \tag{6.26}$$

where η_0 is the viscosity of the suspending fluid. As we have seen, the assumptions involved in the derivation of the Einstein equation do not hold for colloidal systems subject to Brownian forces, electrical interactions and van der Waals forces. Brownian forces result from 'the random jostling of particles by the molecules of the suspending fluid due to thermal agitation and fluctuation on a very short time scale'. The coefficient 2.5 in Einstein's equation (6.26) applies only to spheres; asymmetric particles will produce coefficients greater than 2.5.

Other problems in deriving *a priori* equations result from the polydisperse nature of pharmaceutical suspensions. The particle size distribution will determine η. A polydisperse suspension of spheres has a lower viscosity than its monodisperse equivalent. Structure formation during flow is an additional complication. Structure breakdown also occurs and is evident particularly in clay suspensions, which are generally flocculated at rest. Under flow there is a loss of the structure and the suspension exhibits thixotropy and a yield point. The viscosity decreases with increasing shear stress (Fig. 6.32). Addition of electrolytes to a suspension decreases the thickness of the double layer and reduces electroviscous effects, an effect reflected in the reduced viscosity of the suspension.

6.4.4 Nonaqueous suspensions

Many pharmaceutical aerosols consist of solids dispersed in a nonaqueous propellant. Few studies have

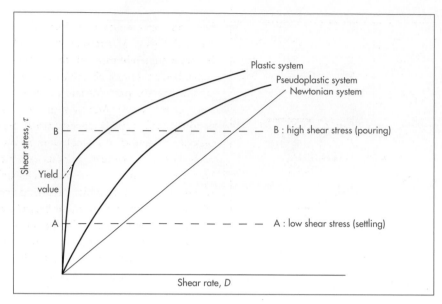

Figure 6.32 A plot of shear stress $\tau = \eta D$ against shear rate D for plastic and pseudoplastic suspensions. As $\eta = \tau/D$, the slope of the line represents the viscosity at each rate of shear; in both the plastic and pseudoplastic systems the viscosity at level A is greater than that at level B.

Modified from Samyn JC, *J Pharm Sci*, 1961; 50: 517.

been published on the behaviour of such systems, although their sensitivity to water is well established. Low amounts of water adsorb at the particle surface and can lead to aggregation of the particles with each other or to deposition on the walls of the container, which adversely affects the product performance.

6.4.5 Electrostatics in aerosols

Aerosol particles can become electrostatically charged as they are projected from the aerosol canister. The net charge is sufficient to affect deposition in the respiratory tract. Positive charges have been found on particles below 0.6 μm and negative charges above that size in Intal Forte, Tilade and Flixotide aerosols, which are suspension formulations with plastic valves. The number of charges on particles ranged from zero to several thousands!

As Schein[11] has written in an article on continuing puzzles in electrostatics, charging of solid surfaces 'remains one of the most poorly understood areas of solid-state physics.' It would be an advance to have charge correlated with the properties of the powders that experience this effect, but the issue in pharmaceuticals is often the presence of excipients. Particle

adhesion, say to plastic components as in spacers, has been thought to be due to electrostatic interactions between the charges on the particles and the resultant induced charges on any surface (Fig. 6.33). But the physical picture is more complex, and appears to be related to the discreteness of the charge, which produces strong electrostatic forces[12].

6.4.6 Adhesion of suspension particles to containers

When the walls of a container are wetted repeatedly, an adhering layer of suspension particles may build up, and this subsequently dries to a hard and thick layer. In Fig. 6.34 three types of wetting are shown. Where the suspension is in constant contact with the container wall, *immersional wetting* occurs, in which particles are pressed up to the wall and may or may not adhere. Above the liquid line, *spreading wetting* of the suspension during shaking or pouring may also lead to adhesion of the particles contained in the spreading liquid. *Adhesional wetting* occurs when a liquid drop remains suspended, like a drop of water on a clothes line. Evidently the surface tension of the suspension plays a part in the spreading and wetting processes.

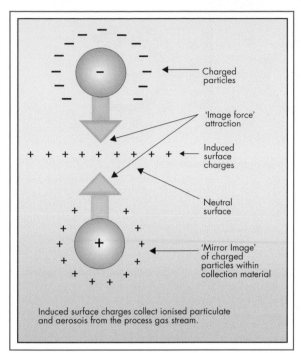

Figure 6.33 Schematic of induced positive charges on surfaces close to a negatively charged aerosol particle, which leads to particle adhesion.

Redrawn from www.verantis.com.

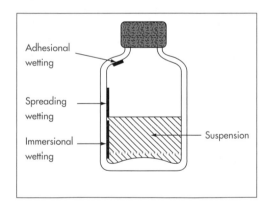

Figure 6.34 Adhesion. (a) Three types of wetting giving rise to adhesion of suspension particles. Suspended particles adhering to the surface of a glass vial can be seen in Fig. 6.26.

Adhesion increases with increase in suspension concentration, and with the number of contacts the suspension makes with the surfaces in question. Additives, especially surfactants, will modify the adhesion of suspension particles. They will act in two ways: (a) by decreasing the surface tension; and (b) by adsorption modifying the forces of interaction between particle and container. The example illustrated in Figs. 6.35 and 6.36 refers to the addition of benzethonium chloride to chloramphenicol suspensions. Benzethonium chloride converts both the glass surface and the particles into positively charged entities (see Fig. 6.35). Adhesion in the presence of this cationic surfactant is concentration-dependent, the process being akin to flocculation. At low concentrations the surfactant adsorbs by its cationic head to the negative glass and to the suspension particle. The glass is thus made hydrophobic. At higher concentrations hydrophobic interactions occur between coated particle and surface (Fig. 6.36). Further increase in concentration results in multilayer formation of surfactant, rendering the surfaces hydrophilic. In this condition the particles repel, reducing adhesion.

6.4.7 Powder processing

We have discussed at some length the interaction of particles with water and surfactants, so it is appropriate to take a look here at powder properties during processing, such as the preparation of granules for tableting where free drug is rarely if ever used. Figure 6.37 shows the steps in converting a powder into a pliant, plastic mass ready to be extruded in the spheronisation process. Clearly there are some complex interactions between the fluid binder phase and the powder. Figure 6.38 shows the steps in spraying binder solution onto a powder mass, the formation of liquid bridges, and then of solid bridges through drying and further agglomeration as well as showing various modes of liquid–particle interactions.

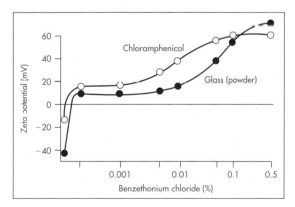

Figure 6.35 Zeta potential of glass (powder) and chloramphenicol in aqueous benzethonium chloride solutions.

Reproduced from Uno H, Tanaka S, *Kolloid Z-Z Polym*, 1972; 250: 238.

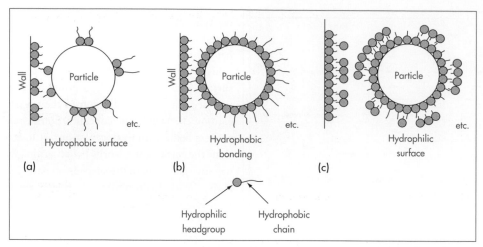

Figure 6.36 Adsorption of benzethonium chloride on particle and wall surfaces creating in (a) hydrophobic surfaces and in (b) hydrophobic bonding between the adsorbed molecules. In (c) further additions of the benzethonium chloride result in the conversion to hydrophilic surfaces.

Modified from Uno H, Tanaka S, *Kolloid Z Z Polym*, 1972; 250: 238.

6.5 Miscellaneous colloidal systems

Several colloidal systems have not been mentioned in this chapter because they are dealt with elsewhere. These include nanoparticle suspensions used in drug delivery and targeting, and vesicular dispersions (liposomes, niosomes, etc.). Variations on the emulsion theme include microsphere-in-water-in-oil systems (s/w/o) and vesicle-in-water-in-oil (v/w/o) formulations. Figure 6.39 shows (a) the appearance of a vesicle-based system and (b) the modes of release of drug encapsulated in the system.

6.6 Applications of colloid stability theory to other systems

There are several colloidal systems other than synthetically produced emulsions and suspensions that are of relevance – blood and other cell suspensions, for example – whose behaviour can now be better understood by application of colloid stability theory. The adhesion of cells to surfaces, the aggregation of platelets, the spontaneous sorting out of mixed cell aggregates and other such phenomena, depend to a large extent on interaction between the surfaces of the objects in question, although the surfaces are frequently more labile and less homogeneous than those encountered in model colloids. The extended circulation in the blood of 'long-life' or 'stealth' liposomes whose surfaces are modified by protruding long surface-bonded hydrophilic chains (usually polyoxyethylene glycols) may also be ascribed to their modified interactions *in vivo* with opsonins and with scavenging cells of the reticuloendothelial system.

Figure 6.37 The stages of powder treatment for the production of spheres in the spheronisation process: mixing, the formation of a plastic mass, extrusion, the formation of wet spheres and then drying to produce the spheres.

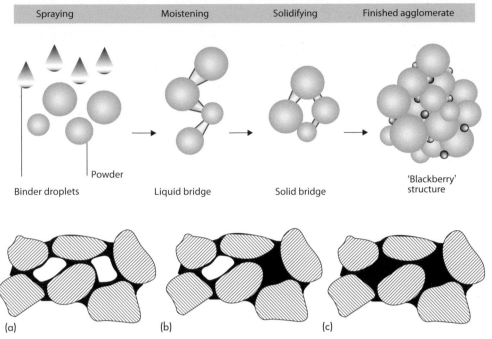

Figure 6.38 Upper panel: the sequence of spraying, moistening, solidifying and agglomeration showing the special part that the aqueous binder plays in achieving the agglomeration of particulates. Lower panel: particles with fluid in the (a) pendular, (b) funicular and (c) capillary states, showing the variety of modes of liquid–particle interactions.

Figure 6.39 (a) Photomicrograph of a vesicle-in-water-in-oil (v/w/o) emulsion. (b) Diagrammatic representation of the modes of release of solutes from the formulation ($\bullet$ = drug).

6.6.1 Cell–cell interactions

A simple way of considering interactions between free-floating cells is to treat the cells as spheres. Adhesion between cells in contact is, however, best considered as interaction between planar surfaces (Fig. 6.40). Cell adhesion and separation occur during the interaction of sperm and egg, in cell fusion and in parasitism; phagocytosis may also have an adhesive component. Cell adhesion can occur with a variety of nonliving materials such as implanted prosthetic devices.

Adhesion is primarily a surface phenomenon. The main factors that act to produce adhesion are:

- Bridging mechanisms
- Electrostatic interactions
- Interactions involving long-range forces

As in suspension flocculation, the bridging agent will be a molecule that combines in some way with both surfaces and thus links them together. Macromolecules may adsorb onto the surface of the particle and, if the length of the molecule is greater than twice the range of the electrostatic forces of repulsion, the other end of the molecule may adsorb on to a second surface. Flexible molecules may adsorb on to the same cell or particle. Alternatively, polyvalent ions may bind to charged groups on the two adjacent surfaces. Brownian motion may provide the means for close approach of the particles, or the polyvalent ion and may so reduce the electrostatic repulsion that the cells can approach each other.

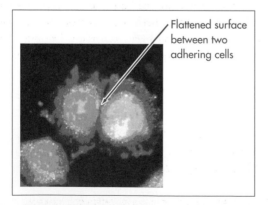

Figure 6.40 Interacting cells with a planar interface formed between them.

Photograph: J. Ivaska, Centre for Biotech, Finland.

Electrostatic forces of attraction will come into play when the surfaces have opposite sign or charge or when the surfaces possess mosaics of charges such that interaction can occur. The long-range forces are those discussed earlier in the chapter. Low pH, high ionic strength and the presence of covalent cations all favour cell–cell adhesion.

It is not possible to discuss all cell–cell interactions rigorously from a purely physical point of view. Often adhesion results in the secretion of complex chemicals that further induce interaction that cannot be treated by any physicochemical model.

6.6.2 Adsorption of microbial cells to surfaces

The contamination of pharmaceutical suspensions for oral use can be a problem. Under some conditions, bacteria may be strongly adsorbed and therefore more resistant to the effects of preservatives. In other cases, the bacteria may be free in the liquid phase of the suspension.

Two distinct phases of bacterial adsorption onto glass have been observed;[13] the first, reversible, phase may be interpreted in terms of DLVO theory. Reversible sorption of a nonmobile strain (*Achromobacter*) decreased to zero as the electrolyte concentration of the medium was increased, as would be expected. The second, irreversible, phase is probably the result of polymeric bridging between bacterial cell and the surface in contact with it. It is obviously not easy to apply colloid theory directly, but the influence of factors such as surface potential, pH and additives can usually be predicted and experimentally confirmed.

In the agglutination of erythrocytes and the adsorption of erythrocytes to virus-infected cells, projections of small radius of curvature have been observed and could well account for the local penetration of the energy barrier and strong adhesion at the primary minimum. The various modes of cell sorption are shown diagrammatically in Fig. 6.41.

Sorption of microbial cells is selective but there is no obvious relation between Gram-staining characteristics and attachment. In Fig. 6.41, bacterial cells are shown adsorbing onto larger solid particles (a) or free in suspension (b); (c) illustrates the opposite effect – small particles are shown adsorbed onto bacterial cells. The bacterial cells are adsorbed onto

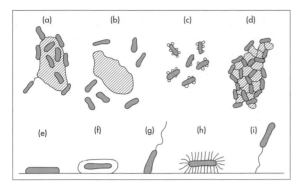

Figure 6.41 Various types of bacterial sorption on solid surfaces (see text).

Reproduced from Zvyagintsev D, *Interaction between Microorganisms and Solid Surfaces*, Moscow: Moscow University Press; 1973.

flocculated particles in (d), onto solid surfaces in (e); (f)–(i) show the more complicated behaviour of bacterial forms with coats, cilia and flagella. The adsorption affects growth partly by masking the cell surface and partly by altering the release of metabolites from the cell.

In addition to the van der Waals and electrical forces, steric forces resulting from protruding polysaccharide and protein molecules affect interactions; specific interactions between charged groups on the cell surface and on the solid surface, hydrogen bonding or the formation of cellular bridges may all occur to complicate the picture.

6.6.3 Blood as a colloidal system

Blood is a non-Newtonian suspension showing a shear-dependent viscosity. At low rates of shear, erythrocytes form cylindrical aggregates (rouleaux), which break up when the rate of shear is increased. Calculations show that the shear rate (D) associated with blood flow in large vessels such as the aorta is about $100\,s^{-1}$, but for flow in capillaries it rises to about $1000\,s^{-1}$. The flow characteristics of blood are similar to those of emulsions except that, while shear deformation of oil globules can occur with a consequent change in surface tension, no change in membrane tension occurs on cell deformation.

Velocity gradients in blood vessels are reduced in cases of retarded peripheral circulation, especially in shock. Under these conditions erythrocytes may aggregate and the discovery of agents that are capable of reducing this structural viscosity is thus of great clinical value. Dextrans and polyvinylpyrrolidones diminish attraction between individual cells in blood and improve flow properties.

Aggregation of platelets involves a contact phase and an adhesive phase, shown diagrammatically in Fig. 6.42. Shearing effects of blood may dislodge platelets. Interest in platelet interaction with simpler surfaces has been stimulated by the increasing use of plastic prosthetic devices which come into contact with blood.

While we do not have a clear idea of the physical and chemical properties of surfaces that are responsible for the attraction of platelets, a relationship between adhesion and the critical surface tension of uncharged hydrophobic surfaces has been demonstrated. The number of platelets adsorbed increases as the critical surface tension increases. There is other evidence that platelets adhere readily to high-energy hydrophilic surfaces and less readily to low-energy hydrophobic surfaces. Thus platelet adhesion to glass is reduced following coating of the latter with dimethylsiloxane.

6.7 Foams

Aqueous foams are formed from a three-dimensional network of surfactant films in air. They are disperse systems with a high surface area. Consequently, foams tend to collapse spontaneously. They can, however, if suitably stabilised, be used as formulations for the delivery of enemas and topical products. Foams that develop in production of liquids or in ampoules are troublesome, hence there is an interest in breaking foams and preventing foam formation. The breaking and prevention of liquid foams is less well understood

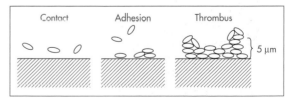

Figure 6.42 Sequence in the formation of a thrombus at a surface, involving three stages: contact, adhesion and thrombus growth.

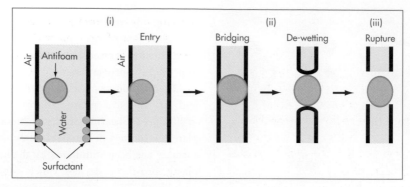

Figure 6.43 A schematic drawing of the antifoaming mechanism of antifoam droplets (i) entering a foam lamella, (ii) bridging– de-wetting and (iii) rupturing the foam wall.

Reproduced from Perry D *et al.*, *Foam Control in Aqueous Coatings*, Dow Corning Corporation; 2001.

than the stabilisation of foams. It is recognised, how- ever, that small quantities of specific agents can reduce foam stability markedly. There are two types of such agent:

- *Foam breakers*, which are thought to act as small droplets forming in the foam lamellae (see Fig. 6.43)
- *Foam preventatives*, which are thought to adsorb at the air–water interface in preference to the surfactants that stabilise the thin films. Once adsorbed, however, they do not have the capacity, to stabilise the foam.

It is well established that pure liquids do not foam. Transient foams are obtained with solutes such as short-chain aliphatic alcohols or acids that lower the surface tension moderately; really persistent foams arise only with solutes that lower the surface tension strongly in dilute solution – the highly surface-active materials such as detergents and proteins. The physical chemistry of the surface layers of the solutions is what determines the stability of the system.

Ordinarily, three-dimensional foams of surfactant solutes persist for a matter of hours in closed vessels. Gas slowly diffuses from the small bubbles to the large ones (since the pressure and hence thermodynamic activity of the gas within the bubbles is inversely pro- portional to bubble radius). Diffusion of gas leads to a rearrangement of the foam structures and this is often

sufficient to rupture the thin lamellae in a well-drained film.

The most important action of an antifoam agent is to eliminate surface elasticity – the property that is responsible for the durability of foams. To do this it must displace foam stabiliser. It must therefore have a low interfacial tension in the pure state to allow it to spread when applied to the foam, and it must be pres- ent in sufficient quantity to maintain a high surface concentration. Many foams can be made to collapse by applying drops of liquids such as ether, or long- chain alcohols such as octanol. Addition of ether, which has a low surface tension, to an aqueous foam will locally produce regions with a low surface tension. These regions are rapidly pulled out by surrounding regions of higher tension. The foam breaks because the ethereal region cannot stretch. Long-chain alcohols also break foams because the surface is swamped by rapidly diffusing molecules so that changes in surface tension are rapidly reversed (that is, elasticity disappears).

Generally more effective and more versatile than any soluble antifoams are the silicone fluids, which have surface tensions as low as $20 \, \text{mN m}^{-1}$. Quantities of the order of 1–60 ppm prevent foaming in fermentation vats, sewage tanks and dyebaths. Antifoam droplets are seen in Fig. 6.43 entering the foam lamella, bridging between the surfaces, de- wetting and then rupturing the foam wall.

Clinical point

X-ray studies have clearly shown the presence of foam in the upper gastrointestinal tract in humans. Silicone antifoaming agents derive their value from their ability to change the surface tension of the mucus-covered gas bubbles in the gut and thus to cause the bubbles to coalesce. A range of polydimethylsiloxanes is available commercially, including Dimethicone 20, 200, 350, 500 and 1000 (the numbers refer to the viscosity of the oil in centistokes). In simple *in vitro* tests, polydimethylsiloxane of molecular weight used in pharmaceutical formulations (Dimethicone 1000) has poor antifoaming properties. The addition of a small percentage (2–8%) of hydrophobic silica, which on its own is a weak defoamer, increases the antifoaming effect, the finely divided silica particles being suspended in the silicone fluid. The product is a simple physical mixture of silica and polydimethylsiloxane.

Some *in vivo* results are listed in Table 6.7. The incorporation of these materials into antacid tablets is widespread; certain antacids have been found, however, to adsorb the polydimethylsiloxane and reduce its antifoaming potential.[14]

Summary

This chapter has covered the topic of pharmaceutical colloids, with a special emphasis on emulsions and suspensions. These have been rather traditional pharmaceutical forms, but they are attracting increasing interest because of increased knowledge of the biodistribution and fate of colloidal particles in the body, and the need to deliver highly lipophilic and often very potent drugs in carriers. Emulsions, microemulsions and solid suspensions are all, therefore, important in modern drug delivery.

The chapter has dealt with the stability and stabilisation of colloidal systems and covered topics such as their formation and aggregation. If the particle size of a colloidal particle determines its properties (such as its viscosity or its fate in the body), then maintenance of that particle size throughout the lifetime of the product is important. The emphasis in the section on

Table 6.7 *In vivo* effects of polydimethylsiloxane (PDMS)[a]

Treatment by mouth	Volume (cm³)	Dose (mg/rat)		Mean percentage reduction[b] in foam height (± SEM).
		PDMS	Silica	
PDMS	0.25	250		19±4
	0.50	500		29±6
	1.00	1000		56±6
	2.00	2000		84±3
PDMS containing 65 w/v silica	0.005	4.7	0.2	45±6
	0.01	9.4	0.6	58±5
	0.02	18.9	1.1	61±5
	0.04	37.7	2.0	87±2

[a] Reproduced from Birtley RDN *et al., J Pharm Pharmacol*, 1973; 25: 859.
[b] 10 rats in each group; foam induced by saponin.

stability is therefore understandable. Various forms of emulsions, microemulsions and multiple emulsions have also been discussed, while other chapters deal with other important colloidal systems, such as protein and polymer micro- and nanospheres and phospholipid and surfactant vesicles. Suspensions also feature in processing technologies, as in the formation of granules and spherules where a powder–liquid mass is the basis for further processing. Some aspects of these systems are discussed and should be read in the light of an understanding of contact angles and solid surface hydrophobicities.

Towards the end of the chapter we point out the biological importance of an understanding of colloid chemistry and several examples of biological importance are covered. Pharmaceutical and biological colloids are often very complex systems, but even so the fundamental principles can be applied to obtain an appreciation of the behaviour of systems such as blood, platelets and microorganisms when they come in contact with inert or biological surfaces. In simplifying the concepts here, we do not pretend that there are no other forces at work. It is nonetheless useful to think of complex systems in a straightforward physicochemical manner, as pointed out in the introduction to the book.

References

1. Suitthimeathegorn O *et al.* Novel anhydrous emulsions: formulation as controlled release vehicles. *Int J Pharm* 2005;298:367–371.
2. Kovarik JM *et al.* Cyclosporine pharmacokinetics and variability from a microemulsion formulation – a multi-center investigation in kidney transplant patients. *Transplantation* 1994;58:658–663.
3. Mueller EA *et al.* Improved dose linearity of cyclosporine pharmacokinetics from a microemulsion formulation. *Pharm Res* 1994;11:301–304.
4. Date AA, Nagarsenker MS. Parenteral microemulsions: an overview. *Int J Pharm* 2008;355:19–30.
5. Ansari MJ *et al.* Microemulsions as potential delivery systems: a review. *PDA J Pharm Sci Technol* 2008;62:66–79.
6. Barry BW. Structure and rheology of emulsions stabilized by mixed emulsifiers. *Rheol Acta* 1971;10:96–105.
7. Whateley TL *et al.* Particle size stability of Intralipid and mixed total parenteral nutrition mixtures. *J Clin Hosp Pharm* 1984;9:113–26.
8. Yamaguchi T *et al.* Distribution of prostaglandin E_1 in lipid emulsion in relation to release rate from lipid particles. *Chem Pharm Bull* 1994;42:646–450.
9. Henderson NL *et al.* Approximate rates of shear encountered in some pharmaceutical processes. *J Pharm Sci* 1961;50:788–791.
10. Costello I *et al. Paediatric Drug Handling.* London: Pharmaceutical Press; 2007.
11. Schein LB. Recent progress and continuing puzzles in electrostatics. *Science* 2007;316:1572–1573.
12. Kwok PCL *et al.* Electrostatic charge characteristics of aerosols produced from metered dose inhalers. *J Pharm Sci* 2005;94:2789–2799.
13. Marshall KC *et al.* Mechanism of the initial events in the sorption of marine bacteria to surfaces. *J Gen Microbiol* 1971;68:337–348.
14. Rezak MJ. *In vitro* determination of deforming inactivation of silicone antacid tablets. *J Pharm Sci* 1966;55:538–539.

7

Polymers and macromolecules

This survey of the pharmaceutical aspects of polymers, copolymers and macromolecules emphasises their use in formulation but also deals with the uses of some polymers such as dextran in therapeutics. It stresses the key features of polymers – their molecular weight distribution and their versatility in terms of their morphology, crystallinity, solubility and performance.

It is convenient to think of polymeric systems as either water-soluble or water-insoluble. This division, while not rigid because some polymers are water-dispersible, is useful in that it separates the two main areas of use that form the basis of this chapter. Water-soluble materials can be used to modify the viscosity of aqueous solutions and to maintain the stability of suspensions, or to form the basis of film coatings and water-soluble matrices. The higher-molecular-weight polyoxyethylene glycols, for example, are used as suppository bases. Water-soluble polymers can be crosslinked electrostatically or covalently to give hydrogels. Crosslinked hydrogels absorb water but do not dissolve. The differences in release of drugs from water-insoluble matrices and from swelling hydrogels should be appreciated.

Bioadhesives are usually water soluble, while pressure-sensitive adhesives used in transdermal patches tend to be insoluble polyacrylates and polysiloxanes. Water-insoluble materials form membranes and matrices. The factors affecting the transport of drugs in these systems should be understood: that is to say, the thickness of the membrane, the solubility of the drug in the membrane and the relationship of this to its lipophilicity generally, copolymer ratios, porosity and the heterogeneity of the mix caused by fillers or plasticisers.

7.1 Pharmaceutical polymers

Natural polymers such as acacia and tragacanth have been used in pharmacy for many years. Mostly they have been replaced by synthetic polymers whose properties are more readily characterised and controlled.

A wide spectrum of polymers are used widely in pharmaceutical systems as suspending and emulsifying agents, flocculating agents, adhesives, packaging and coating materials, and increasingly as components of controlled and site-specific drug delivery systems (Scheme 7.1). The synthesis of polymers with specific properties (e.g. pH-dependent solubility or viscosity, biodegradability, membrane-forming character) offers exciting possibilities, especially as it holds out the hope of obtaining new polymers for drug delivery devices, so essential for the efficient use of many of today's potent and toxic drugs. Polymer biodegradability is an issue in some applications.

7.1.1 Definitions

Polymers are substances of high molecular weight made up of repeating *monomer* units. Substances with short chains containing relatively few monomers are called *oligomers*. Polymers owe their unique properties to their size, their three-dimensional shape and sometimes to their flexibility and asymmetry. The chemical reactivity of polymers depends on the chemistry of their monomer units, but their properties depend to a large extent on the way the monomers are assembled; it is this fact that leads to the versatility of synthetic polymers. Polymer molecules may be linear or branched, and separate linear or branched chains may be joined by crosslinks. Extensive crosslinking leads to a three-dimensional and often insoluble polymer network. Polymers in which all the monomeric units are identical are referred to as *homopolymers*; those formed from more than one monomer type are called *copolymers*. Various arrangements of the monomers A and B in the copolymer molecules (Fig. 7.1) can be produced with consequent effects on the physical properties of the resulting polymer. Synthetic polymers may have their main chains substituted in different ways, depending on the conditions of the reaction, such that atactic (random), isotactic or syndiotactic forms are produced, as diagrammatically represented in Fig. 7.1.

Copolymers may be described as alternating copolymers, block copolymers or graft copolymers. The molecular architecture of copolymers may, however, be more complicated than represented in Fig. 7.1. Block copolymers such as the polyoxyethylene–polyoxypropylene–polyoxyethylene (ABA) systems have both hydrophobic (A) and hydrophilic regions (B); they form an interesting group of surfactants and are discussed in Chapter 5. Homopolymers can be linear, star or branched

Scheme 7.1

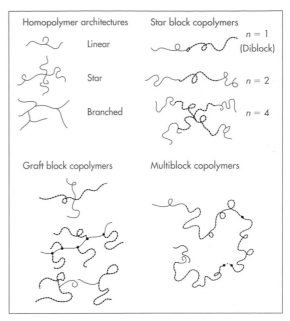

Figure 7.2 The range of structures of homopolymers and star block, graft block and multiblock copolymers.

Figure 7.1 (a) Varieties of copolymer molecular structures attainable though the polymerisation of two different monomers represented by A and B. (b) Representations of random atactic, isotactic and symmetrical copolymers.

materials. It is because of this that synthetic polymers also have an advantage over many variable natural polymers, although many natural derivatives such as cellulosic derivatives are used extensively. Natural materials can be modified chemically, and this approach can lead to useful new products, as with those derived from cellulose or dextran. The structural

(Fig 7.2), giving rise to so-called star block copolymers defined by the number of arms (*n*).

Polymers that have fairly symmetrical chains and strong interchain forces can be drawn into fibres. *Plastics* are polymers with lower degrees of crystallinity that can be moulded. Further down the rigidity scale are *rubbers* and *elastomers*, whose properties are well known.

It is apparent that polymer molecules will have a much wider range of physical properties than small chemical entities. Even when considering one chemical type (for example, polyethylene) its properties may be altered by increasing or decreasing the molecular weight (Fig. 7.3). There is a degree of control over properties that is not present with small organic

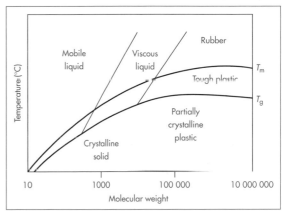

Figure 7.3 Approximate relation between molecular weight, T_g (glass transition temperature), T_m (melting point), and polymer properties.

Reproduced from Billmeyer FW, *Textbook of Polymer Science*, 2nd edn, New York: Wiley; 1971.

formulae of some common macromolecules are given in Table 7.1.

Dendrimers are highly branched polymer constructs formed from a central core that defines their initial geometry.[1] Their branch-like structure (Fig. 7.4) leads to spheres, which in higher generations appear to be the size of micelles, and ultimately nanospheres of small dimensions. They can be functionalised and in this way 'layered' systems can be formed by using different monomers for succeeding reactions (generations); such chemical architecture has virtually no bounds.[2] Dendrons are partial dendrimers, usually having a branched structure coupled to a linear chain.

7.1.2 Polydispersity

Nearly all synthetic polymers and naturally occurring macromolecular substances exist with a range of molecular weights; exceptions to this are proteins and natural polypeptides, each of which occurs with a single well-defined molecular weight. The molecular weight of a polymer or macromolecule is thus an average molecular weight, which may be determined by chemical analysis or by osmotic pressure or light-scattering measurements. When determined by chemical analysis or osmotic pressure measurement a *number-average molecular weight*, M_n, is found, which in a mixture containing $n_1, n_2, n_3, \ldots$ moles of polymer with molecular weights $M_1, M_2, M_3, \ldots$, respectively, is defined by

$$M_n = \frac{n_1 M_1 + n_2 M_2 + n_3 M_3 + \cdots}{n_1 + n_2 + n_3 + \cdots}$$
$$= \frac{\Sigma n_i M_i}{\Sigma n_i} \tag{7.1}$$

The individual molecular weights $M_1, M_2, \ldots$ cannot be determined separately – the equation merely explains the meaning of the value M_n.

In light-scattering techniques, larger molecules produce greater scattering; thus the weight (or more strictly the mass) rather than the number of the molecules is important, giving a weight-average molecular weight, M_w:

$$M_w = \frac{m_1 M_1 + m_2 M_2 + m_3 M_3 + \cdots}{m_1 + m_2 + m_3 + \cdots}$$
$$= \frac{\Sigma n_i M_i^2}{\Sigma n_i M_i} \tag{7.2}$$

In equation (7.2) $m_1, m_2, m_3, \ldots$ are the masses of each species, and m_i is obtained by multiplying the molecular weight of each species by the number of molecules of that weight; that is $m_i = n_i M_i$. Thus the molecular weight appears as the square in the numerator of equation (7.2); the weight-average molecular weight is therefore biased towards larger molecules. Another consequence is that $M_w > M_n$; that is, the average molecular weight of a polymer measured by light scattering must be greater than that obtained by osmotic pressure measurements if the polymer is polydisperse (that is, contains a range of molecular weights). The ratio M_w/M_n expresses the degree of polydispersity. Table 7.2 shows actual values for the number-average and weight-average molecular weights for dextrans, microbial polysaccharides used therapeutically as plasma expanders.

7.1.3 Polymer mixtures or blends

Of course not all polymers are soluble or miscible with each other; some indeed de-mix when added together. The different phase behaviours that are realised with representative molecular architectures are shown in Fig. 7.5. Such mixtures produce solid polymeric structures such as films and membranes with distinctive morphologies and properties. When polymer blends are used as drug delivery matrices or as the basis of micro- and nanoparticles, it is important that polymer–polymer interactions are studied.

7.1.4 Polymer solubility

The solubility of polymeric substances in water is determined by the same considerations that apply to smaller molecules. Those polymers that are sufficiently polar will be able to interact with the water to provide energy to remove individual polymer chains from the solid state.

Water-soluble polymers have an ability to increase the viscosity of solvents at low concentrations, to swell or change shape in solution, and to adsorb at surfaces. These are significant features of their behaviour, which we will deal with briefly.

Insoluble polymers or polymers with a low rate of solution are used more to form thin films, as film-coating materials, surgical dressings or membranes for dialysis or filtration, or to form matrices for enveloping drugs to control their release properties, or simply as packaging materials.

Table 7.1 Structural formulae of some macromolecular compounds

Name	Chain structure	Monomer
Polymers with a carbon chain backbone:		
Polyethylene	$-CH_2-CH_2-CH_2-CH_2-CH_2-$	$CH_2=CH_2$
Polypropylene	$-CH_2-\underset{\underset{CH_3}{\vert}}{CH}-CH_2-\underset{\underset{CH_3}{\vert}}{CH}-CH_2-\underset{\underset{CH_3}{\vert}}{CH}-CH_2-$	$CH_2=\underset{\underset{CH_3}{\vert}}{CH}$
Polystyrene	$-CH_2-CH-CH_2-CH-CH_2-CH-CH_2-$ with phenyl rings	$CH=CH_2$ with phenyl ring
Poly(vinyl chloride)	$-CH_2-\underset{\underset{Cl}{\vert}}{CH}-CH_2-\underset{\underset{Cl}{\vert}}{CH}-CH_2-\underset{\underset{Cl}{\vert}}{CH}-CH_2-$	$CH_2=\underset{\underset{Cl}{\vert}}{CH}$
Polytetrafluoroethylene	$-\underset{\underset{F}{\vert}}{\overset{\overset{F}{\vert}}{C}}-\underset{\underset{F}{\vert}}{\overset{\overset{F}{\vert}}{C}}-\underset{\underset{F}{\vert}}{\overset{\overset{F}{\vert}}{C}}-\underset{\underset{F}{\vert}}{\overset{\overset{F}{\vert}}{C}}-\underset{\underset{F}{\vert}}{\overset{\overset{F}{\vert}}{C}}-\underset{\underset{F}{\vert}}{\overset{\overset{F}{\vert}}{C}}-$	$\underset{\underset{F}{}}{\overset{\overset{F}{}}{C}}=\underset{\underset{F}{}}{\overset{\overset{F}{}}{C}}$
Polyacrylonitrile	$-CH_2-\underset{\underset{CN}{\vert}}{CH}-CH_2-\underset{\underset{CN}{\vert}}{CH}-CH_2-\underset{\underset{CN}{\vert}}{CH}-CH_2-$	$CH_2=\underset{\underset{CN}{\vert}}{CH}$
Poly(vinyl alcohol)	$-CH_2-\underset{\underset{HO}{\backslash}}{CH}-CH_2-\underset{\underset{HO}{\backslash}}{CH}-CH_2-\underset{\underset{HO}{\backslash}}{CH}-CH_2-$	$CH_2=\underset{\underset{OH}{\vert}}{CH}$
Poly(vinyl acetate)	$-CH_2-\underset{\underset{O}{\vert}}{CH}-CH_2-\underset{\underset{O}{\vert}}{CH}-CH_2-\underset{\underset{O}{\vert}}{CH}-CH_2-$ with $\underset{\underset{CH_3}{\vert}}{C=O}$ groups	$CH_2=CH$ with $-O-\underset{\underset{CH_3}{\vert}}{C}=O$
Polyacrylamide	$-CH_2-\underset{\underset{CONH_2}{\vert}}{CH}-CH_2-\underset{\underset{CONH_2}{\vert}}{CH}-CH_2-\underset{\underset{CONH_2}{\vert}}{CH}-CH_2-$	$CH_2=CH$, $O=C-NH_2$
Poly(methyl methacrylate)	$-CH_2-\underset{\underset{COOCH_3}{/}}{\overset{\overset{CH_3}{\vert}}{C}}-CH_2-\underset{\underset{COOCH_3}{/}}{\overset{\overset{CH_3}{\vert}}{C}}-CH_2-\underset{\underset{COOCH_3}{/}}{\overset{\overset{CH_3}{\vert}}{C}}-CH_2-$	$CH_2=\underset{\underset{COOCH_3}{\vert}}{\overset{\overset{CH_3}{\vert}}{C}}$

(continued overleaf)

Table 7.1 *(continued)*

Name	Chain structure	Monomer
Polyvinylpyrrolidone		
Polymers with a heterochain backbone:		
Poly(ethylene oxide)		
Poly(propylene oxide)		
Cellulose (polyglucoside, $\beta \rightarrow 1,4$)		Glucose
Chitosan		
Amylose (polyglucoside, $\alpha \rightarrow 1,4$) (component of starch)		Glucose
Pectinic acid (polygalacturonoside, $\alpha \rightarrow 1,4$) (jelly-forming component of fruits)		Galacturonic acid
Polyethylene glycol terephthalate		

(continued overleaf)

Table 7.1 *(continued)*

Name	Chain structure	Monomer
Polydimethylsiloxane	$$O-\underset{\underset{CH_3}{\mid}}{\overset{\overset{CH_3}{\mid}}{Si}}-O-\underset{\underset{CH_3}{\mid}}{\overset{\overset{CH_3}{\mid}}{Si}}-O-\underset{\underset{CH_3}{\mid}}{\overset{\overset{CH_3}{\mid}}{Si}}-$$	

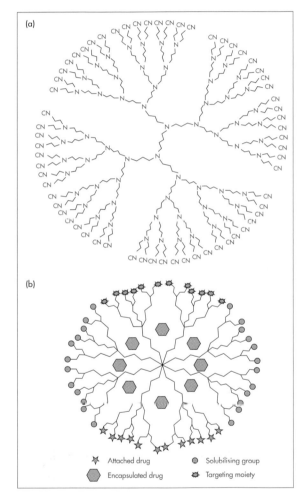

Figure 7.4 (a) A two-dimensional view of a dendrimer with 64 cyano functional groups. It is possible to trap small to medium-size molecules in dendrimers that have pores of appropriate dimensions between the branches of the structure. (b) A diagrammatic representation of possible sites for covalent attachment of drugs, solubilising groups and targeting moieties, and encapsulation of drugs.

(a) Reproduced from Gibson HW, *Nature*, 1994; 371: 106.

Table 7.2 Number- and weight-average molecular weights for dextran fractions[a]

Fraction	M_n	M_w	M_w/M_n
A	41 000	47 000	1.14
B	38 000	50 000	1.31
C	64 000	76 000	1.18
D	95 000	170 000	1.79
E	240 000	540 000	2.25

[a] Reproduced from Wales M *et al., J Polymer Sci*, 1953; 10: 229.

Figure 7.5 Representative polymer–polymer phase behaviour with different molecular architectures. Microphase separation (a) results when thermodynamically incompatible linear homopolymers are mixed. The covalent bond between blocks in a diblock copolymer leads to microphase segregation (c). A mixed architecture of linear homopolymers and the corresponding diblock copolymer produces a surfactant-like stabilised intermediate-scale phase separation (b).

Figure 7.6 illustrates the variety of morphologies that polymeric systems can adopt depending on the nature of the solvent, the polymer concentration and the nature of the polymer itself. Such diversity explains the wide range of uses in pharmacy and medicine.

Key points

- Polymers are substances of high molecular weight made up of repeating *monomer* units; they may be linear or branched, and separate linear or branched chains may be joined by crosslinks. Extensive crosslinking leads to a three-dimensional and often insoluble polymer network.

- Polymers in which all the monomeric units are identical are referred to as *homopolymers*; those formed from more than one monomer type are called *copolymers*. Homopolymers can be linear, star or branched; copolymers may be alternating copolymers, block copolymers or graft copolymers. *Dendrimers* are highly branched polymer constructs formed from a central core.

- There is usually a range of sizes of the polymer chains in solution, i.e. the polymer solutions are *polydisperse*. As a consequence, the measured molecular weight varies depending on the experimental method used: techniques such as light scattering are more influenced by the larger molecules and give a *weight-average* molecular weight, others such as chemical analysis and osmometry give a *number-average* molecular weight.

7.2 Water-soluble polymers

The rate of solution of a water-soluble polymer depends on its molecular weight: the larger the molecule, the stronger are the forces holding the chains

Figure 7.6 Representation of the variety of polymer morphologies in solution and in the gel (or microgel) or solid states. In solution the conformation of the polymer depends on the nature of polymer–solvent interactions and whether or not the polymer chains associate to form micellar aggregates. Crystals of polymer and microcrystals can be prepared, and gels can be formed from covalently crosslinked chains or polymer chains associated by hydrogen bonding or hydrophobic interactions. Listed are the forms in which most polymers can be fabricated: membranes, fibres, composites, matrices; micro-spheres and microcapsules can also feature, as discussed later in this chapter.

together. More energy has to be expended to force the chains apart in the solvent. The greater the degree of crystallinity of the polymer, the lower the rate of solution.

The velocity of penetration (S) of a solvent into the bulk polymer obeys the relationship

$$S = kM^{-A} \tag{7.3}$$

where M is the polymer molecular weight, k and A being constants. The dissolution process, however, is more complicated than with ordinary crystalline materials. It is frequently observed that swollen layers and gel layers form next to the polymer (see Fig. 7.7). If a

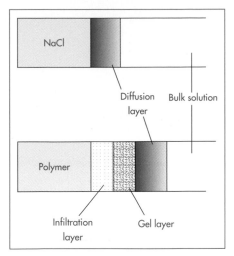

Figure 7.7 Penetration of solvent into (top) soluble crystalline material and (bottom) polymer compared.

drug is embedded in the polymer, the drug has to diffuse through these gel layers and finally through the diffusion layer.

It is the combination of slow solution rate and the formation of viscous surface layers that makes hydrophilic polymers useful in controlling the release rate of soluble drugs (see section 7.5). Choice of appropriate polymer molecular weight controls both the rate of dissolution and the viscosity of its resulting solution. A balance between rate of polymer solution and viscosity of the solution layer must be achieved in controlled-release systems. If the polymer solution rate is too slow, then soluble drug is leached out with little retardation.

The bulk viscosity of polymer solution is an important parameter also when polymers are being used as suspending agents to maintain solid particles in suspension by prevention of settling (see Chapter 6) and when they are used to modify the properties of liquid medicines for oral and topical use.

7.3 General properties of polymer solutions

7.3.1 Viscosity of polymer solutions

The presence in solution of large macromolecular solutes has an appreciable effect on the viscosity of the solution. From a study of the viscosity as a function of polymer concentration it is possible to gain information on the shape or hydration of these polymers in solution and also their average molecular weight. The assumption is made in this section that the solution exhibits Newtonian flow characteristics.

The viscosity of solutions of macromolecules is conveniently expressed by the *relative viscosity*, defined as the ratio of the viscosity of the solution, η, to the viscosity of the pure solvent η_0:

$$\eta_{rel} = \frac{\eta}{\eta_0} \tag{7.4}$$

Another useful expression is the *specific viscosity*, η_{sp}, of the solution, defined by

$$\eta_{sp} = \eta_{rel} - 1 \tag{7.5}$$

For ideal solutions the ratio η_{sp}/c (called the *reduced viscosity*) is independent of solution concentration. In real solutions the reduced viscosity varies with concentration owing to molecular interactions so it is usual to extrapolate plots of η_{sp}/c versus c to zero concentration. The extrapolated value is called the *intrinsic viscosity* $[\eta]$.

Einstein showed from hydrodynamic theory that for a dilute system of rigid, spherical particles

$$\eta_{rel} = 1 + 2.5\phi \tag{7.6}$$

i.e.

$$\lim_{\phi \to 0}(\eta_{sp}/\phi) = 2.5 \tag{7.7}$$

where ϕ is the volume fraction of the particles, defined as the volume of the particles divided by the total volume of the solution.

Departure of the limiting value of η_{sp}/ϕ from the theoretical value of 2.5 may result from either hydration of the particles, or from particle asymmetry, or from both as discussed in Box 7.1.

Shape and solvent effects

As the shape of molecules is to a large extent the determinant of flow properties, change in shape due to changes in polymer–solvent interactions and the binding of small molecules with the polymer may lead to significant changes in solution viscosity. The nature of the solvent is thus of prime importance in this regard. In so-called 'good' solvents, linear macromolecules will be expanded as the polar groups will be solvated. In a 'poor' solvent, the intramolecular attraction

Box 7.1 Effect of shape and hydration on viscosity

Effect of particle shape

A more general form of equation (7.6) allowing for particle asymmetry is

$$\eta_{rel} = 1 + \nu\phi \tag{7.8}$$

where ν is a shape factor related to the axial ratio of an ellipsoid. In the case of non-hydrated spheres ν reduces to 2.5. The volume is usually replaced by the weight concentration, c. For a macromolecule of hydrodynamic volume υ_h and molecular weight M,

$$\phi = \frac{N_A c \upsilon_h}{M} \tag{7.9}$$

and equation (7.8) becomes

$$\eta_{rel} - 1 = \nu\phi = \frac{\nu N_A \upsilon_h c}{M} \tag{7.10}$$

Hydration effects

Consider a hydrated macromolecule containing δ_1 grams of solvent per gram of dry macromolecular material. The specific volume υ_0 (volume per gram) of the entrapped water may be considerably different from that of pure solvent, $\upsilon_1^{\ominus}$. If υ_2 is the average specific volume of the macromolecular material, then the total hydrodynamic volume of the particle, υ_h, is

$$\upsilon_h = \frac{M}{N_A}(\upsilon_2 + \delta_1 \upsilon_1) \tag{7.11}$$

The total volume V of a solution containing g_1 grams of solvent and g_2 grams of dry macromolecular solute is

$$V = \text{volume of solute}$$
$$+\text{volume of water of hydration}$$
$$+\text{volume of free solvent}$$

$$= g_2 \upsilon_2 + g_2 \partial_1 \upsilon_1 + (g_1 - g_2 \partial_1)\upsilon_1^{\ominus} \tag{7.12}$$

Therefore,

$$\bar{\upsilon}_2 = \left(\frac{\partial V}{\partial g_2}\right)_{P,T,g_1} = \upsilon_2 + \partial_1\upsilon_1 - \partial_1\upsilon_1^{\ominus} \tag{7.13}$$

Substituting for υ_2 in equation (7.11) gives

$$\upsilon_h = \frac{M}{N_A}(\bar{\upsilon}_2 + \partial_1\upsilon_1^{\ominus}) \tag{7.14}$$

Substituting for υ_h in equation (7.10),

$$[\eta] = \lim_{c \to 0}\left(\frac{\eta_{rel} - 1}{c}\right) = \nu(\bar{\upsilon}_2 + \partial_1\upsilon_1^{\ominus}) \tag{7.15}$$

If the particle can be assumed to be unhydrated, or if the degree of hydration can be estimated with certainty from other experimental techniques, equation (7.15) may be used to determine the asymmetry of the particle. Alternatively, if the macromolecule may be assumed to be symmetrical or its asymmetry is known from other techniques, then this equation may be used to estimate the extent of hydration of the macromolecule.

between the segments is greater than the segment–solvent affinity and the molecule will tend to coil up (see Fig. 7.6). The viscosity of ionised macromolecules is complicated by charge interactions that vary with polymer concentration and additive concentration. Flexible charged macromolecules will vary in shape with the degree of ionisation. At maximum ionisation they are stretched out owing to mutual charge repulsion and the viscosity increases. On addition of small counterions, the effective charge is reduced and the molecules contract; the viscosity falls as a result. Some of the effects are illustrated later in this chapter in discussion of individual macromolecules.

The viscosity of solutions of globular proteins (which are more or less rigid) is only slightly affected by change in ionic strength. The intrinsic viscosity of serum albumin varies only between 3.6 and 4.1 cm^3 g^{-1} when the pH is varied between 4.3 and 10.5 and the ionic strength between zero and 0.50.

Viscosity in pharmacopoeial specifications

In cases where control of molecular weight is important, for example in the use of dextran fractions as plasma expanders,[3] a viscosity method is specified, for example, in the BP monograph. Staudinger proposed that the reduced viscosity of solutions of linear high polymers is proportional to the molecular weight of the polymer or its degree of polymerisation, p:

$$\frac{\eta_{sp}}{c} = K_m p \qquad (7.16)$$

This empirical law has been modified to

$$\lim_{c \to 0} \frac{\eta_{sp}}{c} = [\eta] = KM^a \qquad (7.17)$$

where a is a constant in the range 0–2, which for most high polymers has a value between 0.6 and 0.8, $[\eta]$ is the intrinsic viscosity as defined previously, and M is the molecular weight of the polymer. For a given polymer–solvent system, K and a are constant. Values of these constants may be determined from measurements on a series of fractions of known molecular weight and hence the molecular weight of an unknown fraction can be determined by measurement of the intrinsic viscosity. The *viscosity-average molecular weight* is essentially a weight average since the larger macromolecules influence viscosity more than the smaller ones. The intrinsic viscosity of Dextran 40 BP is stated to be not

less than $16 \, cm^3 \, g^{-1}$ and not more than $20 \, cm^3 \, g^{-1}$ at 37°C, while that of Dextran 110 is not less than $27 \, cm^3 \, g^{-1}$ and not more than $32 \, cm^3 \, g^{-1}$.

 Key points

- Assuming that the polymer solution exhibits Newtonian flow properties, its viscosity can be expressed by:
  - The *relative viscosity*, η_{rel}, defined as the ratio of the viscosity of the solution, η, to the viscosity of the pure solvent η_0, i.e. $\eta_{rel} = \eta/\eta_0$
  - The *specific viscosity*, η_{sp}, of the solution defined by $\eta_{sp} = \eta_{rel} - 1$
  - The *intrinsic viscosity* $[\eta]$ obtained by extrapolation of plots of the ratio η_{sp}/c (called the *reduced viscosity*) against concentration c to zero concentration.
- If the polymer forms spherical particles in dilute solution then a plot of η_{sp}/ϕ against ϕ the volume fraction) should have an intercept of 2.5; departure of the limiting value from this theoretical value may result from either hydration of the particles, or particle asymmetry, or both.
- A change in shape due to changes in polymer–solvent interactions and the binding of small molecules may lead to significant changes in solution viscosity. In 'good' solvents, linear macromolecules will be expanded as the polar groups will be solvated; in 'poor' solvents, the intramolecular attraction between the segments is greater than the segment–solvent affinity and the molecule will tend to coil up. Flexible charged macromolecules will vary in shape with the degree of ionisation.
- The intrinsic viscosity of solutions of linear high-molecular-weight polymers is proportional to the molecular weight M of the polymer as given by the *Staudinger equation*.

7.3.2 Gel formation

Concentrated polymer solutions frequently exhibit a very high viscosity because of the interaction of polymer chains in a three-dimensional fashion in the bulk solvent. These viscous crosslinked systems are termed *gels*. A gel is a polymer-solvent system containing a three-dimensional network of quite stable bonds that are almost unaffected by thermal motion. If such a polymer network is surrounded by the solvent (the system can be arrived at by swelling of solid polymer or by reduction in the solubility of the polymer in the solution) the system is a gel regardless of whether the network is formed by chemical or physical bonds. When gels are formed from solutions, each system is characterised by a critical concentration of gelation below which a gel is not formed. This concentration is determined by the hydrophile–lipophile balance of the polymer and the degree of regularity of the structure, by polymer–solvent interaction, by molecular weight, and by the flexibility of the chain: the more flexible the molecule, the higher is the critical gelling concentration. The characteristic features of a gel include the considerable increase in viscosity above the gel point, the appearance of a rubber-like elasticity, and, at higher polymer concentrations, a yield point stress. Under small stress the gel should retain its shape, but considerable deformation can occur at higher stress.

Type I and type II gels

Gels can be categorised into two groups, depending on the nature of the bonds between the chains of the network. Gels of type I are irreversible systems with a three-dimensional network formed by covalent bonds between the macromolecules. They include swollen networks, which have been formed by polymerisation of a monomer in the presence of a crosslinking agent.

Type II gels are heat-reversible, being held together by intermolecular bonds such as hydrogen bonds. Sometimes bridging by additive molecules can take place in these type II systems. Poly(vinyl alcohol) solutions gel on cooling below a temperature known as the gel point. The gel point can therefore be influenced by the presence of additives that can induce gel formation by acting as bridge molecules, as, for example, with borax and poly(vinyl alcohol). The gel point of polymers can also be increased or decreased by the addition of solvents that alter the polymer's affinity for the solvent (Table 7.3).

Table 7.3 Gel points of 10% poly(vinyl alcohol)[a]

Solvent	Gel point (°C)
Water	14
Glycerol	64
Ethylene glycol	102

[a] Reproduced from Pritchard JG, *Poly(vinyl alcohol): Basic Properties and Uses*, London: Macdonald; 1970.

Solutions of vinyl alcohol polymers in water are viscous mucilages that resemble those formed by methylcellulose; the viscosity of the mucilage is greatly increased by incorporating sodium perborate or silicate. Because of their gelling properties poly(vinyl alcohol) solutions are used as jellies for application of drugs to the skin. On application, the gel dries rapidly, leaving a plastic film with the drug in intimate contact with the skin. Plastic Film (Canadian Pharmacopoeia) is prepared from poly(vinyl alcohol) and other additives and is intended as a vehicle for acriflavine, benzocaine, ichthammol and other topical drugs.

Depending on the polymer, gelation can occur either with a fall or a rise in the temperature.

Crosslinked polymeric systems

If water-soluble polymer chains are covalently crosslinked, gels will be formed when the dry material interacts with water. The polymer swells in water but cannot dissolve as the crosslinks are stable. This expansion on contact with water has been put to many uses, such as in the fabrication of expanding implants from crosslinked hydrophilic polymers that imbibe body fluids and swell to a predetermined volume. These materials, such as the poly(hydroxyethyl methacrylate)s (poly(HEMA)s), are insoluble and chemically stable because of their three-dimensional structure, (see **I** and **II**) and do not dissolve. Implanted in the dehydrated state, these polymers swell to fill a body cavity or to give form to surrounding tissues. The gels may be used as vehicles for antibiotics, permitting protracted release of drug in the immediate environment of the implant. Antibiotic-loaded gels like this have been used in infections of the middle ear and other sites not readily reached by other methods of administration. Surgical suture material coated with antibiotic-containing hydrophilic gels acquires a chemotherapeutic role as the development of spread of infection along the suture fibre is prevented.

Structure I Poly(HEMA) crosslinked with ethylene glycol dimethacrylate (EGDMA)

Structure II Poly(HEMA) crosslinked with *N,N'*-methylenebisacrylamide (BIS)

Hydrophilic contact lenses (such as Soflens) are made from crosslinked poly(2-hydroxyethyl methacrylates). The emphasis in their development has been on their permeability to oxygen. They have also been used as reservoirs for drug delivery to the corneal surface. Conventional eye drop medication (see Chapter 10) has been modified over the years through the addition to formulations of a variety of viscosity-enhancing agents, polymers such as hydroxypropylmethylcellulose, poly(vinyl alcohol) and silicones. These all prolong contact of drug with the cornea by increasing the viscosity of the medium and retarding the drainage of the tear fluid from the eye via the punctae.

Heterogels

As it is possible to produce macromolecular chains with segments that have different solubilities in a given solvent (copolymers), one would expect that concentrated solutions of such copolymers would behave in a manner different from that of a simple polymer. In block copolymers of the type AAABBBAAA, in which A is water-soluble and B is water-insoluble, the insoluble parts will tend to aggregate. If, for instance, a polystyrene–poly(oxyethylene) copolymer, comprising 41% polystyrene and 59% poly(oxyethylene), is dissolved at 80°C in butyl phthalate (a good solvent for polystyrene), a gel with a microscopic layer structure is formed at room temperature; in nitromethane the form is somewhat different (Fig. 7.8a) as the nitromethane preferentially dissolves the poly(oxyethylene) chains.

Poly(oxyethylene)–poly(oxypropylene)–poly(oxyethylene) block copolymers, known commercially as Pluronic or poloxamer surfactants, are used as emulsifiers. Some form micellar aggregates in aqueous solutions above a critical micelle concentration, in which the hydrophobic central block associates with other like blocks, leaving the hydrophilic poly(oxyethylene) chains to the outside and protecting the inner core. Packing of these micelles in solution of high concentration leads to the reversible formation of gels as shown in Fig. 7.9.

7.3.3 Syneresis

Syneresis is the term used for the separation of liquid from a swollen gel. Syneresis is thus a form

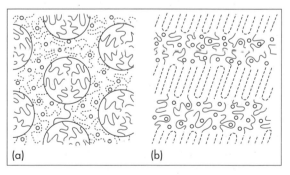

Figure 7.8 Structure of a copolymer of type A–B made from polystyrene and polyoxyethylene (a) in nitromethane (cylindrical structure) and (b) in butyl phthalate (layer structure). Nitromethane dissolves the poly(oxyethylene) part preferentially, but butyl phthalate dissolves the polystyrene part. (——) Polystyrene; (– – –), poly(oxyethylene); (○) solvent. Reproduced from Sadron F, *Angew Chem*, 1963; 2: 248.

of instability in aqueous and nonaqueous gels. Separation of a solvent phase is thought to occur because of the elastic contraction of the polymeric molecules; in the swelling process during gel formation, the macromolecules involved become stretched and the elastic forces increase as swelling proceeds. At equilibrium, the restoring force of the macromolecules is balanced by the swelling forces, determined by the osmotic pressure. If the osmotic pressure decreases, as on cooling, water may be squeezed out of the gel.

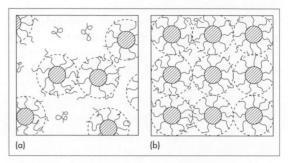

Figure 7.9 ABA-type copolymers: (a) micelles in dilute solution; (b) formation of a cubic-phase gel, by packing of micelles.

Key points

- A gel is a polymer–solvent system containing a three-dimensional network that can be formed by swelling of solid polymer or by reduction in the solubility of the polymer in the solution.
- When gels are formed from solutions, each system is characterised by a critical concentration of gelation below which a gel is not formed.
- Gelation is characterised by a large increase in viscosity above the gel point, the appearance of a rubber-like elasticity, and a yield point stress at higher polymer concentrations.
- Gels can be *irreversible* or *reversible* systems depending on the nature of the bonds between the chains of the network. Gels of *type 1* are irreversible systems with a three-dimensional network formed by covalent bonds between the macromolecules (e.g. poly[HEMA] crosslinked with EGDMA [ethylene glycol dimethacrylate]); these polymers swell in water but cannot dissolve as the crosslinks are stable. *Type II* gels are heat-reversible, being held together by intermolecular bonds such as hydrogen bonds; gelation can be induced either by cooling (e.g. poly(vinyl alcohol)) or heating (e.g. water-soluble methylcelluloses) to the gel point. Solutions of some poly(oxyethylene)–poly(oxypropylene)–poly(oxyethylene) block copolymers form reversible gels by the close packing of their micelles when concentrated solutions are warmed.
- Swollen gels may exhibit *syneresis*, which is the separation of solvent phase from the gel.

7.3.4 Polymer complexes

The varied structure and chemistry of polymers provide ample opportunity for complexes to form in solution. One example occurs when an aqueous solution of high-molecular-weight polyacids is mixed with polyglycols. The viscosity and pH of the solution of the equimolar mixture of polyacid and glycol remain the same with the increase in oligomer chain length up to a critical point. The nature of the interaction is shown in (III); this occurs only when the polyethylene glycol molecules have reached a certain size.

Structure III Polycomplex formed by interaction of polyacid and polyoxyethylene glycol

Such macromolecular reactions are highly selective and strongly dependent on molecular size and conformation. On mixing, some of the macromolecules might be involved in the complex while the rest will be free. The reason for compositional heterogeneity of the products could be the conformational transitions of macromolecules in the course of complex formation.

Interactions between macromolecules can occur in formulations, for example when preparations are mixed. They can be put to good advantage in the synthesis of novel compounds. Polyethyleneimine and poly(acrylic acid) form a polyelectrolyte complex with salt-like bonds as shown in (**IV**). If the complex is heated as a film, interchain amide bonds are formed between the groups that formed electrostatic links. The nonionised COOH and NH groups in the chain are the points of structural defects in the film.

 Clinical point

Dietary fibre from plants binds calcium in proportion to its uronic acid content. This binding by the noncellulosic fraction of fibre reduces the availability of calcium for small-intestinal absorption, although colonic digestion of uronic acids liberates the calcium.[4] The pH dependence of the binding strongly suggests the involvement of carboxylic acid groups. Where daily fibre intakes vary between 50 and 150 g, with perhaps 30–110 mmol uronic acid, the binding capacity of fibre may exceed the total intake of calcium, which may be less than 20 mmol (800 mg) per day.

Structure IV Complex formation between polyethyleneimine and poly(acrylic acid)

7.3.5 Binding of ions to macromolecules

Calcium is coordinated between certain uronic acid-containing polysaccharides (**V**), which can explain the tight binding of calcium and other multivalent ions in polysaccharide structures, and also how bivalent ions can induce gel formation in acidic polysaccharides such as alginic acid solutions.

Structure V Calcium complexed in polysaccharides

It has been found that such interactions have dietary significance.

7.3.6 Interaction of polymers with solvents including water

As a consequence of their size, polymers interact with solvents in a more complex fashion than do smaller crystalline solutes. A given polymer may have no saturation solubility; it usually either dissolves completely or is only swollen by a given liquid. If the polymer is crosslinked, solution cannot occur and the polymer will only swell by imbibition of liquid to form a gel. Swelling decreases as the degree of crosslinking increases. Swelling is also a function of the solubility parameter of the liquid phase, and if the polymer is ionic, swelling will be dependent on the ionic strength of the solution as shown in Fig. 7.10 for crosslinked hyaluronic acid gels. Increasing ionic strength decreases the repulsion between the chains and allows the polymer to shrink.

Highly polar polymers like poly(vinyl chloride) and some cellulose derivatives require polar liquids as solvents, in which dipole interactions or hydrogen bonding between polymer and solvent molecules occur. However, solvation does not necessarily lead to solution because the liquid, if it is to act as a solvent, must dissolve the solvated polymer. This process may be very slow because of the high viscosity of the partially solvated system.

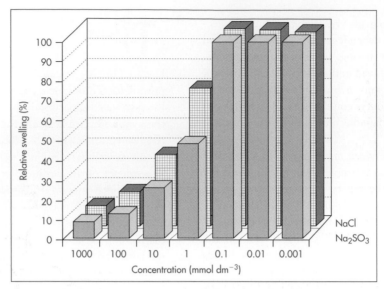

Figure 7.10 Relative swelling of hyaluronic acid hydrogels in different concentrations of NaCl and Na_2SO_3 solutions.
Reproduced from Tomer R *et al.*, *J Control Release*, 1995; 33: 405.

Swelling of hydrogels and drug release

The relative mobility of a drug diffusing in the swelling hydrogel is given by the *swelling interface number*, Sw defined as

$$Sw = \frac{\nu \cdot \delta(t)}{D} \qquad (7.18)$$

where ν is the velocity of the moving front, $\delta(t)$ is the thickness of the rubbery layer (the infiltration and gel layers represented in Fig. 7.7) at time t, and D is the diffusion coefficient of the drug in the matrix.[5] When $Sw \gg 1$, Fickian drug diffusion predominates, whereas when $Sw \ll 1$, zero-order release kinetics are observed. The amount of drug released from a thin slab is expressed as an exponential:

$$\frac{M_t}{M_\infty} = kt^n \qquad (7.19)$$

n varying from -0.5 to >1.0 where M_t/M_∞ is the fraction of drug and k is a constant.

It has been seen in Chapter 6 that the use of macromolecules as dispersion stabilisers depends in part on the osmotic forces arising from the interaction of solvated polymer chains as neighbouring particles approach (see Fig. 6.7). It is thus important to know how factors such as temperature and additives affect this interaction. Flory has given the free energy of dilution (the opposite process to the concentration

effect discussed in section 6.2) as

$$\Delta G_1 = RT(k_1 - \psi_1)\phi_2 \qquad (7.20)$$

where ϕ_2 is the volume fraction of polymer, and k_1 and ψ_1 are heat and entropy parameters, respectively.

It is sometimes convenient to define the temperature at which a polymer of infinite molecular weight just becomes insoluble in a given solvent; this temperature is the *Flory temperature* or *theta temperature*, θ, which may also be defined by

$$\theta = \frac{k_1 T}{\psi_1} \qquad (7.21)$$

so that substituting in equation (7.20) we obtain the relationship between ΔG_1 and temperature:

$$\Delta G_1 = -RT\psi_1\left(1 - \frac{\theta}{T}\right)\phi_2 \qquad (7.22)$$

ΔG_1 is therefore zero at the theta temperature when deviations from ideality vanish, that is, there are no polymer–polymer or polymer–solvent interactions. When $T = \theta$ there can thus be no stabilisation as molecules will interpenetrate without net interaction and will exert no forces on each other.

Not only do most linear polysaccharides tend to form spirals in solution, but in their tendency to associate they may form double helices, as does carrageenan, for instance. Under certain conditions of

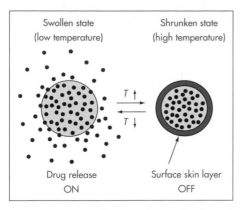

Figure 7.11 On–off switching mechanism for drug release.

Reproduced from Yoshida R *et al., Adv Drug Deliv Rev*, 1993; 11: 85.

concentration and temperature the double helices may associate, forming gels. Possibilities exist for complex gel formation as with carrageenan, or of xanthan gum with locust bean gum. The locust bean gum molecule can associate over part of its length with the helix of xanthan, for example, while the other part of the molecule associates with another xanthan molecule, thereby acting as a bridging agent.

The firmness or strength of gels produced by such interactions will depend on the degree of interaction of the complex with water and the properties of the bridging units.

The ability to change the swelling characteristics of a polymer gel by heat, pH or application of electric current can be valuable in specialised delivery systems, as exemplified in Fig. 7.11, which shows the effect of temperature change on the swelling and de-swelling of a hydrogel, resulting in an on-off 'switching' mechanism.

The relationship between swelling and release in an electrically responsive hydrogel is shown in Fig. 7.12. The mechanism of the current-induced change in volume of the gel is shown in Fig. 7.12b.

Hydrophilic polymers as bulk laxatives

The ability of carbohydrates and other macromolecules to imbibe large quantities of water is put to use both medicinally and industrially; for example in absorbent paper and sanitary towels, incontinence

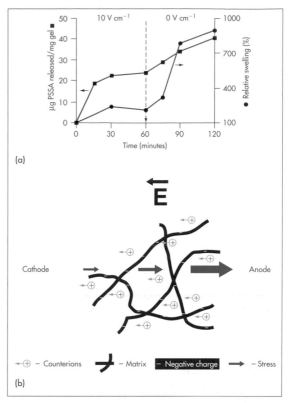

Figure 7.12 (a) Responsive swelling (●) and release (■) from PSSA-loaded HA hydrogels when an electric field of 10 V cm^{-1} was switched off. (b) The effect of an electric field on a polyelectrolyte network. The redistribution of ions causes shrinkage of the gel at the cathode and expansion at the anode.

(a) Reproduced from Tomer R *et al., J Control Release*, 1995; 33: 405.

pads and surgical dressings. Medically, use is made of the swelling properties in the treatment of constipation and in appetite suppression. Three properties are of importance in the *in vitro* evaluation of bulk laxatives:

- The volume of water absorbed in the various media
- The viscosity and texture of the gel formed
- The ability of the gel to retain water

The swelling properties of a sterculia-based preparation (Normacol) in various aqueous media and a comparison of Normacol with two other agents are shown in Fig. 7.13.

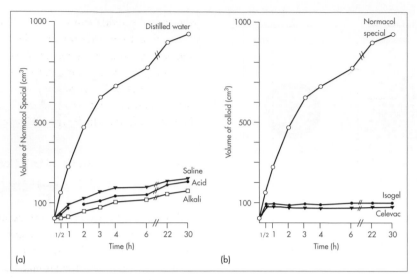

Figure 7.13 (a) The volume attained by 5 g of Normacol Special in various solutions over 30 hours. (b) The volumes attained by 5 g of Normacol Special, Isogel and Celevac in distilled water.

Reproduced from Ireson JD, Leslie GB, *Pharm J*, 1970; 205: 540.

 Clinical point

It is desirable that colloidal bulk laxatives swell in the lower part of the small intestine and in the large intestine to cause reflex peristalsis, rather than in the stomach or duodenum; that is, they should swell in neutral rather than acidic or alkaline conditions. In artificial intestinal juice, psyllium seed gum increased in volume 5–14 times, locust bean gum 5–10 times and methylcellulose 16–30 times in 24 hours. *In vivo* evaluation of methylcellulose and carboxymethylcellulose suggests that they have two advantages over the natural gums. Methylcellulose is more efficient as a bulk laxative because of its greater water-retentive capacity, whereas carboxymethylcellulose gives uniform distribution through the intestinal contents.

7.3.7 Adsorption of macromolecules

The ability of some macromolecules to adsorb at interfaces is made use of in suspension and emulsion stabilisation (see Chapter 6). Gelatin, acacia, poly(vinyl alcohol) and proteins adsorb at interfaces.

Sometimes such adsorption is unwanted, as in the case of insulin adsorption onto glass infusion bottles and poly(vinyl chloride) infusion containers and tubing used in giving sets.

 Clinical point

Adsorption of insulin to glass bottles and plastic IV tubing at slow rates of infusion is well documented. Adsorption ranges from 5% to 3.1% when 20 and 40 units respectively are added to 500 cm^3 of isotonic sodium chloride solution. Plastic IV tubing adsorbed 30% of 20 units and 26% of 40 units added to the same infusion bottles (Fig. 7.14). Adsorption occurs rapidly, within 15 seconds. Addition of albumin to prevent adsorption is now common practice. The albumin adsorbs at the glass or plastic surface and presents a more polar surface to the solution, thus reducing, but not always preventing, adsorption of the insulin (Fig. 7.15). The binding is considered to be a nonspecific phenomenon that may occur on other inert materials such as polyethylene and glass.

Figure 7.14   Amounts of insulin lost by adsorption to glass bottles and plastic intravenous tubing, following injection of 30 units of insulin. The patient receives only 6.36 units.

Reproduced from Petty C, Cunningham NL, *Anaesthesiology*, 1974; 40, 400.

The adsorption of macromolecules at interfaces may be the reason why molecules such as those of hyaluronic acid can act as biological lubricants in joint fluids. In healthy joints only 0.5 cm^3 of synovial fluid is required to provide almost perfect lubrication; in diseased joints there are sometimes faults in this lubrication system and some research has been aimed at producing synthetic substitutes for synovial fluid. Polymer solutions provide one approach as their rheological characteristics more closely approach those of the natural fluid, which is non-Newtonian.

7.4 Water-soluble polymers used in pharmacy and medicine

In this section the properties of some specific polymers used in pharmacy and medicine will be discussed. This cannot be an exhaustive treatment of the subject, so choice of the macromolecular material for this section has been based partly on the degree of use but partly on the generally interesting features they display. The choice of a macromolecular material for a particular pharmaceutical use is often difficult because of the diversity of properties exhibited by the materials available. Figure 7.16 illustrates how the field can be narrowed to some extent by grouping the natural and synthetic materials of interest to the formulator. This is, however, a very general guide, as the properties of individual macromolecules will, as discussed, often vary with pH, temperature, molecular weight and

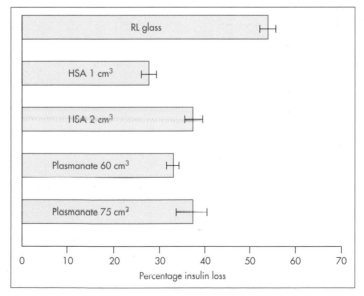

Figure 7.15   Prevention of insulin loss via adsorption by the addition of human serum albumin (HSA) or Plasmanate to 1000 cm^3 of Ringer's lactate (RL) solution in a glass bottle. Insulin (30 units) was injected and measured at 5 minutes. Values represent means $\pm$ SEM. All HSA and Plasmanate values were significantly different from Ringer's lactate solution control ($p < 0.001$).

Reproduced from Petty C, Cunningham NL, *Anaesthesiology*, 1974; 40: 400.

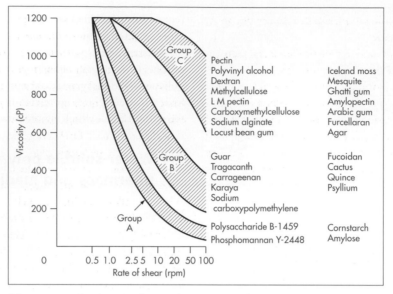

Figure 7.16 Effect of shear rate on the viscosity of gum solutions grouped according to their rheological behaviour.

Modified from Szezesniak AS, Farkas EH, *J. Food Sci*, 1962; 27: 381.

ionic strength. The most readily altered variable is, of course, the concentration of the macromolecule, whose effect on viscosity is illustrated for a range of compounds in Fig. 7.17. The most viscous material shown here is Carbopol 934.

7.4.1 Carboxypolymethylene (Carbomer, Carbopol)

Carboxypolymethylene is used as a suspending agent in pharmaceutical preparations and as a binding agent in tablets, and it is used in the formulation of prolonged-action tablets. It is a high-molecular-weight polymer of acrylic acid, containing a high proportion of carboxyl groups. Its aqueous solutions are acidic; when neutralised the solutions become very viscous with a maximum viscosity between pH 6 and 11. Electrolytes reduce the viscosity of the system and thus high concentrations of the polymer have to be employed in vehicles where ionisable drugs are present. A carbomer gel prolongs the contact time of drugs instilled into the eye.

7.4.2 Cellulose derivatives

Cellulose itself is virtually insoluble in water, but aqueous solubility can be conferred by partial methylation or carboxymethylation of cellulose.

Ethylcellulose is an ethyl ether of cellulose containing 44–51% of ethoxyl groups. It is insoluble in water but soluble in chloroform and in alcohol. It is possible

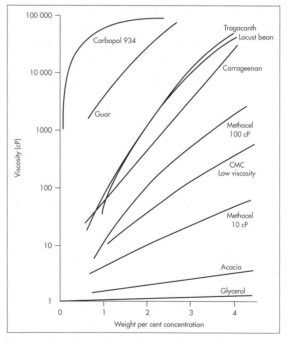

Figure 7.17 Viscosity of solutions of some pharmaceutical polymers and gums compared with glycerol plotted as a function of concentration.

Reproduced from Martin AN *et al.*, *Adv Pharm Sci*, 1964; 1: 1.

to form water-soluble grades with a lower degree of substitution.

Methylcellulose samples are prepared by heterogeneous reaction that is usually controlled to allow substitution of, on average, about one-half of the hydroxyl groups. This leads to a product in which the methylated groups are not evenly distributed throughout the chains; rather, there are regions of high density of substitution (as in structure **VI**) that are hydrophobic in nature, and regions of low density of substitution that are hydrophilic in nature.

Structure VI Highly methylated region of methylcellulose chain

Methylcellulose is thus a methyl ether of cellulose containing about 29% of methoxyl groups; it is slowly soluble in water. A 2% solution of methylcellulose 4500 has a gel point of about 50°C. High concentrations of electrolytes salt out the macromolecules and increase their viscosity; eventually precipitation may occur. Low-viscosity grades are used as emulsifiers for liquid paraffin and other mineral oils. High-viscosity grades are used as thickening agents for medicated jellies and as dispersing and thickening agents in suspensions.

Since methylcelluloses are poorly soluble in cold water, preliminary use of hot water ensures wetting of all portions of the particle prior to solution in cold water. The water-soluble methylcelluloses possess the property of thermal gelation; that is, they gel on heating while the natural gums gel on cooling. Methylcellulose exists in solution as long thread-like molecules hydrated by water molecules. On heating, the water of solvation tends to be lost; the 'lubricating' action of the hydration layer is also lost and the molecules lock together in a gel. Gelation is reversible on cooling. Variation in the alkyl or hydroxyalkyl substitution can be a means of controlling the gel points (Table 7.4). As the methoxyl content is lowered, the temperature of gelation increases and water solubility decreases. Unlike the ionic celluloses, the nonionic alkylcelluloses possess surface activity. As the methoxyl content is reduced, the surface and interfacial activities are also reduced, reflecting the importance of the hydrophobic moiety in determining surface activity.

Ethylhydroxyethylcellulose is an ether of cellulose with both ethyl and hydroxyethyl substituents attached via ether linkages to the anhydroglucose rings. It swells in water to form a clear, viscous colloidal solution. Preparation of solutions of cellulose derivatives requires hydration of the macromolecules, the rate of which is a function of both temperature and pH, as shown in the example in Fig. 7.18.

Hydroxyethylcellulose is soluble in hot and cold water but does not gel. It has been used in ophthalmic

Table 7.4 Gel point and surface activity of cellulose derivatives[a]

Derivative	Percentage —OCH_3	Percentage —$OCH_2CH(OH)CH_3$	Gel point[b] (°C)	Surface tension[c] (mN m^{-1})	Interfacial tension[d] (mN m^{-1})
Methocel MC	27.5–3.2	–	50–55	47–53	19–23
Methocel 60HG	28–30	7–12	55–60	44–50	18–19
Methocel 65HG	27–30	4–7.5	60–65	–	–
Methocel 70HG	24–27	4–8	66–72	–	–
Methocel 90IIG	22–25	6–12	85	50–56	26–28

[a] Reproduced from Windover FE, in: Davidson RL, M. Sittig M, eds, *Water Soluble Resins*, New York: Reinhold; 1962: 52ff.

[b] 2% solution.

[c] Surface tension at 25°C.

[d] Interfacial tension versus paraffin oil at 25°C.

Figure 7.18 Effect of pH and temperature on the hydration time of fast-dissolving grades of hydroxyethylcellulose.

Reproduced from Whistler RL, ed., *Industrial Gums*, 2nd edn, New York: Academic Press; 1973.

solutions. More widely used for the latter, however, is *hydroxypropylmethylcellulose* (hypromellose) which is a mixed ether of cellulose containing 27–30% of OCH_3 groups and 4–7.5% of OC_3H_6OH groups. It forms a viscous colloidal solution. There are various pharmaceutical grades. For example, hypromellose 20 is a 2% solution that has a viscosity between 15 and 25 cSt (centistokes) at 20°C; the viscosity of a 2% hypromellose 15000 solution lies between 12 000 and 18 000 cSt. Hypromellose prolongs the action of medicated eyedrops and is employed as an artificial tear fluid.

Sodium carboxymethylcellulose is soluble in water at all temperatures. Because of the carboxylate group, its mucilages are more sensitive to change in pH than are those of methylcellulose. The viscosity of a sodium carboxymethylcellulose mucilage is decreased markedly below pH 5 or above pH 10.

7.4.3 Natural gums and mucilages

Gum arabic (acacia) has been used traditionally in pharmacy as an emulsifier. It is a polyelectrolyte whose solutions are highly viscous owing to the branched structure of the macromolecular chains; its adhesive properties are also believed to be due to, or in some way related to, this branched structure. Molecular weights between 200 000 and 250 000 Da

(M_n) have been determined by osmotic pressure, values between 250 000 and 3×10^6 Da by sedimentation and diffusion, and values of 10^6 Da by light scattering measurements which also point to the shape of the molecules as short stiff spirals with numerous side-chains. Arabic acid prepared from commercial gum arabic by precipitation is a moderately strong acid whose aqueous solutions have a pH of 2.2–2.7.

Whereas most gums are very viscous in aqueous solution, gum arabic is unusual in that, being extremely soluble, it can form solutions over a wide range of concentrations up to about 37% at 25°C. The marked variation in viscosity means that the gum arabic molecules must be flexible, with the ionic acid carboxyl groups distributed along the chain. At low pH the carboxyl groups are un-ionised. On increase of pH the carboxyl groups become progressively ionised and the folded chains expand owing to repulsion between the charged groups, causing an increase in viscosity. On addition of NaOH to the system the viscosity falls again as the concentration of counterion (Na^+) increases and effectively shields the acidic groups. The molecule then folds on itself. Similar falls in viscosity are exhibited on addition of sodium chloride. The effect of salt addition to the gum at fixed pH reflects the decrease in effective charge on the molecules of gum with resultant contraction and reduction in viscosity.

The gum arabic molecule is, in addition, surface-active; a 4% solution at 30°C has a surface tension of 63.2 mN m^{-1}. Addition of electrolytes makes the molecule more surface-active either by causing a change in conformation of the molecule at the interface, allowing closer packing, or by increasing the hydrophobicity of the molecule. It is an effective emulsifier, the stabilisation of the emulsion being dependent mainly on the coherence and elasticity of the interfacial film, which is by no means monomolecular.

Gum arabic is incompatible with several phenolic compounds; under suitable conditions it forms coacervates (see section 7.6.3) with gelatin and positively charged polyelectrolytes.

Gum tragacanth partially dissolves in water; the soluble portion is called tragacanthin and this can be purified by precipitation from water with acetone or alcohol. Tragacanthin is a highly viscous polyelectrolyte with a molecular weight of 800 000 Da (as determined by sedimentation measurements). It is one of the most widely used natural emulsifiers and thickeners. As its molecules have an elongated shape, its solutions have a high viscosity which, as with gum arabic, is dependent on pH. The maximum viscosity occurs at pH 8 initially, but because of ageing effects the maximum stable viscosity is near pH 5.

It is an effective suspending agent for pharmaceuticals and is used in conjunction with acacia as an emulsifier, the tragacanth imparting a high structural viscosity while the gum arabic adsorbs at the oil–water interface.

Clinical point

Tragacanth is also used in spermicidal jellies, acting by immobilising spermatozoa and as a viscous barrier to spermatozoa.

Alginates. Although the solutions of alginate are very viscous and set on addition of acid or calcium salts, they are less readily gelled than pectin and are used chiefly as stabilisers and thickening agents. Propylene glycol alginate does not precipitate in acid and as it is nontoxic is widely used as a stabiliser for foodstuffs. The molecules are highly asymmetric, with molecular weights in the range 47 000–370 000 Da. Sodium alginate has the structure given in **VII**.

Structure VII Sodium alginate

Pectin is a purified carbohydrate product from extracts of the rind of citrus fruits and consists of partially methoxylated polygalacturonic acid (**VIII**). It has remarkable gelling qualities but is also used therapeutically, often with kaolin, in the treatment of diarrhoea. It has been established that the longer the pectin chains, the greater its capacity for gel formation. The presence of inorganic cations and the

degree of esterification of the carboxyl groups are important factors; in the case of calcium pectate gel it can be assumed that the calcium or indeed other polyvalent cations can interlink the chains by binding through $COO^-...Ca^{2+}...^-OOC$ interactions. Thus a high degree of esterification will disfavour gelation in this case. In the absence of inorganic cations, however, a high degree of esterification aids gelation, suggesting that hydrophobic interactions cause the chains to associate.

Structure VIII Partially methylated chain of poly(galacturonic acid) of pectin

7.4.4 Chitosan

Chitosan is a polymer obtained by the deacetylation of chitin, one of the most abundant polysaccharides. Chitosan, or poly[α-(1,4)-2-amino-2-deoxy-D-gluco-pyranose] has the structure (**IX**). As might be expected, the degree of deacetylation has a significant effect on the solubility and rheological properties of the polymer. At low pH, the polymer is soluble, with the sol–gel transition occurring at approximate pH 7. Chitosan also has film-forming abilities and its gel- and matrix-forming abilities make it useful for solid dosage forms, such as granules or microparticles.[6] The molecular weight, crystallinity and degree of deacetylation are all factors that can be varied to control the release rates from chitosan-based granules.

Structure IX The chemical structure of chitosan. The amine groups on the polymer have a pK_a in the range 5.5–6.5, depending on the source of the polymer

7.4.5 Dextran

Certain fractions of partially hydrolysed dextran are used as plasma substitutes or 'expanders'. Certain strains of *Leuconostoc meserentoides* are cultivated to synthesise dextran (**X**), which is a polymer of anhydroglucose, linked through α-1,6 glucosidic linkages. The chains are branched; on the average, one branch occurs for every 10–12 glucose residues. The intrinsic viscosity $[\eta]$ is related to M by the relationship

$$[\eta] = 10^{-3}M^{1/2} \tag{7.23}$$

in the molecular weight range 20 000–200 000 Da. The dextrans produced by fermentation are hydrolysed and fractionated to give a range of products suitable for injection. Dextran, being a hydrophilic colloid, exerts an osmotic pressure comparable to that of plasma and it is thus used to restore or maintain blood volume. Other substances that have been used in a similar way include hydroxyethyl starch, polyvinylpyrrolidone and gelatin.

 Clinical point

Dextran injections are sterile solutions of dextran with weight-average molecular weights of about 40 000–110 000 Da. Dextrans with a molecular weight of about 50 000 Da or less are excreted in the urine within 48 hours of injection. Dextran molecules with higher molecular weights disappear more slowly from the bloodstream and are temporarily stored in the reticuloendothelial system.

Dextran 70 (70 000 Da) and Dextran 110 (110 000 Da) are used to maintain blood volume, and Dextran 40 is used primarily to prevent intravascular aggregation of blood cells and for assisting capillary blood flow. This latter effect is the result of dextran adsorption and stabilisation of the erythrocyte suspensions. If the higher-molecular-weight fractions exceed about 1% concentration in the blood, rouleaux tend to form.

Structure X Dextran

Figure 7.19 Variation of indices of red-cell aggregation with the concentration of five dextran fractions of different molecular weight: (a) microscopic aggregation index; (b) relative viscosity at a shear rate of $0.1\ s^{-1}$. Note that the maximum of each curve (that is, maximum aggregation of the red cells) corresponds to a well-defined concentration of a particular dextran fraction. Maxima in both indices of aggregation of red cells occur at about the same concentration of dextran fraction.

Reproduced from Chien S, *Bib Anat Basel*, 1973; 11: 244.

The sensitivity of blood to the concentration and molecular weight of dextran is clearly seen in Fig. 7.19, where aggregation and relative viscosity of red-cell suspensions are shown in the presence of varying amounts of five different dextrans. Molecular weight control is thus important and may be exercised by measurement of intrinsic viscosity, $[\eta]$.

Iron–dextran complexes are soluble, nonionic and suitable for injection for the treatment of anaemia; the complex is stable on storage in the pH range 4–11. Aminoethyldextran–methotrexate complexes have been prepared, the object being to influence uptake of the drug selectively into tumour cells. Attachment of the drug to the macromolecule allows selective uptake into malignant cells, as such cells are more active than normal cells in pinocytosis, the mechanism by which macromolecules are taken into many cells.

7.4.6 Polyvinylpyrrolidone

Polyvinylpyrrolidone (PVP) is used as a suspending and dispersing agent, as a tablet binding and granulating agent, and as a vehicle for drugs such as penicillin, cortisone, procaine and insulin to delay their absorption and prolong their action. It forms hard films that are utilised in film-coating processes. Chemically it is a homopolymer of N-vinylpyrrolidone (**XI**). It is available in a number of grades designated by numbers ranging from K15 to K90. The K values represent a function of the mean molecular weight, and can be calculated from

$$\frac{\log \eta_{rel}}{c} = \frac{75K_0^2}{1 + 1.5K_0c} + K_0 \qquad (7.24)$$

where c = concentration in grams per $100\ cm^3$ and η_{rel} is the viscosity relative to the solvent. $K = 1000K_0$. Viscosity is essentially independent of pH over the range 0–10 and aqueous solutions exhibit a high tolerance for many inorganic salts. Its wide solubility in organic solvents is unusual. The viscosity of a range of aqueous solutions of PVP is shown in Fig. 7.20.

Structure XI Polyvinylpyrrolidone

Figure 7.20 Viscosity of polyvinylpyrrolidone (PVP) solutions as a function of molecular weight (PVP K15 (mol wt 40 000 Da) to PVP K90 (mol wt 700 000 Da)) and concentration of the polymer in water.

Reproduced from Azorlosa JL, Martinelli AJ, in: Davidson RL, M. Sittig M, eds, *Water Soluble Resins*, New York: Reinhold; 1962.

PVP forms molecular adducts with many substances. Soluble complexes, called *iodophors*, are formed with iodine: the solubility of iodine is increased from 0.034% in water at 25°C to 0.58% by 1% PVP. The resulting iodophor retains the germicidal properties of iodine. It is thought that the iodine is held in a PVP helix in solution. The influence of two samples of PVP on the solubility of testosterone is shown in Fig. 7.21. The PVP correspondingly increases the rate of solution of the steroid from solid dispersions.

7.4.7 Polyoxyethylene glycols (Macrogols)

Macrogols (polyoxyethylene glycols, PEGs, **XII**) are liquid over the molecular weight range 200–700 Da; the liquid members and semisolid members of the series are hygroscopic. Macrogol 200 has a hygroscopicity 70% of that of glycerol, but this decreases with molecular weight: the comparable value for Macrogol 1540 is only 30%. They are used as solvents for drugs such as hydrocortisone. The macrogols are incompatible with phenols and can reduce the antimicrobial activity of other preservatives. Higher-molecular-weight PEGs are more effective on a molecular basis as complexing agents. Up to four phenol molecules bind to each PEG molecule; the complex formed is of the donor–acceptor type. The semisolid and waxy members of the series may be used as suppository bases; in such cases their potential to interact with medicaments must be borne in mind.

$$HO(CH_2CH_2O)_nH$$

Structure XII Polyoxyethylene glycol

Figure 7.21 The influence of PVP 11500 and PVP 40000 on the aqueous solubility of testosterone at 37°C.

Reproduced from Hoelgaard A, Muller N, *Arch Pharm Chem*, 1975; 3: 34.

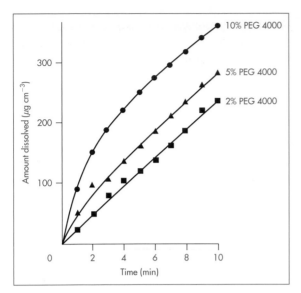

Figure 7.22 Dissolution rates of sulfathiazole (Form I)–polyethylene glycol 4000 physical mixtures.

Reproduced from Niazi S, *J Pharm Sci*, 1976; 65: 302.

Use of polyoxyethylene glycols, and other hydrophilic polymers, in high concentrations in formulations can influence the behaviour of drugs even when the drug is present as a physical mixture with the polymer. For example, combination of polyoxyethylene glycol 4000 with sulfathiazole increases the solution rate of sulfonamides (Fig. 7.22). Probable mechanisms include an increase in drug solubility or increased wetting of the drug surrounded by the hydrophilic polymer. Apart from these uses, the polyoxyethylene glycols have turned out to be one of the most versatile water-soluble polymers. They have been successful in modifying the behaviour of proteins, including monoclonal antibodies, in solution and in the circulation after being grafted to these molecules. The polyoxyethylene glycols also prolong the circulation time of particulate delivery systems such as liposomes and nanoparticles through their adsorption or incorporation into the surface of these carriers, preventing the adsorption of opsonins and reducing uptake by the liver and spleen, as discussed in Chapter 12.

7.4.8 Bioadhesivity of water-soluble polymers

Adhesion between a surface of a hydrophilic polymer, or a surface to which a hydrophilic polymer has been grafted or adsorbed, and a biological surface arises from interactions between the polymer chains and the macromolecules on the mucosal surface. From Fig. 7.23a it is clear that to achieve maximum adhesion there should be maximum interaction

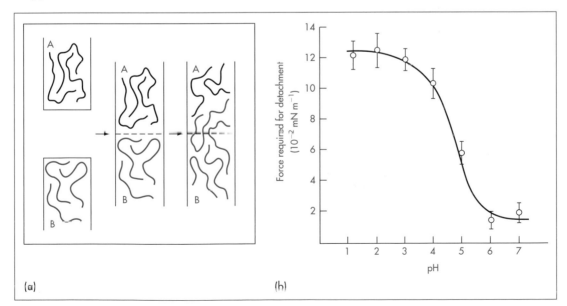

Figure 7.23 (a) Schematic representation of two phases, adhesive (A) and mucus (B), which adhere owing to chain adsorption and consecutive chain entanglement during mucoadhesion. (b) Effect of pH on *in vitro* bioadhesion of polycarbophil to rabbit gastric tissue.

(a) Reproduced from Peppas NA, Mikos AG, in: Gurney R, Junginger HE, eds, *Bioadhesion*, Stuttgart: Wiss. Verlagsgesellschaft; 1990.
(b) From reference 7.

between the polymer chains of the bioadhesive (A) and the mucus (B). The charge on the molecules will be important, and for two anionic polymers maximum interaction will occur when they are not charged. Penetration and association must be balanced. Table 7.5 shows the adhesive performance of a range of polymers, many of which have been discussed in this chapter. Of these, two classes have been approved by the FDA: anionic poly(acrylic acid) (carbophil) derivatives and the cationic chitosans. Polycarbophil and carbomer (Carbopol 934P) have pK_a values of about 4.5 and display maximum mucoadhesivity at pH values where they are mostly undissociated[7] (see Fig. 7.23b).

Table 7.5 Some representative mucoadhesives and their relative mucoadhesivities

Substance	Adhesive performance
Carboxymethylcellulose	Excellent
Carbopol	Excellent
Carbopol and hydroxypropylmethylcellulose	Good
Carbopol base with white petrolatum/ hydrophilic petrolatum	Fair
Carbopol 934 and EX 55	Good
Poly(methyl methacrylate)	Excellent
Polyacrylamide	Good
Poly(acrylic acid)	Excellent
Polycarbophil	Excellent
Homopolymers and copolymers of acrylic acid and butyl acrylate	Good
Gelatin	Fair
Sodium alginate	Excellent
Dextran	Good
Pectin	Poor
Acacia	Poor
Povidone	Poor
Poly(acrylic acid) crosslinked with sucrose	Fair

7.4.9 Polymers as wound dressings

Several polymers are now used in the preparation of synthetic wound dressings. Synthaderm is a 'synthetic skin' of a modified polyurethane foam, hydrophilic on one side and hydrophobic on the other. The hydrophilic side is placed in contact with the wound. The system has been described as an 'environmental dressing'[8] because it (a) maintains a high humidity at the dressing interface, (b) removes excess exudate, (c) allows gaseous exchange and (d) provides insulation; moreover, it is impermeable to bacteria, the outer surface remaining dry, unlike many saturable dressings. Lyofoam is a similar product.[9] According to the SMTL Dressings Datacard[10] it consists of 'a soft, open-cell, hydrophobic, polyurethane foam sheet approximately 8 mm thick. The side of the dressing that is to be placed in contact with the skin or wound has been heat-treated to collapse the cells of the foam, and thus enable it to absorb liquid by capillarity. The dressing is freely permeable to gases and water vapour but resists the penetration of aqueous solutions and wound exudate. In use, the dressing absorbs blood or other tissue fluids, and the aqueous component is lost by evaporation through the back of the dressing'.

Crosslinked dextran gels are insoluble hydrophilic gels that can be partially depolymerised to the required molecular weight. The gel is produced in a bead shape; the degree of crosslinking determines the water uptake and pore size. Dextranomer (Debrisan) is a crosslinked dextran with pores large enough to allow substances with a molecular weight of less than 1000 Da to enter the beads. Each gram of beads abstracts approximately $4 \, cm^3$ of fluid. Applied to the surface of secreting wounds, dextranomer removes by suction various exudates that tend to impede tissue repair, while leaving behind high-molecular-weight materials such as plasma proteins and fibrinogen.

7.4.10 Polymer crystallinity

Polymers form perfect crystals with difficulty simply because of the low probability of arranging the chains in a regular fashion, especially at high molecular weights. Advantage can be taken of defects in crystals in the preparation of microcrystals. Microcrystalline cellulose (Avicel) is prepared by disruption of larger crystals. It is used as a tablet excipient and as a binder-disintegrant. Dispersed in water it forms colloidal gels, and it can be used to form heat-stable o/w emulsions. Spheroids of microcrystalline cellulose with accurately controlled diameters can be prepared and drugs can be incorporated during preparation. The concept of crystallinity is potentially important when considering polymer membranes, as discussed below.

7.5 Water-insoluble polymers and polymer membranes

In defining the properties of polymers for drug formulation, certain characteristics are important. Obviously molecular weight and molecular weight distribution must be known, as these affect solvent penetration and crystallinity. The functionality of the polymer is best described by a series of parameters such as

- Glass transition temperature, T_g
- Tensile strength
- Diffusion coefficient
- Hardness (crystallinity)
- Solubility

Crystallinity defines several features of polymers: rigidity, fluidity, the resistance to diffusion of small molecules in the polymer, and degradation.

In hydrogels T_g can be measured and is a measure of polymer structure, crosslinking density, solvent content and polymer–solvent interactions, as can be seen from Table 7.6.

Table 7.6 Effect of hydrogel structure and characteristics on T_g

Feature	Effect on T_g
Presence of flexible groups in main chain	↓
Bulky, inflexible side-chains	↑
Flexible side-chains	↓
Increase in main chain polarity	↑
Increase in crosslinking	↑
Plasticiser content	↓

7.5.1 Permeability of polymers

Hydrophobic polymers also play an important role in pharmacy. When these materials are used as membranes, containers or tubing material, their surfaces may come into contact with solutions. The surfaces of insoluble polymers are not as inert as might be thought. The interaction of drugs and preservatives with plastics depends on the structure of the polymer and on the affinity of the compound for the plastic. The latter is determined by the degree of crystallinity of the polymer, as permeability is a function of the degree of amorphous content of the polymer. The crystalline regions of the solid polymer present an impenetrable barrier to the movement of most molecules. Diffusing molecules thus have to circumnavigate the crystalline islands, which act as obstructions. The greater the volume fraction of crystalline material (ϕ_c) the slower the movement of molecules.

Diffusion

Diffusion in a nonporous solid polymer is of course a more difficult process than in a fluid because of the necessity for the movement of polymer chains to allow passage of the drug molecule, and it is therefore slower. The equation that governs the process is Fick's first law (see section 2.6, equation 2.92):

$$J = -D\frac{dc}{dx} \tag{7.25}$$

where J is the flux, D is the diffusion coefficient of the drug in the membrane, and dc/dx is the concentration gradient across the membrane. If the membrane is of thickness l, and Δc represents the difference in solution concentration of drug at the two faces of membrane,

$$J = \frac{DK\Delta c}{l} \tag{7.26}$$

where K is the distribution coefficient of the permeant towards the polymer. Therefore, alteration of polymer/membrane thickness, coupled with appropriate choice of polymer, can give rise to the desired flux. Within a given polymer, permeability is a function of the degree of crystallinity, itself a function of polymer molecular weight. If P is the permeability of drug in a partially crystalline polymer (see Fig. 1.17, Chapter 1), the volume fraction of the crystalline regions being ϕ_c, and P_a is the permeability in an amorphous sample, then

$$\frac{P}{P_a} = (1 - \phi_c)^2 \tag{7.27}$$

Permeation of drug molecules through the solid polymer, which may be acting as a drug depot, is a function of the solubility of the drug in the polymer as

$$P = DK \tag{7.28}$$

Addition of inorganic fillers in which the drug is insoluble alters the overall solubility of the drug in the polymer and hence alters the permeation characteristics. The equation for overall solubility (S) is given by

$$S = S_f \phi_f + S_p \phi_p \tag{7.29}$$

where f refers to filler and p to polymer. Thus, when $S_f \rightarrow 0$, as happens when inorganic fillers such as zinc oxide are employed, an obstruction-type equation may be written:

$$\frac{S}{S_p} = 1 - \phi_f \tag{7.30}$$

The natural permeabilities of polymers vary over a wide range and this widens the choice, provided one can select a polymer that is compatible with the tissues with which it comes into contact. Once a polymer has been chosen that gives a flux of drug sufficient to provide adequate circulating levels, use of fillers and plasticisers can give fine control of permeability (Table 7.7).

The method of preparation also influences the properties of the film. Cast films of varying properties can be prepared by variation *inter alia* of the solvent power of the casting solution containing the polymer, although the complex processes involved in film formation are not yet fully understood. It is clear, however, that the conformation of the polymer chains in concentrated solution just prior to solvent evaporation will determine the density of the film, and the number and size of pores and voids. Drug flux through dense (nonporous) polymer membranes is by diffusion; flux through porous membranes will be by diffusion and by transport in solvent through pores in the film. With porous films, control can be exercised on porosity, and hence overall permeability, by the use of swelling agents. Dense membranes can be subjected to certain post-formation treatments such as thermal annealing that modify their structural and performance characteristics.

The solubility of sterilising gases in polymers is important in determining the retention of residues that may, as in the case of ethylene oxide residues, be toxic. The quality control problems of polymers and plastics are considerable. Both the chemical and physical natures of the material have to be taken into account, as well as purity.

Permeability of polymers to gases

The permeability of polymers to the gaseous phase is of importance when the use of polymers as packaging materials is considered. Figure 7.24 shows oxygen penetration through a wide range of plastic materials ranging from Teflon to dimethylsilicone rubber, which has the highest permeability. Ether, nitrous oxide, halothane and cyclopropane diffuse through silicone rubbers, and general anaesthesia in dogs has been achieved by passing the vapours of these substances through a coil of silicone rubber tubing, each end of which is placed in an artery or vein. Aspects of the permeability of polymeric films of interest pharmaceutically include the process of gas diffusion, water sorption and permeation and dialysis processes. With few exceptions, there is an inverse relationship between water-vapour transmission and oxygen permeability. Water-vapour permeability has been shown to be dependent on the polarity of the polymer. More polar films tend to be more ordered and less porous, hence less oxygen-permeable. The less polar films are more porous, permitting the permeation of oxygen but not necessarily of the larger water molecules. Being more lipophilic, the less polar films have less affinity for water. Because of the importance of water as a solvent and permeant species, much work has been directed towards the synthesis of polymeric membranes with controlled hydrophilic/hydrophobic balance. The

Table 7.7 Factors that influence diffusivity in polymers	
Factor	**Net effect on D**
Increased polymer molecular weight	↓
Increased degree of crosslinking	↓
Diluents and plasticisers	↑
Fillers	↓
Increased crystallinity of polymers	↓
Increased drug molecular size	↓

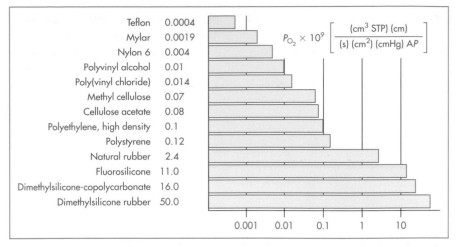

Figure 7.24 Permeation of oxygen through several polymer films. This illustrates the diversity of the properties of available polymers and shows the relatively high permeability of polydimethylsiloxane, a common component of prolonged-action drug devices.

Reproduced from Kesting R, *Synthetic Polymeric Membranes*, New York: McGraw-Hill; 1971.

hydrophilicity of the cellulose acetates is directly proportional to their —OH content and inversely proportional to the hydrophobic acetyl content (Table 7.8). Alternative approaches to alteration of characteristics of water permeability include the use of block copolymers where one can alter the ratio of hydrophilic polymer to increase transport rates of polar materials.

The affinity of drugs for plastics

Drugs may adsorb onto the surface of plastics or they may diffuse into the interior of the material. The affinity of drugs for plastics will vary with the structure of the drug: proteins, polypeptides and other hydrophilic or amphipathic molecules may adsorb, and smaller hydrophobic molecules *sorb*, that is enter the plastic. Chlorpromazine, for example, has a very high affinity for some materials used as tubing (Table 7.9). Silicone is actually very

Table 7.8 Effect of hydroxyl and acetyl content on water permeability and sorption of moisture by cellulose acetates[a]

Hydroxyl content (%)	Acetyl content (%)	Moisture sorption (%) at 95% relative humidity at 25°C	Water permeability D_1C_1 (10^{-7} g cm s^{-1})
7.2	34	19	12
5.9	36	17	7
4.6	38	14.7	4
3.3	40	12.6	2.5
2.0	42	10.5	1.5

[a] Reproduced from Reid C, Breton E, *J Appl Polymer Sci*, 1959; 1: 133.

Table 7.9 Concentration of chlorpromazine in buffer solution after shaking with various polymers for 1 h at 22°C (original concentration 100 μmol dm^{-3})[a]

Material	Chlorpromazine concentration (μmol dm^{-3})
Silicone tubing	1 ± 0.4
Latex tubing	16 ± 4.7
PVC tubing	14 ± 1.0
Polyethylene tubing	60 ± 2.0
Polyethylene test-tube	70 ± 3.8
Polyethylene stopper	77 ± 5.3
Plexiglass chippings	74 ± 4.3
Teflon chippings	81 ± 4.4
Polystyrene test-tube	89 ± 1.2

[a] Reproduced from Krieglstein G *et al.*, *Arzneim Forsch*, 1972; 22: 1538.

permeable to hydrophobic molecules and this can be put to good use in other areas, such as in controlled-release systems. The downside is that some drugs, e.g. steroids, are adsorbed from solutions passing through polyethylene tubing. In analytical chemistry such interactions can also be important in defining the accuracy of the method. Glyceryl trinitrate, which has a high affinity for lipophilic plastics, migrates from tablets in contact with plastic liners in packages, causing a reduction of the active content of many tablets to zero. This peculiar migratory behaviour is due to the volatility of the drug; normally the drug molecules would only be able to be significantly affected by such transfer when in the solution state.

7.5.2 Ion-exchange resins

Synthetic organic polymers comprising a hydrocarbon crosslinked network to which ionisable groups are attached have the ability to exchange ions attracted to their ionised groups with ions of the same charge present in solution (Fig. 7.25). These substances, usually prepared in the form of beads, are ion-exchange resins and are insoluble in water, the aqueous phase diffusing into the porous resin beads. Because ions must diffuse into and out of the resin for exchange to occur, ions larger than a given size may be excluded from reaction by altering the nature of the crosslinks in the polymer. The resins may be either cation

exchangers in which the resin ionisable group is acidic, for example, sulfonic, carboxylic (**XIII**) or phenolic groups, or anion exchangers in which the ionisable group is basic, either amine or quaternary ammonium groups.

Sulfonic acid ion-exchange resin

Carboxylic acid ion-exchange resin

Structure XIII Sulfonic acid and carboxylic acid ion-exchange resins

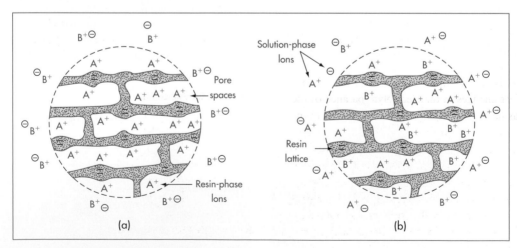

Figure 7.25 Schematic diagram of a cation-exchange resin framework with fixed exchange sites prior to and following an exchange reaction: (a) initial state prior to exchange reaction with cation B^+; (b) equilibrium state after exchange reaction with cation B^+.

Modified from Weber WJ, *Physicochemical Processes for Water Quality Control*, New York: Wiley, 1972.

The equations describing the equilibria involved are

Cation-exchange resin

$$POL - (SO_3^-)A^+ + B^+ \rightleftharpoons POL - (SO_3^-)B^+ + A^+$$

Anion-exchange resin

$$POL - N(CH_3)_3^+ X^- + Y^- \rightleftharpoons POL - N(CH_3)_3^+ Y^- + X^-$$

The equilibrium constant for the cation exchange resin is

$$K_{cation} = \frac{[POL - B^+][A^+]}{[POL - A^+][B^+]} \qquad (7.31)$$

However, application of equation (7.31) is impossible because of the inaccessibility of the terms [POL-B$^+$] and [POL-A$^-$]. Some estimation of a resin's affinity for ions can be made using a standard ion such as lithium for cation exchange resins. A selectivity coefficient, k, may be defined as

$$k = \frac{[B^+]_{resin}[A^+]_{solution}}{[A^+]_{resin}[B^+]_{solution}} \qquad (7.32)$$

Even here there is a problem arising from the difficulty in the determination of the activity of the ions in the resin (because of the complexity of the environment) and the overall concentration of ion is generally used instead.

The ability of a resin to exchange one ion for another depends on its affinity for the ion and the concentration of ions in solution. Cation-exchange resins tend to have affinity in decreasing order for calcium, potassium, sodium, ammonium and hydrogen ions.

Clinical point

Administered orally, cation-exchange resins effect changes in the electrolyte balance of the plasma by exchanging cations with those in the gut lumen. In the ammonium form, cation-exchange resins are used in the treatment of retention oedema and for the control of sodium retention in pregnancy. Depletion of plasma potassium can be prevented by including a proportion of resin in the form of the potassium salt. These resins are also used (as calcium and sodium forms) to treat hyperkalaemia.

Anion-exchange resins such as polyamine methylene resin and polyaminostyrene have been used as antacids.

Some pharmaceutical ion exchangers are listed in Table 7.10.

Apart from these medical uses, ion-exchange resins are used in the removal of ionised impurities from water and in the prolongation of drug action. Purified water may be obtained by passing through two columns containing a strong cation exchanger and a strong anion exchanger, respectively, or a column containing mixed resins. Anionic impurities in the water are replaced by OH$^-$ from the anion exchanger and cations by H$^+$ from the cation-exchange resin. Dissolved salts are thus removed and replaced by H$_2$O molecules, but of course nonionic impurities and colloidal material are not removed. Regeneration of the resins is accomplished using NaOH and HCl for the anion and cation exchangers, respectively.

In the prolongation of drug action, ion-exchange resins are employed to form complexes with drug substances, especially basic drugs such as ephedrine, pholcodine (**XIV**) and phenyltoloxamine (**XV**) (an isomer of diphenhydramine). Pholtex is a sustained-action liquid utilising a sulfonic acid ion-exchange resin with pholcodine and phenyltoloxamine as resin complexes.

Structure XIV Pholcodine

Structure XV Phenyltoloxamine

Ion-exchange resin (Amberlite IRP-69 resin) has been used with betaxolol as an ophthalmic suspension. This formulation with 0.25% betaxolol gave levels of

Table 7.10 Ion exchangers used in pharmacy

Name	Type	Comments	Trade name
Ammonium polystyrene sulfonate	Cation exchanger	Each gram exchanges 2.5 mEq Na^+	Katonium
Polycarbophil	Cation exchanger	Synthetic hydrophilic resin copolymer of acrylic acid, loosely crosslinked with divinyl glycol. Marked water-binding capacity	–
Calcium polystyrene sulfonate	Cation exchanger	Each gram exchanges about 1.3 mEq K^+	Calcium Resonium
Colestyramine	Anion exchanger	The chloride of a strongly basic anion-exchange resin containing quaternary ammonium groups attached to styrene-divinylbenzene copolymer	–
Polyamine–methylene resin	Anion exchanger	Effects a temporary binding of HCl + pepsin in the stomach, later released in the intestine	–
Sodium polystyrene sulfonate	Cation exchanger	Each gram exchanges 2.8–3.5 mEq K^+	Resonium A
Polyaminostyrene	Weak anion exchanger		–

drug in the aqueous humour virtually identical to those with the 0.5% control.[11] The rate of release of basic drugs from cation-exchange resins depends on the diameter of the resin beads, on the degree of crosslinking within the resin, and on the pK_a of the ionisable resin group. The resin–drug complex may be tableted and administered orally; resin complexes have been used to mask the taste of bitter drugs and to reduce the nausea produced by some irritant drugs. Some types, such as polacrilin potassium (Amberlite IRP 88, sulfonated polystyrene resin) are used as tablet disintegrants because of the high degree of swelling the dry resins undergo on interaction with water.

7.5.3 Silicone oligomers and polymers

The silicones are examples of hydrophobic liquid polymers, although in high molecular weight they exist as waxes and resins. Silicones are polymers with a structure containing alternate atoms of silicon and oxygen; the dimethicones are fluid polymers with the general formula (**XVI**) in which each unit has two methyl groups and an oxygen atom attached to the silicon atom in the chain. The viscosity range extends from 0.65 cSt to 3×10^6 cSt. The dimethicones 20, 200, 350 and 1000 (the number representing the average viscosity in centistokes at $25°C$) have rheological properties that allow them to be used in ophthalmology and in rheumatoid arthritis. Dimethicone 200 has been used as a lubricant for artificial eyes and to replace the degenerative vitreous fluid in cases of retinal detachment. It can also act as a simple lubricant in joints. More common uses are as barrier substances, silicone lotions and creams acting as water-repellent applications protecting the skin against water-soluble irritants. Methylphenylsilicone is used as a lubricant for hypodermic syringes. Glassware which has been treated with a thin film of silicone is rendered hydrophobic; solutions and aqueous suspensions thus drain completely from such vessels.

Structure XVI Dimethicone

Activated dimethicone (activated polymethylsiloxane) is a mixture of liquid dimethicones containing finely divided silica to enhance the defoaming properties of the silicone. The mechanism by which dispersion of colloidal silica antifoams improves their action is not well understood.

By varying the amounts of polymer in resin a variety of products, catheters, tubing materials for reconstructive surgery and membranes for drug reservoirs can be formed.

The release of lipophilic steroids from silicone elastomer matrices is dependent on the crosslinking density of the polymer and the content of filler, but also on the lipophilicity of the drug. A relationship between the solubility parameters of a number of drugs and their release rate is shown in Fig. 7.26.

An interesting application of the silicone fluids is their coformulation with adhesives to increase 'tack' and in elastomers to soften the product. Pressure-sensitive silicone adhesives are formed from the most highly crosslinked systems based on the structure **XVI**.

Other pressure-sensitive adhesives used in transdermal delivery device include those shown in Table 7.11.

Figure 7.26 Comparative release rates of different drugs from a pressure-sensitive silicone matrix as a function of their solubility parameter.

Reproduced from Clauss LC, in: *Proceedings of the International Conference on Pharmaceutical, Ingredients and Intermediates (1990)*, Maarssen: Expoconsult; 1991: 116.

Table 7.11 Pressure-sensitive adhesives in transdermal patches[a]

Adhesive class	Adhesive polymer
$\left[CH_2-\underset{\underset{CH_3}{\mid}}{\overset{\overset{CH_3}{\mid}}{C}} \right]_x$	Polyisoprene Polybutene Polyisobutylene
$\left[CH_2-\underset{\underset{\underset{O}{\overset{\mid}{}}}{\overset{H}{\underset{\mid}{C}}}\overset{\mid}{\underset{C=O}{}} \right]_x$	Ethyl acrylate 2-Ethylhexyl acrylate Isooctyl acrylate
$\left[\underset{\underset{CH_3}{\mid}}{\overset{\overset{CH_3}{\mid}}{O-Si}} \right]_x OH$	Polydimethylsiloxane Polysilicate resin Siloxane blends

[a] Reproduced from Pfister WR *et al.*, *Pharm Tech*, 1992; 16(1): 42.

Key points

- Water-soluble (hydrophilic) polymers are widely used in pharmacy, for example as suspending agents, emulsifiers, binding agents in tablets, thickeners of liquid dosage forms and in film coating of tablets. Important examples include: carboxypolymethylene (Carbomer, Carbopol), cellulose derivatives (methylcellulose, hydroxypropylmethylcellulose), natural gums and mucilages (acacia and tragacanth gums, alginates, pectin), chitosan, PVP, and polyethylene glycols.
- Water-insoluble (hydrophobic) polymers are mainly used in packaging material and tubing, and in the fabrication of membranes and films. Important examples include ion-exchange resins and silicones (e.g. dimethicone).
- Important properties of hydrophobic polymers that affect their suitability for use in pharmacy are their permeability to drugs and gases and their tendency to adsorb drugs.

7.6 Some applications of polymeric systems in drug delivery

Control of the rate of release of a drug when administered by oral or parenteral routes is aided by the use of polymers that function as a barrier to drug movement.

7.6.1 Film coating

Polymer solutions allowed to evaporate produce polymeric films that can act as protective layers for tablets or granules containing sensitive drug substances or as a rate-controlling barrier to drug release. Film coats have been divided into two types; those that dissolve rapidly and those that dissolve very slowly and behave as dialysis membranes, allowing slow diffusion of solute or some delayed diffusion by acting as gel layers. Materials that have been used as film formers include shellac, zein, glyceryl stearates, paraffins and a range of anionic and cationic polymers such as the Eudragit polymers (**XVII** to **XX**). Newer materials used for the same purpose include cellulose acetate phthalate.

Different film coats applied to tablet surfaces can lead to quite different rates of solution. In Fig. 7.27, hydroxypropylmethylcellulose, an acrylic derivative and zein are compared for their effect on sodium chloride dissolution from discs. Two plasticisers have been used: glycerin and diethyl phthalate. Times for 50% dissolution range from a few minutes to 450 minutes, indicating the scope of the technique for retard formulations, and the possibility of unwittingly extending dissolution times by the injudicious choice of coating material.

The process of film coating generally involves spraying the chosen polymer solution onto a bed of tablet cores. Several physical properties are important, for example, the viscosity and surface tension of the solutions will determine the droplet size and might also influence the spreading of the polymer on the tablet surfaces as well as its adhesion to the substrate. Additives are used to modify the native properties of the polymer solutions; in one example the addition of microcrystalline cellulose allowed a greater interaction with the tablet surface, probably through interaction with the same material in the tablet formulation. Polymer blends are used to tailor release rates of drugs from coated tablets. As with many pharmaceutical processes, matters are far from simple. Blended polymers may be incompatible, polymer dispersions may flocculate and plasticisers migrate. Ultimately the coated systems must be tested rigorously, with respect to their main functions, control of drug release rate, reduction of water permeability into the core and reduced oxygen permeability to minimise degradation.

Structure XVII Poly(methacrylic acid, methyl methacrylate) 1:1 copolymer (Eudragit L12.5, L100)

Structure XVIII Poly(ethylacrylate, methacrylic acid) 1:1 (Eudragit L 30 D, L 100-55).

Structure XIX Poly(butylmethacrylate, 2-dimethylaminoethyl methacrylate, methyl methacrylate) 1:2:1 (Eudragit E 100, E 12.5)

Structure XX Poly(ethylacrylate, methyl methacrylate) 2:1 (Eudragit E 30 D).

Figure 7.27 Dissolution of sodium chloride from tablets coated with hydroxypropylmethylcellulose (○), a vinyl polymer (●) and zein (⊙) with glycerin as an additive, and the same polymers with diethyl phthalate as additive (□, ■, and ⊡ respectively).

Reproduced from Laguna O et al., Ann Pharm Franc, 1975; 33: 235.

Stents are tiny wire mesh tubular devices that enlarge diseased arteries. A relatively new form of drug delivery has appeared in the form of coated stents in which polymer coatings are used to deliver drugs direct to tissues. Some designs use several polymers in several layers to control drug release, as in the diagram below (Fig. 7.28)

7.6.2 Matrices

The use of a barrier film coating is only one of several procedures that can be adopted to control release of drugs (Fig. 7.29). Various methods are shown schematically in Table 7.12. If hydrophobic water-insoluble polymers are used, the mechanism of release is the passage of drug through pores in the plastic, or by leaching or slow diffusion of drug through the polymer wall (Fig. 7.29b), as discussed earlier in this chapter. Release may also be effected by erosion of the polymer (Fig. 7.29c). When water-soluble polymers are employed, for example as hydrophilic matrices, the entry of water into the polymer is followed by swelling and gelation and the drug must diffuse through the viscous gel, a process obviously slower than diffusion through plain solvent.

Release of drugs from matrices

Equations describing the rate of drug release from hydrophobic and hydrophilic matrices are useful in determining which factors may be altered to change the measured release rate of drug. Higuchi[12] proposed the following equation for the amount of drug, Q, released per unit area of tablet surface in time t, from an insoluble matrix:

$$Q = \left[\frac{D\varepsilon}{\tau}(2A - \varepsilon C_s)C_s t\right]^{1/2} \quad (7.33)$$

D is the diffusion coefficient of the drug in the release medium, C_s is the solubility of drug in the medium, ε is the porosity of the matrix, τ is the tortuosity of the matrix, and A is the total amount of drug in the matrix per unit volume.

If the same matrix is saturated with a solution of the drug (as in medicated soft contact lenses) the appropriate equation becomes, if C_0 is the concentration of drug solution:

Figure 7.28 A diagrammatic representation of a polymer coated stent (the Infinitum stent). The stent structure is coated with three different layers of polymers that have different functions from the outermost coat, which contains no drug but protects the underlying structures.

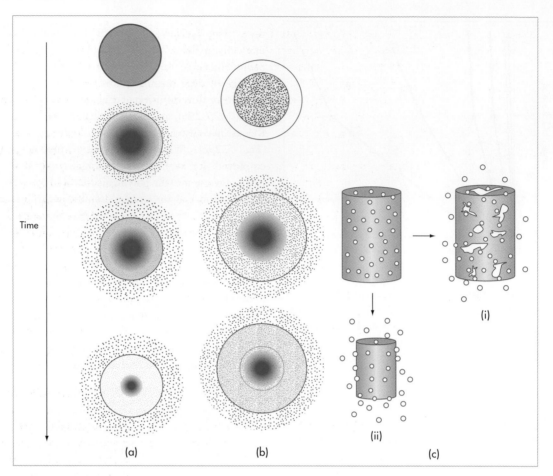

Figure 7.29 (a) Drug delivery from a matrix delivery device showing diagrammatically the depletion of drug from the system and the release of the drug. (b) Release from a typical reservoir system with a membrane controlling release from the internal store of drug. (c) Illustrating release from (i) a bulk-eroding system and (ii) a surface-eroding system.

After Brannon-Peppas L, *Medical Plastics and Biomaterials*, 1997(Nov.): 34.

$$Q = 2C_0\varepsilon\left(\frac{Dt}{\tau\pi}\right)^{1/2} \tag{7.34}$$

That is, for a given drug in a given matrix, $Q \propto t^{1/2}$. The more porous the matrix, the more rapid the release. The more tortuous the pores, the longer the path for diffusing molecules, the lower is Q. More-soluble drugs diffuse more quickly from the matrix.

The extension of these equations to hydrophilic matrices is difficult because the conditions in a hydrophilic matrix change with time as water penetrates into it. If the polymer does not dissolve but simply swells and if the drug has not completely dissolved in the incoming solvent, diffusion of drug commences from a saturated solution through the gel layer, and

$$Q = \frac{D\varepsilon}{\tau}\left[\left(\frac{2W_0}{V} - \varepsilon C_s\right)tC_s\right]^{1/2} \tag{7.35}$$

Equation (7.35) is similar to equation (7.33) except that the effective volume V of the hydrated matrix is used as this is not a fixed quantity. W_0 is the dose of the drug in the matrix. If the drug completely dissolves on hydration of the matrix, an analogue of equation (7.34) is used:

$$Q = \frac{2W_0}{V}\left(\frac{Dt}{\tau\pi}\right)^{1/2} \tag{7.36}$$

In the initial stages of the process the rate of movement of water into the matrix may be important in determining release characteristics. When a homogeneous barrier wall is present diffusion through the

Table 7.12 Depot forms employing polymeric films and matrices[a]

Type	Materials[b]	Diagrammatic representation	Mechanisms
1 Barrier coating	Beeswax, glyceryl monostearate, ethylcellulose, nylon (Ultramid IC), acrylic resins (Eudragit retard)	drug / coating	Diffusion
2 Fat embedment	Glycerol palmitostearate (Precirol), beeswax, glycowax, castorwax, aluminium monostearate, carnauba wax, glyceryl monostearate, stearyl alcohol	drug / fat	Erosion, hydrolysis of fat, dissolution
3 Plastic matrix	Polyethylene Poly(vinyl acetate) Polymethacrylate Poly(vinyl chloride) Ethylcellulose	drug / polymer	Leaching, diffusion
4 Repeat action	Cellulose acetylphthalate	enteric coat	Dissolution of enteric coat
5 Ion exchange	Amberlite Dowex		Dissociation of drug–resin complex
6 Hydrophilic matrix	Carboxymethylcellulose Sodium carboxymethylcellulose Hydroxypropylmethylcellulose	hydrophilic polymer / drug	Gelation, diffusion
7 Epoxy resin beads	Epoxy resins	epoxy resin bead or microcapsule	Dissolution of resin or swelling, diffusion
8 Microcapsules	Polyamides, gelatin		
9 Soft gelatin depot capsules	Shellac–PEG Poly(vinyl acetate)–PEG		Diffusion

[a] Modified from Ritschel WA, in: Ariens AJ, ed., *Drug Design*, vol. IV, New York: Academic Press; 1974.

[b] Materials are not all polymeric. The waxes are included for completeness; these depend on conferring a hydrophobic layer on the drug, tablet or granule to prevent access of solvent.

walls has to take place and equations in section 7.5 apply.

7.6.3 Microcapsules and microspheres

Microencapsulation is a technique that, as its name suggests, involves the encapsulation of small particles of drug, or solution of drug, within a polymer film or coat. Microspheres, on the other hand, are solid but not necessarily homogeneous particles that can entrap drug. Although the terms tend to be used interchangeably, we retain the distinction here. Microspheres can be prepared also by a variety of techniques discussed briefly below. Typical photomicrographs of poly(ε-caprolactone) microspheres are shown in Fig. 7.30. Three main processes can be considered:

- *Coacervation* of macromolecules around the core material, this being induced by temperature change, solvent change or addition of a second macromolecule of appropriate physical properties.
- *Interfacial* polymerisation of a monomer around the core material by polymerisation at the interface of a liquid dispersion.
- *Spray coating and other methods* in which larger particles may be coated in suspension.

Any method that will cause a coherent barrier to deposit itself on the surface of a liquid droplet or a solid particle of drug may be applied to the formation of microcapsules. Many so-called microencapsulation procedures result in the formation of macroscopic 'beads', which are simply coated granules.

Coacervation

Coacervation is the term used to describe the separation of macromolecular solutions into colloid-poor and colloid-rich (coacervate) phases when the macromolecules are desolvated. The liquid or solid to be encapsulated is dispersed in a solution of a macromolecule (such as gelatin, gum arabic, carboxymethylcellulose or poly(vinyl alcohol)) in which it is immiscible. A nonsolvent, miscible with the continuous phase but a poor solvent for the polymer, under certain conditions will induce the polymer to form a coacervate (polymer-rich) layer around the disperse phase. This coating layer may then be treated to give a rigid coat of capsule wall. This is the process of *simple coacervation*. Successful application of the technique relies on the determination of the appropriate conditions for coacervate deposition, which can be achieved not only by the addition of nonsolvents such as ethanol and isopropanol and salts (sodium and ammonium sulfates) but also by the choice of macromolecules incompatible under selected conditions with the first species. The latter process is termed *complex coacervation*. In both simple and complex coacervation utilising hydrophilic macromolecules it is the decrease in solubility that results in deposition of the macromolecule layer at the particle–solution interface.

Desolvation of water-insoluble macromolecules in nonaqueous solvents leads to the deposition of a coacervate layer around aqueous or solid disperse droplets. Table 7.13 lists both water-soluble and

Figure 7.30 Scanning electron micrographs of bovine serum albumin-loaded microspheres prepared from a ternary blend of poly(ε-caprolactone). Protein entrapment efficiency and mean particle size were 28.6% and 2.9 μm, respectively.

Reproduced from Huatan H *et al*, *J Microencapsul*, 1995; 12: 557.

water-soluble macromolecules that have been used in coacervation processes. Desolvation, and thus coacervation, can be induced thermally and this is the basis of some preparative techniques. Conditions for phase separation are best obtained using phase diagrams.

For example, in the region of pH 6, gelatin will be positively charged and gum arabic negatively charged. In admixture, complex coacervates will form under the conditions described in Fig. 7.31, which shows the partial phase diagram of the ternary system gum arabic–gelatin–water. The hatched area at the top of the phase diagram is the restricted region in which coacervation occurs. At higher concentrations of the macromolecules, macroscopic precipitates of the complex will occur.

Interfacial reaction

Reactions between oil-soluble monomers and water-soluble monomers at the oil–water interface of w/o or

Table 7.13 Materials used in coacervation microencapsulation

Water-soluble macromolecules	Water-insoluble macromolecules
Arabinogalactan	Cellulose acetate phthalate
Carboxymethylcellulose	Cellulose nitrate
Gelatin	Ethylcellulose
Gum arabic (acacia)	Poly(ethylene vinyl acetate)
Hydroxyethylcellulose	Poly(methyl methacrylate)
Poly(acrylic acid)	
Polyethyleneimine	
Poly(vinyl alcohol)	
Polyvinylpyrrolidone	
Methylcellulose	
Starch	

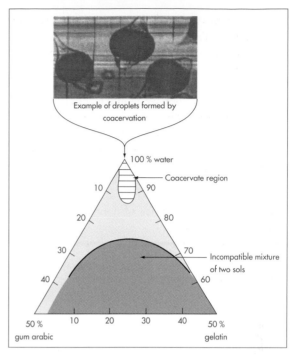

Figure 7.31 Ternary diagram showing complex coacervation region for mixtures of gum arabic and gelatin at pH 4.5; below the curved line the mixture separates into two sols (US Patent 2800457). Insert: Typical droplets formed by coacervation (Ronald T. Dodge).

o/w dispersions can lead to *interfacial polymerisation* resulting in the formation of polymeric microcapsules, the size of which is determined by the size of the emulsion droplets. Alternatively, reactive monomer can be dispersed in one of the phases and induced to polymerise at the interface, or to polymerise in the bulk disperse phase and to *precipitate* at the interface owing to its insolubility in the continuous phase. There are many variations on this theme. Probably the most widely studied reaction has been the interfacial condensation of water-soluble alkyl diamines with oil-soluble acid dichlorides to form polyamides. Representative examples of other wall materials are polyurethanes, polysulfonamides, polyphthalamides and poly(phenyl esters). The selection of polymer is restricted to those that can be formed from monomers with the requisite preferential solubilities in one phase so that polymerisation takes place only at the interface.

Physical methods of encapsulation

Various physical methods of preparing microcapsules such as spray drying and pan coating are available.

Pan coating application of films to particles can only be used for particles greater than 600 μm in diameter. The process has been applied in the formation of sustained-release beads by application of waxes such as glyceryl monostearate in organic solution to granules of drug.

The *spray drying* process involves dispersion of the core material in a solution of coating substance and spraying the mixture into an environment that causes the solvent to evaporate. In an analogous *spray congealing* process the coating material is congealed thermally or by introducing the core coat mixture into a nonsolvent mixture. Both processes can produce microcapsules in the size range 5000–6000 μm.

Spray polycondensation is a variant based on the polycondensation of surface-active monomers on a melamine–formaldehyde base on the surface of suspended particles during spray drying. A dispersion of the core material is prepared in a continuous phase containing aminoplast monomers or precondensates of relatively low molecular weight, in addition to other film-forming agents and catalyst. The reactive monomers derived from hexamethylol melamine derivatives are selectively adsorbed at the surface of the disperse phase. Spray drying at 150–200°C results in vaporisation of the water and causes simultaneous polycondensation of the monomers and precondensates by acid catalysis.

The preparation and properties of particles in the nano size range are discussed in Chapter 8.

General considerations

In all techniques discussed there are several factors which are of importance in relation to the use of the product as a drug delivery vehicle or carrier.

- The efficiency of encapsulation of the active ingredient
- The effect of the encapsulation process on the properties of the encapsulated agent
- The presence of potentially toxic residue (e.g. monomer, salts) in the final product
- The reproducibility of the process and ease of separation
- The biocompatibility of the encapsulating agent
- The biodegradability of the material (in some cases)
- The properties of the microcapsule in relation to use, size distribution, porosity and permeability of the wall

Biodegradable polymers cannot always be induced to form microcapsules and a polymer found to be degradable in solid or film form may not be degradable when formed into microcapsules if the polymer chains are crosslinked. In their application in medicine, the permeability of the capsule wall is probably the most important feature of the product. The effects of the various parameters relating to wall material, capsule and environment on permeability are outlined in Table 7.14.

Protein microspheres

Aqueous solutions of proteins such as albumin can be emulsified in an oil and induced to form microspheres, either by crosslinking the protein molecules with glutaraldehyde or other agents or by coagulating the protein by heating. Incorporation of a drug within the

Table 7.14 General parameters affecting capsule wall permeability[a]

Parameter	For lower permeability
Properties of wall polymer	
Density	Increase
Crystallinity	Increase
Crosslinking	Increase
Plasticiser content	Decrease
Fillers	Increase
Solvents used in film formation	Use good solvents versus poor
Properties of capsule	
Size	Increase
Wall thickness	Increase
Treatment	Utilise (e.g. crosslinking, sintering)
Multiple coatings	Utilise
Environmental properties	
Temperature	Decrease

[a] Reproduced from Vandegaer JE, ed., *Microencapsulation, Processes and Applications*, New York: Plenum Press; 1974.

initial protein solution results in drug-laden microspheres that are biodegradable. The particle size of the microspheres (generally 0.2–300 μm diameter) is determined by the size distribution of the initial emulsion.

Protein microspheres have been used for physical drug targeting, i.e. the entrapment of carrier and therefore drug in, for example, the capillaries of the lung. Microspheres greater than about 7 μm in diameter will be physically trapped in capillary beds. On intra-arterial injection of large microspheres, the blood supply to an organ is reduced; the process of chemo-embolisation involves both blockage and delivery of drugs to the organ. External control over intravenously administered protein microspheres has been achieved by incorporation of magnetite (Fe_3O_4) particles into the microspheres, which then respond to an externally applied magnetic field.

7.6.4 Rate-limiting membranes and devices

The use of rate-limiting membranes to control the movement of drugs from a reservoir has been referred to above. Implants of silicone rubber or other appropriate polymeric material in which drug is embedded can be designed by choice of polymer, membrane thickness and porosity, to release drug at preselected rates. The Progestasert device (Fig. 7.32c) is designed to be implanted into the uterine cavity and to release there 65 µg progesterone per day to provide contraceptive cover for one year. The Ocusert device and the Transiderm therapeutic system (also shown in Fig. 7.32), which are discussed in Chapter 10, are products of the Alza Corporation (USA) and rely on rate-limiting polymeric membranes to control drug release. The opportunities for prolonged release of drugs given by the oral route are fewer. The aim in oral dosage forms is for controlled rather than prolonged release, so that dosage frequency can be reduced or so that side-effects resulting from fast dissolution of drug can be minimised. Ion-exchange resin–drug complexes have also been used, and drugs may also be embedded in hydrophilic or hydrophobic matrices.

7.6.5 Eroding systems

Release of drug by erosion of the polymeric or macromolecular matrix in which a drug is dissolved or dispersed provides another mechanism for controlling drug absorption. Erosion of course demands some degree of solubility of the matrix to allow enzymes and other agents to penetrate. A typical bioerodible system would be that achieved by the molecular association of a cellulose acetate phthalate (CAP) (a carboxylic acid polymer) with a poloxamer block copolymer such as Pluronic L101. This interaction is between the proton-donating CAP and the proton-accepting poloxamer. By varying the ratio of CAP to poloxamer, the erosion periods can be controlled from hours to days. Figure 7.33 shows the relationship between the percentage polymer eroded and

Figure 7.32 Examples of drug-delivery systems employing polymeric membranes. (a) Ocusert system for the eye with two rate-controlling membranes. (b) Transiderm system for transdermal medication with one rate-controlling layer. (c) The Progestasert device for intrauterine insertion in which the body of the device serves as the rate-controlling barrier. (d) The oral Oros device in which the membrane is a semipermeable membrane that prevents drug transport, allowing water ingress only.

Figure 7.33 Characteristics of *in vivo* polymer erosion and metronidazole (MTZ) release from 50/50 CAP/Pluronic L101 films (with 10% metronidazole loading) in a dorsal rat model.

Reproduced from Gates KA *et al., Pharm Res*, 1994; 11: 1605.

the release of drugs from a $50:50$ mixture of the polymers containing 10% of the drug metronidazole.

Computer simulation of eroding matrices (Fig. 7.34) can give an accurate representation of the process and can predict the position of the erosion front and the weight of the matrix.

More precise control of release than is possible with matrices has recently been achieved by the application of several features of polymer physical chemistry, as discussed below.

7.6.6 Osmotic pumps

A variety of osmotic pumps have been described in the patent literature.[13,14] In the oral osmotic pump (Oros or Osmet) the drug is mixed with a water-soluble core material. This core is surrounded by a water-insoluble semipermeable polymer membrane in which is drilled a small orifice. Water molecules can diffuse into the core through the outer membrane to form a concentrated solution inside. An osmotic gradient is set up across the semipermeable membrane with the result that drug is pushed out of the orifice (Fig. 7.35).

The core may be a water-soluble polymer, an inert salt or, as in the case of metoprolol fumarate,[15] the drug itself, whose saturated solution has an osmotic pressure of 32.5 atm. The osmotic tablet of nifedipine is described in detail in Fig. 7.36, which shows the semipermeable cellulose acetate coating, the swellable

$t \times \lambda_a = 0.042$

$t \times \lambda_a = 0.104$

$t \times \lambda_a = 0.339$

Figure 7.34 Theoretical representation of a polymer matrix: changes during erosion (dark pixels = nondegraded areas, white pixels = degraded areas), where λ_a (a rate constant) = $2.7 \times 10^{-7}\,\text{s}^{-1}$ for a sample containing 50% polyanhydride CPP.

Reproduced from Göpferich A *et al.*, in: Cleland JL, Langer R, eds, *Formulation and Delivery of Proteins and Peptides*, ACS Symposium Series no. 567, Washington DC: American Chemical Society; 1994.

hydrogel layer of polyoxyethylene glycol and hydroxypropylmethylcellulose (HPMC), and the drug chamber containing nifedipine in HPMC and PEG.

For simple osmotic systems the initial zero-order delivery rate (dm/dt) is given by

$$\frac{dm}{dt} = \frac{A}{H} k(\pi_f - \pi_e) S_d \qquad (7.37)$$

where S_d is drug concentration in the system, π_f is the osmotic pressure of the formulation, π_e is the osmotic pressure of the environment (7.7 atm for isotonic saline at 37°C), k is the membrane permeability to water, H is the thickness of the membrane and A is its area. Calculated and experimental release rates are shown in Fig. 7.37.

One problem is that of controlling the transit of the device down the gastrointestinal (GI) tract, as individual subjects vary considerably in GI transit times. If the system is designed to release drug over a period of 10 hours and total transit time in the gut is 5 hours, bioavailability will obviously be reduced.

7.6.7 Transdermal delivery systems

Several transdermal systems ostensibly dependent on rate-controlling membranes are available for the delivery of glyceryl trinitrate, hyoscine, estradiol, fentanyl and other drugs. The word 'ostensibly' is used as there is a debate about whether the barrier membrane in these devices is the rate-limiting step in

Figure 7.35   Low-power scanning electron micrographs of an oral osmotic pump (Osmet). (a) A section showing the semipermeable membrane, the osmotic core and the laser-drilled orifice. (b) The same 8 hours after immersion in water. (c) The laser-drilled orifice. (d) Another view of the tablet via the orifice after 24 hours of immersion.

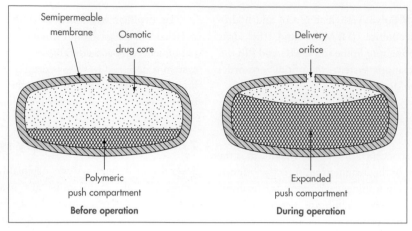

Figure 7.36 Cross-section of the 'push–pull' osmotic pump for nifedipine.

Reproduced from Zaffaroni A, *Ann N Y Acad Sci*, 1991; 618: 405.

absorption. The barrier properties of skin are so variable, however, that one advantage of rate-controlling systems is that they prevent too rapid dosing in patients with highly permeable skin. In those with less permeable skin, the systems probably act only as reservoirs. The now wide range of systems is listed in Table 7.15, which includes a reference to the pressure-sensitive adhesives discussed earlier in this chapter.

Some of the devices and the bases of their design are shown in Fig. 7.38 (the Transiderm system is also shown in Fig. 7.32). There are two groups: membrane and matrix systems. Membrane systems generally consist of a reservoir, a rate-controlling membrane and an adhesive layer. Diffusion of the active principle through the controlling membrane governs release rate. The active principle is usually present in suspended form; liquids and gels are used as dispersion media. In matrix systems the active principle is dispersed in a matrix that consists either of a gel or of an adhesive film.

In Transiderm Nitro, the rate-controlling membrane is composed of a polyethylene–vinyl acetate copolymer having a thin adhesive layer (membrane type) (see Table 7.15). The reservoir contains glyceryl trinitrate dispersed in the form of a lactose suspension in silicone oil. The Nitro-Dur system consists of a hydrogel matrix (composed of water, glycerin, poly(vinyl alcohol) and polyvinylpyrrolidone) in which a glyceryl trinitrate–lactose triturate is homogeneously dispersed.

In Nitro Disc, glyceryl trinitrate is distributed between microscopically small liquid compartments and a crosslinked silicone matrix. In the approximately 10–200 μm sized micro compartments there is active ingredient also in the form of a lactose triturate, in an aqueous solution of PEG 400. The system is secured to the skin with the aid of a circular adhesive disc having a centrally located silicone matrix, not coated with adhesive. The system is termed a 'micro sealed drug delivery system'. The basis of the Deponit system[16] is shown in detail in Fig. 7.39.

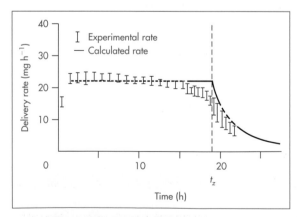

Figure 7.37 *In vitro* release rate of potassium chloride from elementary osmotic pumps in water at 37°C.

Reproduced from Theeuwes F, *J Pharm Sci*, 1975; 64: 1987.

Table 7.15 Some transdermal drug-delivery devices[a]

Product	Drug	Adhesive	Adhesive use[b]	Marketing company
Anti-anginal				
Nitrodisc	GTN[c]	Acrylic	Rim	G. D. Searle
Nitro-Dur I	GTN	Acrylic	Rim	Schering-Plough
Nitro-Dur II	GTN	Acrylic	Matrix	Schering-Plough
Diafusor	GTN	Acrylic	Matrix	Lab Pierre Fabre Med
Minitran	GTN	Acrylic	Matrix	3M Riker
Transiderm-Nitro	GTN	Silicone	Face	Novartis
Nitroderm TTS	GTN	Silicone	Face	Novartis
Nitrol patch	GTN	Acrylic	Rim	Adria Lab.
NTS patch	GTN	Acrylic	Rim	Bolar, Major, Qualitest, Bio-Line, Goldline, Geneva, Rugby
Transdermal-NTG	GTN	Acrylic	Rim	Warner Chilcott Lab.
Nitrocine	GTN	Acrylic	Rim	Kremer Urban
Deponit	GTN	Polyisobutylene	Matrix	Schwarz/Wyeth
Frandol Tape	Isosorbide dinitrate	Acrylic	Matrix	Toaeiyo, Yamanouchi Pharm.
Motion sickness				
Trasiderm-Scop	Hyoscine	Polyisobutylene	Matrix	Novartis
Kimite-patch	Hyoscine	Polyisobutylene	Matrix	Myun Moon Pharm. Co.
Hypertension				
Catapress-TTS	Clonidine	Polyisobutylene	Matrix	Boehringer Ingelheim
Estrogen therapy				
Estraderm	Estradiol	Polyisobutylene	Face	Novartis
Analgesia				
Duragesic	Fentanyl	Silicone	Face	Jansen Pharm.
Smoking cessation				
Nicotinell	Nicotine	Acrylic	Matrix	Novartis
Nikofrenon	Nicotine	Acrylic	Matrix	Novartis

[a] Reproduced from Foster WP *et al.*, *Pharm Tech*, 1992; 16(1): 42.
[b] Indicated as an adhesive laminated to an overlying backing substrate forming a rim around the matrix (rim): a drug-containing adhesive matrix laminated to a backing substrate (matrix); or an adhesive laminated to the face of a rate-controlling membrane (face).
[c] GTN = glyceryl trinitrate.

Figure 7.38 The structures of some commercial transdermal membrane-controlled and matrix systems (the structure of the Deponit TTS is shown in Fig. 7.39).

 Key points

- Polymers may be used to control the rate of release of a drug when administered by oral or parenteral routes. Materials such as shellac, zein, cellulose acetate phthalate, glyceryl stearates, cellulose acetate phthalate, and a range of anionic and cationic polymers (Eudragits) form *film coats*, allowing slow diffusion of solute or delaying diffusion by acting as gel layers. *Matrices* may be formed by (i) hydrophobic water-insoluble polymers (e.g. PVC, PVA, ethylcellulose) that release drug by slow diffusion through pores or through the polymer wall, or by erosion of the polymer and (ii) water-soluble polymers (e.g. carboxymethylcellulose, HPMC) that swell in water to form viscous gels (hydrophilic matrices), from which drug is released by slow diffusion.

- Drug may also be slowly released from *microcapsules*, which encapsulate the drug as small particles or as a drug solution in a polymer film or coat, and *microspheres*, which are solid polymeric spheres that entrap drug. Microcapsules can be prepared by coacervation, by interfacial polymerisation or by spray coating.
- Rate-limiting membranes may be used to control the movement of drugs from a reservoir as in the Progestasert device designed to release progesterone into the uterine cavity, the Ocusert device for delivery to the eye, and the Transiderm therapeutic system for transdermal medication
- In oral *osmotic pumps* (Oros or Osmet) an osmotic gradient is set up across a semipermeable polymeric membrane that encloses a solution of drug in a water-soluble core material; the osmotic pressure developed as water diffuses into the core pushes the drug out of a small orifice drilled in the membrane.

Figure 7.39 Cross-section of Deponit TTS. Deponit contains glyceryl trinitrate directly embedded in a lactose-containing adhesive film approximately 0.3 mm thick. In cross-section, the Deponit transdermal system, closely resembling a plaster, consists of three components in macroscopic proportions, the ratios of which are as given in the figure. The adhesive film is both a store of active ingredient and the release-controlling matrix.

Reproduced from reference 16.

Summary

Although there is no strict boundary line, we have divided polymers into water-soluble polymers and water-insoluble systems, typified respectively by materials used to prepare viscous solutions and those that function as barrier membranes or containers. In the first case we have considered the factors controlling their properties: the influence of molecular weight (distribution), branching, charge, flexibility, ionic strength and pH on solution properties. In the case of water-soluble polymers, the main concern has been with solute transport through the polymer bulk. Equations dealing with viscosity and with diffusion have been cited. The variety of pharmaceutical uses of polymers has been described, and the variety of morphologies that polymers can adopt has been emphasised: solutions, gels, microcrystals, crystals, fibres and dendrimers.

When a polymer is being characterised for pharmaceutical use, therefore, much more than its molecular weight distribution should be determined. Its end use will, of course, determine the tests to be applied.

References

1. Svenson S, Tomalia DA. Dendrimers in biomedical applications – reflecting on the field. *Adv Drug Deliv Rev* 2005;57:2106–2129.
2. Menoge AR *et al*. Dendrimer based drug and imaging conjugates: design considerations for nanomedical applications. *Drug Discov Today* 2010;15:171–185.
3. McCahon R, Hardman J. Pharmacology of plasma expanders. *Anesth Intensive Care Med* 2007;8:79–81.
4. James WP *et al*. Calcium binding by dietary fiber. *Lancet* 1978;1:638–639.
5. Peppas NA, Khare AR. Preparation, structure and diffusional behavior of hydrogels in controlled release. *Adv Drug Deliv Rev* 1993;11:1–35.
6. Chaubal M. Using chitosan as an excipient for oral drug delivery. *Drug Deliv Technol* 2003;3:32–34,36.
7. Lueßen HL *et al*. Bioadhesive polymers for the peroral delivery of peptide drugs. *J Control Release* 1994;29:329–338.
8. Turner TD. Synthaderm – an 'environmental' dressing. *Pharm J* 1982;228:206–208.
9. Myers JA. Lyofoam – a versatile polyurethane foam surgical dressing. *Pharm J* 1985;235:270.
10. SMTL. *Alphabetical list of dressings data cards*. www.dressings.org/dressings-datacards-by-alpha.html. (accessed 18 January 2011).
11. Jani R *et al*. Ion exchange resins for ophthalmic delivery. *J Ocul Pharmacol* 1994;10:57–67.
12. Higuchi T. Mechanism of sustained-action medication. Theoretical analysis of rate of release of solid drugs dispersed in solid matrices. *J Pharm Sci* 1963;52:1145–1149.
13. Santus G, Baker RW. Osmotic drug delivery: a review of the patent literature. *J Control Release* 1995;35:1–21.
14. Gupta BP *et al*. Osmotically controlled drug delivery systems with associated drugs. *J Pharm Pharm Sci* 2010;13:571–588.
15. Theeuwes F *et al*. Osmotic delivery systems for the alpha-adrenoceptor antagonists metoprolol and oxyprenolol: design and evaluation of systems for once-daily administration. *Br J Clin Pharmacol* 1985;19(Suppl):69S–76S.
16. Wolff M *et al*. *In vitro* and *in vivo* release of nitroglycerin from a new transdermal therapeutic system. *Pharm Res* 1985;2:23–29.

Further reading

Liechty WB *et al*. Polymers for drug delivery. *Annu Rev Chem Biomol Eng* 2010;1:149–173.
Wilson CG *et al*. Ocular contact time of a carbomer gel (GelTears) in humans. *Br J Ophthalmol* 1998;82:131–134.
Khan H *et al*. The influence of additives on the spreading coefficient and adhesion of a film coating formulation to a model tablet surface. *Int J Pharm* 2001;227:113–119.
Siepmann F *et al*. Polymer blends for controlled release coatings. *J Control Rel* 2008;125:1–15.

8

Pharmaceutical nanotechnology

This chapter provides an introduction to the characteristics of nanosystems, especially those that are used as drug carriers for targeting and delivery. Wherever possible the preparation, properties and uses of the nanoparticles are related here to issues already discussed in other chapters. The preparation of nanoparticles often means solvent change, supercritical states, emulsion formation and solvent diffusion and evaporation. Many of the biological attributes of nanocarriers depend on their physical chemistry, such as their surface charge, diameter, hydrophilicity or hydrophobicity. Their movement in cells, tissues and complex media (e.g. mucus) is largely dependent on the laws of diffusion and hence size. We will discuss their diffusion, the adsorption of proteins onto their surfaces, as well as their physical stability. Aggregation of nanoparticles in blood or elsewhere *in vivo* negates the advantage of small and controlled size.

Introduction

Nanotechnology deals mainly with particles or constructs that have dimensions ranging from several nanometres to around 150nm. Nanopharmacy or pharmaceutical nanotechnology generally covers the manipulation and processing of systems, their physicochemical characterisation, their applications and biological evaluation. The principal pharmaceutical interest in nanoparticles at present is their potential as carriers for drugs and other active entities. In this role drugs are encapsulated in, or attached to, the particles and the fate of the nanoparticles determines to a large extent the fate of the drug itself, but they have many potential uses, not least as excipients. Colloid science (see Chapter 6) and pharmaceutical nanotechnology overlap considerably as nanoparticles are of course colloidal in nature.

Although the descriptor *nanotechnology* came to the fore in the late 1980s it has a somewhat longer pedigree in pharmacy, since, in fact, Professor Peter Speiser and his colleagues[1,2] in Zurich prepared and investigated 'nanoparts' and 'nanocapsules' a decade earlier.[3] Surfactant micelles (Chapter 5) have diameters of some 1–3 nm; they have also been studied for many decades as solubilisers of poorly water-soluble drugs and can be considered to be nanosystems. Microemulsions, a name coined in 1959,[4] are used in pharmacy, as in the ciclosporin concentrate Neoral, which on dilution forms droplets in the size range 10–100 nm, well within the nano range.

Typical nanosized pharmaceutical carrier systems therefore include nanoparticles formed from polymers or lipids, or drugs themselves as nanosuspensions, nanoemulsions (usually termed microemulsions), dendrimers, fullerenes and carbon nanotubes as well as the smallest liposomes. Some are represented in Fig. 8.1.

Clearly a main focus in pharmaceutical nanotechnology is how to characterise nanosystems. This includes investigation of drug loading capacity, drug release rate and the chemical and physical stability of both drug and carrier (Fig. 8.2). Particle size is a key property, and surface charge and character (whether the surface is hydrophilic or hydrophobic) are other defining properties. Biological evaluation of nanosystems involves knowledge of the absorption, distribution and excretion of both the drug and the carrier along with its load of encapsulated or attached drug.

8.1 Particle size

The whole nanotechnology topic is defined to a large extent by the size (or more usually, the size range) of the systems used. Dendrimers are an exception as they are synthesised as discrete chemical entities of identical size. Small size brings with it both advantages and disadvantages. Rates of release may be rapid, because of the large surface area per unit weight and because diffusional path lengths within the particles are small. Particle size influences many of the properties and behaviour of nanoparticles as demonstrated in Fig 8.3.

- *Drug release*: the larger surface area per unit weight of nanoparticles leads to potentially high release rates compared to the same weight of larger particles, as solvent penetration will be a function of $n\pi r^2$, where n = number of nanoparticles per unit weight and r is the particle radius.
- *M-cell uptake*: although we state in Chapter 9 that drugs must be in their molecular form to be taken up by epithelial cells, there is a mechanism for particle uptake. The main site involves the

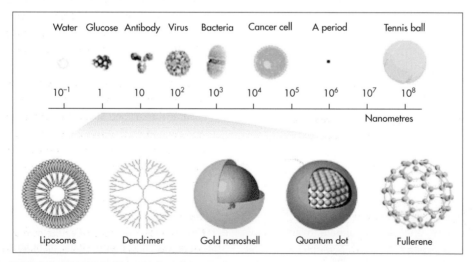

Figure 8.1 Typical nanocarriers and imaging systems in the size range 1–100 nm (not drawn to scale), which will be increasingly used in pharmacy as carriers of drugs and diagnostic agents in comparison with molecules, viruses, bacteria, cancer cells and a full stop in printing.

Figure 8.2 Pharmaceutical nanotechnology's main areas of focus, namely, applications, manipulation and processing, physicochemical characterisation, and biological evaluation. An understanding of the relevance of the physicochemical properties of these systems and biological barriers and environments is essential. Absorption, distribution, metabolism and toxicology refer to both the drug once released from the delivery system and the delivery system itself, the two being intertwined.

membranous epithelial cells (M-cells) of the gut-associated lymphoid tissue (GALT), which can more readily take up smaller particles (i.e. those 5–150 nm) than larger particles (>300 nm). Particles above a certain size will not be absorbed, at least not intact.

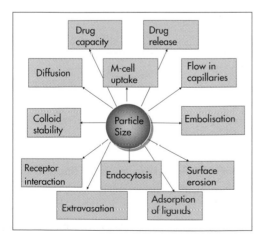

Figure 8.3 Particle size and its bearing either directly or indirectly on the behaviour and fate of nanoparticles. For examples see the text.

- *Flow in capillaries*: once injected, nanoparticles flow in the blood and particle diameter is clearly important.
- *Embolisation*: nanoparticles are too small to block blood vessels and capillaries, but if they aggregate then such blockage (embolisation) can occur.
- *Surface erosion* is involved in many degradation and drug release processes, and will be a function of surface area.
- *Adsorption of ligands*: adsorption of proteins, whether from the blood or deliberately engineered to alter the surface properties of nanoparticles, will depend on the available surface area per particle, the area/molecule of the adsorbing molecule, the charge and hydrophobicity of the surface.
- *Endocytosis* (uptake of particles by cells) is size dependent.
- *Extravasation* (escape of particles from the circulation into target cells or tissues) occurs more readily with small particles.
- *Physical (colloid) stability* is dependent on radius, the nature of the material, its charge, and the presence of any adsorbed molecules (see Chapter 6).

- *Diffusion* is important in the translocation of nanoparticles and their transport through mucus and tissues, as well as in tumours and other targets. In a simple fluid medium the influence of particle radius on diffusion coefficient can be recognised from equation (8.1).

$$D = \frac{kT}{6\pi\eta r} \qquad (8.1)$$

Movement in complex media, e.g. cells and gels, will be represented by more complex equations (see section 8.9)

8.2 Physicochemical characterisation of nanosystems

The key physicochemical properties of nanoparticles are listed in Table 8.1 under two headings: those of importance in relation to use, and those important in relation to their preparation and properties.

8.3 Nanoparticles in pharmacy

8.3.1 Nanoparticles as drug carriers

The rationale for the encapsulation of drugs in nanoparticles or in some cases the adsorption of, for example, therapeutic proteins onto the nanoparticles is twofold.

- First, the active is protected to a greater or lesser degree from the external environment until such time as it is released. Once released, the drug behaves as free drug, although it might have been deposited in the liver and spleen by the carrier.
- Second, the nature, destination and fate of the nanoparticles, rather than the characteristics of the drug, determine at least the initial fate of the drug as the body 'sees' the carrier rather than the drug.

It is important to distinguish between the *pharmacokinetics* of drug released from the carrier and the kinetics of the particles themselves, a subject that is termed *particokinetics*.[5] Size is particularly important in determining the ability of nanoparticles to access

Table 8.1 Key physical and chemical properties of nanoparticles as drug carriers

In relation to use
Surface area
Shape
Drug release rate
Biodegradation processes including rate of degradation
Diffusion (e.g. in tissues and mucus)
Aggregation and flocculation (*in vitro* and *in vivo*)
Adsorption (e.g. to biological and polymer membranes)
Deposition (e.g. on surfaces)
Rheology (e.g. in blood)
Elasticity (to aid progress in capillary networks)
In relation to preparation and properties
Drug–polymer interactions and compatibility (e.g. important in loading drug into systems)
Polymer–polymer interactions (e.g. when two polymers are used to fabricate particles)
Hydrophobicity and hydrophilicity of surfaces
Surface charge
Surface adsorption of macromolecules

sites that are out of bounds to larger particles. There is, however, a continuum of diameters and one of the great challenges in drug delivery and targeting is the production of nanosystems with narrow size distributions. Nature achieves this in the case of low-density lipoproteins (the natural carrier of cholesterol to dividing cells), which have a mean diameter of 26.7 nm and a size range of only 25.8–28.2 nm in young healthy females and 25.5–28.1 nm in males.[6] Small size at the limit where the drug molecules approach the size of the carrier (as with dendrimers in the 2–10 nm range) means a carrier/drug ratio of ~1. Some nanoparticles, such as drug nanocrystals, on the other hand, consist virtually only of drug as discussed in section 8.6.

8.3.2 Application of nanoparticles in drug delivery

One pharmaceutical problem is to design and formulate systems that are stable *in vitro* but can also survive their dilution in blood, and the mixing and shearing forces in flow. There are many changes in the particle environment as it passages through tissues, one of which is a change in surface characteristics brought about by opsonin adsorption, a precursor of uptake by the reticuloendothelial system (RES) and hence loss from the circulation.

As shown in Fig. 8.4:

- The compatibility of drug and carrier system is vital to the even distribution of drug throughout the nanoparticle and to avoid premature release that occurs when the drug migrates to the particle surface.

- The loading of the drug into the particles depends on the nature of the drug and the nature of the carrier material.

- The intravenous route results in mixing of the nanoformulation with blood, perhaps particle adsorption onto erythrocytes, opsonisation (which is the adsorption of the proteins or opsonins onto the surface of the nanoparticles, which then cause the particles to be recognised as foreign and taken up by the liver and spleen), partial escape from the circulation by extravasation, and interaction with the receptor before a cascade of events such as internalisation and diffusion with tissues.

Nanoparticles can potentially be used to deliver drugs, genes and radiolabels by a variety of routes, including the ocular, oral, intravenous, intraperitoneal, intraluminal, subcutaneous, intramuscular, nasal, respiratory and intratumoral routes. Sometimes nanoparticle-based delivery depends not on any single property. With ocular delivery to the cul-de-sac of the eye, nanoparticles can prolong the action of a drug both by slow release characteristics and by slowing the loss via the punctae when compared with a solution. The adhesive qualities of some nanosystems can also enhance site-specific activity.[7] Bioadhesive nanoparticles have been advocated to assist adhesion of the carriers to the mucosa and thus increase the probability of arrest, as well as to provide time for the transfer of drug from the carriers or the particles themselves into the gut wall.

To be successful therapeutically, systems must have optimal size and surface characteristics, high loading capacity efficiency, and a high degree of chemical and physical stability, as well as appropriate release characteristics at the target site and be biodegradable and biocompatible. Not all drug (active)–polymer (carrier) combinations can be readily formulated, sometimes because of the low affinity of the drug for the carrier or indeed incompatibility between drug and carrier. For example, protein drugs do not always mix with polymers without phase separation:

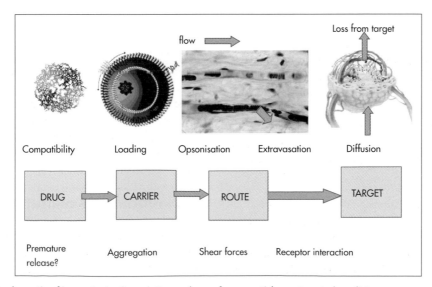

Figure 8.4 A schematic of issues in the formulation and use of nanoparticles as targeted medicines.

see Chapter 7 for a discussion of some of these issues. Formulations in which drug and carrier material phase-separate (that is, do not produce an isotropic mixture) or whose production process leads to a movement of drug towards the surface of the particles usually demonstrate *burst (initial fast) release* effects. Size polydispersity can also lead to ambiguous results, as it complicates the achievement of targeting through potentially different fates of the particles of different sizes.

The importance of the lymphoid tissue in the gut, the gut-associated lymphoid tissue (GALT), is crucial to the understanding of some of these possibilities. The M-cells and lymphoid tissues of other anatomical regions can be important in particle delivery; for example, the nasal lymphoid tissue (NALT), the bronchial tissue (BALT) and other sites (omentum, OALT) provide the possibility of access of particles in small quantities, which may be sufficient for immunisation with vaccines.

Hard and soft systems

While size defines all nanosystems, they can differ in their material properties, their chemistry and their physics. It is useful, for reasons that are apparent in relation to movement of nanoparticles *in vivo*, to divide nanosystems into two types namely 'hard' and 'soft'.

- *Soft systems* include nanoemulsions and polymeric micelles.
- *Hard systems*, which are neither flexible nor elastic, include polymeric nanoparticles, nanosuspensions or nanocrystals, dendrimers and carbon nanotubes.

Hard systems may block spaces and fenestrae that have the same dimensions as the particles, whereas soft systems can by definition deform and reform (erythrocytes and many liposomes fall into this category). They are thus better able to navigate constricted capillary beds and tissue extracellular spaces.

 Key points

- Nanosystems have a size range of several nanometres up to about 150 nm.
- Typical nanosized carrier systems include 'soft systems' such as micelles and

nanoemulsions (microemulsions) and 'hard systems' such as polymeric nanoparticles, dendrimers, fullerenes, microtubes, and nanosuspensions or nanocrystals of drugs themselves.

- Their main pharmaceutical interest is as carriers for drugs, which may be encapsulated in or attached to the nanoparticles. This provides two main advantages: the drug is protected from the external environment until it is released, and the fate of the drug *in vivo* is determined by the fate of the carrier rather than the characteristics of the drug itself.
- The important characteristics of nanoparticles are their size and surface characteristics. The size influences a wide range of properties including drug release, M-cell uptake, capillary flow, embolisation, surface erosion, adsorption of ligands, endocytosis, extravasation, physical stability and diffusion.
- Their formulation requires an investigation of the drug loading capacity, drug release rate and the chemical and physical stability of both the carrier and encapsulated drug. An important requirement of the formulation is that it should have a narrow size distribution with an even distribution of drug throughout the carrier; it should be stable *in vitro* and be able to survive dilution in blood and the passage through tissues.
- Their biological fate requires knowledge of the absorption, distribution and excretion of both the drug and the carrier.

8.4 Nanoparticle manufacturing methods

There is a large number of methods to prepare nanoparticulate systems, as can be seen from Table 8.2. These depend to a large extent on the material that

Table 8.2 Methods of manufacturing polymeric or protein nanoparticles

Method	Relevant physical events
1. Solvent displacement	Mixing of solvents
2. Salting-out	Reducing solvency
3. Emulsion diffusion	Diffusion of solvent from globules
4. Emulsion-solvent evaporation	Evaporation of solvents
5. Supercritical fluid technology	Solvent phase behaviour
6. Complexation, coacervation	Macromolecular interactions
7. Reverse micellar methods	Solubilisation of monomers
8. *In situ* polymerisation	Growth of polymers in suspension
9. Synthesis (e.g. dendrimers)	Covalent growth from a core molecule

Some of the above are outlined in the text. A fuller account can be found in Florence AT, Pharmaceutical aspects of nanotechnology, in: Florence AT, Siepmann J, eds, *Modern Pharmaceutics*, 5th edn, Volume 2, Chapter 12, New York: Informa Healthcare; 2009.

Figure 8.5 Comminution (size reduction) versus molecular assembly, polymerisation and solvent change and hence precipitation in the preparation of nanosystems. Methods are listed in Table 8.2.

will form the basis of the carrier, which can include polymers, proteins, metals (gold) or ceramics.

One can consider four main approaches to the manufacture of nanoparticles, shown in Fig 8.5:

1 *Comminution* (milling in the case of solids, and emulsification in the case of liquids)
2 *Molecular self-assembly* (such as occurs with polymeric surfactants to form polymeric micelles, or dendrons forming dendrimer aggregates)
3 *Precipitation* from a solution of the polymer
4 *Polymerisation* of monomers dissolved in either micelles or emulsion droplets

8.4.1 Solvent displacement

The method of solvent displacement (Fig. 8.6) is perhaps the simplest means of preparing polymeric nanoparticles. Here the polymer is dissolved along with the drug to be encapsulated in commonly used water-miscible solvents – ethanol, acetone or methanol. The polymer solution is then diluted in the presence of stabilisers such as poly(vinyl alcohol) (PVA) or the surfactant polysorbate 80, and forms nanoparticles with narrow size distributions.

8.4.2 Salting-out

A variant on the above technique includes a polymer + drug dissolved in a water-miscible organic solvent that is added to a stirred aqueous gel containing a

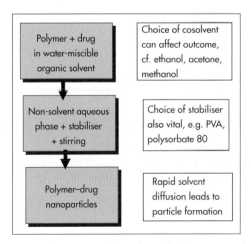

Figure 8.6 A summary of the solvent displacement method. The PVA or polysorbate 80 stabilises the particles as they precipitate following the dilution of the nonaqueous solvents. The rapid diffusion of solvent from the polymer phase allows rapid formation and hence a small size distribution.

salting-out agent and a stabiliser. The polymer–drug combination is salted out as nanoparticles.

8.4.3 Emulsion-diffusion

A different approach is illustrated in Fig. 8.7. A *partly* water-miscible solvent in which the drug and polymer is dissolved forms an emulsion on dilution in an aqueous phase containing a stabiliser. Because of the partial miscibility of the first solvent, it diffuses from the dispersed drops into the bulk to provide polymer nanoparticles containing drug.

8.4.4 Emulsion-solvent evaporation

Figure 8.8 illustrates a different approach with the emulsion-solvent evaporation technique. It involves the dissolution of the drug–polymer mix in an organic solvent that is immiscible with water, so that on addition to an aqueous phase an emulsion is formed in the presence of emulsifiers. On heating, the internal organic phase can be evaporated in a controlled fashion leaving the polymer–drug nanoparticles, whose size is dependent on the nature of the emulsion.

In a variant of this process the drug and the polymer (or protein such as albumin) is dissolved in water, and this is then added to an organic phase. A water-in-oil emulsion is formed initially, from which the water

Figure 8.8 A process similar to that in Fig. 8.7. The polymer/drug organic solution is emulsified in water as an oil-in-water system, or the polymer and drug are dissolved in an aqueous phase, which when added to an organic phase forms a water-in-oil emulsion. The internal phase in both cases is evaporated leaving the polymer–drug particles

is removed by evaporation. The oily phase is later 'washed' off.

8.4.5 Supercritical fluid technologies

A supercritical fluid (SCF) is a substance at a temperature and pressure above its thermodynamic *critical point* (T_c) (see Fig. 8.9a). In this state it can diffuse through solids like a gas, and dissolve materials like a liquid. Carbon dioxide and water are the most commonly used supercritical fluids. Supercritical fluid technologies deserve a special mention as they are less commonly applied at a laboratory scale in the preparation of nanoparticles. A drug and polymer are dissolved in an organic solvent or carbon dioxide. Under certain conditions of pressure and temperature (see Fig. 8.9) the liquid phase is transformed into the supercritical state, which for CO_2 occurs at pressures >74 bar (atmospheric pressure = 1.013 bar (101.3 kPa)) and temperatures >31°C (T_c). The rapid expansion of this supercritical solution on exposure to atmospheric pressure causes the formation of microspheres or nanospheres.

8.4.6 Coacervation and complexation techniques

A coacervate is a gel-like liquid state of matter that can be treated to produce solid microparticles or

Figure 8.7 Schematic of the emulsion technique wherein the drug and polymer are dissolved in a partly water-miscible solvent. This is then added to an aqueous phase in the presence of surfactant or other stabiliser. Emulsion particles are formed. The solvent, being partly miscible in the water phase, diffuses from the emulsion droplets to form nanoparticles.

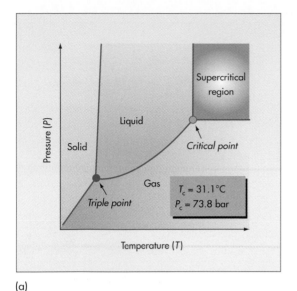

(a)

(b)

Figure 8.9 (a) The pressure–temperature phase diagram of CO_2 showing the T_c and P_c at the supercritical region. (b) Schematic of the process of producing nanoparticles using supercritical fluid technology. (See, for example, Byrappa K et al., Nanoparticle synthesis using supercritical fluid technology – towards biomedical applications, *Adv Drug Del Rev*, 2008; 60: 299–327.)

nanoparticles. There are several possibilities: one is *complex coacervation* in which positively charged macromolecules are mixed with negatively charged macromolecules. Under certain conditions of temperature and relative concentration and ionic strength, there will be a phase separation whereby a coacervate

Figure 8.10 A phase diagram of PEGylated chitosan as a function of TPP (tripolyphosphate) concentration showing the region where 'nanogel' coacervate nanoparticles form.

Reproduced from Wu Y, *Int J Pharm*, 2005; 295: 235–245 with permission of Elsevier.

forms (see Fig. 8.10). In *simple coacervation* with single macromolecules of either charge, solvent change and salting-out create the conditions for the formation of coacervate particles.

8.4.7 *In situ* polymerisation

In this mode of synthesis of polymeric nanoparticles (e.g. of polybutylcycanoacrylates PBCA), monomeric materials (e.g. butylcyanoacrylate) are dispersed in a suitable solvent and emulsified. An initiator is generally added to the system and the monomers condense to form a polymeric matrix. In the case of the alkyl cyanoacrylates, no initiator is required as the aqueous medium itself acts as the initiator of polymerisation.

8.5 Nanocrystal formation

Nanocrystals of poorly water-soluble drugs are important in pharmacy as their greatly reduced particle size increases the surface area per unit weight and hence increases the rate of dissolution of the drug, all things being equal. The Noyes–Whitney equation (see also Chapter 1) relates the change of weight, dw, with time, dt:

$$dw/dt = (DA/\delta)(c_s - c) \qquad (8.2)$$

where A is the surface area of the material, D is the diffusion coefficient, δ is the diffusion layer thickness and c_s is the saturation solubility, c being the concentration of agent in the solution at any given time t. There may be a degree of supersaturation, but the equilibrium solubility is unaffected by particle size until very small particle sizes are reached as shown in Fig. 8.11. The critical value depends, as can be seen, on the surface energy of the material in question. The combination of increased intrinsic solubility and increased surface area has the potential to change solution, and hence absorption properties dramatically. If the absorption of the drug is dissolution rate-limited this will assist in the extent of absorption; enhanced solubility has the potential to increase concentration gradients across the biological membrane.

A review of the topic can be found in reference 8.[8] Modes of preparation of nanocrystalline suspensions include precipitation, homogenisation, sonochemical techniques (e.g. for azithromycin[9]) and combinations of these technologies. Figure 8.12 demonstrates the effect on the plasma level versus time plots of danazol of a nanosized suspension over a conventional suspension. It can be seen that nanocrystal formation leads to results equivalent in this case to the effect of solubilisation in a cyclodextrin.

Figure 8.12 Danazol is a drug with a solubility of $10\,g\,mL^{-1}$. Plasma drug levels are plotted as a function of time after administration of three forms of the drug including a nanoparticulate dispersion and a hydroxypropyl-β-cyclodextrin complex, using a suspension with a mean particle size of $10\,m$ as a comparator.

Reproduced from reference 10 with permission of Elsevier.

Nanoparticles of all descriptions can be used not only as suspensions but also as freeze-dried powders for reconstitution, they can be incorporated into liposomes, used as aerosols, incorporated in gels or in microspheres (e.g. gelatin), adsorbed onto microparticles, dispersed in soft gelatin capsules, or used as mini-depot tablets.

Figure 8.11 The solubility enhancement S/S_0 as a function of particle diameter for three hypothetical compounds with surface energies of 50, 75 and $100\,mN\,m^{-1}$ (dyne cm^{-1}). It can be seen that where S_0 is the solubility of a large crystal, and S is the solubility of the crystal of a specific size, the solubility enhancement (S/S_0) does not increase significantly until particle diameters reach below around 75 nm.

Reproduced from Kipp JE, *Int J Pharm*, 2004; 284: 109–122 with permission of Elsevier.

Key points

- The general approaches to the manufacture of nanoparticles include: comminution, as in the milling of solids or the emulsification of liquids; molecular self-assembly, as in the formation of some dendrimers and polymeric micelles; precipitation from solution; and polymerisation of monomers dissolved in micelles or emulsion droplets. The choice of method is influenced by the nature of the material that forms the basis of the carrier.

- The main methods of manufacture include
  - Solvent displacement
  - Salting-out
  - Emulsion-diffusion
  - Emulsion-solvent evaporation
  - Use of supercritical fluid technologies
  - Coacervation and complexation techniques
  - *In situ* polymerisation
  - Nanocrystal formation

8.6 Drug targeting with nanoparticles – particle flow[11]

Drug targeting using nanoparticulate carriers depends on many factors to achieve accumulation in target sites. Particles must translocate from the site of injection to distant organs. To an extent, therefore, this depends on the flow patterns of nanoparticles in the blood and then in interstitial spaces. The theoretical advantage of nanosystems is that their small size allows freer movement than that of, say, microspheres in the circulation, lymph and tissues. Flow rates are important also in the determination of the possibility and success of interaction of nanoparticles with endothelial receptors prior to internalisation. What is the influence, for example, of nanoparticle *size* on particle flow in the circulation? What is the influence of *shape* on flow and fate? Nanoparticles *in vivo* are driven by the blood flow to distant sites. Particle velocities can be size dependent because the flow rates across the diameter of the vessels are not constant and hence particle segregation in polydisperse systems might occur as shown in Fig. 8.13. Flow results in shearing forces at the point of interaction between nanoparticles and the target receptors; smaller particles suffer lower forces likely to dislodge them from receptor surfaces. This is illustrated in Fig. 8.14. Any aggregation of particles, which might even be flow induced, will alter flow patterns and interactions with receptors.

Larger particles close to the walls of the vessels experience greater shearing forces because of the nature of the flow patterns shown. Adhesion, seen as a prerequisite to cellular uptake from blood and interstitial fluids, is not a foregone conclusion. The determining factors include particle diameter, flow rate, the density of receptors and the force of attraction between particle and receptor.

Figure 8.14 simply reinforces previous points and considers in greater detail the forces involved in nanoparticle interaction with biological surfaces. Particles have to be close to the surface to experience the force of attraction, which allows initial contact with membranes. This diagram again should clearly

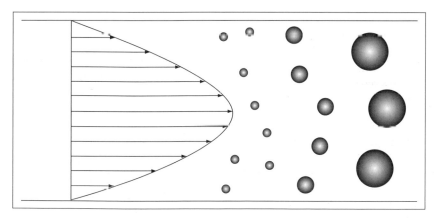

Figure 8.13 Diagram of the velocity pattern in a tube of flowing liquid showing particles of different sizes separating according to their diameter. The large particles, being unable to approach close to the capillary wall, experience the faster fluid streamlines towards the centre and hence move more rapidly.

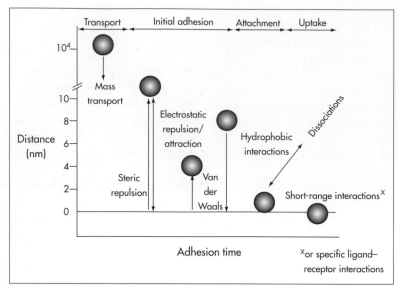

Figure 8.14 Processes occurring in the deposition of nanoparticles in flow conditions as a function of the range of interaction of forces (nanometres) and adhesion times. At the start, mass transport to the surface occurs, initial adhesion occurring through electrostatic attractions and van der Waals forces. Hydrophobic interactions can play their part as well as specific receptor–ligand interactions, which are short-range interactions. Physical adsorption of ligands to the surface of nanoparticles or covalent attachment of ligands changes the nature of the primary surface and may influence each of the forces referred to here.

Drawn after reference 12 with kind permission from Springer Science and Business Media.

demonstrate the importance of physical phenomena in the biological environment.

8.7 Aggregation

Given their large surface to volume/weight ratios, nanoparticles are prone to aggregate. The formulation of a stable nanoparticle suspension in the laboratory is one thing; the maintenance of the monodisperse state *in vivo* is another. Particles will have moved from an aqueous medium (of the formulation) to a more complex situation in blood or tissues. There are biological consequences because opsonins adsorb from the plasma onto the surface of the nanoparticles, which leads to uptake by the reticuloendothelial system (RES). (An opsonin is any molecule that acts as a binding enhancer for the process of phagocytosis, for example, by coating the surface of injected particles and other foreign objects.) In terms of the pharmaceutics of the nanosystems, the potential of the particles to aggregate is critical. Aggregation changes the hydrodynamic size of the particles, decreases their diffusion, restricts extravasation and reduces the effective surface area for interactions with receptors.

8.8 PEGylated nanoparticles

PEGylation involves the covalent attachment of polyoxyethylene glycol (PEG) chains to the surface of the particles. PEGylation (Fig. 8.15) of course creates a hydrated surface on hydrophobic particles, which allows for both steric and enthalpic stabilisation. It also reduces opsonin adsorption, this leading to increased circulation times and the enhanced statistical possibility of nanoparticle uptake after multiple passages through the circulation. PEGylation changes the nature of the surface, turning hydrophobic surfaces into hydrophilic ones. The effect of PEG depends on its chain length.[13] PEG 5000 has a greater effect than PEG 2000 or PEG 750, as predicted by calculations of enthalpic and entropic stabilisation.

8.9 Nanoparticle diffusion

The Stokes–Einstein equation (Chapter 2) relates the diffusion coefficient, D, to continuous phase viscosity η and the radius of the particle, r, as was discussed earlier in the chapter, in the form $D = kT/6\pi\eta r$.

(a)   (b)

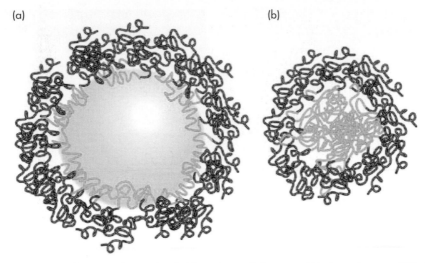

Figure 8.15 A representation of (a) a particle PEGylated with a polyoxyethylene-based block copolymer and (b) a block copolymer micelle with the external hydrophilic chains. The hydrophilic polymer chains on adjacent particles provide both a physical and thermodynamic barrier to aggregation. See Chapter 6.

In any one liquid medium, e.g. water, the diffusion coefficient of spherical particles is inversely related to their radius. This alone is important in thinking of the translocation of nanoparticles towards their targets in tissues. Diffusion is important in free solution, in cell culture media, in the gel-like interior of cells, even perhaps in the cell nucleus and in the extracellular matrix. In the brain, for example, diffusion of drugs from nanoparticles or implants is slow and the radius of spread of a drug like paclitaxel after release from implants or nanoparticles is of the order of only millimetres. Gels have been used as models for diffusion of nanoparticles in complex media: the Stokes–Einstein equation applies and the ratio of diffusion in the gel (D) to diffusion in water (D_0) can be calculated. In gels the viscosity in the equation is not the bulk viscosity but the so-called *microscopic viscosity*[14], η_0, which is actually close to that of water, as it is the viscosity of the medium in which nanoparticles move between the entangled chains of the macromolecular gels. When the diameter of the particles reaches a critical size in gels, a size approaching the nominal diameter of the pores, diffusion asymptotically approaches zero.

Diffusion within cells is even more complex than within simple gels; first the cytoplasm is a molecularly crowded zone, a complex gel with structural obstacles such as actin and myosin fibrils and strands. There is the additional tortuosity that occurs in gels as the moving particle avoids the regions of the macromolecular chains and the obstruction effects from the impenetrable regions of the cytoplasm. If we designate by D_e the effective diffusion coefficient and by D_0 the coefficient in water we can write, where τ is the tortuosity factor and ε is the void fraction available to the diffusing solute:

$$\frac{D_e}{D_0} = \frac{\varepsilon}{\tau} \tag{8.3}$$

$\varepsilon = (1 - \phi_p)$ and ϕ_p is the volume fraction of the polymer or other materials that are in the path of the diffusing material. D_G (the diffusion coefficient in the gel) can be written as a ratio with the coefficient in water:[15]

$$\frac{D_G}{D_0} = \frac{(1 - \phi_p)^2}{(1 + \phi_p)^2} \tag{8.4}$$

If $\phi_p = 0.5$, D_G is 0.111 times that in water. When $\phi_p = 0.8$, $D_G \sim 0.012 D_0$. The binding of particles to actin reduces the number of free particles and hence further reduces flux.

Nanoparticle size is important in diffusion in complex media because the diffusional space may be restricted when the diameter of the particle exceeds the 'pore' diameter of the membrane. The diffusion coefficients of 6 nm dendrimers in the cytoplasm of Caco2 cells and SK/MES-1 cells[16] were determined to be 9.8×10^{-11} cm^2 s^{-1} and $\sim 6 \times 10^{-11}$ cm^2 s^{-1}, respectively, some 1000 times lower than that in water. Adsorption, obstruction and entrapment occur, and at a certain particle radius diffusion virtually ceases.

Key points

Physicochemical properties are important in determining the biological fate of nanoparticles:

- The particle size of the nanoparticle influences its flow in blood and interstitial spaces. Polydispersity of size may lead to particle segregation during flow; particle aggregation may be induced by flow, which will alter flow patterns and interaction with receptors. Particle size, flow rate, forces of interaction between particles and receptors, and the density of receptors can all influence the adhesion of the nanoparticles onto receptors.

- Particle aggregation increases the hydrodynamic size of the particles, decreases their diffusion, restricts extravasation, and reduces the effective surface area for interaction with receptors.

- Covalent attachment of PEG chains to the nanoparticle surface allows for steric and enthalpic stabilisation and reduces opsonin adsorption.

- The diffusional properties of the nanoparticles are important in their translocation towards their targets in tissues. Diffusion within complex media such as cells is not only determined by the diameter of the nanoparticle but is also strongly influenced by the tortuosity of its path through the cytoplasm, the void volume available for diffusion, and any adsorption or entrapment of the particles. Gels have been used as models of diffusion through such complex environments.

8.10 Regulatory challenges: characterisation

Regulatory challenges generally have evolved for good reasons to ensure reproducibility and quality *in vitro* and *in vivo*. Parameters that must be closely defined for nanosystems include those in Table 8.3.

Table 8.3 Parameters and questions that must be addressed before clinical use of nanosystems

- Particle size determination is key: can there be a standardised procedure for measuring mean particle diameter and size distribution?
- Is there assurance of stability of size *in vitro*, that is, lack of aggregation/flocculation?
- Standardisation of surface characteristics: what specific methodology is used (zeta potential measurements may be nonspecific)?
- The distribution on surfaces and properties of ligands on the surfaces of targeted systems.
- Determination or prediction of stability *in vivo* (*esp.* of particle diameter).
- Measurement and validation of the release rate of active from the systems and the choice of suitable experimental media.
- Biocompatibility: is the system compatible with blood?
- Biodegradability: is there evidence of biodegradation of the system to nontoxic products?
- Toxicity of nanosystems: what are reasonable predictive animal or tissue culture tests?

N.B. Targeted systems congregate in specific organs hence can alter the toxicological balance.

Summary

This chapter covers some of the physicochemical principles of the preparation and the use of nanoparticles as drug delivery vectors. It should be clear from this chapter that physical and chemical properties of nanoparticles are important in determining their biological fate and success. In targeting it should be remembered that even decorated particles with specific ligands may not reach the site of action because transport to most sites of action is a stochastic process with many complications and barriers in the way. Nonetheless, continuing research will ensure that nanosystems will play a large part in the future of pharmaceuticals – as therapeutic carriers, as carriers of imaging agents or as excipients that are more precise than those that exist today.

References

1. Kreuter J. Nanoparticles and nanocapsules – new dosage forms in the nanometer size range. *Pharm Acta Helv* 1978;53:33–29.

2. Couvreur P *et al.* Nanocapsules: a new type of lysosomo-tropic carrier. *FEBS Lett* 1977;84:323–326.

3. Kreuter J. Nanoparticles – a historical perspective. *Int J Pharm* 2007;331:1–10.

4. Schulman JH *et al.* Mechanism of formation and structure of microemulsions by electron microscopy. *J Phys Chem* 1959;63:1677–1680.

5. Teeguarden JG *et al.* Particokinetics in vitro: dosimetry considerations for in vitro nanoparticle toxicity assessments. *Toxicol Sci* 2007;95:300–312.

6. Ambrosch A *et al.* LDL size distribution in relation to insulin sensitivity and lipoprotein patterning in young and healthy subjects. *Diabetes Care* 1998;21:2077–2084.

7. De TK *et al.* Polycarboxylic acid nanoparticles for ophthalmic drug delivery: an ex vivo evaluation with human cornea. *J Microencapul* 2004;21:841–855.

8. Rabinow BE. Nanosuspensions in drug delivery. *Nat Rev Drug Discov* 2004;3:785–796.

9. Pi Z *et al.* Preparation of ultrafine particles of azithromycin by sonochemical method. *Nanomedicine* 2007;3:86–88.

10. Liversidge GG, Cundy KC. Particle size reduction for improvement of oral bioavailability of hydrophobic drugs: absolute oral bioavailability of nano-crystalline danazol in beagle dogs. *Int J Pharmac* 1995;125:91–97.

11. Florence AT. Nanoparticle flow: implications for drug delivery. In: Torchilin VP, ed. *Nanoparticulates as Drug Carriers*. London: Imperial College Press; 2006: 9–27.

12. Vacheethanasee K, Marchant RE. Non-specific *Staphylococcus epidermidis* adhesion: contributions of bacterial hydrophobicity and charge. In: An YH, Friedman RJ, eds. *Handbook of Bacterial Adhesion: Principles, Methods and Applications*. Totowa, NJ: Humana Press; 2000: 73–90.

13. Mori A *et al.* Influence of the steric barrier of amphipathic poly(ethyleneglycol) and ganglioside GM1 on the circulation time of liposomes and on the target binding of immunoliposomes in vivo. *FEBS Lett* 1991; 284:263–266.

14. Ruenraroengsak P, Florence AT. The diffusion of latex nanospheres and the effective (microscopic) viscosity of HPMC gels. *Int J Pharm* 2005;298:361–366.

15. Mackie JS, Meares P. The diffusion of electrolytes in a cationic membrane. I. Theoretical. *Proc Roy Soc Lo A Math Phys Sci* 1955;232:498–509.

16. Ruenraroengsak P *et al.* Cell uptake, cytoplasmic diffusion and nuclear access of a 6.5 nm diameter dendrimer. *Int J Pharm* 2007;331:215–219.

9

Drug absorption and the oral route

This chapter provides basic information on the physicochemical mechanisms of drug absorption and how the processes of absorption are affected by the physicochemical properties of the drug and its formulation, and importantly by the interaction of the drug with the aqueous phase. The nature of the barrier membranes varies, however, and while they share the same basic structures, differences in detail can determine the extent of absorption at different sites in the gastrointestinal (GI) tract. The oral route, as the most frequently used and most acceptable route of drug administration, is discussed here in some detail. The influence of the following intertwined parameters in determining bioavailability should become clear:

- The rate and extent of dissolution of the drug, an essential prelude to absorption
- The rate of gastric emptying and its importance in the dynamics of the absorption process
- The site of absorption, especially in relation to the influence of pH

The pH of the contents of the GI tract and the effect of pH on the ionisation of the drug (discussed also in section 4.2.4) are crucial. The application of the so-called pH-partition hypothesis – and its limitations – should be understood, so that the effects of the nature of the drug and the medium on absorption can be assessed. In the case of the oral route, the effect of concomitant medication (e.g. H_2 antagonists, antacids), which might alter the pH of the gut contents, can be approximated by calculating the change in the drug ionisation. The word 'approximated' is used deliberately because the multiple factors involved in absorption from the GI tract means that the theoretical equations can only explain each process in part.

Absorption, whether it is from the GI tract, the buccal mucosa or the rectal cavity, generally requires the passage of the drug in a molecular form across one or more barrier membranes and tissues. Most drugs are presented to the body as solid or semisolid dosage forms and obviously these must first release the drug contained within them. Tablets or capsules will disintegrate, and the drug will then dissolve either completely or partially and at a greater or lesser rate. Many tablets contain granules or drug particles that deaggregate to facilitate the solution process. If the drug has the appropriate physicochemical properties, it will pass by passive diffusion from a region of high concentration to a region of low concentration across the membrane separating the site of absorption from tissues containing the blood supply. Soluble drugs can, of course, also be administered as solutions, but it should be remembered that drugs can precipitate from solution formulations as they interact with biological fluids.

The special features of the different routes of administration are dealt with in Chapter 10. A brief summary of the general properties of biological membranes and drug transport, knowledge of which is important in understanding all absorption processes, is given here. Where attempts have been made to quantify absorption, equations are presented, but the derivations of most equations have been omitted.

9.1 Biological membranes and drug transport

Biological membranes confine the aqueous contents of cells and separate them from an aqueous exterior phase. To achieve this, membranes are lipoidal in nature. To allow nutrients to pass into the cell and waste products to move out, biological membranes are selectively permeable. Membranes have specialised transport systems to assist the passage of water-soluble materials and ions through their lipid interior. Lipid-soluble substances can pass by passive diffusion through the membrane from a region of high concentration to one of low concentration. Biological membranes differ from polymer membranes in that they are composed of small amphipathic molecules, phospholipids

(see Fig. 9.1) with two hydrophobic chains and cholesterol or other related structures, which associate into lipoidal bilayers in aqueous media. Embodied in the matrix of lipid molecules are proteins, which are generally hydrophobic in nature, embedded in the matrix of lipid molecules. Glycoproteins provide a hydrophilic element to the external membrane; cells have a net negative surface charge.

Cholesterol is a major component of most mammalian biological membranes. Cholesterol forms complexes with phospholipids and its presence reduces the permeability of phospholipid membranes to water, cations, glycerol and glucose. The shape of the cholesterol molecule allows it to fit closely in bilayers with the hydrocarbon chains of unsaturated fatty acids (Fig. 9.1). Cholesterol condenses and rigidifies membranes without

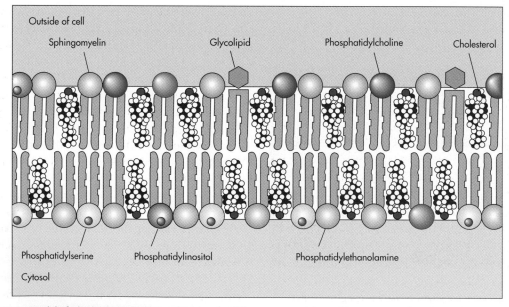

Figure 9.1 Model of a biological membrane showing the different compositions of the interior and exterior sides. Glycolipids are seen on the outside, while phosphatidylserine and phosphatidylinositol predominate on the cytosolic side. See Figure 9.2 for an impression of the membrane surface appearance.

solidifying them. Its removal causes the membrane to lose its structural integrity and to become highly permeable. The flexibility of biological membranes is one of their important features, giving them their ability to re-form and to adapt to changed environments, a vital part of their function. The dynamic characteristics of biological membranes are due to their unique construction from small amphipathic molecules. On stretching (as with a soap film), the molecules at the surfaces become less concentrated in the bilayer but then are rapidly replenished from the bulk phase to maintain the original tension. That is, they are dynamic structures. Figure 9.2 shows a diagram of the 'fluid mosaic' model of a biological membrane.

Although most of the data on permeation of non-electrolytes across biological membranes can be explained on the basis of the membrane behaving as a continuous hydrophobic phase, a fraction of the membrane may be composed of aqueous channels. These are effectively pores that offer a pathway parallel to the diffusion pathway through the lipid. In the absence of flow of water in one direction or the other, these pores play a minor part in the transfer of most drugs, although in the case of ions and charged drugs such as the quaternary ammonium compounds the pore pathway must be important. The fluid mosaic model of membranes allows the protein–lipid complexes to form either hydrophilic or hydrophobic 'gates' to allow transport of materials with different characteristics.

Overall, membrane permeability is controlled by the nature of the membrane, its degree of internal bonding

Figure 9.2 Representation of the 'fluid mosaic' model of a biological membrane, showing embedded protein and protruding glycoproteins.
From Funhouse Films.

and rigidity, its surface charge and the nature of the drug (solute) being transported. There are some similarities between solute transport in biological membranes and in synthetic membranes. As we have discussed in Chapter 7, the permeation of drugs and other molecules through hydrophobic membranes made of polydimethylsiloxane, for example, depends primarily on the solubility of the drug in the membrane. Drugs with little affinity for the membrane are unlikely to permeate, although in porous membranes, such as those of cellophane or collagen, even drugs with little affinity for the polymer may be transported through the pores.

Most biological membranes bear a surface negative charge, so one would imagine that this might influence permeation. Membranes with un-ionised surfaces (such as cellophane) or positively charged surfaces such as collagen have different permeability characteristics for ionic drugs. Crucially, anionic solutes permeate faster than cationic solutes. With amphoteric drugs such as sulfisomidine and sulfamethizole, a similar order of permeation may be observed depending on the pH of the medium, namely: un-ionised > anionic > cationic form. In acidic media the membrane is positively charged and cationic drugs will therefore be repelled from the surface.

In biological membranes, one might expect some preference for cationic drugs, other things being equal, but we have to remember that biological membranes are more complex and more dynamic than synthetic membranes and there are many confounding factors. One of these, which is outside the scope of this book, is the existence of efflux mechanisms centred on P-glycoproteins (P-gp) 'pumps'. Some drugs are ejected from cells by the efflux pump, so that these drugs have a lower apparent absorption than predicted on physicochemical grounds. Some excipients (e.g. surfactants such as polysorbate 80) interact with these proteins, so both drug and excipients must be studied for their effect on the efflux pump activity.

In Chapter 4 we examined some relationships between the lipophilicity of drugs and their activity, controlled by their ability to pass across lipid barriers. Although of the same basic construction, biological membranes in different sites in the body serve different functions and thus one might expect them to have different compositions and physicochemical properties, as indeed they do. Tissues derived from the ectoderm (the epidermis, the epithelium of nose and mouth and the anus, and the tissues of the nervous system) have protective and sensory functions. Tissues evolved from the endoderm, such as the epithelium of the gastrointestinal (GI) tract, have evolved mainly to allow absorption.

9.1.1 Lipophilicity and absorption

If one measures the absorption of a sufficiently wide range of substances in a series, one generally finds that there is an optimal point in the series for absorption. In other words, a plot of percentage absorption versus $\log P$ would be parabolic with the optimum value designated as $\log P_o$ (Fig. 9.3). By noting the values of optimal partition coefficient for different absorbing membranes and surfaces, one can deduce something about their nature. Some values are given in Table 9.1.

The parabolic nature of activity–$\log P$ plots is due to a combination of factors: with drugs with high $\log P$ values, protein binding, low solubility and binding to extraneous sites cause a lower measured activity than if it were possible to take the drug and place it at the receptor without it having to traverse the various lipid and aqueous hurdles that it has to overcome on its way to the site of action.

Molecular weight and drug absorption

The larger drug molecules are, the poorer will be their ability to traverse biological membranes. The change of permeability with increasing molecular size is shown in Fig. 9.4.

Table 9.1 Ideal lipophilic character of drugs ($\log P_o$) in different regions of the body

System	Solute or drug	Log P_o (octanol/ water) for maximal transport
Buccal cavity (human)	Bases	5.52 (undissociated)
		3.52 (dissociated)
	Acids	4.19 (undissociated)
Epidermis (human)	Steroids	3.34
Whole skin (rabbit)	Non-electrolytes	2.55
Small intestine (rat)	Sulfonamides	2.56–3.33
Stomach (rat)	Barbiturates	2.01
	Acids	1.97
Cornea (rabbit)	Steroids	2.8
Biliary excretion	Sulfathiazoles	0.60
Milk/plasma	Sulfonamides	0.53
Prostatic/plasma ratio	Sulfonamides	0.23

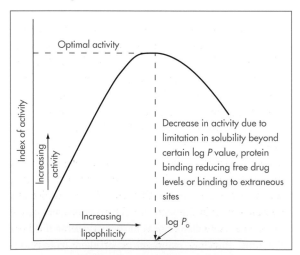

Figure 9.3 Parabolic nature of a typical activity–$\log P$ plot: the decrease in biological activity beyond the optimal $\log P_o$ is probably due to the factors listed.

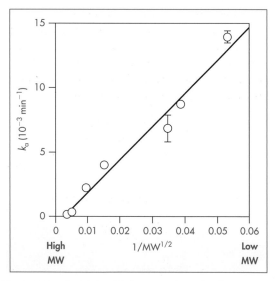

Figure 9.4 The relationship between the molecular weight of compounds and absorption rate constant. The membrane studied is the rat kidney surface, but similar plots hold for other sites.

Reproduced from Nishida K *et al.*, *Eur J Pharm Biopharm*, 2004; 58, 705–711.

In a survey of over 2000 drugs only 11% had molecular weights above 500 Da, and only 8% had molecular weights above 600 Da. Lipinski[1] devised the so-called 'Rule of 5' which refers to drug-like properties of molecules. It states that *poor* oral absorption is more likely when the drug molecule:

- Has more than five hydrogen-bond donors (−OH groups or −NH groups)
- Has a molecular weight >500 Da
- Has a log $P > 5$
- Has more than 10 H-bond acceptors

Note that all the numbers are factors of 5, hence the name of the rule. Compounds that are substrates for transporters are exceptions to the rule.

9.1.2 Permeability and the pH-partition hypothesis

If, in the first instance, the plasma membrane is considered to be a strip of lipoidal material, homogeneous in nature and with a defined thickness, one must assume that only lipid-soluble agents will pass across this barrier. As most drugs are weak electrolytes it is to be expected that the un-ionised form (U) of either acids or bases, the lipid-soluble species, will diffuse across the membrane, while the ionised forms (I) will be rejected. This is the basis of the *pH-partition hypothesis* in which the pH dependence of drug absorption and solute transport across membranes is considered. The equations of Chapters 2 and 4 are relevant here.

For weakly acidic drugs such as acetylsalicylic acid (aspirin) and indometacin, the ratio of ionised to un-ionised species is given by the equation

$$pH - pK_a = \log \frac{[\text{ionised form}]}{[\text{un-ionised form}]}$$

$$= \log \frac{[I]}{[U]} \tag{9.1}$$

For weak bases the equation takes the form

$$pK_a - pH = \log \frac{[\text{ionised form}]}{[\text{un-ionised form}]}$$

$$= \log \frac{[I]}{[U]} \tag{9.2}$$

One can calculate from these equations (and equations 2.71 and 2.72) the relative amounts of absorbable and nonabsorbable forms of a drug

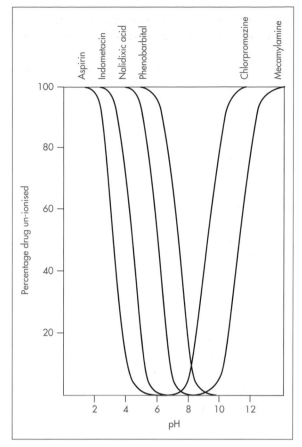

Figure 9.5 Plot of percentage drug un-ionised (that is, in its lipid-soluble form) as a function of solution pH, for the acidic drugs aspirin, indometacin, nalidixic acid and phenobarbital, and for the basic drugs chlorpromazine and mecamylamine.

substance ([U] and [I], respectively), given the prevailing pH conditions in the lumen of the gut or the site of absorption. The profiles for un-ionised drug (%) versus pH for several drugs are given in Fig. 9.5. In very broad terms, one would expect acids to be absorbed from the stomach and bases from the intestine.

A comparison of the intestinal absorption of several acids and bases at various pH values (Table 9.2) indicates the expected trend. Surprisingly, however, it will be seen that salicylic acid is absorbed from the rat intestine at pH 8, although with a pK_a of 3.0 it is virtually completely ionised at this pH. There are two explanations: one is that absorption and ionisation are both dynamic processes and that the small amount of un-ionised drug absorbed is replenished; the second is that the bulk pH is not the actual pH at the membrane. Nevertheless, instilling solutions of different pH directly into the lumen of the rat stomach indicates the correct qualitative trends of absorption (62% absorption at pH 1 for salicylic acid and 13% at pH 8). Similarly, Box 9.1 shows that the absorption of acetylsalicylic acid is much greater than one would expect from a calculation of the pH dependency of its ionisation.

In attempts to explain away discrepancies between theoretical prediction and observed results we have already hinted that a local pH exists at the membrane surface that differs from the bulk pH (see below). This local pH is due to the attraction of hydrogen ions by the negative groups of membrane components so that, in the intestine, while the bulk pH is around 7 the surface pH is nearer 6. A 'virtual' surface pH can be calculated, which will allow results such as those in Table 9.2 to be explained. If we take as another example salicylic acid, again calculating the percentage of un-ionised species by equation (9.1), we obtain the following figures (taken from Table 9.2):

pH	4	5	7	8
Percentage un-ionised	9.09	0.99	0.0099	0.001
Percentage absorbed	64	35	30	10

Table 9.2 Intestinal absorption of acids and bases in the rat at several pH values[a]

Acid/base	pK_a	Perentage absorption			
		pH 4	pH 5	pH 7	pH 8
Acids					
Salicylic acid	3.0	64	35	30	10
Acetylsalicylic acid (aspirin)	3.5	41	27	–	–
Benzoic acid	4.2	62	36	35	5
Bases					
Amidopyrine	5.0	21	35	48	52
Quinine	8.4	9	11	41	54

[a] Reproduced from Brodie BB, in: Bonns, ed., *Absorption and Distribution of Drugs*, Edinburgh: Livingstone; 1964.

Box 9.1 Calculation of percentage ionisation

Absorption values for acetylsalicylic acid at pH 4, 5, 7 and 8 are quoted in Table 9.2. The amount of drug in the un-ionised form at these pH values is obtained from equation (9.1). For example, at pH 4,

$$4 - 3.5 = \log \frac{[I]}{[U]}$$

$$\therefore \frac{[I]}{[U]} = 3.162$$

Percentage un-ionised

$$= \frac{[U] \times 100}{[U] + [I]} = \frac{100}{1 + \frac{[I]}{[U]}}$$

$$= \frac{100}{1 + 3.162} = \frac{100}{4.162} = 24.03\%$$

In the same way, we find 3.07% un-ionised at pH 5; 0.032% at pH 7; and less than 0.009% un-ionised at pH 9. Absorption is much greater than one would expect, being 41% at pH 4 and 27% at pH 5, although the trend is as predicted.

To have 30% of this compound in its un-ionised form when the bulk pH is 7 would require a surface pH of about 3.4, which is lower than anticipated. Again, however, we must remember that absorption and ionisation processes are dynamic processes. As the un-ionised species are absorbed, so the level of [U] in the bulk falls and, because of a shift in equilibrium, more of the un-ionised species appears in the bulk. In fact, if a pH of 5.3 is taken as the pH of the absorbing surface, the results in Table 9.2 become more explicable, as we discuss in the next section.

9.1.3 Problems with the quantitative application of the pH-partition hypothesis

There are several reasons why the pH-partition hypothesis cannot be applied quantitatively in practical situations. Some are discussed here.

Variability in pH conditions

The variation in the stomach pH in human subjects is remarkable, bearing in mind that each pH unit represents a 10-fold difference in hydrogen ion concentration. While the normally quoted range of stomach pH is 1–3, studies using pH-sensitive radiotelemetric capsules have shown a greater spread of values, ranging up to pH 7 as seen in Fig. 11.2 in Chapter 11. This means that the dissolution rate of many drugs will vary markedly in individuals – this is indeed one of the reasons for individual-to-individual variation in drug availability.

The scope for variation in the small intestine is less, although in some pathological states the pH of the duodenum may be quite low owing to hypersecretion of acid in the stomach. Table 9.3 lists the normal pH of the blood and of different regions of the GI tract.

pH at membrane surfaces

Data on the relationship between absorption and pH of the intestinal contents on the one hand, and the percentage of drug in the un-ionised state on the other, can generally be rationalised if the apparent pH is reduced below the pH of the intestine. As described above, this pH 'shift' is due to the existence of a pH at the membrane surface lower than that of the bulk pH. One might expect that the hydrogen ion concentration at the surface would be greater (and hence pH lower) at the membrane surface as hydrogen ions would accumulate near anionic groups, leading to an effect that can be quantified by the equation

$$[H^+]_{surface} = [H^+]_{bulk} \exp \frac{-F\zeta}{RT} \qquad (9.3)$$

where F is the Faraday constant, R is the gas constant, T is absolute temperature and ζ is the zeta potential of the surface (see Chapter 6). Thus, in terms of pH,

Table 9.3 pH of blood and contents of the human alimentary tract[a]	
Sample	**pH**
Blood	7.35–7.45
Buccal cavity	6.2–7.2
Stomach	1.0–3.0
Duodenum	4.8–8.2
Jejunum and ileum	7.5–8.0
Colon	7.0–7.5

[a] Reproduced from Bowman WC et al., Textbook of Pharmacology, London: Blackwell; 1967

$$pH_{surface} = pH_{bulk} + \frac{\zeta}{60} \qquad (9.4)$$

where ζ is expressed in millivolts.

The secretion of acidic and basic substances in many parts of the gut wall is also a complicating factor, as the local pH in the region of the microvilli of the small intestine will undoubtedly influence the absorption of weak electrolytes. A drug molecule in the bulk will diffuse towards the membrane surface and so meet different pH conditions from those in the bulk phase. Whether or not this influences the extent of absorption will depend on the pH changes and the pK_a of the drug in question. The negative charge on the membrane will attract small cations towards the surface and small anions will be repelled; one might thus expect some selectivity in the absorption process. The existence of this 'microclimate' has been questioned, but experimental evidence for its existence has been obtained from the use of micro-electrodes, which revealed the existence of a layer on the (rat) jejunum with a pH of 5.5 when the pH of the bathing buffer was 7.2. The existence of this more acid layer has also been demonstrated on the surface of the human intestine.

Other complications include convective water flow and unstirred layers, discussed below.

Convective water flow

The movement of water molecules into and out of the GI tract will affect the rate of passage of small molecules across the membrane. The reasons for water flow are the differences in osmotic pressure between blood and the contents of the lumen, and differences in hydrostatic pressure between lumen and perivascular tissue, resulting, for example, from muscular contractions. It can be appreciated that the absorption of water-soluble drugs will be increased if water flows from the lumen across the mucosa to the blood side, provided that drug and water are using the same route. Water movement is greatest within the jejunum.

Unstirred water layers

A layer of relatively unstirred water lies adjacent to all biological membranes. The boundary between the bulk water and this unstirred layer is indistinct but, nevertheless, it has a real thickness. During absorption, drug molecules must diffuse across this layer and then on through the lipid layer. The overall rate of transfer is the result of the resistance in both water layer and lipid layer. The flux, J, for a substance across the unstirred layer is given by the expression

$$J = (C_1 - C_2)\frac{D}{\delta} \qquad (9.5)$$

where C_1 and C_2 are the concentrations of the substance in the bulk water phase and in the unstirred water layer, respectively, D is the diffusion coefficient and δ is the effective thickness of the unstirred layer. The flux of molecules that pass by passive diffusion through the lipid membrane can be written as

$$J = C_2 P_c \qquad (9.6)$$

where P_c is the permeability coefficient. The rate of absorption must equal the rate of transport across the unstirred layer; that is,

$$J = (C_1 - C_2)\frac{D}{\delta} = C_2 P_c \qquad (9.7)$$

The rate of movement across the unstirred layer, as can be seen from the equations, is proportional to D/δ; the rate of absorption is proportional to P_c. Compounds with a large permeability coefficient may be able to penetrate across cell membranes much faster than they can be transported through the unstirred layer. Under these circumstances diffusion through the water layer becomes the rate-limiting step in the absorption process. Neglect of the unstirred layer causes errors in the interpretation of experimental flux data.

Effect of the properties of the drug

Drugs must be in their molecular form before diffusional absorption processes take place. We would expect bases to be more soluble than acids in the stomach, but it is impossible to generalise in this way. Although the basic form of a drug as its hydrochloride salt should be soluble to some extent in this medium, this is not always so. Indeed the free bases of, for example, chlortetracycline, dimethylchlortetracycline and methacycline are more soluble than their corresponding hydrochlorides in the pH range of the stomach (see Chapter 4). It has been shown that mean plasma levels following administration of the free base and the hydrochloride of these tetracyclines reflect the

differences in solubility, the bases giving higher levels. The reason is most likely that discussed in section 4.7.2, namely the influence of high ionic strength on the solubility of the drug substance (the common ion effect). As absorption of the tetracyclines takes place mainly from the duodenum, it is vital that they reach the intestine in a dissolved or readily soluble form, as their solubility is low at the pH conditions prevailing in the duodenum (pH 4–5).

The presence of buffer components in the formulation also creates a pH microenvironment around dissolving particles that may aid drug dissolution. If dissolution is the rate-limiting step in the absorption process, this will be significant in determining absorption. Bulk pH will then give little help in calculating the solution rate on the basis of a knowledge of saturation solubilities in bulk conditions.

Other complicating factors

The very high area of the surface of the small intestine also upsets the calculation of absorption based on considerations of theoretical absorption across identical areas of absorbing surface. The sheer complexity of the situation precludes mathematical precision, yet the pH-partition hypothesis is useful especially in predicting what follows from a change in bulk pH – for example, on ingestion of antacids or drugs such as histamine receptor antagonists (H_2 blockers) that reduce gastric acid secretion. The extent of the change in pH after administration of one of the first in the class, cimetidine, can be seen from the diagram in Fig. 9.6, which shows a rise in resting pH from below 2 to near neutrality. The effect in turn depends on the formulation used. The fact that aspirin, an acid with a pK_a of 3.5, is absorbed from the small intestine is due partly to the massive surface area available for absorption which allows significant absorption to occur, even though the percentage of absorbable species is very low, and partly to the dynamics of the process referred to earlier.

A warning, however, about other complications: drugs that (1) are unstable in the GI tract (for example, erythromycin), (2) are metabolised on their passage through the gut wall, (3) are hydrolysed in the stomach to active forms (namely prodrugs), and (4) bind to mucin or form complexes with bile

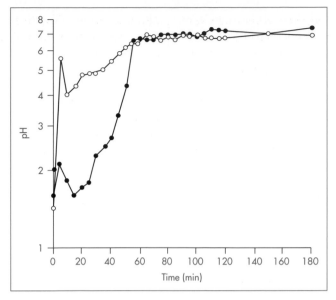

Figure 9.6 Intragastric pH after administration of (○) effervescent cimetidine and (●) standard cimetidine, plotted as median values from 13 patients with gastro-oesophageal reflux given 800 mg orally of the preparations.

Reproduced from Ström M *et al.*, *Lancet*, 1991; 337: 433.

salts may not always be absorbed in the manner expected.

Ion pairing

The interaction of drugs in the charged form with other ions to form absorbable species with a high lipid solubility is a possible explanation for the ability of molecules such as quaternary ammonium compounds, ionised under all pH conditions, to be usefully absorbed. The origin of the ions that pair with drug ions is not clear, but there is evidence that ion-pair formation will aid absorption.

One could assume that small organic ions are absorbed through water-filled pores or channels in the membrane, but the effective diameter of such pores means that large drug ions would be excluded from this route. Although membranes are impermeable to large organic ions, nevertheless ion-pairing between a drug ion and an organic ion of opposite charge forming an absorbable neutral species is possible.

Two ionic species A^+ and B^- may exist in solution in several states:

A : B	⇌	A^+, B^-	⇌	$A^+ B^-$	⇌	$A^+ + B^-$
undissociated		'tight'		'loose'		free ions
species		ion pair		ion pair		

The formation of tight or loose ion pairs will depend on solvent–ion interactions: hydrophobic ions might be encouraged to form ion pairs by the mechanism of *water-structure enforced ion pairing* in which the water attempts to minimise the disturbance on its structuring, and achieves this end by reducing the polarity of the species in solution by ion-pair formation. Ion pairing in highly structured solvents, then, is due not to an electrostatic interaction but to a solvent-mediated effect. The significance of the phenomenon is that ion pairs have the property of being almost neutral species, so that the ion pair can partition into an oily phase when its parent ionic species cannot, a property that is important in drug absorption and drug extraction procedures, and that is put to use in chromatography.

The two reactions below are examples of (i) a quaternary amine pairing with a weak acid, and (ii) an alkyl sulfate with a weak base, both under pH conditions in which the solute is charged:

(i) $RCOO^- + N^+(C_4H_9)_4 \rightleftharpoons RCOON(C_4H_9)_4$

(ii) $RNH_3^+ + {}^- O_3SO(CH_2)_{11}CH_3 \rightleftharpoons$
$$RNH_3 O_3 SO(CH_2)_{11}CH_2$$

hydrophilic   ion-pair agent

solute   hydrophobic pair

Figure 9.7 shows clearly the effect of chloride ion and other anions such as methane sulfonate on the apparent partition coefficient of chlorpromazine. The nature of the anion significantly affects the partitioning of the drug. Ion pairing in the GI tract obviously could influence absorption.

Key points

- Biological membranes are composed primarily of phospholipids and cholesterol forming a lipoidal bilayer in which proteins are embedded; as a consequence they have a hydrophilic negatively charged exterior and a hydrophobic interior. They are selectively permeable, allowing nutrients to pass into the cell and waste products to move out.

- Lipid-soluble agents can cross the membrane by passive diffusion; in addition there are pores that offer an alternative diffusion pathway that is particularly important for the transference of ions and charged drugs such as the quaternary ammonium compounds. Overall, the permeability is controlled by the nature of the membrane, its degree of internal bonding and rigidity, its surface charge and the nature of the solute being transported.

- A plot of percentage absorption versus $\log P$ for drugs within a series is generally parabolic; optimum absorption occurs at $\log P_o$. A relationship between the properties of a drug and its extent of absorption was devised by Lipinski, the 'Rule of 5'. **Poor** absorption is likely when the drug has a molecular weight >500 Da, more than 5 H-bond donors, a $\log P > 5$, and more than 10 H-bond acceptors.

- The pH-partition hypothesis assumes that only lipid-soluble agents will cross the membrane, which for simplicity is considered to be a strip of lipoidal material. It is therefore expected that un-ionised forms of either acidic or basic drugs will diffuse across the membrane, while the ionised forms will be rejected.

- Absorption is sometimes much greater than predicted from the pH-partition hypothesis. There are several possible reasons for this:
  - The pH of the stomach may be higher than the normally quoted range of 1–3.
  - The pH at the membrane surface is lower than the bulk pH; there may also be secretion of acidic and basic substances in parts of the gut wall.
  - The movement of water molecules, due to differences in osmotic pressure between blood and the contents of the lumen and differences in hydrostatic pressure between the lumen and the perivascular tissue, affects the rate of absorption of small molecules.
  - A layer of unstirred water lies adjacent to the membrane, which is an additional barrier across which molecules must diffuse during their absorption.
  - Although we would expect that bases would be more soluble than acids in the stomach, this may not always be the case because, for example, of the common ion effect.
  - A variety of other factors may complicate the absorption process, including the complex nature and very high area of the surface of the small intestine and the properties of the drug, for example its stability in the GI tract, its binding to mucin or complexation with bile salts, and the formation of ion pairs.

Figure 9.7 Apparent partition coefficients for chlorpromazine between *n*-octanol and aqueous buffers at pH 3.9, in the presence of various anions at 30°C: ○, chloride; ●, propanesulfonate; ⊗, ethanesulfonate; △, methanesulfonate.

Reproduced from Murthy LS, Zografi G, *J Pharm Sci*, 1970; 59: 1281.

9.2 The oral route and oral absorption

9.2.1 Drug absorption from the gastrointestinal tract

The oral route is the most popular and convenient route of drug administration for those drugs that can survive the acid of the stomach, that are resistant to enzymatic attack, and that are absorbed across GI membranes. The functions of the GI tract are the digestion and absorption of foods and other nutrients and it is not easy to separate these two functions from that of drug delivery. Indeed, the natural processes in the gut frequently influence the absorption of drugs. This is not surprising when it is considered that on average approximately 500 g of solid and up to 2.5 litres of fluid are ingested each day. As well as this oral intake, an estimated 30 litres of endogenous fluid are excreted each day into the intestine.

The pH of the gut contents and the presence of enzymes, foodstuffs, bile salts, fat and the microbial flora will all influence drug absorption. The complexity of the absorbing surfaces means that a simple physicochemical approach to drug absorption remains an approach to the problem and not the complete picture, as described above. Whatever the limitations

of theory – and one should not expect simple theories to hold in the complex and dynamic circumstances that are involved in drug absorption – theory provides a starting point in rationalising the behaviour of drugs in the GI tract. While most drugs are absorbed by passive diffusion across the lipid membranes separating the gut contents from the rest of the body, certain molecules that resemble naturally occurring substances are actively transported by special mechanisms.

We first consider the physiological situation that might impinge on passive drug absorption. The delivery of macromolecules, including peptides and proteins, is treated in Chapter 12.

Particulate absorption from the gut

While the general rule is that only drugs in solution are absorbed from the GI tract, colloidal particles, some viruses, bacteria and prion proteins can gain entry in low amounts to the lymphatic system after absorption by specialised cells (M-cells) in the gut-associated lymphoid tissue (GALT). A discussion of this route of uptake is outside the scope of this book, but it is a route that is likely to be increasingly explored as a means of delivering proteins and perhaps genes in carrier nanoparticles and for oral vaccination. It has yet to fulfil its promise.[2]

9.2.2 Structure of the gastrointestinal tract

We first consider the physiological situations and the structure and function of the GI tract that might impinge on passive drug absorption.

Figure 9.8 diagrammatically represents the GI tract and some of the factors involved in the process of drug absorption from this complex milieu. The stomach is not an organ that has evolved for absorption; the main site of absorption is the small intestine.

The stomach may be divided into its two main parts: (i) the body of the stomach which is in effect a receptacle or hopper, which includes pepsin- and HCl-secreting areas, and (ii) the pyloris (a churning chamber), the mucus-secreting area of the gastric mucosa. The stomach varies its luminal volume with the content of food and this is one reason why food intake can be so important in relation to drug absorption; the stomach of adults may contain a few millilitres or a litre or more of fluid. Hydrochloric acid is liberated

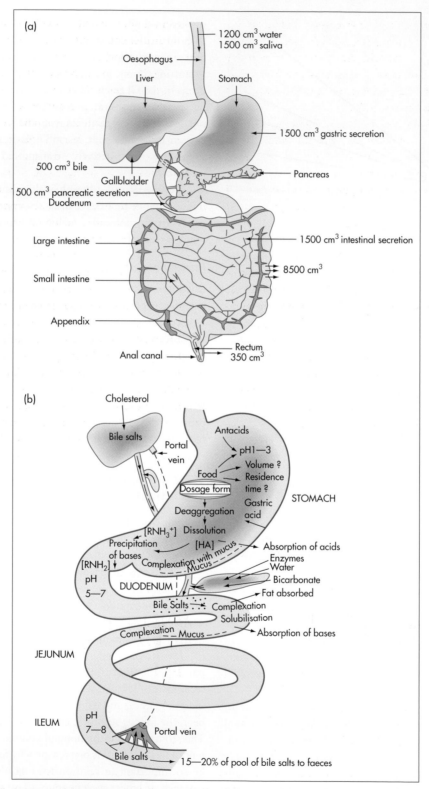

Figure 9.8 Representation of the processes occurring along the gastrointestinal tract, and of the factors that must be taken into account in considering drug absorption.

from the parietal cells at a concentration of 0.58%, or 160 mmol dm^{-3}. The gastric glands produce some 1000–1500 cm^3 of gastric juice per day. It is in this somewhat chaotic environment that pharmaceutical dosage forms find themselves. Some of the events that result are shown in Fig. 9.8b.

The small intestine is divided anatomically into three sections: duodenum, jejunum and ileum. Histologically there is no clearly marked transition between these parts. All three are involved in the digestion and absorption of foodstuffs, absorbed material being removed by the blood and the lymph. The absorbing area is enlarged by surface folds in the intestinal lining that are macroscopically apparent: the surfaces of these folds possess villi and microvilli (Fig. 9.9). It has been calculated that with a maximum of 3000 microvilli per cell in the epithelial brush border (so called because of its physical appearance) the number of microvilli in the small intestine mucosa, even of the rat, is 2×10^8 per mm^2. Although one would expect organic acids to be absorbed only from the stomach where they will exist in the un-ionised lipid-soluble and membrane-diffusible form, the enormous surface area in the intestine allows significant absorption of acidic drugs from the intestine even though (as noted earlier) the fraction of un-ionised molecules is very small.

Over the entire length of the large and small intestines and the stomach, the brush border has a uniform coating (3 nm thick) of mucopolysaccharides that consist of multibranched polymeric chains. This coating layer appears to act as a mechanical barrier to bacteria, cells or food particles, or as a filter. Whatever its function, the weakly acidic, sulfated mucopolysaccharides influence the charge on the cell membrane and complicate the explanations of absorption.

The goblet cells of the epithelium form mucus; secretions are stored in granule form in the apical cell region and are liquefied on contact with water to form mucus, which is composed of protein and carbohydrate and acts as a protective mechanism for the gut surface. Its role in the absorption of drugs is unclear.

The large intestine is concerned primarily with the absorption of water and the secretion of mucus to aid the intestinal contents to slide down the intestinal 'tube'. Villi are therefore completely absent from the large intestine, but there are deep crypts distributed over its surface.

Differences in the absorptive areas and volumes of gut contents in experimental animals are important when comparing experimental results on drug absorption in various species and in humans.[3] The all-important extrapolation to the human animal is complex. The human small intestine has a calculated active surface area of approximately 100 m^2. No analogous

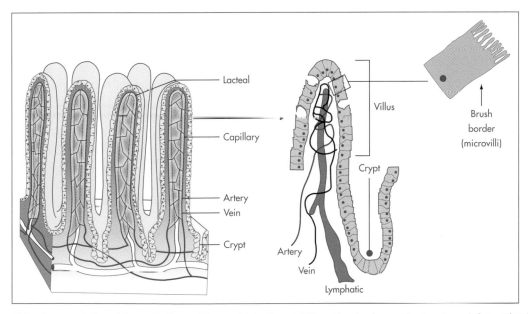

Figure 9.9 Representation of the epithelium of the small intestine at different levels of magnification. From left to right: the intestinal villi and microvilli that comprise the brush border.

calculations are available for the most commonly used laboratory animals, although the surface area of the small intestine of the rat is estimated to be 700 cm^2.

Passive transport, carrier-mediated transport and specialised transport

In discussing the pH-partition hypothesis, it has been considered that drugs are absorbed by passive diffusion through epithelial cells – the enterocytes of the GI tract for example. In fact there is the possibility of some passage of drugs by way of the tight junctions (the paracellular route) and there are transcellular carrier-mediated uptake mechanisms as well as endocytosis. Figure 9.10 summarises these.

9.2.3 Bile salts and fat absorption pathways

Fat is absorbed by special mechanisms in the gut. The bile salts that are secreted into the jejunum are efficient emulsifiers and disperse fat globules, allowing the action of lipase at the much increased globule surface. Medium-chain triglycerides are thought to be directly absorbed. Long-chain triglycerides are hydrolysed, and the monoglycerides and fatty acids produced form mixed micelles with the bile salts and are absorbed either directly in the micelle or, more probably, brought to the microvillus surface by the micelle and transferred directly to the mucosal cells, the bile salts remaining in the lumen. The bile salts are reabsorbed in the ileum and transported via the portal vein back into the bile salt pool.

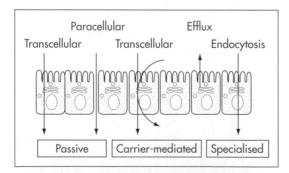

Figure 9.10 GI membrane transport. Transport through the enterocyte barrier can be divided into active, passive and specialised transport; and into the paracellular and transcellular routes. Efflux mechanisms can reduce absorption by these routes.

There have been suggestions that lipid-soluble drugs may be absorbed by fat absorption pathways. Certainly, administration of drugs in an oily vehicle can significantly affect absorption, increasing it in the case of griseofulvin and ciclosporin, but decreasing it in the case of vitamin D.

9.2.4 Gastric emptying, motility and volume of contents

The volume of the gastric contents will determine the concentration of a drug that finds itself in the stomach. The time the drug or dosage form resides in the stomach will determine many aspects of absorption. If the drug is absorbed lower down the gut, the residence time will determine the delay before absorption begins; if the drug is labile in acid conditions, longer residence times in the stomach will lead to greater stability; if the dosage form is non-disintegrating then retention in the stomach can influence the pattern of absorption. Gastroretentive dosage forms are designed to achieve that control.

The stomach empties liquids faster than solids. The rate of transfer of gastric contents to the small intestine is retarded by the activity of receptors sensitive to acid, fat, osmotic pressure and amino acids in the duodenum and the small intestine, and stimulated by material that has arrived from the stomach. Gastric emptying is a simple exponential or square-root function of the volume of a test meal – a pattern that holds for meals of variable viscosity. To explain the effect of a large range of substances on emptying, an osmoreceptor has been postulated that shrinks in hypertonic solutions and swells in hypotonic solutions.

Acids in test meals have been found to slow gastric emptying; acids with higher molecular weights (for example, citric acid) are less effective than those, such as HCl, with very low molecular weights. Natural triglycerides inhibit gastric motility, linseed and olive oils being effective. The formulation of a drug may thus influence drug absorption through an indirect physiological effect. The nature of the dose form – whether solid or liquid, whether acid or alkaline, whether aqueous or oily – may thus influence gastric emptying. The question of gastric emptying and transit down the GI tract has assumed further importance in relation to the design and performance of sustained-release preparations. The transit of pellets of different densities,[4,5] for

Figure 9.11 Gastric emptying of pellets of different density with various sizes of meal.
Reproduced from Wilson CG, Washington N, *Physiological Pharmaceutics*, Chichester: Ellis Horwood; 1989.

example, is shown in Fig. 9.11 and illustrates the influence of both density and food intake.

Food, then, affects not only transit but also pH. The effect of a meal on the hydrogen ion concentration of the stomach contents is shown in Fig. 9.12; the effect of two antacids on gastric volume and pH is shown in Table 9.4. When considering the effect of an antacid, therefore, the effect of volume change and pH change and the effect on gastric emptying must all

be considered. In designing delivery systems all these factors have ideally to be taken into account.

Key points

- The oral route is the most convenient route of drug administration for those drugs that can survive the acid of the stomach, that are resistant to enzymatic attack, and that are absorbed across GI membranes. Prediction of absorption rates is complicated, however, by the complexity of the absorbing surfaces, and the presence of enzymes, foodstuffs, bile salts, fat and microbial flora.
- Absorption is influenced by the volume of the gastric contents, the rate of gastric emptying, and the effect of food on the pH of the stomach contents.
- Although most drugs are absorbed by passive diffusion through epithelial cells, there is also the possibility of absorption by passage through tight junctions (paracellular absorption), by transcellular carrier-mediated uptake mechanisms and by endocytosis.
- Special mechanisms operate for the absorption of fat that involve mixed micelle formation with bile salts.

Figure 9.12 Hydrogen ion concentrations (C_{H^+}) at intervals after a test meal (mean results are shown ± 2SEM); the zero samples were taken just before the meal was begun, and the 1-hour sample just before 45 cm^3 of water.
Modified from Fordtran J, *N Engl J Med*, 1966; 274: 921.

Table 9.4 Effects of antacids on gastric volume and pH in the rat[a,b]

	Water	Maalox	Amphojel
Volume (cm³)	0.29 ± 0.03	1.8 ± 0.3	4.0 ± 0.2
pH	2.2 ± 0.2	7.4 ± 0.1	4.7 ± 0.2

[a] Reproduced from Hava M, Hurwitz A, *Eur J Pharmacol*, 1973; 22: 156.
[b] Ten rats per group. Measurements on gastric contents made 20 minutes after the third hourly dose of 1 cm³ water or antacid by gastric intubation.

9.3 Oral dosage forms

A variety of modified-release oral dosage forms are discussed in other chapters of this book. Here we briefly touch on the conventional delivery systems used in the great majority of cases, namely tablets, capsules, suspensions and liquids. In the main, conventional – that is to say fast-release – products are used as a means of administering large and small doses of drugs in convenient forms, to provide stable systems and reliable dosing. For very low-dose drugs (such as oral contraceptives) there is the problem even today of ensuring that the drug is dispersed evenly in the bulk powder or granules used for tableting, because of the phenomenon of particle segregation. On the other hand, it is possible by appropriate design of the dosage form to alter the pharmacokinetics that the drug would otherwise exhibit. Modified-, sustained-, delayed- or controlled-release forms (these descriptors are used interchangeably) can be used by the oral route to prolong the release and thus the action of drugs, so reducing the frequency of dosing with drugs having a short intrinsic half-life. One of the oldest forms of delayed-release product is the enteric-coated tablet or capsule. These have a polymer coat whose solubility is pH-dependent, this becoming porous or soluble in the lower intestine or colon. Other film coats and non-disintegrating matrix forms are dealt with in Chapter 7.

The preparation and formulation of tablets and capsules can be either straightforward or complex depending on the nature of the drug and the excipients. Particular problems arise with labile drugs that might be affected by moisture, low-dose drugs, and dose forms containing more than one active ingredient, with the potential for the interaction between the drugs themselves or with the excipient materials. A cartoon of a typical coated tablet is drawn in Fig. 9.13, which in a simple way illustrates the potential for problems.

9.3.1 The Biopharmaceutical Classification System (BCS)[6]

With the plethora of drugs now available and being tested, there was a need to assist drug developers to make decisions about the manner in which to deliver drugs by the oral route. Through the work of Gordon

Figure 9.13 A cartoon of a conventional film-coated tablet, showing just some of the ingredients commonly found and the range of possibilities for interactions such as drug–excipient, excipient–excipient, and changes in the polymer film coat.

Table 9.5 The four BCS Drug Classes	
Class I: High solubility, high permeability	Class II: Low solubility, high permeability
Class III: High solubility, low permeability	Class IV: Low solubility, low permeability

Key points

- Conventional oral delivery systems such as tablets, capsules, suspensions and liquids are fast-release formulations. The release of drug can be prolonged in order to reduce the frequency of dosing by enteric coating or the use of non-disintegrating matrix forms.
- Particular problems arise in the formulation of oral dosage forms containing labile drugs that might be affected by moisture, low-dose drugs, and dose forms containing more than one active ingredient, with the potential for the interaction between the drugs themselves or with the excipient materials.
- The Biopharmaceutical Classification System (BCS)[6] is a valuable aid in choosing a strategy for the formulation of oral dosage forms. Drugs are classified as high solubility, high permeability (Class I); low solubility, high permeability (Class II); high solubility, low permeability (Class III); and low solubility, low permeability (Class IV).

Amidon and colleagues, a valuable classification system was developed to relate drug intestinal absorption to the physical properties of drugs. Drugs were characterised into four types or classes, as shown in Table 9.5. The ideal drugs fall within Class I. Different strategies must be adopted to formulate drugs in other classes to achieve efficient oral absorption.

There are, of course, drugs that are at the boundaries of these classifications: it is clear too that properties will vary widely within classes. The commonly seen grid is as shown in Fig. 9.14, where GI permeability is plotted not against drug solubility itself but against the *dose/solubility ratio*. Very poorly soluble drugs may be therapeutically effective orally if their dose is very low. High-dose drugs with a low solubility present the greatest pharmaceutical challenge. The figure also shows some of the stratagems to be adopted to achieve better absorption.

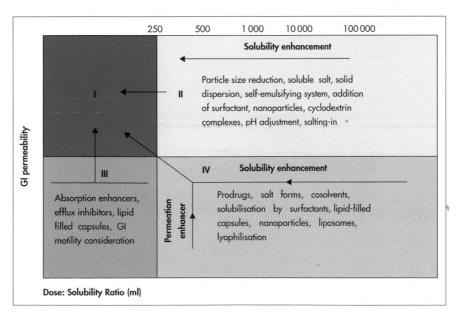

Figure 9.14 A BCS type plot of the four classes of drug with suggested techniques to enhance absorption. Class II compounds benefit from particle size reduction, soluble salt formation, solubilisation by surfactants, etc; Class III drugs require absorption enhancers and efflux inhibitors *inter alia*; Class IV drugs require a range of techniques to attempt to enhance absorption as shown.

9.4 Buccal and sublingual absorption

Mouthwashes, toothpastes and other preparations are introduced into the oral cavity for local prophylactic and therapeutic reasons. It is not known to what extent components of these formulations are absorbed and give rise to systemic effects. The absorption of drugs through the oral mucosa, however, provides a route for systemic administration that avoids exposure to the GI system. Drugs absorbed in this way bypass the liver and have direct access to the systemic circulation. The sublingual, buccal and gingival tissues are shown diagrammatically in Fig. 9.15. The oral mucosa functions primarily as a barrier, however, and it is not a highly permeable tissue, resembling skin more closely than the gut in this respect. Table 9.6 lists some commercially available sublingual and buccal delivery systems. Mucosal adhesive systems have been studied for administration of buprenorphine through the gingiva.

9.4.1 Mechanisms of absorption

The oral mucosa comprises

- A mucus layer over the epithelium
- A keratinised layer in certain regions of the oral cavity
- An epithelial layer
- A basement membrane
- Connective tissue
- A submucosal region

While cells of the oral epithelium and epidermis are capable of absorbing material by endocytosis, it does not seem likely that drugs or other solutes would be transported by this mechanism across the entire stratified epithelium. It is also unlikely that active transport processes are operative in the oral mucosa. There is considerable evidence that most substances are absorbed by simple diffusion. The linear relationship between percentage absorption through the buccal epithelium and $\log P$ of a homologous series is seen in Fig. 9.16. For example, the buccal absorption of some basic drugs increases (Fig. 9.17), and that of acidic drugs decreases, with increasing pH of their solutions.

Nicotine in a gum vehicle when chewed is absorbed through the buccal mucosa; nicotine levels obtained are lower than those obtained by smoking cigarettes and the high peak levels are not seen. Buccal glyceryl trinitrate has been found to be an effective drug. The buccal route has the advantages of the sublingual route – the buccal mucosa is similar to sublingual mucosal tissue – but a sustained-release tablet can be held in the cheek pouch for several hours if necessary. Mucosal adhesive formulations can have obvious advantages.

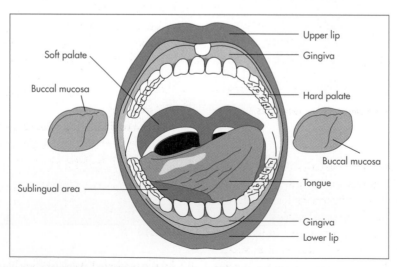

Figure 9.15   The anatomy of the oral cavity including the buccal, sublingual and gingival cavities.

From Kunth K *et al., Adv Drug Deliv Rev*, 1993; 11: 137.

Table 9.6 Commercially available drug-delivery systems for systemic delivery by the oral mucosal route[a]

Mucosal site	Drug	Proprietary name	Dosage form
Sublingual	Glyceryl trinitrate	Nitrostat	Tablets
		Lenitral spray	Spray
		Susadrin	Bioadhesive tablets
	Isosorbide dinitrate	Risordan	Tablets
		Sorbitrate	Chewable tablets
		Isocard spray	Spray
	Erythritol trinitrate	Cardiwell	Tablets
	Nifedipine	Adalat	Tablets
	Buprenorphine	Temgesic	Tablets
	Apomorphine HCl	Apomorphine	Tablets
Buccal	Prochlorperazine	Buccastem	Bioadhesive tablets
		Tementil	Solution
	Phloroglucinol	Spasfon-Lyoc	Lyocs
	Oxazepam	Seresta Expidet	Lyophilised tablets
	Lorazepam	Temesta Expidet	Lyophilised tablets
	Methyltestosterone	Metandren	Tablets
	Nicotine	Nicorette	Chewing-gum

[a] Modified from Ponchel G, *Adv Drug Deliv Rev*, 1994; 13: 75.

Experiments with some analgesics showed that the highly lipid-soluble etorphine was absorbed several times more rapidly from the buccal cavity than the less lipid-soluble morphine.[7] Impressive absorption has been obtained with glyceryl trinitrate (which exerts its pharmacological action 1–2 minutes after sublingual administration), methacholine chloride, isoprenaline, some steroids such as desoxycortisone acetate[8]

and 17β-estradiol (at one-quarter of its normal oral dose), morphine, captopril and nifedipine.

It has been claimed that an oil/water partition coefficient in the range 40–2000 (log P of 1.6–3.3) is optimal for drugs to be used by the sublingual route. Drugs with a log P greater than 3.3 are so oil-soluble that it is difficult for sufficiently high levels of drug to be soluble in the aqueous salivary fluids. Drugs less lipophilic than those with a log P of 1 would not be absorbed to any great extent and would thus require large doses by this route. A comparison of the sublingual/subcutaneous dose ratio serves as an index of the usefulness of the route.[9] For example, cocaine with a P of 28 requires a sublingual/subcutaneous dosage ratio of 2 to obtain equal effects; atropine with a P of 7 requires 8 times the subcutaneous dose; and for codeine ($P \sim 2$) over 15 times the subcutaneous dose must be given sublingually.

 Key points

- Absorption of drugs through the oral mucosa provides a route for systemic administration that avoids exposure of the drug to the GI tract, and also metabolism in the liver.
- The oral mucosa functions primarily as a barrier and is not highly permeable. Most drugs are absorbed by simple diffusion.
- There is a linear relationship between percentage absorption through the buccal epithelium and log P for a homologous series of drugs. Buccal absorption of basic drugs increases and that of acidic drugs decreases with increasing pH of their solutions.
- The optimum log P for drugs to be administered by the sublingual route is between 1.6 and 3.3

Summary

We have considered the basic mechanisms of absorption that apply to all routes of administration, dealing

Figure 9.16 Relationship between the log P of solute and the percentage absorption through the buccal mucosa of human subjects for bases (○) and acids (●).

Plotted from data from Lien E *et al., Drug Intell Clin Pharm*, 1971; 5: 38.

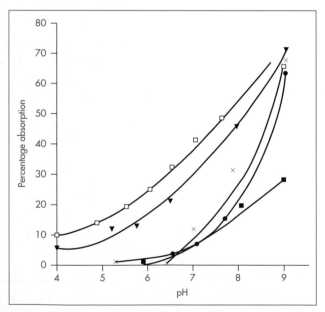

Figure 9.17 Buccal absorption of some basic drugs. The drugs were dissolved in buffered solutions of different pH and placed in the mouth of human subjects; absorption rates were determined from the decrease of drug concentration in expelled solutions: □, chlorphenamine (pK_a = 8.99); ▼, methadone (pK_a = 8.25); ×, amfetamine (pK_a = 9.94); ●, pethidine (pK_a = 8.72); ■, nicotine (pK_a = 8.02).

Reproduced from Beckett AH, Triggs EJ, *J Pharm Pharmacol*, 1976; 19: 31S.

with the factors that depend on the drug itself, its chemical and physicochemical characteristics, the nature of the medium and the subtle differences in biological barriers that drugs experience. While the equations that relate to many of the processes are given, it is emphasised that the dynamic processes of drug absorption, dynamic in two senses in that the drug is moving down the GI tract at the same time as it is being absorbed, deny us a physicochemical 'theory of everything'. Nonetheless, estimates are valuable in understanding what is going on.

The emphasis on the oral route of delivery and sublingual and buccal delivery provided details of the underlying processes. The following chapter considers parenteral (non-oral) routes of drug administration. In all of these the actual processes of absorption of drug once it reaches the absorbing surface are the same as those discussed in the present chapter. Sometimes the route to that surface, such as after inhalation, is very tortuous, and sometimes as with topical preparations there is a more direct contact between the formulation and the barrier to be overcome. In all, there are at least three important factors: the drug, the route and the formulation.

References

1. Lipinski CA *et al*. Experimental and computational approaches to estimate solubility and permeability in drug discovery and development settings. *Adv Drug Deliv Rev* 2001;46:3–26.
2. Florence AT. Nanoparticle uptake by the oral route: fulfilling its potential? *Drug Discov Today: Technology* 2005;2:75–81.
3. Kararli TT. Comparison of the gastrointestinal anatomy, physiology, and biochemistry of humans and commonly used laboratory animals. *Biopharm Drug Dispos* 1995; 16:351–380.
4. Davis SS *et al*. Transit of pharmaceutical dosage forms through the small intestine. *Gut* 1986;27:886–892.
5. Davis SS *et al*. The effect of food on the gastrointestinal transit of pellets and an osmotic device (Osmet). *Int J Pharm* 1984;21:331–340.
6. Amidon GL *et al*. A theoretical basis for a biopharmaceutical classification system: the correlation of *in vitro* drug product dissolution and *in vivo* bioavailability. *Pharm Res* 1995;12:413–420.
7. Dobbs EH *et al*. Uptake of etorphine and dihydromorphine after sublingual and intramuscular administration. *Eur J Pharmacol* 1969;7:328.
8. Gibaldi M, Kanig JL. Absorption of drugs through the oral mucosa. *J Oral Ther Pharmacol* 1965;31:440–450.
9. Speirs CF. Oral absorption and secretion of drugs. *Br J Clin Pharm* 1977;4:97–100.

References

10

Parenteral routes of drug administration

In Chapter 9 we discussed the basic mechanisms of drug absorption across biological membrane barriers. Whatever route of delivery and absorption, the basic principles are the same in terms of the determinants of drug transport across membranes. These are dependent on the physical chemistry and nature of the drug, the environment in which the drug finds itself and the nature of the membrane. In this chapter we look at a range of other routes used to administer formulations for both systemic and local use. We deal here with the particular issues with the following routes:

- Intravenous (IV) and intra-arterial (IA)
- Subcutaneous (SC) and intramuscular (IM)
- Topical
- Ocular
- Aural
- Vaginal
- Rectal
- Respiratory
- Nasal, and
- Intrathecal

Factors affecting drug absorption after delivery of the drug by these routes, often in special formulations are important, particularly with regard to the comparative advantages and disadvantages of the different routes.

10.1 Intravenous and intra-arterial administration

The venous route is used for several reasons: it is the most direct route into the blood and thus in emergencies rapid administration of life-saving drugs such as streptokinase is by intravenous (IV) injection. It is of course used in all clinical studies where possible, as the baseline for bioavailability studies. Bioavailability is measured against the values obtained by the IV route. Antibiotics may be given by this route, often over a period of time. It is also the mode of administration of drugs that cannot be given orally, such as many cytotoxic drugs that are toxic to the gut epithelium and proteins that are not absorbed by the oral route. The main physicochemical issues of the route revolve around (a) the physical and chemical stability of drugs given by infusion in admixture with common fluids such as dextrose; (b) the stability of admixtures when drugs are combined in the same giving set; and (c) tonicity and haemolytic activity. Aqueous solutions, suspensions and emulsions may be employed intravenously. There is a limiting size for any particulate system, which is below 1 µm. The issue of stability is frequently one of physical stability, such as arises with a pH-dependency of solubility (discussed in Chapter 4) and with drug–drug interactions (Chapter 11).

Intra-arterial (IA) drug administration can be used when venous access cannot be established, as in paediatric patients. It also has a use in cancer chemotherapy, and is sometimes employed in conjunction with IV therapy. Injection into an artery leading directly to an organ such as the liver provides the rationale for its use in cancer chemotherapy.

 Clinical point

Intra-arterial injection of BCNU (carmustine; bis-chloronitrosourea) in the treatment of malignant glioma results in levels of drug that are four times greater than those following IV infusion, but arguments persist about the relative clinical risks and of the benefits of IA administration of this drug. The rationale in liver cancer treatment for IA administration is that liver tumours derive their blood supply from the hepatic artery, unlike normal tissue. Two commonly used drugs are 5-FU (fluorouracil) and FUDR (floxuridine).

Microspheres loaded with drugs such as doxorubicin have been used experimentally to optimise delivery by this route.

Implantable infusion pumps

Such devices are implanted under the skin in the lower abdomen and designed to deliver infusate containing the appropriate drug at a constant rate (usually 1 cm³ per day) into an artery or vein. The Infusaid implantable pump was originally devised for the long-term administration of heparin but has since found application for a wide variety of drugs.[1] The device consists of a relatively small (9×2.5 cm) titanium disc that is divided into two chambers by cylindrical titanium bellows that form a flexible but impermeable barrier between the compartments (Figure 10.1). The outer compartment contains Freon (chlorofluorocarbon propellants); the inner compartment contains the infusate and connects via a catheter to a vein or artery through a series of filters and flow-regulating resistance elements. The vapour pressure above the liquid propellant remains constant because of the relatively constant temperature of the body, and hence a constant pressure is exerted on the bellows, ensuring a constant rate of delivery of infusate into the blood stream. The propellant is replenished as required by a simple percutaneous injection through the skin.

Key points

- The venous route is the most direct route into the blood and is used in emergencies for rapid administration of life-saving drugs; it is also the base-line for bioavailability studies and the mode of administration of drugs that cannot be given orally, e.g. many cytotoxic drugs that are toxic to the gut epithelium, and proteins.
- Aqueous solutions, suspensions and emulsions may be employed intravenously, but there is a limiting size for any particulate system, which is below 1 μm.
- Intra-arterial drug administration can be used when venous access cannot be established, as in paediatric patients. It also has use in cancer chemotherapy.

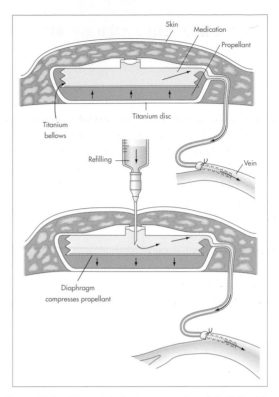

Figure 10.1 Diagrammatic representation of the Infusaid implantable infusion pump during operation (top) and during refilling (bottom).

Reproduced from Blackshear PJ, Rhode TH, in: Burk SD, ed., *Controlled Drug Delivery*, vol. 2, *Clinical Applications*, CRC Press: Boca Raton, FL; 1983: 11.

10.2 Intramuscular and subcutaneous injection

The intramuscular and subcutaneous routes of administration have long been regarded as efficient because they bypass the problems encountered in the stomach and intestine. Early views that subcutaneous (SC) and intramuscular (IM) administration of drugs resulted in only local action at the site were dispelled by Benjamin Bell, who wrote in 1858 in the *Edinburgh Medical Journal* that 'absorption from the enfeebled stomach may not be counted on; we possess in subcutaneous injections a more direct, rapid and trustworthy mode of conveying our remedy in the desired quantity to the circulatory blood'. We now know that not all drugs are efficiently or uniformly released from IM or SC sites. Some of the drugs that are not fully absorbed from their IM sites are listed in Table 10.1.

Where differences in bioavailability between IM, SC, oral or IV delivery occur, the clinical importance is most significant when the route of administration is changed from one to another. Such changes are most important in drugs with a low therapeutic index such as digoxin and phenytoin.

Table 10.1 Widely used drugs that may be incompletely absorbed after intramuscular injection

Ampicillin	Digoxin[a]
Cefaloridine	Insulin[a]
Cefradine	Phenylbutazone
Chlordiazepoxide	Phenytoin[a]
Diazepam	Quinidine
Dicloxacillin	

[a] Clinically important problems have been demonstrated with these.

The various regions into which injections are given are shown in Fig. 10.2. The subcutaneous region has a good supply of capillaries, although it is generally agreed that there are few, if any, lymph vessels in

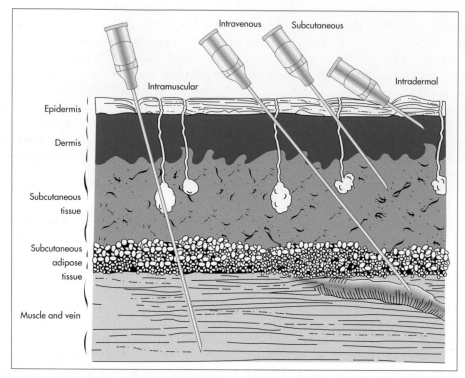

Figure 10.2 Routes of parenteral medication, showing the tissues penetrated by intramuscular, intravenous, subcutaneous and intradermal injections; the needles, with bevel up, penetrate the epidermis (cuticle) consisting of stratified epithelium with an outer horny layer, the corium (dermis or true skin) consisting of tough connective tissue, elastic fibres, lymphatic and blood vessels, and nerves, the subcutaneous tissue (tela subcutanea) consisting of loose connective tissue containing blood and lymphatic vessels, nerves, and fat-forming cells, the fascia (a thin sheet of fibrous connective tissue), and the veins, arteries and muscle.

Drawing modified after Quackenbush DS, in: Martin EW, ed., *Techniques of Medication*, Philadelphia: Lippincott; 1969.

muscle proper. Drugs with the optimal physicochemical characteristics can diffuse through the tissue and pass across capillary walls and thus enter the circulation by way of the capillary supply.

If it is reasonably assumed that drug absorption proceeds by passive diffusion of the drug, it can be considered to be a first-order process. Thus the rate of absorption is proportional to the concentration, C, of drug remaining at the injection site:

$$\frac{dC}{dt} = -k_a C \tag{10.1}$$

where k_a is the first-order rate constant. The half-life of the absorption process is

$$t_{0.5} = \frac{0.693}{k_a} \tag{10.2}$$

Drug absorption is 90% complete when a time equivalent to three times the half-life has elapsed.

Both dissolution and diffusion are important parameters in defining bioavailability of species by the IM or SC routes. Soluble neutral compounds disperse from intramuscular sites according to size: Table 10.2 shows that mannitol, a small molecule, rapidly diffuses from the site of injection; inulin disperses less rapidly; and dextran (molecular weight 70 000 Da), as might be expected, disperses more slowly.

Table 10.2 Influence of molecular size on clearance from intramuscular sites

Substance	Molecular weight	Fraction cleared (5 min)
Mannitol	182	0.70
Inulin	3 500	0.20
Dextran	70 000	0.07

With smaller molecules, those with molecular weights in the range 100–1000 Da, molecular size is a factor but a minor one in controlling release of drugs, but it assumes greater importance with proteins and other macromolecules, as discussed in Chapter 12. To achieve slow release of low-molecular-weight drugs they may be attached to a macromolecular backbone. Hydrophilic molecules such as those listed in Table 10.2 will be transported to the blood after diffusing through muscle fibres and then through the pores in the capillary walls, being incapable of absorption through the lipid walls. The transport through the capillary wall is the rate-limiting step in most cases; the larger the molecule, the more slowly it diffuses (as seen from equation 2.93) and the greater difficulty it has in traversing the aqueous pore in the capillary walls or the cell junction. The pores account for only 1% of the available surface of the capillary wall.

Absorption of weak electrolytes across the capillary walls follows the expected patterns, uptake of more lipid-soluble agents being relatively fast. Hydrophobic drugs may bind to muscle protein, leading to a reduction in free drug and perhaps to prolongation of action. Dicloxacillin is 95% bound to protein, while ampicillin is bound to the extent of 20%; as a consequence, dicloxacillin is absorbed more slowly from muscle than is ampicillin.

The significance of the diffusion phase through muscle tissue was demonstrated by Duran Reynolds who, in 1928, observed that dye solutions injected together with hyaluronidase spread out more rapidly and over a greater distance in the tissue than in the absence of the enzyme. The enzyme achieves its effect by breaking down the hyaluronic acid in intercellular spaces, thus leading to a decrease in viscosity and so easing the passage of small molecules in the matrix.

10.2.1 The importance of site of injection

The region into which the injection is administered is complex, being composed of both aqueous and lipid components. Muscle tissue is more acidic than normal physiological fluids. Measurement of percutaneous muscle surface pH (pH_m) using microelectrodes indicate values of 7.38; patients with peripheral vascular disease demonstrated a mean pH_m of 7.16. pH_m reflects the intramuscular ion concentrations but is stated to be higher than the actual intramuscular pH, which may be as low as 6.4. The pH of the region will determine whether drugs will dissolve in the tissue fluids or precipitate from formulations. In some cases precipitation will occur and may be the cause of the pain experienced on injection (see Chapter 11). The rate of solution here, as in many other routes, therefore determines how quickly the drug begins to act or, in some cases, over which period of time it acts. The deliberate reduction of the solubility of a drug achieves prolonged action by both routes.

10.2.2 Vehicles

Many drugs for IM administration are formulated in water-miscible solvents such as polyethylene glycol (PEG) 300 or 400, propylene glycol or ethanol mixtures. Dilution by the tissue fluids may cause the drug to precipitate. Drugs formulated as aqueous solutions by adjustment of pH will only transiently alter the pH at the injection site. Three main types of formulation are used for IM and SC injections: aqueous solutions, aqueous suspensions and oily solutions. Rapid removal of aqueous vehicles is to be expected, the drug being left perhaps as a precipitate. If the vehicle is nonaqueous and is an oil such as sesame oil, or another vegetable or a mineral oil, the oil phase disperses as droplets in the muscle and surrounding tissue, and is eventually metabolised.

The rate-determining step in the absorption of drug esters such as fluphenazine decanoate (which has an aqueous solubility of about 1 part per million) is the hydrolysis of the drug at the surface of the oil droplet. Hydrolysis of the fluphenazine decanoate to its soluble alcohol therefore depends on the state of dispersion and surface area of the droplets.

 Clinical point

Dispersing the droplets by rubbing the site of injection or by vigorous exercise can result in excessive dosage, with toxic effects. Exercise also causes increased blood flow and, as absorption is a dynamic process requiring the sweeping away of the drug from the localised absorption site, this increased flow increases the rate of drug dispersal.

10.2.3 Blood flow in muscles

Different rates of blood flow in different muscles mean that the site of IM injection can be crucial. Resting blood flow in the deltoid region is significantly greater than in the *gluteus maximus* muscle; flow in the *vastus lateralis* is intermediate. The difference between blood flow in the deltoid and gluteus is of the order of 20% and is likely to be the reason why deltoid injection of lidocaine has been found to give higher blood levels than injection into the lateral thigh. Therapeutic plasma levels for the prevention of arrhythmia with a dose of 4.5 mg kg^{-1} of a 10% solution of lidocaine were achieved only following deltoid injection.

 Clinical point

The age of the patient should influence the behaviour of the injection as ageing affects vascular blood flow and fatty deposits, but age has not been specifically isolated as a factor in studies to date. In some disease states it is possible to predict that the outcome of an IM injection might be different from that in other patients. For example, in patients with circulatory shock, hypotension, congestive heart failure and myxoedema, where blood flow to skeletal muscle is decreased, one might anticipate lower bioavailability.

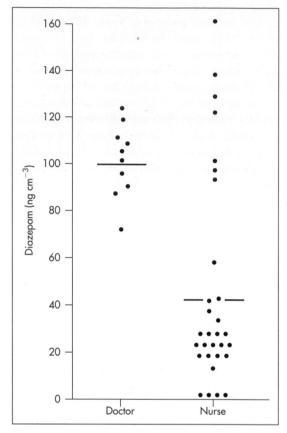

Figure 10.3 Plasma diazepam levels 90 minutes after intramuscular injection by one doctor and several nurses, showing the importance of technique and site of injection, which was variable in the latter group (individual values; horizontal lines denote average levels).

Redrawn with permission from Dundee JW *et al.*, *Lancet*, 1974; 2: 1461.

10.2.4 Formulation effects

Crystalline suspensions of fluspirilene, some steroids and procaine benzylpenicillin can be prepared in different size ranges to produce different pharmacokinetic profiles following IM or SC injection. Variability in response to a drug, or differences in response to a formulation from different manufacturers, can be the result of the nature of the formulation. Some years ago, in one trial diazepam as Valium (Roche) produced plasma levels ranging from about zero to 160 ng cm^{-3} 90 minutes after injection into muscle (see Fig. 10.3). The formulation contained diazepam dissolved in an ethyl alcohol–propylene glycol mixture. Upon injection, this solvent is absorbed and the drug precipitates (see Chapter 11). Injection of the formulation into the fatty tissue of the buttock can result in poor dispersal of drug, as the drug would have little opportunity for dissolution in that environment. Accordingly, the depth of the injection is significant. If, in addition, the blood supply to the region is limited, there will be an additional restriction to rapid removal. An alternative formulation of diazepam (Stesolid) containing a surface-active agent as a solubiliser has a greater bioavailability than a nonaqueous solution form of the drug (Diapam).

Clinical point

Additives can influence dispersion, the solubiliser undoubtedly in this case reducing precipitation at the site of injection and increasing the rate of solution. Reports of marked difference in side-effects and adverse reactions to diazepam formulations are undoubtedly due to the additives present, either indirectly or directly.

Controlled delivery from SC or IM sites may be achieved by dissolving a lipophilic drug in an oil phase as discussed above, or encapsulating the drug in liposomes, niosomes or biodegradable microspheres. These techniques are discussed in Chapters 6 and 7.

10.2.5 The case of insulin

Insulin is a classic example of what can be achieved by manipulation of the properties of a drug and its formulation. Modification of the crystallinity of insulin allows control over its solubility and duration of action. An acid-soluble formulation of insulin was introduced for clinical use in 1923. It had a short duration of action and attempts were then made to prolong the action. In 1936, Hagedorn and his colleagues found that insulin complexed with zinc and protamine from the trout (*Salmo irideus*) to form an amorphous precipitate at neutral pH. When injected subcutaneously, the insulin was slowly released from the complex into the blood and was active for about 36 hours. The prolonged-acting insulins introduced since the advent of protamine-zinc insulin (PZI) have been designed to have intermediate durations of action (Table 10.3).

The long-acting insulins in use today are mainly protamine insulin and zinc insulins. Protamine insulins are the salt-like compounds formed between the acid polypeptide (insulin) and the polypeptide protamine, which consists primarily of arginine. They are used in the form of neutral suspensions of protamine insulin crystals (isophane insulin).

Isophane insulin is produced by titration of an acidic solution of insulin with a buffered solution of

Table 10.3 Pharmaceutical injections of insulin BP[a]

Preparation	pH	Buffer	Description	Onset (h)	Duration of effect (h)
Insulin injection	3.0–3.5	–	Solution	~0.5–1	6–8
Neutral injection	6.6–7.7	Acetate	Solution	~0.5–1	6–9
Protamine zinc	6.9–7.4	Phosphate	Amorphous particles; rod-shaped crystals	~5–7	36
Globin zinc	3.0–3.5	–	Solution	~2	18–24
Isophane	7.1–7.4	Phosphate	Rod-shaped crystals (about 20 μm long)	~2	28
Zinc suspension (amorphous) 'Semilente'	7.0–7.5	Acetate	Amorphous particles (2 μm diameter)	~1	12–16
Zinc suspension 'Lente'	7.0–7.5	Acetate	Amorphous particles (30%) Rhombohedral crystals (70%)	~2	24
Zinc suspension (crystalline) 'Ultralente'	7.0–7.5	Acetate	Rhombohedral crystals (about 20 μm across)	~5–7	36
Biphasic	6.6–7.2	Acetate	Insulin in solution (25%) Rhombohedral crystals (75%)	~1	18–22

[a] Modified from Stewart GA, *Analyst*, 1974; 99: 913.

protamine at neutral pH until so-called isophane precipitation occurs; that is, no insulin or protamine is present in the supernatant. Under these conditions the precipitate consists of rod-shaped crystals. Crystalline forms of insulin free from foreign protein were developed in 1951. Under conditions of high zinc ion concentration (ten times that normally used to crystallise insulin) and in the absence of citrate and phosphate ions, rhombohedral crystals of insulin are formed in acetate buffer (IZS crystalline). By adjustment of the pH during the crystallisation stage, the insulin is produced as an amorphous precipitate (IZS amorphous) that has a duration of action of up to 16 hours. Various mixtures can be used providing modified durations of actions, as in biphasic insulin. Insulin zinc suspensions are incompatible with PZI and isophane insulin, both of which act as a buffer that destroys the zinc complex.

Figure 10.4 is a diagrammatic representation of the events following SC administration of a soluble human insulin existing initially as a hexameric zinc–insulin complex.

The use of insulins in solution obviates the potential source of error that arises when drawing a suspension into a syringe, but soluble insulins have the drawback that they must be stored at acid pH. Figure 10.5 shows the solubility–pH profiles for

Clinical points

1   Variable insulin activity may result from the mixing of PZI and soluble insulin in a syringe prior to administration. It has been suggested that this variability is due to the combination of the soluble insulin with excess protamine. As a general rule, insulin formulations of different pH should not be mixed.

2   Absorption of insulin is faster from injections administered subcutaneously in the arms than into the thighs. Insulin absorption in some patients may be poor because the subcutaneous tissue can act as a mechanical barrier to diffusion and as an active site of degradation.

soluble insulin and a trilysyl derivative. Injected subcutaneously, the insulin precipitates as amorphous particles. The pH of insulin preparations influences their stability, solubility and immunogenicity.

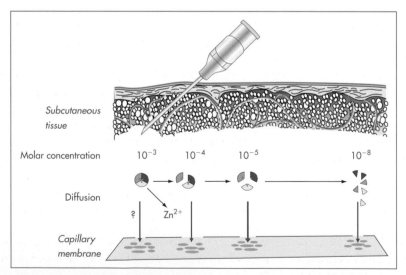

Figure 10.4 Suggested scheme of events after the SC administration of soluble human insulin: the concentration of hexameric zinc-insulin, which is the predominant form of insulin in soluble insulin (40 Unit or 100 Unit – i.e. 0.6 mmol dm^{-3}), decreases as diffusion of insulin occurs and as a result the hexamer dissociates into smaller units; to achieve monomeric insulin requires a 1000- fold dilution. The importance of the association state is that the larger species have more difficulty dispersing and passing through the capillary membrane.

Reproduced with permission from Brange J *et al.*, *Diabetes Care*, 1990; 13: 923.

Clinical points

1   After IM administration, short-acting insulin is absorbed about twice as rapidly as after SC injection, and therefore the IM route is used in the management of ketoacidosis in those cases where continuous IV infusion cannot be established. After SC injection, absorption of short-acting insulin varies considerably depending in particular on the site of injection. Patient-to-patient variability is as great with these preparations as the variations in the absorption rate of intermediate-acting insulins. This can lead to difficulty in control.

2   Flocculation of Humulin N insulin and of NPH insulin leads to changes in the appearance of vials (a frosting) and signals a problem, that of loss of potency and thus control. In affected samples it was found that the insulin concentration ranged from 6 to 64 U/mL, where in normal samples within narrow margins the concentration was 110 U/mL (see Further Reading, see Benson *et al*. 1987).

Key points

- The intramuscular and subcutaneous routes avoid problems encountered in the stomach and intestine; however, not all drugs are efficiently or uniformly released from IM or SC sites.
- Drugs with the optimal physicochemical characteristics can diffuse through the subcutaneous tissue and enter the circulation by way of the extensive capillary supply in this region.
- Drug absorption proceeds by passive diffusion and can be considered to be a first-order process, the rate of absorption being proportional to the concentration of drug remaining at the injection site.
- The bioavailability of species by the IM or SC routes is influenced by dissolution and diffusion. The rate of dispersion of soluble neutral molecules from the injection site and their transport through the capillary wall (the rate-limiting step in most cases) is determined by molecular size: the larger the molecule, the more slowly it diffuses.
- Hydrophilic molecules are incapable of absorption through the lipid walls and enter the blood stream through the pores in the capillary walls. Hydrophobic drugs may bind to muscle protein, leading to a reduction in free drug and perhaps to prolongation of action.
- The pH at the injection site will determine whether drugs will dissolve in the tissue fluids or precipitate from formulations; precipitation may be the cause of the pain experienced on injection.
- The main types of formulation used for IM and SC injections are aqueous solutions, aqueous suspensions and oily solutions, from which drugs can diffuse slowly for long action. Many drugs for IM administration are formulated in water-miscible solvents such as polyethylene glycol (PEG) 300 or 400, propylene glycol or ethanol mixtures; dilution by the tissue fluids may cause the drug to precipitate.
- The site of IM injection can be crucial because of different rates of blood flow in different muscles.
- The nature of the formulation can cause variability in response to a drug, or differences in response to a formulation from different manufacturers.

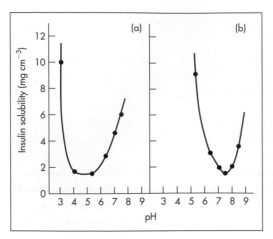

Figure 10.5 The solubility dependence of (a) insulin and (b) trilysyl insulin, a chemically modified insulin with an isoelectric point of 7.4 compared with the isoelectric point of unmodified insulin of 5.3.

Reproduced from Fishel-Ghodsian F, Newton JM, *J Drug Targeting*, 1993; 1: 67.

10.3 Transdermal delivery

A comprehensive account of the pharmaceutics and biopharmaceutics of topical preparations is not possible here. This section is restricted in scope to the physicochemical principles involved in the process of treating the skin or in systemic medication by the *transdermal* or *percutaneous* route. Formulation of topical vehicles for the potent drugs applied to the skin is now a more exact art. It is readily demonstrated that the vehicle in which the drug is applied influences the rate and extent of absorption. However, topical formulations can change rather rapidly once they have been spread on the skin, and absorption of some excipients and evaporative loss of water cause the breakdown of original structures.

Before any drug applied topically can act either locally or systemically it must penetrate the barrier layer of the skin, the *stratum corneum* (Fig. 10.6). This behaves like a passive diffusion barrier with no evidence of metabolic transport processes, drugs being absorbed by transcellular or intercellular pathways.

Penetration of water and low-molecular-weight nonelectrolyte solutes through the epidermis is proportional to their concentration, and to the partition

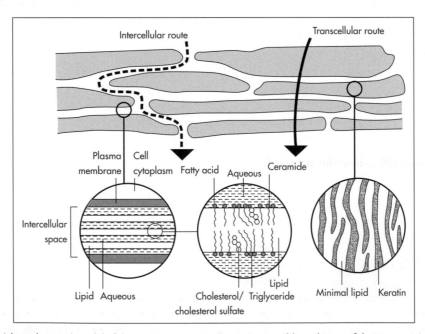

Figure 10.6 'Bricks and mortar' model of the stratum corneum, illustrating possible pathways of drug permeation through intact stratum corneum (transcellular and tortuous intercellular pathways) and the lamellar structure of intercellular lipids.

Reproduced from Moghimi HR *et al.*, *Int J Pharm*, 1996; 131: 117.

coefficient of the solute between tissue and vehicle. A form of Fick's law describes steady-state transport through the skin:

$$J = \frac{DP}{\delta}\Delta C_V \qquad (10.3)$$

where J is the solute flux, D is the solute diffusion coefficient in the stratum corneum (values range from 1×10^{-12} to $1 \times 10^{-17}\,m^2\,s^{-1}$ for human stratum corneum), P is the solute partition coefficient between skin and vehicle and δ is the thickness of the stratum corneum. ΔC_v is the difference in solute concentration between vehicle and tissue. This relation is obtained as shown in Box 10.1.

Box 10.1 Derivation of equation (10.3)

Fick's law of diffusion shows that (for a given vehicle)

$$J \propto \Delta C_v$$

A proportionality constant κ_p may be added. Thus

$$J = \kappa_p \Delta C_v$$

where κ_p is the permeability constant, which provides a means of expressing absorption measurements for comparing different vehicles and conditions. The units of a permeability constant are $m\,s^{-1}$, the concentration term being mol m^{-3}, so that J has the correct units of mol $m^{-2}\,s^{-1}$. It has been shown that

$$\kappa_p = \frac{PD}{\delta}$$

so that equation (10.3) is readily obtained.

Before steady-state penetration is achieved, the rate builds up over a period of time and a lag phase will be apparent (Fig. 10.7). The lag time, τ, does not indicate the point at which steady-state is achieved, which, as shown in Fig. 10.7, is obtained by extrapolation. The linear portion of the graph can be described by an equation relating the total amount absorbed at time t, Q_t, to $\Delta C, P, \delta, t$ and D. From equation (10.3), as $Q_t = Jt$,

$$Q_t = \frac{DP\Delta C_V}{\delta}t \qquad (10.4)$$

But from Fig. 10.7 it is obvious that the time to be substituted is the time over which steady-state flux has been maintained; namely, $t - \tau$. Thus we write

$$Q_t = \frac{DP\Delta C_V}{\delta}(t - \tau) \qquad (10.5)$$

As the lag time, τ, has been shown to be equal to $\delta^2/6D$, the drug's diffusion coefficient D is readily obtained from data such as those shown in Fig. 10.7. Values of τ range from a few minutes to several days, so lag times are of obvious clinical relevance.

10.3.1 Routes of skin penetration

Drug molecules may penetrate the skin not only through the stratum corneum but also by way of the hair follicles or through the sweat ducts, but these offer only a comparatively minor route because they represent such a small fraction of the surface area. Only in the case of molecules that move very slowly through the stratum corneum may absorption by these other routes predominate. Passage through damaged skin is increased over normal skin. Skin with a disrupted epidermal layer will allow up to 80% of hydrocortisone

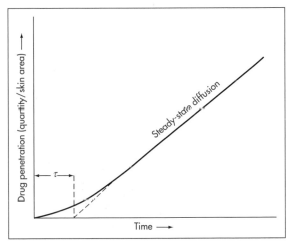

Figure 10.7 Drug penetration–time profile for an idealised drug diffusing through human skin; once steady-state diffusion occurs Q_t can be obtained using equation (10.4) where $t -$ (time elapsed $- \tau$).

to pass into the dermis, whereas only 1% is absorbed through intact skin.

The physicochemical factors that control drug penetration include the hydration of the stratum corneum, temperature, pH, drug concentration, and the molecular characteristics of the penetrant and the vehicle. The stratum corneum is a heterogeneous structure containing about 40% protein (keratin, a disulfide-crosslinked linear polypeptide), about 40% water and 18–20% lipids (principally triglycerides and free fatty acids, cholesterol and phospholipids). Hydration of the stratum corneum is one determinant of the extent of absorption: increased hydration decreases the resistance of the layer, presumably by causing a swelling of the compact structures in the horny layer.

 Clinical point

Occlusive dressings increase the hydration of the stratum corneum by preventing water loss by perspiration; certain ointment bases are designed to be self-occluding. The use of occlusive films can increase the penetration of corticosteroids by a factor of 100 and of lower-molecular-weight drugs up to 5-fold.

In the idealised model of the stratum corneum shown in Fig. 10.8, L represents the lipid-rich interstitial phase and P the proteinaceous phase. If $\rho = P_L/P_P$ (the ratio of the partition coefficients of the drug between vehicle and the L and P phases), and D_L and

D_P are the diffusion coefficients of the drug in these phases, the flux through stratum corneum of average thickness (40 μm) is found to reduce to

$$J = 0.98\rho \frac{D_L}{D_P} \ (\mu g\,cm^{-2}\,h^{-1}) \qquad (10.6)$$

when $\rho(D_L/D_P)$ is very small. When $\rho(D_L/D_P)$ is very large, the flux becomes

$$J = (2.3 \times 10^{-4})\rho \frac{D_L}{D_P} \ (\mu g\,cm^{-2}\,h^{-1}) \qquad (10.7)$$

which emphasises the importance of both the partition coefficient and diffusion coefficient of the drug in the absorption process.

10.3.2 Influence of the drug

The diffusion coefficient of the drug in the skin will be determined by factors such as molecular size, shape and charge; the partition coefficient will be determined not only by the properties of the drug but also by the vehicle as this represents the donor phase, the skin being the receptor phase. The quantity ρ can be approximated by experimentally determined oil/water partition coefficients. Substances that have a very low oil solubility will have lower rates of penetration.

The major pathway of transport for water-soluble molecules is transcellular, involving passage through cells and cell walls. The pathway for lipid-soluble molecules is presumably the endogenous lipid within the stratum corneum, the bulk of this being intercellular. Increase in the polar character of the molecule decreases permeability, as seen from the data on steroids in Table 10.4, in which progesterone and

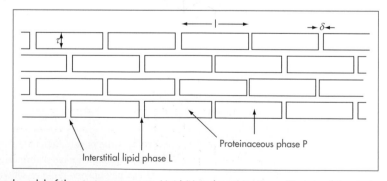

Figure 10.8 Idealised model of the stratum corneum. Lipid (L) and proteinaceous (P) parts of the stratum corneum are represented; this model is used to derive model equations for drug transport across this layer (see text).

Reproduced from Michaels AS et al., A I Chem J, 1975; 21: 985.

hydroxyprogesterone and deoxycortone and cortexolone should be compared. Each pair differs only by a hydroxyl group. The lipid/water partition coefficients of the drugs in Table 10.4 decrease as the number of hydroxyl groups increases, but a simple lipid/water partition coefficient is not an ideal guide, as the stratum corneum is a complex system as described above. If a substance is more soluble in the stratum corneum than in the vehicle in which it is presented, however, the concentration in the first layer of the skin may be higher than that in the vehicle. If depletion of the contact layers of the vehicle occurs, then the nature of the formulation will dictate how readily these are replenished by diffusion and, therefore, will dictate the rate of absorption.

The penetration rates of four steroids through intact abdominal autopsy skin were, in the order of their physiological activity, betametasone (betamethasone) 17-valerate (I) > desonide > triamcinolone acetonide (II) > hydrocortisone (III).

Table 10.4 Permeability constants of steroids[a]

Steroid	Structure	Permeability constant, κ_P (10^{-6} cm^{-2} h^{-1})
Progesterone		1500
Hydroxyprogesterone		600
Desoxycortone		450
Cortexolone		75

[a] Reproduced from Scheuplein R, *J Invest Dermatol*, 1976; 67: 672.

Structure I Betamethasone 17-valerate

Structure II Triamcinolone acetonide

Structure III Hydrocortisone

Clinical point

Note that the order of systemic and transdermal biological activities can be quite different. And of course the esters of certain steroids can results in startling differences in activity.

1   Triamcinolone is five times more active systemically than hydrocortisone, but has only one-tenth of its topical activity.
2   Betamethasone is 30 times as active as hydrocortisone systemically but has only four times the topical potency.
3   Triamcinolone acetonide has a topical activity 1000 times that of the parent steroid because of its favourable lipid solubility.

Of 23 esters of betamethasone (**IV**), the 17-valerate ester possesses the highest topical activity. The vasoconstrictor potency of betamethasone 17-valerate is 360 (fluocinolone acetonide $= 100$), that of betamethasone 0.8, of its 17-acetate 114, of the 17-propionate 190, and of the 17-octanoate 10. The peak activity coincides with an optimal partition coefficient, one that favours neither lipid nor aqueous phase.

Structure IV Betamethasone

10.3.3 Influence of the vehicle

Consideration of equation (10.3) shows immediately that the vehicle has an influence on the absorption of the drug; if the vehicle is changed so that the drug becomes less soluble in it, P increases and so permeability increases. The vehicle is more dominant in topical therapy than in most routes of administration because the vehicle remains at the site, although not always in an unchanged form. Evaporation of water from a w/o base would leave drug molecules immersed in the oily phase. Oil-in-water emulsion systems may invert to water-in-oil systems, in such a way that the drug would have to diffuse through an oily layer to reach the skin. Volatile components are driven off, probably altering the state of saturation of the drug and hence its activity. Drug may precipitate owing to lack of remaining solvent. This all means that theoretical approaches very much represent the simplest or in thermodynamic terms 'ideal' cases.

Formulations

Many modern dermatological formulations are washable oil-in-water systems. Simple aqueous lotions are also used as they have a cooling effect on the skin. Ointments are used for the application of insoluble or oil-soluble medicaments and leave a greasy film on the skin, inhibiting loss of moisture and encouraging the hydration of the keratin layer. Aqueous creams combine the characteristics of the lotions and ointments. A classification of semisolid bases is given in Fig. 10.9.

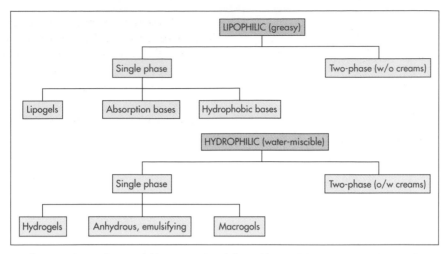

Figure 10.9 Classification of topical semisolid bases into lipophilic and hydrophilic systems in either single-phase or two-phase forms.

The descriptions 'ointment' and 'cream' have no universally accepted meaning and generally refer to the completed formulation. Ointments are generally composed of single-phase hydrophobic bases, such as pharmaceutical grades of soft paraffin or microcrystalline paraffin wax.

'Absorption' bases have an alleged capacity to facilitate absorption by the skin, but the term also alludes to their ability to take up considerable amounts of water to form water-in-oil emulsions. Lipogels are gels prepared by dispersion of long-chain fatty acid soaps such as aluminium monostearate in a hydrocarbon base. Hydrogels prepared from Carbopols or cellulose derivatives are discussed in Chapter 7.

Thermodynamic activity in topical products

The complexity of many of the topical bases means that a physicochemical explanation of their influence on the release of medicament is not always possible. It is not difficult, however, to ascertain this influence and to highlight the problem. The interactions between the physical properties of the base and the drug are exemplified by the effect of propylene glycol in simple bases shown in Fig. 10.10, where the percentage of the glycol acting as a solvent for the drug significantly affects permeation.

The thermodynamic activity of the drug is the ultimate determinant of its biological activity. If the solubility of the drug in the base is increased by addition of propylene glycol, then its partition coefficient, P, towards the skin is reduced. On the other hand, increasing the amount that can be incorporated in the base is an advantage and the concentration (C_v) gradient is increased. It is apparent that there will be an optimum amount of solubiliser. The optimum occurs at the level of additive that just solubilises the medicament. Addition of excess results in desaturation of the system, and a decrease in thermodynamic activity. As the total amount of drug in the vehicle is increased from 0.5 to $1.0\,\mathrm{mg\,g}^{-1}$ (Fig. 10.10b) more propylene glycol has to be added to cause a decrease in C_vP. From Fig. 10.10b one could postulate that threefold dilution of a formulation containing $1.0\,\mathrm{mg\,g}^{-1}$ and 60% solubiliser with a base with no solubiliser would cause the thermodynamic activity to increase. The vehicle affects penetration only when the release of drug is rate-limiting.

In situations where all of the activity gradient is in the applied phase, skin properties play no part. In these cases drug concentration in the vehicle, the diffusion coefficient of the drug in the system and the solubility of the drug are the significant factors. Where these factors are not important, the only significant factor involving the vehicle is the thermodynamic activity of the drug contained in it. Using the simplest model, for a solution of concentration C applied to an area A of the skin, the steady-state rate of penetration, $\mathrm{d}Q/\mathrm{d}t$, is given by

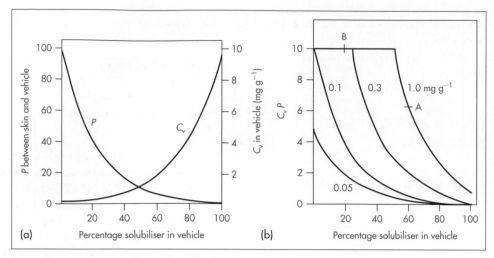

Figure 10.10 (a) Drug partition coefficient and solubility dependence on vehicle composition for the 'ideal' case. (b) Predicted relative steady-state penetration (C_vP) as a function of vehicle composition for the 'ideal' case. Point A represents a formulation containing $1.0\,\text{mg g}^{-1}$ and 60% solubiliser. On 3-fold dilution with a base containing no solubiliser, point B is arrived at where C_vP is higher.

Reproduced from Poulsen BJ, in: Ariens EJ, ed., *Drug Design*, vol. 4, New York: Academic Press; 1973.

$$\frac{\mathrm{d}Q}{\mathrm{d}t} = \frac{PCDA}{\delta} \tag{10.8}$$

δ being the thickness of the barrier phase. An equivalent form of this equation expresses release in terms of the thermodynamic activity, a, of the agent in the vehicle:

$$\frac{\mathrm{d}Q}{\mathrm{d}t} = \frac{a}{\gamma}\frac{DA}{\delta} \tag{10.9}$$

where γ is the activity coefficient of the agent in the skin barrier phase. Ointments containing finely ground particles of drug where the thermodynamic activity is equal to that of solid drug will have the same rate of penetration, provided that the passage of the drug in the barrier phase is rate-limiting.

Drug release from complex vehicles

In more complex vehicles the activity a is impossible to determine and other approaches must be adopted. For example, in emulsions the relative affinity of drug for the external and internal phases of the emulsion is an important factor. A drug dissolved in an internal aqueous phase of a w/o emulsion must be able to diffuse through the oily layer to reach the skin. Three cases can be considered: solution, suspension and emulsion systems.

1. Release from *solutions* is most readily understood and quantified by equations of the form

$$\frac{\mathrm{d}Q}{\mathrm{d}t} = C_0\left(\frac{D}{\pi t}\right)^{1/2} \tag{10.10}$$

$$Q = 2C_0\left(\frac{Dt}{\pi}\right)^{1/2} \tag{10.11}$$

where C_0 is the initial medicament concentration in solution, D is the diffusion coefficient, and t is the time after application of the vehicle. As D is inversely proportional to the viscosity of the vehicle, one would expect that drug release would be slower from a viscous vehicle.

2. If a drug in *suspension* is to have any action it must have a degree of solubility in the base used. An aged suspension of a drug will therefore have a saturated solution of the drug present in the continuous phase. Release of medicament in these conditions is given by

$$\frac{\mathrm{d}Q}{\mathrm{d}t} = \kappa_{\mathrm{sp}}\left(\frac{C_0C_sD}{2t}\right)^{1/2} \tag{10.12}$$

where C_s is the total solubility of the drug in the vehicle and C_0 is the concentration in the vehicle. This equation applies only when $C_s \ll C_0$. Only material in solution penetrates the stratum corneum and the depleted layer in the vehicle is replenished only by solution of particles and diffusion of the drug molecules to the depleted layer.

3. The equations for *emulsion-type* vehicles are discussed in Chapter 6.

10.3.4 Dilution of topical steroid preparations

Clinical point

Inappropriate dilution of carefully formulated creams and ointments may result in changes in stability and the effectiveness. An example would be clobetasol propionate formulated in a base containing the optimum amount of propylene glycol. The solubilities of the steroid as a function of propylene glycol concentration are shown in Fig. 10.11. A 1 in 2 dilution of a 0.05% cream, with a vehicle containing water and no propylene glycol, will precipitate a large proportion of the steroid. The same principles apply to steroids presented in a fatty acid propylene glycol base.

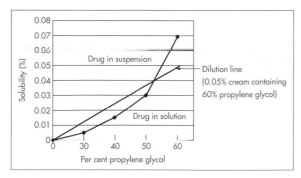

Figure 10.11 A diagram showing the solubility of clobetasol propionate as a function of propylene glycol concentration. The dilution line shows that if a 0.05% cream containing 60% propylene glycol is diluted with a base not containing the glycol, the drug will be precipitated.

Data from Busse M, *Pharm J*, 1978; 220: 25.

10.3.5 Transdermal medication: patches and devices

The ease with which some drugs can pass through the skin barrier into the circulating blood means that the transdermal route of medication is a possible alternative to the oral route. Theoretically there are several advantages:

- For drugs that are normally taken orally, administration through the skin can eliminate the vagaries that influence gastrointestinal absorption, such as pH changes and variations in food intake and intestinal transit time.
- A drug may be introduced into the systemic circulation without initially entering the portal circulation and passing through the liver.
- Constant and continuous administration of drugs may be achieved by a simple application to the skin surface.
- Continuous administration of drugs percutaneously at a controlled rate should permit elimination of pulse entry into the systemic circulation, an effect that is often associated with side-effects.
- Absorption of medication can be rapidly terminated whenever therapy must be interrupted.

Not all drugs are suitable for transdermal delivery. The limitations of the route are indicated in Table 10.5, which compares the percutaneous absorption of a range of drugs, from aspirin (only 22% of which is absorbed even after 120 hours) to chloramphenicol, of which only 2% is absorbed. The transdermal route is now routinely used for a range of drugs, oestrogens, clonidine and nicotine included. The four basic forms of patch systems are shown in Fig. 10.12.

Maximum flux from a saturated aqueous system of several drugs was estimated to be $300\,\mu g\,cm^{-2}\,h^{-1}$ and from a mineral oil system $250\,\mu g\,cm^{-1}$. Using a 'patch' with a rate-limiting polymeric membrane (see section 8.6.4), delivery is controlled to $40–50\,\mu g\,cm^{-2}\,h^{-1}$; that is, it is presented to the skin at that rate. A $10\,cm^2$ device will therefore deliver $0.4–0.5\,mg\,h^{-1}$. Control of release can be exercised by altering the membrane's properties and by changing the pH of the reservoir solution for a drug such as hyoscine (Fig. 10.13).

Table 10.5 Percutaneous absorption of a range of drugs in humans[a]

Drug	Percentage dose absorbed (120 h)
Aspirin	22
Chloramphenicol	2
Hexachlorophene	3
Salicylic acid	23
Urea	6
Caffeine	48

[a] Reproduced from Beckett AH *et al.*, *J Pharm Pharmacol*, 1972; 24: 65P.

Figure 10.12 The four main types of transdermal patch: matrix, reservoir, multilaminate and drug-in-adhesive designs. The matrix and reservoir systems are cut away to show the drug.

Illustration courtesy of 3M.

Iontophoresis

Iontophoresis is the process by which the migration of ionic drugs into tissues such as skin is enhanced by the use of an electric current, a technique that has found application favour in facilitating the delivery of peptides and proteins. A typical iontophoretic device is shown in Fig. 10.14.

Current can be applied in a continuous manner using either direct current (e.g. $0.1 \, \text{mA cm}^{-2}$) or pulsed ($0.1 \, \text{mA cm}^{-2}$; 2000 Hz) to either solutions or gels of a drug. Enhancement of migration results from several possible sources of which two are:

- Convective flow (electro-osmosis)
- Current-induced increases in skin permeability

The flux of drug can be increased by increasing current density. Movement of small (mol wt < 500 Da) neutral and charged compounds increases linearly with current density; with larger drugs (mol wt > 1000 Da), the fraction of total current flowing that is carried by the drugs is small because of competition for smaller ions. Electro-osmosis probably plays a greater role here. Figure 10.15 shows the effect of pH, osmolality and current density on the transport of the nonapeptide buserelin through stratum corneum.

10.3.6 Ultrasound and transdermal penetration

Therapeutic ultrasound has been found[2] to first expand and then collapse air bubbles in the stratum

Figure 10.13 The effect of hyoscine concentration and pH on the flux of hyoscine across a membrane; increasing the pH increases the flux as ionisation is decreased.

Reproduced from Michaels AS *et al.*, *A I Chem J*, 1975; 21: 985.

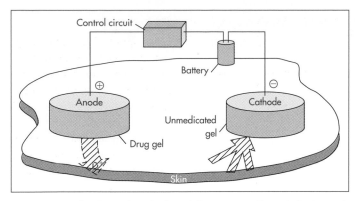

Figure 10.14 The major components of an iontophoretic drug-delivery system. To optimise iontophoretic transdermal drug delivery, the drug should be charged. It should be applied under an electrode of the same polarity, and a counterelectrode opposite in charge to the drug must be placed at an indifferent site on the body. Electric current must be allowed to flow for an appropriate duration at a level minimising skin irritation. Iontophoresis can deliver neutral drugs by inducing solvent flow (electro-osmosis) that results from the migration of ionic species in the applied field. Drug candidates for iontophoretic transdermal delivery must usually be in a salt form with adequate aqueous solubility, be stable in an aqueous environment, and be sufficiently potent to allow therapeutic doses to be delivered at an acceptable current density.

Reproduced from Lattin GA *et al.*, *Ann N Y Acad Sci*, 1991; 618: 450.

corneum (the process of cavitation) (Fig 10.16). Cavitation tends to liquefy the solid fats and allows molecules such as insulin to pass through the skin at levels that in diabetic rats cause blood sugar lowering. The permeability of the skin was found to increase as the frequency of ultrasound decreased and no long-term damage was caused.

10.3.7 Jet injectors

Invented in 1947 as a needle-free method of delivering drugs to the skin,[3] jet injection techniques have received renewed attention recently. They perhaps have not lived up to recent promise, because of a certain unreliability of drug penetration, drug collection or pooling on the skin[4] and rebound of particles from the skin surface. The systems are based on the high-velocity ejection of particles from the injector, through an orifice. Drug delivery is then due to either or both of skin 'failure' and flow through the skin.[4] The theoretical maximum velocity (v) of the jet is related to the pressure (P) in the nozzle and the density (ρ) of the liquid by

$$v = \left(\frac{2P}{\rho}\right)^{1/2} \tag{10.13}$$

but the velocity is affected by diameter of the orifice and is reduced by turbulence and friction.

10.3.8 Topical treatment of the nails: trans-ungual therapy

Treatment of fungal infections of the nail requires special topical approaches. It is a subject that has been the subject of several reviews. The same basic parameters hold for ensuring delivery via the nail as through the skin, but Murdan in her review[5] concludes:

'The permeability of the compact, highly keratinised nail plate to topically applied drugs is poor and drug uptake into the nail apparatus is extremely low. Topical therapy is worth pursuing, however, as local action is required in many nail disorders.' Research aimed at enhancing ungual drug uptake following topical application may be divided into three approaches[6]: (i) understanding the physicochemical factors that influence drug permeation into the nail plate; (ii) the use of chemical enhancers which cause alterations in the nail plate, thus assisting drug permeation; and (iii) the use of drug-containing nail lacquers which are brushed onto nail plates and which act as a drug depot from which drug can be continuously released into the nail.

(a)

(b)

Figure 10.15 (a) The influence of donor pH and ionic strength of the donor medium on buserelin (a nonapeptide) permeation. (b) Continuous iontophoresis and release of buserelin through the stratum corneum, showing the effect of increasing the current.

Reproduced from Knoblauch P, Moll F, *J Control Release*, 1993; 26: 203.

 Key points

- The barrier layer of the skin is the stratum corneum, which behaves like a passive diffusion barrier. The physicochemical factors that control drug penetration include the hydration of the stratum corneum, temperature, pH, drug concentration, and the molecular characteristics of the penetrant and the vehicle.
- Penetration of water and low-molecular-weight nonelectrolyte solutes through the epidermis is proportional to their concentration, and to the partition coefficient of the solute between tissue and vehicle; solute flux can be calculated using a form of Fick's law.
- The major pathway of transport for water-soluble molecules is *transcellular*, involving passage through cells and cell walls. The pathway for lipid-soluble molecules is the endogenous lipid within the stratum corneum, the bulk of this being *intercellular*. Increase in the polar character of the molecule decreases permeability by this route. Drug molecules may penetrate the skin not only through the stratum corneum but also by way of the hair follicles or through the sweat ducts, but these offer only a comparatively minor route.

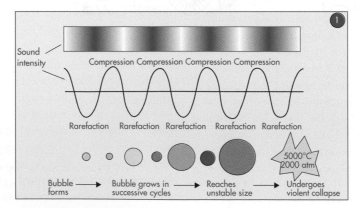

Figure 10.16 The process of cavitation leading to bubble collapse and change in fat structures and expulsion of drug.

- The vehicle in which the drug is applied influences the rate and extent of absorption; formulations can change rapidly once they have been spread on the skin, with absorption of some excipients and evaporative loss of water.
- Many dermatological formulations are washable oil-in-water systems. Simple aqueous lotions are also used as they have a cooling effect on the skin. Ointments are used for the application of insoluble or oil-soluble medicaments; aqueous creams combine the characteristics of the lotions and ointments. Other vehicles such as suspensions and emulsions may be used and equations predicting drug release from these have been given.
- In addition, transdermal medication may be achieved using patches (matrix, reservoir, multilaminate or drug-in-adhesive) and jet injectors, and may be enhanced by iontophoresis or by ultrasound.

10.4 Medication of the eye and the eye as a route for systemic delivery

The eye is not, of course, a conduit for the administration of drugs to the body, although it has been explored for the systemic delivery of peptides and proteins such as insulin. It is considered here because absorption of drugs does occur from medication applied to the eye, producing sometimes toxic systemic effects, although often the desired local effect is on the eye or its component parts. We will consider the factors affecting drug absorption from the eye, and those properties of formulations that affect drug performance. A wide range of drug types are placed in the eye, including antimicrobials, antihistamines, decongestants, mydriatics, miotics and cycloplegic agents.

Drugs are usually applied to the eye in the form of drops or ointments for local action. The absorbing surface is the cornea. Drug absorbed by the conjunctiva enters the systemic circulation. It is useful to consider some of the properties of the absorbing surfaces and their environment.

10.4.1 The eye

The eye (Fig. 10.17) has two barrier systems: a blood–aqueous barrier and a blood–vitreous barrier. The

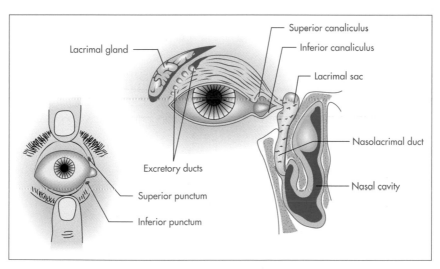

Figure 10.17 Diagrams of parts of the eye of importance in medication: the superior and inferior punctae are the drainage ports for solutions and tear fluids, and medicaments can drain via the canaliculi into the nasolacrimal duct and then to the nasal cavity, from whose surfaces absorption can occur.

Modified from Robinson JR, ed., *Ophthalmic Drug Delivery Systems*, Washington DC: American Pharmaceutical Association; 1980.

former is composed of the ciliary epithelium, the epithelium of the posterior surface of the iris, and blood vessels within the iris. Solutes and drugs enter the aqueous humour at the ciliary epithelium and at blood vessels. Many substances are transported out of the vitreous humour at the retinal surface. Solutes also leave the vitreous humour by diffusing to the aqueous humour of the posterior chamber.

Figure 10.17 is a diagrammatic representation of those parts of the eye involved in drug absorption. The cornea and the conjunctiva are covered with a thin fluid film, the tear film, which protects the cornea from dehydration and infection. Cleansed corneal epithelium is hydrophobic, physiological saline forming a contact angle of about 50° with it, and it has, in this clean condition, a critical surface tension of 28 mN m^{-1}. The aqueous phase of tear fluid is spread by blinking.

Tears

Tears comprise inorganic electrolytes – sodium, potassium and some calcium ions, chloride and hydrogencarbonate counterions – as well as glucose. The macromolecular components include some albumin, globulins and lysozyme. Lipids that form a monolayer over the tear fluid surface derive from the Meibomian glands, which open on to the edges of the upper and lower lids. This secretion consists mainly of cholesteryl esters with low melting points (35°C) due to the predominance of double bonds and branched-chain structures.

Clinical point

Tear fluid lies on the surface of the cornea and its importance lies in the possibility that components of formulations or drugs themselves can so alter the properties of the corneal surface, or interact with components of the tear fluid, that tear coverage of the eye is disrupted. When this occurs the so-called dry-eye syndrome (xerophthalmia) may arise, characterised by the premature break-up of the tear layer resulting in dry spots on the corneal surface.

10.4.2 Absorption of drugs applied to the eye

The cornea, which is the main barrier to absorption, consists of three parts: the epithelium, the stroma and the endothelium. Both the endothelium and the epithelium have a high lipid content and, as with most membranes, they are penetrated by drugs in their unionised lipid-soluble forms. The stroma lying between these two structures has a high water content, however, and thus drugs that have to negotiate the corneal barrier successfully must be both lipid-soluble and water-soluble to some extent (Fig. 10.18).

Tears have some buffering capacity so, as we noted before, the pH-partition hypothesis has to be applied with some circumspection. The acid-neutralising power of the tears when 0.1 cm^3 of a 1% solution of a drug is instilled into the eye is approximately equivalent to 10 µL of a 0.01 mol dm^{-3} strong base. The pH for either maximum solubility (see Chapter 4) or maximum stability (see Chapter 3) of a drug may well be below the optimum in relation to acceptability and activity. Under these conditions it is possible to use a buffer with a low buffering capacity to maintain a low pH adequate to prevent change in pH due to alkalinity of glass or carbon dioxide ingress from the air. When such drops are instilled into the eye, the tears will participate in a fairly rapid return to normal pH.

Clinical point

In agreement with the pH-partition hypothesis, raising the pH from 5 to 8 results in a 2- to 3-fold increase in the amount of pilocarpine reaching the anterior chamber. It is also found, however, that glycerol penetration increases to the same extent. The clue to why this should be so lies in the effect of the buffer solutions on lacrimation. Increased tear flow reduces the concentration of drug in the bathing fluid; loss of drug solution through the punctae and nasolacrimal ducts does not affect concentration, as the whole fluid drains away.

Solution concentration is reduced only by diffusion of drug across the cornea or conjunctiva or by

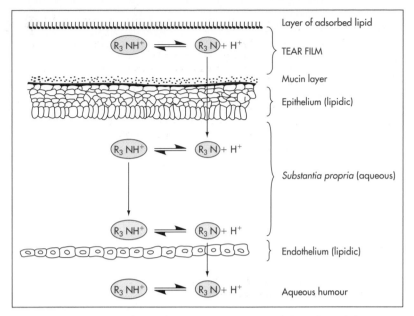

$R_3NH^+ \rightleftharpoons R_3N + H^+$ — Layer of adsorbed lipid — TEAR FILM

Mucin layer

Epithelium (lipidic)

$R_3NH^+ \rightleftharpoons R_3N + H^+$

Substantia propria (aqueous)

$R_3NH^+ \rightleftharpoons R_3N + H^+$

Endothelium (lipidic)

$R_3NH^+ \rightleftharpoons R_3N + H^+$ — Aqueous humour

Figure 10.18 Diagrammatic representation of a tear film and the penetration of a base through the cornea; in this example R_3N represents a drug such as homatropine.

Modified from Moses RA, *Adler's Physiology of the Eye*, 5th edn, St Louis: Mosby; 1970.

tear inflow. The pH 5 solution induced more tear flow than the pH 8 solution; thus the concentration gradient is reduced and transport of both ionised and non-ionic drugs is less at pH 5. At pH 11, absorption of pilocarpine is reduced because of the irritant effects of this solution on the eye.[7] Mechanical irritation can produce the same effects and this can override the influence of other formulation factors.

Aqueous humour

As the examples above have shown, both water-soluble and lipid-soluble drugs can enter the aqueous humour. The pH-partition hypothesis thus accounts only imperfectly for different rates of entry into the aqueous humour. Sucrose and raffinose pass through the leaky ciliary epithelium and reach steady-state aqueous/plasma concentration ratios of 0.2 and 0.3, respectively. Lipid-soluble drugs, including chloramphenicol and some tetracyclines can achieve higher concentrations as they can enter by both pathways. Penicillins, however, reach only low aqueous/plasma concentration ratios because they are removed from aqueous humour by absorption through the ciliary epithelium. Proteins are excluded, so that protein binding of ophthalmic drugs limits their absorption.

10.4.3 Influence of formulation

Pilocarpine activity has been compared in various formulations. Figure 10.19 shows some of the results on formulations, including results on ointments designed to prolong the contact of the drug with the cornea. One of the most difficult problems is to design vehicles that will retard drainage and prolong contact. Viscous polymer vehicles help to some extent but are not the complete answer. The rate of drainage of drops decreased as their viscosity increased and these factors contribute to an increased concentration of the drug in the precorneal film and aqueous humour.[8] The magnitude of the concentration increase was small considering the 100-fold change in the viscosity, and it was concluded that the viscosity of the solution is not as important a factor in bioavailability as was previously thought.

The results of incorporating pilocarpine (**V**) (a relatively water-soluble drug) and fluorometholone (a lipophilic drug) into a water-in-oil ointment base can be compared in Fig. 10.20. Pilocarpine is thought to be released only when in contact with aqueous tear fluid, whereas the steroid, being soluble in the base, can diffuse through the base to replenish the surface concentrations and thus produce a sustained effect.

Structure V Pilocarpine ($pK_a = 7.05$)

Polymeric vehicles

Hydrophilic polymeric vehicles, such as poly(vinyl alcohol) (PVA) and hydroxypropylmethylcellulose (HPMC), are used in ophthalmic formulations.[9] PVA increases the effectiveness of the drug substance, most likely by slowing the drainage rate of the eye drops. The viscosity of Newtonian fluids should be greater than 4.4 cP to influence drainage times, with a maximum effect at 100 cP. HPMC has been found to enhance the activity reduce the effective dose of neomycin sulfate required to prevent infection of corneas of experimental animals (Table 10.6).

Figure 10.19 Aqueous humour levels of pilocarpine after dosing with 10^{-2} mol dm^{-3} ointment and solution in intact and abraded eyes. ●, 25 mg of ointment, intact eyes; ○, 25 mg of ointment, abraded eyes; ■, 25 mm^3 of solution, intact eyes; □, 25 mm^3 of solution, abraded eyes; all points represent an average of 8–16 eyes.

Reproduced from reference 7.

> ✚ Clinical point
>
> Eye drops are often formulated to be isotonic with tear fluid, but deviations from tonicity do not cause major problems, although hypertonicity may cause stinging of the eye and hypotonicity may increase the permeability of the cornea. Some ingredients may increase the permeability of the cornea. Surfactants are known to interact with membranes to increase the permeability: benzalkonium chloride has surfactant properties and may well have some effect on corneal permeability, although its primary purpose is as a bacteriostat and bactericide. Chlorhexidine acetate and cetrimide, both of which are surface-active, are also used.

Figure 10.20 Aqueous humour levels after dosing with pilocarpine and fluorometholone in ointment and aqueous solution. ●, 10^{-2} mol dm^{-3} pilocarpine solution; ○, 10^{-2} mol dm^{-3} pilocarpine ointment; ▲, saturated fluorometholone solution; △, 0.1% fluorometholone ointment.

Reproduced from reference 7.

Log P

The influence of log P of beta-blockers (Table 10.7) on their permeation coefficients into conjunctiva and cornea is shown in Fig. 10.21. In humans, the conjunctiva has 17 times the surface area of the cornea and therefore it absorbs significant amounts of drug. Work has centred on increasing corneal permeability or retention

Table 10.6 Calculated effective dose (ED_{50}) of neomycin sulfate required to prevent infection in 50% of rabbit corneas when incorporated into various vehicles[a]

Vehicle	Derived values (mg base per cm³)	
	ED_{50}	95% confidence limits
HPMC, 0.5%	0.50	0.403–0.620
PVA, 1.4%	1.00	0.750–1.330
PVP, 1.4%	1.10	0.89–1.35
Distilled water	1.03	0.84–1.27

[a] Reproduced from Bach FC *et al.*, *Am J Ophthalmol*, 1970; 69: 659.

of the drug (or product) in the conjunctiva sac. Appropriate doses of drug can achieve a degree of corneal or conjunctival selectivity, represented in Fig. 10.21c by the ratio *C/J*. Increasing lipophilicity increases the *C/J* ratio from <0.1 to approximately 0.5. The locus of the drug is important in understanding adverse reactions. With increasing lipophilicity, the uptake of beta blockers into the choroid–retinal pigment epithelium, iris–ciliary body, sclera and cornea increased. However, the levels of drug in the retina, vitreous fluid and lens decreased.

The prodrug approach

Attempts have been made to improve the performance of drugs used in the eye. One approach has been to modify the drug substance to increase its ability to penetrate the corneal barrier. In Fig. 10.22, the results of application of 0.5% epinephrine (adrenaline) (**VI**) and 0.16% of the dipivoyl derivative of epinephrine (dipivefrine) (**VII**) are shown. The more hydrophobic derivative is absorbed to a greater extent and is then hydrolysed to the active parent molecule in the aqueous humour.

Structure VI Epinephrine (adrenaline)

Structure VII Dipivoyl epinephrine (dipivefrine; compare with Structure VI)

Derivatives of pilocarpine such as the hexadecanoyloxymethylene chloride (**VIII**) similarly show the advantages of the epinephrine prodrug.

R^1 = H, CH₃
R^2 = (CH₂)ₙCH₃
n = 10–16

Structure VIII Pilocarpine derivatives

Reservoir systems

Since the advent of soft contact lenses, attempts have been made to use these as drug reservoirs;[10] a drug such as pilocarpine is imbibed from solutions into the polymer matrix and when this is placed in the eye the drug leaches out, generally over a period of up to 24 hours. Levels of prednisolone applied in a copolymer of 2-hydroxyethyl methacrylate and N-vinyl-2-pyrrolidone were compared with levels in aqueous humour, cornea and iris after applications of prednisolone in solution. When the drug was incorporated into the lens, aqueous and corneal levels of the drug were 2- to 3-fold higher 4 hours after insertion.

The Ocusert device (Fig. 10.23) releases controlled amounts of pilocarpine over a period of 7 days and is designed for the treatment of glaucoma. It comprises a drug reservoir in which pilocarpine is embedded in an alginic acid matrix, and this is bounded by two rate-controlling membranes of polymer (vinyl acetate–ethylene copolymer). It is inserted into the lower conjunctival sac of the eye. The rate-controlling membranes are subject to strict quality control during manufacture and their thicknesses adjusted to give the appropriate flux of drug, either 20 or 40 µg h⁻¹. The difference between the two available systems is effected

Table 10.7 Log *P* values of beta-blockers (in increasing order of lipophilicity)

Compound		Log *P*
Sotalol		−0.62
Atenolol		0.16
Nadolol		0.93
Pindolol		1.75
Acebutolol		1.77
Metoprolol		1.88
Timolol		1.91
Oxprenolol		2.07
Levobunolol		2.40
Labetalol		2.55
Alprenolol		2.61
Propranolol		3.21
Betaxolol		3.44

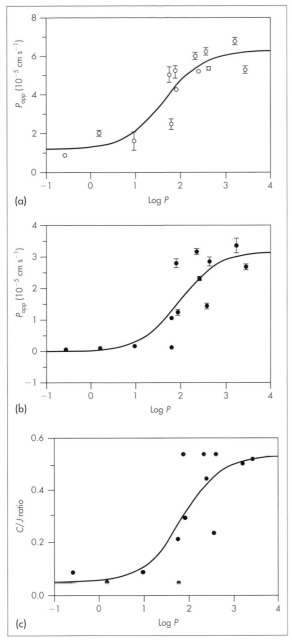

Figure 10.21   Influence of drug lipophilicity (log P) on the permeability coefficients (P_{app}) of beta blockers across (a) the conjunctiva and (b) the cornea of the pigmented rabbit. Plot (c) shows the influence of log P on the ratio of the corneal (C) and conjunctival (J) permeability coefficients.

Reproduced from Wong W *et al., Curr Eye Res*, 1991: 6: 571.

by altering the amount of di-(2-ethylhexyl)phthalate in the polymer; increasing the concentration of this plasticiser increases the permeability to pilocarpine.

10.4.4 Systemic effects from eye-drops

Most of the dose applied to the eye in the form of drops reaches the systemic circulation and typically less than 5% acts on ocular tissues.

 Clinical point

Atropine toxicity resulting from the use of the eye-drops to dilate the pupil has been reported,[11] as has a rise in blood pressure in premature infants following the use of 10% phenylephrine eye-drops in preparation for ophthalmoscopy.[12] The mucosa in the eye, nose and mouth of infants is much thinner and more permeable to a drug than is, say, the skin. Drugs placed in the eye, nose or mouth, moreover, may bypass the metabolic transformations which may inactivate the drug given orally. Reduction in exercise tachycardia in normal volunteers is induced following administration of 0.5% timolol eye-drops, showing the significant effects of beta blockers.

 Key points

- Drugs (including antimicrobials, antihistamines, decongestants, mydriatics, miotics and cycloplegic agents) are usually applied to the eye in the form of drops or ointments for local action.
- The eye has two barrier systems: a blood–aqueous barrier and a blood–vitreous barrier.
- The absorbing surface is the cornea, which comprises an epithelium, a stroma and an endothelium; the epithelium and endothelium have high lipid contents and are penetrated by drugs in their un-ionised form, the stroma lying between the two other structures has a high water content. Thus drugs that have to negotiate the corneal barrier successfully must be both

Figure 10.30 Longitudinal view of the Rotahaler.

Reproduced from Hallworth GW, *Br J Clin Pharmacol*, 1977; 4: 689.

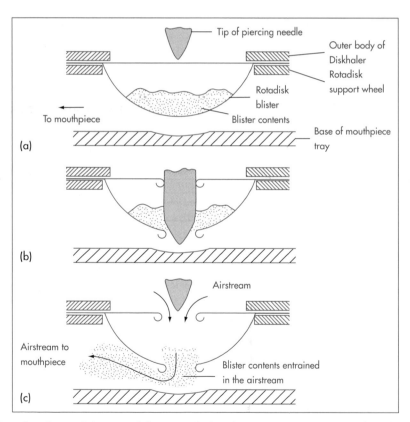

Figure 10.31 Dispersion of Ventodisk or Becodisk contents by breath actuation: a cross-section of a Diskhaler is shown with a disc located on the support wheel. (a) A disc is located beneath an aperture in the body of the Diskhaler through which a piercing needle enters. (b) The needle penetrates the upper and lower surfaces of the blister. (c) The patient inhales through the device and pierced blister, entraining the blister contents into the airstream.

Reproduced from Farr SJ *et al.*, in: Florence AT, Salole EG, eds., *Routes of Drug Administration*, London: Wright; 1990.

Table 10.9 Physicochemical properties of hydrofluoroalkanes[a]

Propellant	Molecular formula	Molecular weight	Boiling point (°C) at 1.013 bar (1 atm)	Gauge vapour pressure (psig) at 20°C
HFA 134a	$C_2H_2F_4$	102.0	−26.5	68.4
HFA 227	C_3HF_7	170.0	−17.3	56.0

[a] Data from reference 16.

where p_i is the partial vapour pressure of a component i in the vapour phase, x_i is the mole fraction of that component in solution and $p_i^\ominus$ is the vapour pressure of the pure component. Its application to this type of aerosol system is illustrated in Example 10.1.

Example 10.1 Calculation of the vapour pressure of a mixture of hydrofluoroalkanes

Assuming ideal behaviour, calculate the vapour pressure at 20°C above an aerosol mixture consisting of 30% w/w of HFA 134a (tetrafluoroethane, molecular weight 102 Da) with a vapour pressure of 68.4 psig and 70% w/w of HFA 227 (heptafluoropropane, molecular weight 170 Da) with a vapour pressure of 56.0 psig. Convert the pressure into pascals using the relationship between the various units of pressure shown in Box 10.2.

Answer

For the two propellants HFA 134a and HFA 227 with respective vapour pressures $p_{134}^\ominus$ and $p_{227}^\ominus$ we have

$$p_{134} = p_{134}^\ominus x_{134}$$

$$p_{227} = p_{227}^\ominus x_{227}$$

where p_{134} and p_{227} are the partial pressures of components HFA 134a and HFA 227 respectively, and x_{134} and x_{227} are the mole fractions of these components in the liquid phase.

Amount of HFA 134a in mixture = 30/102 = 0.2941 mole
Amount of HFA 227 in mixture = 70/170 = 0.4118 mole
$x_{134} = 0.2941/0.7059 = 0.4166$
$x_{227} = 0.4118/0.7059 = 0.5834$

From Dalton's law of partial pressures, the total vapour pressure P is the sum of the partial pressures of the component gases, assuming ideal behaviour. Thus,

$$p = p_{134}^\ominus x_{134} + p_{227}^\ominus x_{227}$$

and hence

$$P = (68.4 \times 0.4166) + (56.0 \times 0.5834) = 61.17 \, \text{psig}$$

Converting pressures into pascals (Pa) using

$$\text{psia} = \text{psig} = 14.7 \quad \text{and} \quad 1 \, \text{psia} = 6894.76 \, \text{Pa}$$

we obtain

$$P = 5.23 \times 10^5 \, \text{Pa}$$

Box 10.2 Pressure units

In practice, pressure is expressed in terms of a wide range of units. The SI unit is the pascal (Pa) where $1\ Pa = 1\ N\ m^{-2}$. Pressure should usually be converted to this unit before substitution into equations. The relationship of other commonly used pressure units to the pascal is as follows:

$1\ bar = 10^5\ Pa$
$1\ mmHg = 1\ torr = 133.32\ Pa$
$1\ atmos = 1.013 \times 10^5\ Pa$
$1\ psi* = 6894.76\ Pa$

Standard atmospheric pressure is $760\ mmHg = 760\ torr = 1.013\ bar = 1.013 \times 10^5\ Pa$.

*It is common to report vapour pressure of propellants as pounds per square inch gauge, psig. Gauge pressure uses the actual atmospheric pressure as the zero point for measurement and hence atmospheric pressure (14.7 psi at sea level) must be added to measurements quoted in psig to obtain the absolute pressure in pounds per square inch, psia, i.e.

psia = psig + 14.7

Binary mixtures of hydrofluoroalkanes show behaviour that approaches ideality.[17] Figure 10.32a shows the vapour pressure–composition plots for a mixture of the propellants HFA 134a (tetrafluoroethane) and HFA 227 (heptafluoropropane); the linearity of the plots indicates that Raoult's law is obeyed over the temperature range examined. It is frequently necessary to include a cosolvent such as alcohol in the aerosol formulation to enhance the solvent power of the propellant blend.[18] Figure 10.32b shows large positive deviations from Raoult's law due to interactions between the components of the formulation. In practical terms such behaviour is beneficial as it enables substantial addition of ethanol without reduction in vapour pressure and aerosol performance.

Optimisation of vapour pressure, drug stability, solubility and spray patterns take place during the design stage. Other ingredients of the formulation can include surfactants to act as solubilisers, stabilisers or lubricants to ease the passage of the particles when emitted from the valve.

The Autohaler has been devised as a breath-activated pressurised inhaler system because of the difficulty experienced by some patients in coordinating manual operation of an aerosol with inhalation. The Autohaler is activated by the negative pressure created during the inhalation phase of respiration and is specifically designed to respond to shallow inhalation in those with restricted pulmonary capacity.

Nebulisers[19]

Modern nebulisers for domestic and hospital use generate aerosols continuously for chronic therapy of respiratory disorders. A Venturi-type system is shown in Fig. 10.33a and an ultrasonic device in Fig. 10.33b. The particle size distribution and hence efficiency of such systems varies with the design and sometimes with the mode of use. Hence adequate monitoring of particle size is important. *In vitro* analysis of the particle size distribution of aerosols and nebulisers is discussed in Chapter 13.

Key points

- The respiratory tract epithelium has permeability characteristics similar to those of the classical biological membrane, so lipid-soluble compounds are absorbed more rapidly than lipid-insoluble molecules.
- Compared with the gastrointestinal mucosa, the pulmonary epithelium possesses a relatively high permeability to water-soluble molecules.
- The efficiency of inhalation therapy is often low because of the difficulty in targeting particles to the sites of maximal absorption.
- The major processes that influence deposition of drug particles in the respiratory tract are interception, impaction, gravitational settling, electrostatic attractions and Brownian diffusion.

Figure 10.32 (a) Plots of vapour pressure versus mole fraction of HFA 227 for propellant systems composed of HFA 134a and HFA 227 at 6, 16, 25 and 42°C showing ideality of mixing (Raoult's law obeyed). (b) Plots of vapour pressure of HFA 134a (circles) and HFA 227 (squares) versus mole fraction of ethanol at 21.5°C. Solid symbols represent experimental data; open symbols represent theoretical values calculated assuming ideal (Raoult's law) behaviour.

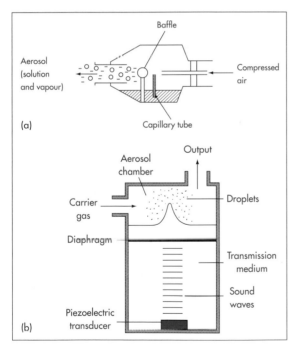

Figure 10.33 Schematic diagrams of (a) a Venturi-type nebuliser and (b) an ultrasonic nebuliser.

Modified from Egan DF, *Fundamentals of Respiratory Therapy*, 3rd edn, New York: Mosby; 1977.

- Deposition of particles in the various regions of the respiratory tract is dependent on particle size and size distribution; this will be affected by the nature of the aerosol-producing device and the formulation. Particles of hygroscopic materials are removed from the airstream more effectively than are non-hygroscopic particles because of their growth through uptake of water from the moist air in the respiratory tract.
- Delivery devices include pressurised aerosols and nebulisers.

10.8 The nasal route

Two main classes of medicinal agents are applied by the nasal route:

- Drugs for the alleviation of nasal symptoms
- Drugs that are inactivated in the gastrointestinal tract following oral administration and where the route is an alternative to injection, such as for peptides and proteins

Figure 10.34 The vascular network of the nasal mucous membrane in the inferior turbinate.

Intranasal beclometasone dipropionate in a dose as low as 200 µg daily is a useful addition to the therapy of perennial rhinitis. Considerable attention is being paid to the delivery by the nasal route of peptides and proteins such as insulin, luteinising hormone-releasing hormone (LHRH) analogues such as nafarelin, as well as vasopressin, thyrotropin-releasing hormone (TRH) analogues and adrenocorticotropic hormone (ACTH).

A diagram of the structures involved in delivery by the nasal route is given in Fig. 10.34. Formulations have to be efficiently delivered to the epithelial surfaces: what physical factors affect the utility of this route? Factors such as droplet or particle size that affect deposition in the respiratory tract are involved if administration is by aerosol, but formulations may also be applied directly to the nasal mucosa. The physiological condition of the nose, its vascularity, and mucus flow rate are therefore of importance. So too is the formulation used – the volume, concentration, viscosity, pH and tonicity of the applied medicament can affect activity.[20] As the condition of the nasal passages changes with changes in the environment, temperature and humidity, it is clearly not an ideal route for absorption of drugs or vaccines, but may be the only feasible route for some agents. As with all routes, however, absorption decreases with the increasing molecular weight of the active, as seen in Fig. 10.35 for a series of model molecules.

The air passages through the nasal cavity begin at the nares (nostrils) and terminate at the choanae (posterior nares). Immediately above the nares are the vestibules, lined by skin that bears relatively coarse hairs and sebaceous glands in its lower portion. The hairs curve radially downward, providing an effective barrier to the entry of relatively large particles. The division of the nasal cavity exposes the air to maximal surface area. As in the other parts of the respiratory tree, sudden changes in the direction of airflow cause

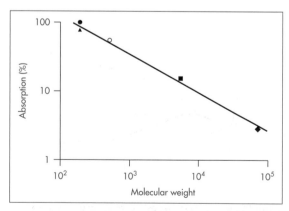

Figure 10.35 Correlation between the percentage dose absorbed after nasal administration and molecular weight: ●, 4-oxo-4*H*-1-benzopyran-2-carboxylic acid (chromocarb); ▲, *p*-aminohippuric acid; ○, sodium cromoglicate; ■, inulin; ◆, dextran; $r = -0.996$.

Reproduced from Fisher AN *et al.*, *J Pharm Pharmacol*, 1987; 39: 357.

impingement of large particles through inertial forces. The respiratory portion of the nasal passage is covered by a mucous membrane that has a mucous blanket secreted in part by the goblet cells. The ciliary streaming here is directed posteriorly so that the nasal mucus is transported towards the pharynx. Figure 10.36 shows the fractional deposition of inhaled particles in the nasal chamber as a function of their particle size. A diameter of not less than 10 μm minimises the loss of drug to the lung. In the external nares, removal of particles occurs on nasal hairs; further up inertial deposition takes place; and in the more tortuous upper passages deposition is assumed to be by inertia and sedimentation.

Comparison of the nasal route with other routes has been made in some instances. Desmopressin (1-desamino-8-d-arginine vasopressin) administered as 20 μg dose elicits a response equivalent to approximately 2 μg administered by IV injection. A greater dose of virus is required to obtain an equivalent response to a nasal vaccine than when administered by other routes. The role of the intranasal route for the delivery of peptides and proteins has been widely researched (see also Chapter 12); as can be inferred from above, the bioavailability of desmopressin acetate ranges from 9% to 20% in humans, buserelin 6% and salmon calcitonin 3% when compared with the IM route. Penetration enhancers can lead to increases in uptake, but insulin's bioavailability in human subjects ranges from only 3% to 13% depending on the study involved.

In the treatment of nasal symptoms the patient adjusts the dose so that, perhaps, the theoretical bases of droplet and particle retention are less vital. Although formulation of the nasal drops, or sprays from plastic squeeze-bottles must obviously influence the efficiency of medication, little work has in the past been carried out relating formulation to the effect of intranasal medicines. Microsphere delivery systems have received some attention, however, with special interest being directed to bioadhesive microsphere carriers.

10.9 Rectal absorption of drugs

Drugs administered by the rectal route in suppositories are placed in intimate contact with the rectal mucosa, which behaves as a normal lipoidal barrier. The pH in the rectal cavity lies between 7.2 and 7.4, but the rectal fluids have little buffering capacity. As with topical medication, the formulation of the suppository can have marked effects on the activity of the drug. Factors such as retention of the suppository for a sufficient duration of time in the rectal cavity also influence the outcome of therapy; the size and shape of the suppository and its melting point may also determine bioavailability.

The once traditional suppository base cocoa butter (theobroma oil) is a variable natural product that undergoes a polymorphic transition on heating. It is primarily a triglyceride. Four polymorphic forms exist: γ, m.p. 18.9°C; α, m.p. 23°C; β′, m.p. 28°C; and the stable β form, m.p. 34.5°C. Heating above 38°C converts the fat to a metastable mixture solidifying at 15–17°C instead of 25°C, and this subsequently melts at 24°C instead of at 31–35°C. Reconversion to the stable β-form takes 1–4 days depending on storage conditions.

Modern bases include polyoxyethylene glycols of molecular weight 1000–6000 Da and semisynthetic vegetable fats. The appropriate bases must be selected carefully for each substance. The important features of excipient materials are melting point, speed of crystallisation and emulsifying capacity. If the medicament dissolves in the base, it is likely that the melting point of the base will be lowered, so that a base with a melting point higher than 36–37°C has to be chosen.

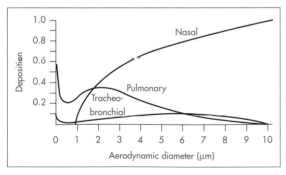

Figure 10.36 Regional deposition of inhaled particulate matter as a function of particle size; nose breathing at 15 respirations per minute and 730 cm³ tidal volume (the 'pulmonary compartment' refers to deposition beyond the terminal bronchiole).

Reproduced from Muir CDF, *Clinical Aspects of Inhaled Particles*, London: Heinemann; 1972.

If the drug substance has a high density, it is preferable that the base crystallises rapidly during production of the suppositories to prevent settling of the drug. Preservatives, hardening agents, emulsifiers, colouring agents and materials which modify the viscosity of the base after melting are common formulation additives.

The rectal cavity

The rectum is the terminal 15–19 cm of the large intestine. The mucous membrane of the rectal ampulla, with which suppositories and other rectal medications come into contact, is made up of a layer of cylindrical epithelial cells, without villi.

Figure 10.37 shows the blood supply to the rectal area. The main artery to the rectum is the superior rectal (haemorrhoidal) artery. Veins of the inferior part of the submucous plexus become the rectal veins, which drain to the internal pudendal veins. Drug absorption takes place through this venous network. Superior haemorrhoidal veins connect with the portal vein and thus transport drugs absorbed in the upper part of the rectal cavity to the liver; the inferior veins enter into the inferior vena cava and thus bypass the liver. The particular venous route the drug takes is affected by the extent to which the suppository migrates in its original or molten form further up the gastrointestinal tract, and this may be variable. The rectal route therefore does not necessarily, or even reproducibly, avoid the liver.

A schematic representation of the processes occurring following insertion of a suppository into the rectum is shown in Fig. 10.38. Cocoa butter suppositories usually liquefy within a few minutes, but the drug is not necessarily released from solution or suspension, as the fat in this case is not emulsified or absorbed. Surfactants may be required to aid dispersal of the fat and thus when this base is used the physicochemical properties of the drug are important. The rate-limiting step in drug absorption for suppositories made from a fatty base is the partitioning of the dissolved drug from the molten base, not the rate of solution of the drug in the body fluids.

The influence of the aqueous solubility on *in vitro* release from fat-based suppositories is shown in Fig. 10.39, the results being collated from the study of 35 drugs grouped into classes I–V in decreasing order of water solubility. The results may be explained as follows. The water-soluble active substances will be insoluble in the fatty base, while the less water-soluble material will tend to be soluble in the base, and will thus diffuse from the base more slowly. Water-soluble

Figure 10.37 Blood supply to the rectum and anus. The significance of the location of the superior and the inferior rectal veins is discussed in the text.

Reproduced from Tondury G, *Topographical Anatomy*, Stuttgart: Thieme; 1959.

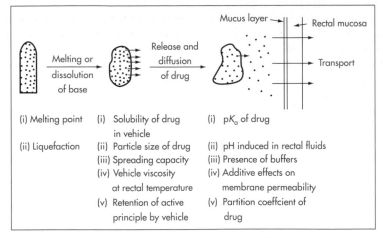

Figure 10.38 Schematic representation of rectal absorption of an active principle from a suppository, and the factors at each stage likely to affect the bioavailability of the drug.

Modified from Jaminet F, in: Guillot BR, Lombard AP, eds., *The Suppository*, Paris: Maloine; 1973.

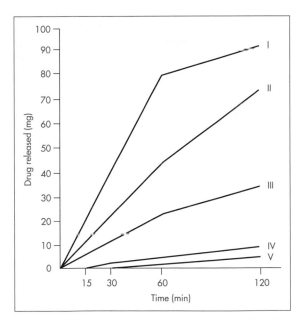

Figure 10.39 Release of drugs of varying solubilities from fat-based suppositories of equal active agent content.

Type	Solubility in water
I	1 in 1
II	1 in 10
III	1 in 10 to 1 in 100
IV	1 in 100 to 1 in 1000
V	1 in 1000 to 1 in 10 000

Modified from Voigt R, Falk G, *Pharmazie*, 1968; 23: 709.

drugs are better absorbed from a fatty excipient than from a water-soluble one, and ethyl nicotinate, for example, which is lipid-soluble, is absorbed faster from a water-soluble excipient.

In a study of the various physical properties of suppositories, the most important parameter for the bioavailability of paracetamol was found to be their rheological properties at 37°C. The relationship between the excretion of paracetamol (APAP; N-acetyl-p-aminophenol) and the rheology of the excipient drug suspension is shown in Fig. 10.40. The greater the limiting shear stress, τ, of the system, the lower the bioavailability of the drug.

Apparatus for studying the many variables in suppository formulation has been designed to measure rates of release *in vitro*. Both a circulating dissolution apparatus and a dialysis device utilising an aqueous and a nonaqueous phase have been described, and are discussed in Chapter 13. As the suppository base is heated before moulding, certain effects can be noted that are unique to this type of medication. Testosterone dissolves when hot in the semisynthetic excipient Witepsol H, to give, on cooling, crystals of about 2–3 μm in diameter. After dissolution in theobroma oil, the drug does not crystallise on cooling but remains dissolved as a solid solution. In the former case, high absorption rates are obtained, while in the latter poor absorption is achieved.

Figure 10.40 Variation of the excretion of APAP (paracetamol) in the urine 2 hours after rectal administration of a formulation as a function of the limiting shear stress, τ, of the excipient–drug mixture at 37°C.

Modified from Moës A, *J Pharm Belg*, 1974; 29: 319.

Absorption from the rectum depends on the concentration of drug in absorbable form in the rectal cavity and, if the base is not emulsified, on the contact area between molten excipient and rectal mucosa. Addition of surfactants may increase the ability of the molten mass to spread and tends to increase the extent of absorption. Significant increases in absorption can be obtained with polyoxyethylene sorbitan monostearate (polysorbate 60), sodium lauryl sulfate and cetyltriethylammonium (cetrimonium) bromide. Surfactants increase wetting and spreading and may increase the permeability of the rectal mucosal membrane.

A study of the effect of polyoxyethylene glycols on the rectal absorption of un-ionised sulfafurazole demonstrated the importance of the affinity of the drug substance for base and for rectal mucosa. As the amount of Macrogol 4000 (polyoxyethylene glycol 4000) was increased, the partition coefficient (lipid/vehicle) fell and absorption decreased correspondingly, because the affinity of the drug for the suppository base increased and its tendency to partition to the rectal lipids decreased. In a similar way, incorporation

of water-soluble drug into a water-in-oil emulsified suppository base tends to decrease bioavailability as the drug is transferred in dispersed aqueous droplets in the molten base.

 Clinical point

The hygroscopicity of some hydrophilic bases such as the polyoxyethylene glycols (each oxygen can interact with up to 4 water molecules under certain circumstances) results in the abstraction of water from the rectal mucosa. This causes a stinging sensation and discomfort and probably affects the passage of drugs across the rectal mucosa. The hygroscopicity of the glycols decreases as the molecular weight increases. The problem may be overcome by the incorporation of water into the base, although the presence of water may affect drug stability. Glycerogelatin bases are also hygroscopic.

Deliberate incorporation of water into a formulation gives rise to the possibility that, on storage, water will be lost by evaporation and drug may crystallise as a result. Reactions between components of the formulation are more likely to occur in the presence of moisture than in its absence.

Incompatibility between base and drug

Various incompatibilities have been noted with polyoxyethylene glycol bases. Phenolic substances complex with glycol, probably by hydrogen-bonding between the phenolic hydroxyl group and the glycol ether oxygens. Polyoxyethylene glycol bases are incompatible with tannic acid, ichthammol, aspirin, benzocaine, clioquinol and sulfonamides. High concentrations of salicylic acid alter the consistency of the bases to a more fluid state.

Glycerogelatin bases are prepared by heating together glycerin, gelatin and water. Although primarily used *per se* as an intestinal evacuant, the glycerogelatin base may be used to deliver drugs to the body. For this purpose the USP XVIII specified two types of gelatin to avoid incompatibilities. Type A is acidic and cationic with an isoelectric point between pH 7 and 9; type B is less acidic and anionic with an isoelectric point between pH 4.7 and 5. Use of untreated gelatin renders the base incompatible with acidic and basic drugs.

10.10 Intrathecal drug administration

Administration of drugs in solution by intrathecal catheter provides an opportunity to deliver drugs to the brain and spinal cord. Relatively hydrophilic drugs such as methotrexate ($\log P = -0.5$) that do not cross the blood–brain barrier in significant amounts have been infused intrathecally to treat meningeal leukaemia, and baclofen ($\log P = -1.0$) to treat spinal cord spasticity. High lumbar CSF concentrations are achieved as a result. Figure 10.41 shows the anatomy of the epidural space and routes of drug transport. The spinal CSF has a small volume ($70\,\text{cm}^3$) and a relatively slow clearance (20–$40\,\text{cm}^3\,\text{h}^{-1}$) of hydrophilic drugs.

The intrathecal route is more invasive than IV, IM or SC routes. Both percutaneously implanted catheters

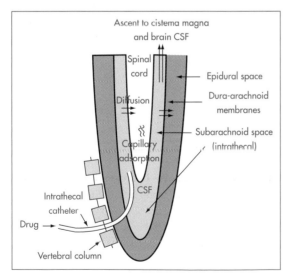

Figure 10.41 Anatomical structures and pathways of drug movement important in intrathecal drug administration; the lower part (sacral, lumbar) of the spinal cord is shown in this diagram.

Reproduced from Kroin JS, *Clin Pharmacokinet*, 1992; 22: 319.

and subcutaneously implantable pumps have been used to reduce the risk of infection on repeated puncture.

Diffusion of the drug following administration intrathecally is critical in determining activity. The CSF pharmacokinetics of three drugs (morphine, $\log P = 0.15$; clonidine, $\log P = 0.85$; and baclofen, $\log P = -1.0$) were found to be similar, leading to the suggestion that bulk flow mechanisms may be the dominant factor in determining distribution.

Summary

The routes discussed in this chapter are sometimes simpler, and perhaps sometimes more complex than the oral route. In several of those we have covered there is a more intimate contact between the formulation and the absorbing surface – as in the topical and rectal routes – so the formulation and the thermodynamic activity of the drug in the vehicle becomes more directly important. In essence:

- Each route has its own special characteristics. Administration of the same dose of drug by different routes usually produces significantly different pharmacokinetics.
- The optimal lipophilicity of a drug to traverse the barrier membrane depends on the nature of the membrane.
- Some barriers as in the eye are complex, having the characteristics of typical lipid barriers, interspersed with more aqueous hurdles.
- In some cases, as with intramuscular injections, the nature of the tissue into which the drug is injected, whether fatty or aqueous, is key to the process of transferring drug into the blood.
- No one equation can yet predict the pharmacokinetic profile of a drug delivered by a particular route in a particular formulation, but the equations presented in this chapter help to show the effect of key parameters.
- The overriding importance of lipophilicity is clear when drug is absorbed in molecular form.
- When drug is delivered as a suspension (as in an aerosol), the paramount importance of particle size in first getting the drug to the site of action is clear; once it has reached that site, its rate of solution and its lipophilicity are again important.

References

1. Balch CM *et al.* Continuous regional chemotherapy for metastatic colorectal cancer using a totally implantable infusion pump. A feasibility study in 50 patients. *Am J Surg* 1983;145:285–90.
2. Mitragotri S *et al.* Ultrasound-mediated transdermal protein delivery. *Science* 1995;269:850–853.
3. Figge FHJ, Barnett DJ. Anatomic evaluation of a jet injection instrument designed to minimise pain and inconvenience of parenteral therapy. *Am Pract* 1948; 3:197–206.
4. Shramm J, Mitragotri S. Transdermal drug delivery by jet injectors: energetics of jet formation and penetration. *Pharm Res* 2002;19:1673–1679.
5. Murdan S. Drug delivery to the nail following topical application. *Int J Pharm* 2002;236:1–26.
6. Elkeeb R *et al.* Transungual drug delivery: current status. *Int J Pharm* 2010;384:1–8.
7. Sieg JW, Robinson JR. Vehicle effects on ocular drug bioavailability II: Evaluation of pilocarpine. *J Pharm Sci* 1977;66:1222–1228.
8. Chrai SS, Robinson JR. Binding of sulfisoxazole to protein fractions of tears. *J Pharm Sci* 1976;65:437–439.
9. Snell JW. Ophthalmic drug delivery systems. *Drug Del Res* 1985;6:245–261.
10. Hull DS *et al.* Ocular penetratin of prednisolone and the hydrophilic contact lens. *Arch Ophthalmol* 1974;92:413–416.
11. German E, Siddiqui N. Atropine toxicity from eyedrops. *N Engl J Med* 1970;282:689.
12. Borromeo-McGrail V *et al.* Systemic hypertension following ocular administration of 10% phenylephrine in the neonate. *Paediatrics* 1973;51:1032–1036.
13. Benziger DP, Edelson J. Absorption from the vagina. *Drug Metab Ther* 1983;14:137–68.
14. Kunth K *et al.* Hydrogel delivery systems for vaginal and oral applications. Formulations and biological considerations. *Adv Drug Deliv Rev* 1993;11:137–167.
15. Cox JSG *et al.* Disodium cromoglycate (Intal). *Adv Drug Res* 1970;5:115–196.
16. McDonald KJ, Martin GP. Transition to CFC-free metered dose inhalers-into the new millennium. *Int J Pharm* 2000;201:89–107.
17. Williams RO, Lie L. Influence of formulation additives on the vapor pressure of hydrofluoroalkane propellants. *Int J Pharm* 1998;166:99–103.
18. Vervaet C, Byron P. Drug–surfactant–propellant interactions in HFA-formulations. *Int J Pharm* 1999;186:13–30.
19. O'Callaghan C, Barry PW. The science of nebulised drug delivery. *Thorax* 1997;52(Suppl2):S31–S44.
20. Constantino HR *et al.* Intranasal delivery: physicochemical and therapeutics aspects. *Int J Pharm* 2007;337:1–14.

Further reading

Benson EA *et al.* Flocculated humulin insulin. *N Engl J Med* 316, 1027–1028 (1987). [See also J.H. Anderson, E.H. Massey, *N Engl J Med* 316, 1028 (1987)].

Dolovich MB, Dhand R. Aerosol drug delivery: developments in device design and clinical use. *Lancet* 2011; 377: 1032–1045.

Kadam RS, Kompella UB. Influence of lipophilicity on drug partitioning into sclera, choroid-retinal pigment epithelium, retina, trabecular meshwork and optic nerve. *J Pharmacol Exp Ther* 2010;332(3):1107–1120.

Playan J *et al.* Flocculation of NPH insulin. *Rev Clin Esp* 1994;194:20–22.

Zhu H, Chauhan A. Effect of viscosity on tear drainage and ocular residence time. *Optom Vis Sci* 2008;85:715–725.

11

Physicochemical drug interactions and incompatibilities

This chapter deals with some practical consequences of the physical chemistry of drugs, especially their interactions with each other, with solvents and with excipients in formulations. Sometimes the interaction is beneficial and sometimes not. In this chapter you will appreciate that there are several physicochemical causes of interactions. These include:

- pH effects – changes in pH that may lead to precipitation of the drug
- Change of solvent characteristics on dilution, which may also cause precipitation
- Cation–anion interactions in which complexes are formed
- Salting-out and salting-in – the influence of salts in decreasing or increasing solubility, respectively
- Chelation – in which a chelator molecule binds with a metal ion to form a complex
- Ion-exchange interactions – in which ionised drugs interact with oppositely charged resins
- Adsorption to excipients and containers – causing loss of drug
- Interactions with plastics – another source of loss of material
- Protein binding – through which the free concentration of drugs *in vivo* is reduced by binding to plasma proteins

The chapter discusses the topic of drug interactions from a physicochemical rather than a pharmacological or pharmacodynamic viewpoint. Many drug interactions *in vitro* are, not surprisingly, readily explained by resorting to the physical chemistry discussed in earlier chapters of this book. There is no reason why the same forces and phenomena that operate *in vitro* cannot explain many of the observed interactions that occur in the body, although of course the interplay of physicochemical forces and physiological conditions makes a fascinating exercise. Interactions such as protein binding, adsorption of drugs onto surfaces, chelation and complexation, all occur in physiological conditions and are predictable to a large degree. We can also observe drug–drug and drug–excipient interactions.

Drug–drug or drug–excipient interactions can take place before administration of a drug. These may result in precipitation of the drug(s) from solution, loss of potency, or chemical instability. Under some circumstances they can occur even in the solid state. With the decline in traditional forms of extemporaneous dispensing, this aspect of pharmaceutical incompatibility may seem to have decreased somewhat in importance. However, extemporaneous preparation still exists, for example in the form of addition of drugs to intravenous fluids where interactions can be critical, and which should be carried out with pharmaceutical oversight, particularly with new drugs and new formulations and especially during clinical trials.

An *incompatibility* occurs when one drug is mixed with other drugs or agents and produces a product unsuitable for administration either because of some modification of the effect of the active drug, such as increase in toxicity, or because of some physical change, such as decrease in solubility or stability. Some drugs designed to be administered by the intravenous route cannot safely be mixed with all available intravenous fluids. If, as discussed in Chapter 4, the solubility of a drug in a particular infusion fluid is low, crystallisation may occur sometimes very slowly when the drug and fluid are mixed. Microcrystals may be formed that are not immediately visible. When infused, these have potentially serious effects. The mechanism of crystallisation from solution will often involve a change in pH; the problem is a real one because the pH of commercially available infusion fluids can vary within a pH range of perhaps 1–2 units. Therefore, a drug may be compatible with one batch of fluid and not another. The proper application of the equations relating pH and pK_a and solubility discussed in section 4.2.4 should allow additions of drugs to be made safely or to be avoided.

We now discuss, in turn, some of the potential interactions that can occur.

11.1 pH effects *in vitro* and *in vivo*

The pH of a medium, whether in a formulation or in the body, can be a primary determinant of drug behaviour. For convenience we here discuss separately pH effects in the laboratory and in the body.

11.1.1 *In vitro* pH effects

Chemical, as well as physical, instability may result from changes in pH, buffering capacity, salt formation or complexation. Chemical instability may give rise to the formation of inactive or toxic products. Although infusion times are generally not greater than 2 h, chemical changes following a change in pH may occur rapidly. pH changes often follow from the addition of a drug substance or solution to an infusion fluid, as shown in Table 11.1. This increase or decrease in pH

may then produce physical or chemical changes in the system.

Table 11.1 Changes in pH of 5% dextrose (1000 cm^3) following addition of three drugs[a]

Drug	Quantity	ΔpH	Final pH
Aminophylline	250 mg	+4.2	8.5
	500 mg	+4.2	8.5
Cefalothin sodium	1 g	+0.1	4.2
	2 g	+0.2	4.3
Oxytetracycline hydrochloride	500 mg	−1.25	2.9
	1 g	−1.45	2.7

[a] Reproduced from Edwards M, *Am J Hosp Pharm*, 1967; 24: 440.

The titratable acidity or alkalinity of a system may be more important than pH itself in determining compatibility and stability. For example, an autoclaved solution of dextrose may have a pH as low as 4.0, but the titratable acidity in such an unbuffered solution is low, and thus the addition of a drug such as benzylpenicillin sodium, or the soluble form of an acidic drug whose solubility will be reduced at low pH, may not be contraindicated. As seen from Table 11.1, the additive may itself change the pH of the solution or solvent to which it is added. As little as 500 mg of ampicillin sodium can raise the pH of 500 cm^3 of some fluids to over 8, and carbenicillin or benzylpenicillin may raise the pH of 5% dextrose or dextrose saline to 5.6 or even higher. Both drugs are, however, stable in these conditions.

The solubility of calcium and phosphate in total parenteral nutrition (TPN) solutions is dependent on the pH of the solution. TPN solutions are, of course, clinically acceptable only when precipitation can be guaranteed not to occur. Dibasic calcium phosphate,

for example, is soluble only to the extent of 0.3 g dm^{-3}, whereas monobasic calcium phosphate has a solubility of 18 g dm^{-3}. At low pH the monobasic form predominates, while at higher pH values the dibasic form becomes available to bind with calcium and precipitates tend to form.

Calcium solubility curves for TPN solutions containing 1.5% (w/v) amino acid and 10% (w/v) dextrose at pH 5.5 are shown in Fig. 11.1. The broken straight lines show the calcium and phosphate concentrations at 3 : 1 and 2 : 1 ratios. The dotted curve for Aminosyn solutions shows the concentrations at which precipitation occurs after 18 hours at 25°C followed by 30 minutes in a water bath at 37°C. The full curve is for TrophAmine solutions, and represents calcium or phosphate concentrations at which visual or microscopic precipitation or crystallisation occurs. Compositions to the left of the curves represent physically compatible solutions. The compatibility and stability of additives in parenteral nutrition mixtures is discussed in a review by Allwood and Kearney.[1]

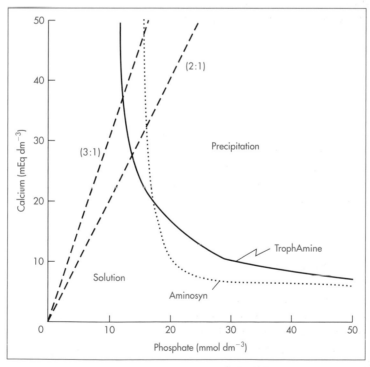

Figure 11.1 Solubility curves for TPN solutions containing amino acid (15 g dm^{-3}) and 10% dextrose at pH 5.5. Dotted line: Aminosyn. Solid line: TrophAmine. Dashed lines: relative calcium-to-phosphate ratios.
Modified with permission from Fitzgerald KA, MacKay MW, *Am J Hosp Pharm*, 1986; 43: 88–93.

11.1.2 *In vivo* pH effects

The sensitivity of the properties of most drugs to changes in the pH of their environment means that the hydrogen-ion concentration will be an important determinant of solubility, crystallisation and partitioning. Gastric pH is 1–3 in normal subjects, but the measured range of pH values in the human stomach is wide, as can be seen in Fig. 11.2. Remembering that pH is a logarithmic scale, the order of the change in the gut and its effect on aqueous and lipid solubility in particular can be appreciated. Changes in the acid–base balance therefore have a marked influence on the absorption and thus on the activity of drugs.

Ingestion of antacids, food, and weak electrolytes will all change the pH of the stomach. Weakly acidic drugs, being un-ionised in the stomach, will be absorbed from the stomach by passive diffusion. One might expect, therefore, that concomitant antacid therapy would delay or partially prevent absorption of certain acidic drugs. The main mechanism would be an increase in pH of the stomach, increasing ionisation of the drug and reducing absorption. A problem in generalisations of this kind is that the acid-neutralising capacity of antacids is very variable, as the results quoted in Table 11.2 show. Some acidic drugs, listed in Table 11.3, are also known to be absorbed in the

intestine, in which case the co-administration of an antacid is not necessarily prohibited, as its effects may be transitory.

Clinical point

The effects of antacids are not always clear-cut, as pointed out at the beginning of this chapter. There are contradictory reports of the effect of antacids on the absorption of levodopa, as one example. Levodopa is metabolised within the gastrointestinal tract and more rapidly degraded in the stomach than in the intestine, so the rate at which the drug is emptied from the stomach can affect its availability. It has been suggested that when an antacid is administered prior to the drug, serum levodopa concentration is increased because it is transferred to the intestine more rapidly.

The use of ranitidine, nizatidine, famotidine and other H_2-antagonists has given rise to the possibility of a drug interaction involving the increase in gastric pH, as these drugs inhibit gastric acid secretion. A few subjects have transient achlorhydria after oral cimetidine, so increased absorption of acid-labile drugs is a predictable side-effect, as breakdown is reduced.

Sodium bicarbonate (sodium hydrogen carbonate) is one of the most effective antacids in terms of neutralising capacity. It can greatly depress the absorption of tetracycline – the mean amount of drug appearing in the urine of patients receiving only drug was 114 mg at 48 hours and was 53 mg for those also given sodium bicarbonate. Chelation (see section 11.5) is not possible with the monovalent Na^+ ion as it is with the multivalent components of other antacids, nor does adsorption occur. If the drug is dissolved prior to administration, the antacid does not affect the excretion of the antibiotic, suggesting that in normal dosage forms it is the rate of dissolution of the drug that is affected by the antacid, as explained below in the case of tetracycline.

The aqueous solubility of tetracycline at pH 1–3 is 100-fold greater than at pH 5–6. Consequently, its

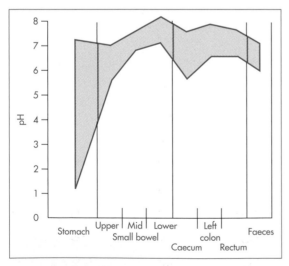

Figure 11.2   pH profile in the gut as measured by radiotelemetric capsule; the shaded area represents extremes of values observed in 9 subjects.

Reproduced from Meldrum SJ *et al., Br Med J,* 1972; 2: 104.

Table 11.2 Amounts of various antacids required to neutralise 50 mEq HCl[a]

Antacid	Neutralising capacity of 1 g or 1 cm^3		Dose required to neutralise 50 mEq	Weight of tablet (g)	No. of tablets
	cm^3 0.1 mol dm^{-3} HCl	mEq HCl			
Powders					
NaHCO$_3$	115	11.5	4.4 g		
MgO	85	8.5	5.9 g		
CaCO$_3$	110	11.0	4.5 g		
Magnesium trisilicate	10	1.0	50 g		
MgCO$_3$	8	0.8	63 g		
Suspensions					
Al(OH)$_3$ gel	0.7	0.07	715 cm^3		
Milk of Magnesia	27.7	2.8	17.8 cm^3		
Titralac	24	2.4	20.6 cm^3		
Aludrox	1.7	0.17	294 cm^3		
Oxaine	2.4	0.24	208 cm^3		
Mucaine	1.7	0.17	294 cm^3		
Kolantyl gel	3.4	0.34	147 cm^3		
Tablets					
Gastrogel	5.0	0.5	100 g	1.08	93
Gastrobrom	15.0	1.5	33.3 g	1.48	23
Glyzinal	2.5	0.25	200 g	0.72	278
Actal	7.7	0.77	65 g	0.60	109
Amphotab	2.5	0.25	200 g	1.04	192
Gelusil	2.5	0.25	200 g	1.36	147
Nulacin	10.0	1.0	50 g	3.12	17
Kolantyl wafer	5.0	0.50	100 g	1.64	61
Titralac	42.5	4.25	11.8 g	0.65	18
Almacarb	3.0	0.3	167 g	1.28	130
Dijex	4.6	0.46	109 g	1.65	66

Note that proprietary preparations available in different countries may not have the same formulation.

[a] Reproduced from Piper DW, Fenton BH, *Gut*, 1964; 5: 585.

Table 11.3 Drugs whose absorption may be affected by antacid administration

Drug whose activity would be reduced	Drug whose activity would be potentiated
Tetracyclines	Theophylline
Nalidixic acid	Chloroquine
Nitrofurantoin	Mecamylamine
Benzylpenicillin	Amfetamine
Sulfonamides	Levodopa

Figure 11.3 Mean plasma concentrations ($\mu g\,cm^{-3}$) of naproxen in 14 male volunteers with and without intake of sodium bicarbonate, magnesium oxide or aluminium hydroxide.
Modified from Segre EJ *et al.*, *N Engl J Med*, 1974; 291: 582.

rate of solution, dc/dt, at this lower pH is greatly reduced as, according to equation (11.1),

$$\frac{dc}{dt} = kc_s \qquad (11.1)$$

where c_s is the solubility. A 2 g dose of $NaHCO_3$ will increase the intragastric pH above 4 for a period of 20–30 minutes, sufficient time for 20–50% of the undissolved tetracycline particles to be emptied into the duodenum where the pH (at 5–6) is even less favourable for solution to occur. The fraction of drug absorbed is therefore decreased.

Effects of antacids other than directly on pH

The effect of antacids on gastric emptying rate is a factor that makes difficult a direct physicochemical analysis of the problem. The difficulty in predicting the effect of antacids is clearly shown by studies with naproxen, a weakly acidic nonsteroidal anti-inflammatory with a pK_a of 4.2. Several textbooks of drug interactions state that antacids decrease the absorption of acidic drugs such as nalidixic acid, nitrofurantoin and benzylpenicillin (as indicated in Table 11.3), but antacids both increase and decrease the absorption of naproxen. Magnesium carbonate, magnesium oxide and aluminium hydroxide decrease absorption and, as these are insoluble agents, adsorption effects that reduce the quantity of free drug in solution are suspected (see Fig. 11.3). On the other hand intake of Maalox, which contains magnesium and aluminium hydroxides, slightly increased the area under the curve. The extent to which Al^{3+} and Mg^{2+} ions chelate with

nalidixic acid is not clear, but the structure of the drug suggests it has chelating potential (see section 11.5).

 Clinical point

Even though gastric emptying tends to become more rapid as the gastric pH is raised, antacid preparations containing aluminium or calcium are prone to retard emptying, and magnesium preparations to promote it. The caution about the co-administration of antacids containing divalent or trivalent metals and tetracyclines should be extended to antacids containing sodium bicarbonate or any substance capable of increasing intragastric pH.

Similar principles can be applied to intestinal absorption, although here the pH gradients between the contents of the intestinal lumen and capillary blood are smaller. Sudden changes in the acid–base balance may, none the less, change the concentration of drugs able to enter cells, providing that the pH change does not alter binding of the drug to protein, or drug excretion, which of course it invariably does.

Accurate prediction of the effect of a change in the acid–base balance on the activity of any drug requires a knowledge of its site of action and the potential effect of pH changes on its excretion and biotransformation, and requires knowledge of the extent of pH changes throughout the body.

Clinical point

Ingestion of some antacids over a period of 24 hours will increase urinary pH and hence affect renal resorption and handling of some drugs. For example, administration of sodium bicarbonate with aspirin reduces blood salicylate levels by about 50%, probably owing to its increased excretion in the urine. Although high doses of alkalising agents that raise the pH of the urine will increase the renal excretion of free salicylate and result in lowering of plasma salicylate levels, in some commercial buffered aspirin tablets (such as Bufferin) there is insufficient antacid to cause a change in the pH of the gastric fluids. The small amount of antacid is sufficient, however, to aid the dissolution of the acetylsalicylic acid and this leads to more favourable absorption rates.

The importance of urinary pH

Change in the pH of urine will change the rate of urinary excretion (as represented in Fig. 11.4). When a drug is in its un-ionised form it will more readily diffuse from the urine to the blood. In an acidic urine, acidic drugs will diffuse back into the blood from the urine. Acidic compounds such as nitrofurantoin are excreted faster when the urinary pH is alkaline. Amfetamine, imipramine and amitriptyline are excreted more rapidly in acidic urine. The control of urinary pH in studies of pharmacokinetics is thus vital. It is difficult, however, to find compounds to use by the oral route for deliberate adjustment of urinary pH. Sodium bicarbonate and ammonium chloride may be used but are unpalatable. Intravenous administration of acidifying salt solutions presents one approach,

especially for the forced diuresis of basic drugs in cases of poisoning.

Clinical point

Urinary pH can be important in determining drug toxicity more directly. A preparation containing the urinary antiseptic methenamine mandelate and sulfamethizole caused turbidity in the urine of 9 out of 32 patients. The turbidity was higher in acidic urine, and was caused by precipitation of an amorphous sulfonamide derivative containing 63% sulfamethizole. The efficacy of both agents is reduced by precipitation and the danger of renal blockade is, of course, increased.[2]

Precipitation of drugs in vivo

Pain on injection may be the result of precipitation of a drug at the site of injection brought about either by solvent dilution or by alteration in pH. Precipitation of drugs from formulations used intravenously can, of course, lead to thromboembolism. The kinetics of precipitation under realistic conditions must be appreciated, since a sufficiently slow rate of infusion may obviate problems from this source as the drug precipitates and then redissolves. A simple but important equation[3] yields the flow rate (Q) of blood or normal saline required to maintain a drug in solution during its addition to an IV fluid:

$$Q = \frac{R}{S_m} \tag{11.2}$$

where R is the rate of injection of drug in $mg\,min^{-1}$ and S_m is the drug's apparent maximum solubility in the system ($mg\,cm^{-3}$). Using diazepam and normal saline as an example, if R is $5\,mg\,min^{-1}$, S_m is approximately $0.3\,mg\,cm^{-3}$, so Q would have to exceed $17\,cm^3\,min^{-1}$ to prevent observable precipitation. As this is a high rate of infusion, it is evident that the administration of diazepam through the tubing of an IV drip is likely to result in precipitate formation.

Figure 11.4 (a) A highly simplified diagram of a kidney tubule to illustrate the filtration and secretion of drugs from the blood into the tubular filtrate, and their subsequent reabsorption or loss in the urine. (b) Schematic representation of the influence of urinary pH on the passive reabsorption of a weak acid and a weak base from the urine in the renal tubules; at a high pH the passive reabsorption of the weak base and the excretion of the weak acid are enhanced, while at a low pH value the reabsorption of the weak acid and the excretion of the weak base are enhanced.

 Clinical point

Too rapid injection of the diazepam preparation directly into the venous supply might result in precipitation; slow venous blood flow would contribute to the effect. This would perhaps explain a finding that thrombophlebitis occurs less frequently when smaller veins are avoided and when injection of diazepam is followed by rigorous flushing of the infusion system with normal saline.[4]

11.2 Dilution of mixed solvent systems

In several cases the special nature of a formulation will preclude dilution by an aqueous infusion fluid. Injectable products containing phenytoin, digoxin and diazepam may come into this category if they are formulated in a nonaqueous but water-miscible solvent (such as an alcohol–water mixture) or as a solubilised (e.g. micellar) preparation. Addition of the formulation to water may result in precipitation of the drug, depending on the final concentration of the drug and solvent. It has been suggested that precipitation of the relatively insoluble diazepam may account for the high (3.5%) incidence of thrombophlebitis that occurs when diazepam is given intravenously.

Other additives in formulations may give rise to subtle problems that are not immediately obvious. One diazepam injection contains 40% propylene glycol and 10% ethanol; it is buffered with sodium benzoate and benzoic acid and preserved with benzyl alcohol. Addition of this formulation to normal saline results in the formation of a precipitate; a precipitate also forms on the addition of the diazepam solution to human plasma.

A graphical technique has been described to predict whether a solubilised drug system will become supersaturated and thus have the potential to precipitate. When a drug dissolved in a cosolvent system is diluted with water, both drug and cosolvent are diluted. The logarithm of the solubility of a drug in a cosolvent system generally increases linearly with the percentage of cosolvent present (Fig. 11.5a). On dilution, the drug concentration falls linearly with a fall in the percentage of cosolvent. The aim of the graphical method is to plot dilution curves and solubility curves on the same graph. This is achieved in Fig. 11.5b, where the dilution curves have been plotted semilogarithmically for three systems containing initially 1, 2 and 3 $mg\,cm^{-3}$ of drug substance (plots I, II and III, respectively). With solution III, dilution below about 30% cosolvent causes the system to be supersaturated; with solution II, below 20% cosolvent the solubility line and the dilution line touch. Only with solutions containing 1 $mg\,cm^{-3}$ can be diluted without precipitation.

11.3 Cation–anion interactions

The interaction between a large organic anion and an organic cation may result in the formation of a relatively insoluble precipitate. Complexation, precipitation or phase separation can occur in these circumstances, the product being affected by changes in ionic strength, temperature and pH. Examples of

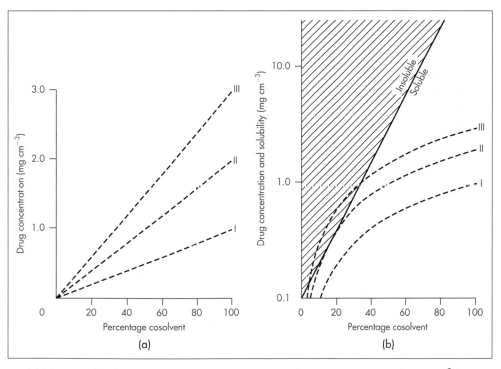

Figure 11.5 (a) Dilution profiles for three solutions (I, II and III) in pure cosolvent containing 1, 2 and 3 $mg\,cm^{-3}$ drug, respectively. (b) Curves from (a) plotted on semilog scale along with typical solubility line.

Reproduced from Yalkowsky SH, Valvani S, *Drug Intell Clin Pharm*, 199; 11: 417.

cation–anion interactions include those between procainamide and phenytoin sodium, procaine and thiopental sodium, and hydroxyzine hydrochloride and benzylpenicillin (Scheme 11.1). The nature of many of these interactions has not been studied in detail. In the absence of this it is necessary to predict possible incompatibilities from a knowledge of the physical properties of the drug and other components in the formulation. Sometimes, as when chlorpromazine and morphine injections are mixed, the incompatibility is not due to an interaction between the two drugs but to drug–bactericide interaction; the chlorocresol contained in the morphine injection precipitates with the chlorpromazine, possibly by an anion–cation interaction. Nitrofurantoin sodium must be diluted prior to use with 5% dextrose or with sterile water for injection; alkyl p-hydroxybenzoates (parabens), phenol or cresol, all of which tend to precipitate the nitrofurantoin, must be absent.

Phase diagrams such as that shown in Fig. 11.6 are useful in determining regions of incompatibility and compatibility in cation–anion mixtures because admixture is not always contraindicated. The example shown here is for mixtures of disodium cromoglicate (DSCG, sodium cromoglicate) which is a di-anionic drug with a cationic surfactant, tetradecyldimethylammonium bromide $(C_{14}BDAC)$. As can be seen, the interaction is strongly concentration dependent. In some regions, below the line AB, the two ions coexist. Ion pairs (see below) form in the shaded region below AB. Above this solubility product line, turbidity occurs in the hatched region. On increasing the concentration of surfactant, the complex is solubilised so that the interaction is masked.

The incompatibility of organic iodide contrast media and antihistaminic drugs (added to reduce anaphylactic reactions) is due to the acidity of the

ACIDS

Phenytoin sodium

BASES

Procainamide

Thiopental sodium

Procaine

Benzylpenicillin sodium

Hydroxyzine dihydrochloride

Scheme 11.1

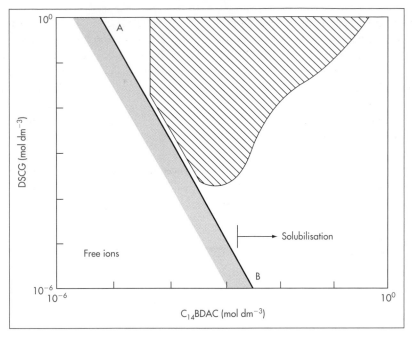

Figure 11.6 Phase diagram for mixtures of disodium cromoglicate (DSCG, sodium cromoglicate) and tetradecyldimethylammonium bromide (C_{14}BDAC).
Reproduced from Tomlinson E, *Pharm Int*, 1980; 1: 156–158.

antihistamine solutions, resulting in the precipitation of the organic iodide.[5] One of the antihistamines, promethazine, reacted strongly with all the contrast media, probably because its solution had the lowest pH of the drugs studied. It is not only with intravenous fluids that such interactions may occur. Examples have been quoted of the inadvisable mixture of syrups; for example, immediate precipitation in a prescribed mixture of a syrup containing cloxacillin sodium and a syrup containing the bases codeine and promethazine. Precipitation was followed by a 20% loss in antibiotic activity in 5 hours and 99% loss in 5 days. The double-decomposition reactions involved are likely to be those shown in Fig. 11.7.

Complexes that form are not always fully active. A well-known example is the complex between neomycin sulfate and sodium lauryl sulfate that will form when Aqueous Cream BP is used as a vehicle for neomycin sulfate. Aqueous cream comprises 30% emulsifying ointment, which itself is a mixture of emulsifying wax that contains 10% of sodium lauryl sulfate or a similar anionic surfactant.

Interactions are also not always visible. The formation of visible precipitates depends to a large extent on the insolubility of the two combining species in the particular mixture and the size to which the precipitated particles grow.

Interactions between drugs and ionic macromolecules are another potential source of problems. Heparin sodium and erythromycin lactobionate are contraindicated in admixture, as are heparin sodium and chlorpromazine hydrochloride or gentamicin sulfate. Tables of incompatibilities abound with such examples. Interference with the sulfate groups reduces the anticoagulant activity of heparin.

Ion-pair formation

Ion-pair formation may be responsible for the absorption of highly charged drugs such as the quaternary ammonium salts and sulfonic acid derivatives, the absorption of which is not explained by the pH-partition hypothesis. Ion pairs may be defined as neutral species formed by electrostatic attraction between oppositely charged ions in solution, which are often sufficiently lipophilic to dissolve in nonaqueous solvents. The formation of an ion pair (Fig. 11.8) results

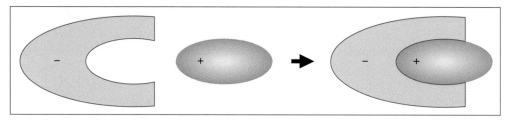

Figure 11.7 The interaction of cloxacillin sodium with promethazine hydrochloride, codeine phosphate and ephedrine hydrochloride.

Figure 11.8 Representation of an organic ion-pair – the anion is shown here interacting with a cationic molecule of complementary shape (purely schematic), thus masking the exposure of the charge to the aqueous environment.

in the 'burying' of charges and alteration to the physical properties of the drug. Interactions between charged drug species and appropriate lipophilic ions of opposite charge may constitute a drug interaction and may occur *in vitro* or *in vivo*.

11.4 Polyions and drug solutions

The extensive clinical use of polyionic solutions for intravenous therapy means that drugs are frequently

added to systems of a complex ionic nature. Reduction in the solubility of both weak electrolytes and non-electrolytes can occur through salting out, a phenomenon discussed in section 4.2.3.

Most physicochemically based drug interactions can take place in the body, or outside it, or during concomitant drug administration, so it is probably not profitable to consider them separately. Some interactions, such as complexation, which are probably more important *in vivo* than *in vitro* are discussed below.

Clinical point

Sodium sulfadiazine and sulfafurazole diolamine in therapeutic doses (1 mg) added to 5% dextrose and 5% dextrose and saline solution have been found to be compatible, yet when added to commercial polyionic solutions (such as Abbott Ionosol B, Baxter electrolyte No.2) both rapidly form heavy precipitates. pH and temperature are two vital parameters, but the pH effect is not simply a solubility-related phenomenon. Polyionic solutions of a lower initial pH (4.4–4.6) cause crystallisation of sulfafurazole at room temperature within 2.5 hours, the pH values of the admixtures being 5.65 and 5.75 respectively.

Other solutions with slightly higher initial pH levels (6.1–6.6) formed crystals only after preliminary cooling to 20°C at pH values from 4.25 to 4.90. If the temperature remains constant, the intensity of precipitation varies with the composition and initial pH of the solution used as a vehicle.[6]

and acts as a bidentate (two-toothed) ligand. When a drug forms a metal chelate, the solubility and absorption of both drug and metal ion may be affected, and drug chelation can lead to either increased or decreased absorption. Tetracyclines have similar chelating groups in their structure. Therapeutic chela2-tors are used in syndromes where there is metal ion overload. Deferiprone (I) chelates iron. EDTA (ethylenediaminetetraacetic acid) (II) as the monocalcium disodium salt is used in treatment of lead poisoning.

Structure I   Deferiprone shown as chelate with iron

Structure II   EDTA

11.5 Chelation

The term chelation (derived from the Greek *chele* meaning lobster's claw) relates to the interaction between a metal atom or ion and another species, known as the *ligand*, by which a heteroatomic ring is formed. Chelation changes the physical and chemical characteristics both of the metal ion and the ligand. It is simplest to consider the ligand as the electron-pair donor and the metal the electron-pair acceptor, the donation establishing a coordinate bond. Many chelating agents act in the form of anions that coordinate to a metal ion. For chelation to occur there must be at least two donor atoms capable of binding to the same metal ion, and ring formation must be sterically possible. For example ethylenediamine (1,2-diamino-ethane, $NH_2CH_2CH_2NH_2$) has two donor nitrogens

Tetracyclines

Probably the most widely quoted example of complex formation leading to decreased drug absorption is that of tetracycline chelation with metal ions. Polyvalent cations such as Fe^{2+} and Mg^{2+}, and anions such as the trichloracetate or phosphate interfere with absorption in both model and real systems. Figure 11.9 shows the effect of a dose of 40 mg ferrous ion on the serum levels following 300 mg of tetracycline. As can be seen from this figure, the nature of the iron salt ingested is important. Ferrous sulfate has the greatest inhibitory effect on tetracycline absorption, perhaps because it dissolves in water more quickly than organic iron compounds. The ability of the various iron compounds to

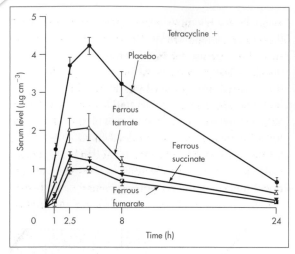

Figure 11.9 The effect of simultaneous ingestion of various iron salts (dose equivalent to 40 mg elemental iron) and tetracycline hydrochloride (500 mg) on serum levels of tetracycline (mean levels in 6 patients).
Reproduced from Neuvonen PJ, Turakka H, *Eur J Clin Pharmacol*, 1974; 7: 357.

Clinical point

The complexing of tetracyclines with calcium poses a problem in paediatric medicine. Discoloration of teeth results from the formation of a coloured complex with the calcium in the teeth; the deposition of drug in the bones of growing babies can lead to problems in bone formation.[7]

Table 11.4 shows that there is no correlation between the binding capacity of a tetracycline with iron and that with calcium, suggesting different modes of complexation. The *in vitro* data are simpler to interpret: the serum levels are the result of two processes, the chelation of the tetracycline and the partitioning of the chelate. Clinical studies have shown that the absorption of doxycycline is not significantly affected by milk in conditions where the absorption of tetracycline itself is reduced.

liberate ferrous or ferric ions in the upper part of the gastrointestinal tract before tetracycline is absorbed would seem to be an essential step in the interaction. The order of activity of the different iron salts in the chelation process *in vivo* turns out to be the same as the order of the intestinal absorption of these iron compounds. All the active tetracyclines form stable chelates with Ca^{2+}, Mg^{2+} and Al^{3+}. The antibacterial action of the tetracyclines depends on their metal-binding activity, as their main site of action is on the ribosomes, which are rich in magnesium.

The tetracyclines have an avidity for divalent metals similar to that of glycine (**III**) but they have a greater affinity for the trivalent metals, with which they form 3 : 1 drug–metal chelates. Therapeutically active tetracyclines form 2 : 1 complexes with cupric, nickel and zinc ions while inactive analogues form only 1 : 1 complexes.

Structure III The 1 : 1 copper–glycine chelate

Table 11.4 Relative calcium-binding capacities of tetracycline derivatives and decreases in serum levels after 200 mg ferrous sulfate

Tetracycline	Calcium binding[a] (%)	Decrease in serum concentration (%) after 200 mg ferrous sulfate
Demeclocycline	74.5	n.s.[b]
Chlortetracycline	52.7	n.s.[b]
Tetracycline	39.5	40–50
Methacycline	39.5	80–85
Oxytetracycline	36.0	50–60
Doxycycline	19–22	80–90

[a] Percentage of dissolved antibiotic (5 mg/50 cm³ H_2O) bound to calcium phosphate after overnight shaking. From the *US Dispensatory*, 27th edn, p. 1155ff.
[b] n.s. = not studied.

The structures of some tetracyclines are reproduced in Table 11.5, together with their pK_a values; from these data it should be possible to determine something of the relative affinities of the tetracyclines for metal ions. One piece of evidence relating to the site of chelation is that isochlortetracycline, which lacks the C-11,C-12 enolic system, does not chelate with Ca^{2+} ions.

The decreased aqueous solubility of chelates suggests increased lipophilicity but, in the case of the tetracycline chelates, precipitation would decrease the biological activity of the drug as it would be less

available for transp
molecular volume of
easy absorption in the i

Complex formation o
occurs between magnesium io
mulations. In this case the forma
able species is indicated since
bishydroxycoumarin are elevated in
magnesium hydroxide but are unaffected
hydroxide; neither antacid influenced warfa
tion.[8] A magnesium–bishydroxycoumarin ch
ing the structure (**IV**) has been isolated. Adsc

Table 11.5 Structures and pK_a values for some tetracyclines

	R¹	R²	R³	R⁴	pK_{a1}	pK_{a2}	pK_{a3}
Chlortetracycline	Cl	Me	OH	H	3.27	7.43	9.33
Oxytetracycline	H	Me	OH	OH	3.5	7.6	9.2
Tetracycline	H	Me	OH	H	3.33	7.7	9.5
Demeclocycline	Cl	H	OH	H	3.3	7.16	9.25
Doxycycline	H	Me	H	OH	3.4	7.7	9.7

Structure IV   Suggested form of the bishydroxycoumarin-Mg chelate

Figure 11.11 Concentrations of ciprofloxacin in the urine following administration of 50 mg to 12 healthy volunteers in a three-way randomised crossover design by RW Frost *et al.* (*Antimicrob Agents Chemother*, 1992; 36: 830), who write: 'The precise conditions required for ciprofloxacin to form chelate complexes with other cations have not been fully elucidated, but the carboxyl group seems to be the most likely site for chelation. Thus, the gastric pH would need to be elevated sufficiently to ionise the carboxyl group. Therefore, the lack of interaction with dairy products might be attributable to a gastric pH that was not elevated sufficiently to ionise the carboxyl group. Alternatively, it could be due to a decrease in the availability of calcium to chelate ciprofloxacin because of a lipid barrier.'

...g interactions and incompatibilities | *

...orp-
...ox-
...his
...e

...art across membranes; the larger
...the chelate would also prevent
...act form.
...of a coumarin derivative
...s present in antacid for-
...ion of a more absorb-
...plasma levels of
...the presence of
...by aluminium
...rin absorp-
...ate hav-
...ption

...o-
...sorp-
...e metals
...not receiv-
...er trace metals by
...ed in the increased absorption
...estinal lumen.

Desferrioxamine (as the mesylate) is used as a drug to sequester iron in iron poisoning or chronic iron overload; penicillamine is similarly used to aid the elimination of copper in Wilson disease. Chelation is also used for the safe delivery of toxic ions such as gadolinium (Gd^{3+}), which is used as a magnetic resonance imaging enhancing agent. One such preparation is gadobenic acid (**XI**) which is a gadolinium–BOPTA (**XIa**) octodentate chelate.

Figure 11.10 Plasma levels of bishydroxycoumarin (BHC), also known as dicoumarol, in 6 subjects after a 300 mg oral dose with water (solid line), magnesium hydroxide (dotted line) or aluminium hydroxide (dashed line). Closed data points represent a significant difference from control.
Reproduced from Ambre JJ, Fischer LF, *Clin Pharm Ther*, 1973; 14: 231–237.

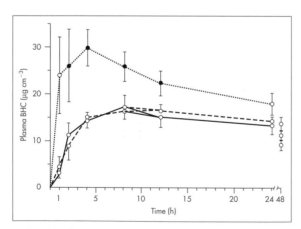

Structure V Ciprofloxacin

Structure VI Nalidixic acid

Structure VII Ofloxacin

Structure VIII   Enoxacin

Structure IX   Norfloxacin

5, 7 - diiodo-8-hydroxyquinoline

Structure X   Suggested form of the chelate of zinc–diiodohydroxyquinolone

11.6 Other complexes

Molecular complexes of many types may be observed in systems containing two or more drug molecules. Generally, association follows from attractive interactions (hydrophobic, electrostatic or charge-transfer interactions) between two molecules. In the charge transfer system one component is usually an aromatic compound; the second may be a saturated moiety containing an electron lone pair (donor atom) or a weakly acidic hydrogen (acceptor atom). The interaction therefore takes place between electron-rich donors and electron-poor acceptors. Interactions between aromatic rings in which there is a parallel overlap of π-systems fall into this category, as in the following example involving nicotinamide (acceptor) and the indole moiety of tryptophan (donor) (**XII**).

The imidazole moiety (**XIII**) is involved in many interactions; it is regarded as aromatic and the molecule is planar. Not surprisingly, caffeine (**XIV**) and theophylline (**XV**) are frequently implicated in interactions with aromatic species. Caffeine not only increases the solubility of ergotamine but also that of benzoic acid. The marked difference in the solubilising properties of caffeine and dimethyluracil (**XVI**) towards substances such as benzoic acid suggests that the imidazole ring of the xanthine nucleus is the portion involved in the interaction. In the main, 1 : 1

Structure XI   Gadobenic acid as the meglumine salt

Structure XIa   BOPTA (benzyloxypropionic tetraacetate)

Structure XII Example of donor–acceptor interaction between tryptophan (donor) and nicotinamide

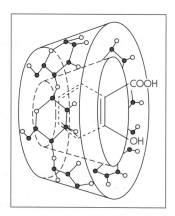

can accept protons (moderately strong base)

can lose proton (weakly acidic)

Structure XIII Imidazole

Structure XIV Caffeine

Structure XV Theophylline

Structure XVI Dimethyluracil

complexes are formed but 2 : 1 drug–caffeine complexes may also be found. Hydrophobic interactions are also implicated in the interaction since caffeine has a greater solubilising capacity than theophylline, which, as can be seen, lacks the NCH_3 group in the imidazole nucleus.

11.6.1 Interaction of drugs with cyclodextrins

Compounds that have interior cavities large enough to incarcerate organic 'guest' molecules have been named molecular container compounds.

Over the last decade there has been growing interest in the interaction of drugs with one group of container compounds, the β-cyclodextrins (cyclic D-glucose oligomers) and their now myriad derivatives. The cyclodextrin molecules have cyclic structures with internal diameters of 0.6–1 nm (see section 4.6). The interior cavity of the cyclodextrin ring is hydrophobic in nature and binds a hydrophobic portion of the 'guest' molecule, usually forming a 1 : 1 complex. The possible structure of β-cyclodextrin complexes of aspirin is shown in Fig. 11.12.

COOH

OH

Figure 11.12 Schematic drawing of an aspirin–β-CD complex.
Reproduced from Loftsson T, Masson M, *Int J Pharm*, 2001; 225: 15–30.

Inclusion of some drugs (including peptides) into cyclodextrins increases their solubility, chemical stability and absorption. The solubilising effect of β-cyclodextrin on flufenamic acid suggests that a 1 : 1 complex is formed in aqueous solution. A relationship between the oil/water partition coefficient of a drug and its tendency to form inclusion complexes has generally been found.[9] This indicates that the hydrophobic cavity of the cyclodextrin 'eye' is more attractive to lipophilic guest molecules. The formation constants for mefenamic acid were, however, lower than expected from the Me or Cl *ortho* substituent. α-Cyclodextrin showed no appreciable interaction with the anti-inflammatory acids, mefenamic acid and meclofenamic acid, suggesting that its cavity is not large enough to contain the drug molecules.[10]

The altered environment of the drug molecules leads to changes in stability. The cyclodextrins

catalyse a number of chemical reactions such as hydrolysis, oxidation and decarboxylation. Although interactions between drugs and cyclodextrins have been mostly the result of deliberate attempts to modify the behaviour or properties of the drug, they are included here to illustrate an additional mode of interaction with other components that may well occur inside the body as well as in the laboratory.

11.6.2 Ion-exchange interactions

Ion-exchange resins are now being used medicinally and as systems for modified release of drugs (see Fig. 11.13). Colestyramine and colestipol are insoluble quaternary ammonium anion-exchange resins that, when administered orally, bind bile acids and increase their elimination because the high-molecular-weight complex is not absorbed. As bile acids are

Figure 11.13 The basis of the ion-exchange process in drug delivery with factors affecting the therapeutic efficacy of the system at each stage. R and a blue circle represents resin; a minus sign depicts the integral ion of the resin, and A^+ is the counterion. D is the drug ion, X^- is the ion associated with drug cation and H^+Cl^- is hydrochloric acid. Ions inside and outside the resin indicate ions adsorbed at the surface, as well as in the interior, of the resin structure.

Reproduced from Anand V *et al.*, *Drug Discov Today*, 2001; 6: 905–915.

Structure XVII   Phenylbutazone

Structure XVIII   Warfarin

Structure XIX   Chlorothiazide

Table 11.6 The effect of colestyramine administration on sodium fusidate levels[a]

Resin dose (mg kg⁻¹)	Mean serum conc. (μg cm⁻³)
0	3.7
72	2.5
215	1.9
356	0.8

[a] Reproduced from Johns WH, Bates TR, *J Pharm Sci*, 1972; 61: 735.

converted *in vivo* into cholesterol, colestyramine is used as a hypocholesteraemic agent. When given to patients receiving other drugs as well, the resin would conceivably bind anionic compounds and reduce their absorption. Phenylbutazone (**XVII**), warfarin (**XVIII**), chlorothiazide (**XIX**) and hydrochlorothiazide are bound strongly to the resin *in vitro*.

Colestyramine had no effect in animal experiments on the blood levels of these drugs. However, 95% of both warfarin and phenylbutazone were bound and peak blood levels of the latter were halved, although the same total amount was eventually absorbed. A single dose of resin did not significantly reduce the pharmacological effect of warfarin. Nevertheless, it is prudent to administer drugs orally a short time before colestyramine to preclude delay in the action of the drug through adsorption and slow leaching. Table 11.6 shows the effect of very high resin levels on the serum concentration of sodium fusidate.

Since the binding is pH-dependent (Table 11.7), an ion-exchange resin can bind any drug with an appropriate charge under pH conditions in which both species are ionised. Decreased drug absorption caused by colestyramine or colestipol in the main has been reported with thyroxine, aspirin, phenprocoumon, warfarin, chlorothiazide, cardiac glycosides and ferrous sulfate as a consequence of binding. Absorption of vitamin K and vitamin B_{12} is decreased indirectly by competition of the resin for binding sites on intrinsic factor molecules.[11,12]

The influence of buffer ions on the binding of the drug in Table 11.7 indicates one of the problems of making *in vitro* measurements and attempting to assess the biological significance of the results. Binding of cefalexin, clindamycin (**XX**) and the components of co-trimoxazole to colestyramine has been measured; *in vivo* absorption of these substances in the presence of the resin is delayed and somewhat reduced, but the changed pattern of absorption is unlikely to affect therapeutic efficacy,

Table 11.7 Binding of acetylsalicylic acid (aspirin) *in vitro* to colestyramine[a]

	Percentage binding			
	pH 2	**pH 3**	**pH 5**	**pH 7.5**
Buffer	5	–	6	6
Water	51	95	98	97

[a] Reproduced from Halin K-J *et al.*, *Eur J Clin Pharmacol*, 1972; 4: 142.

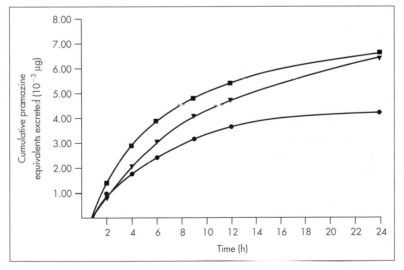

Structure XX   Lincomycin (R = OH) and clindamycin (R = Cl)

except perhaps with cefalexin where it is more pronounced.

11.7 Adsorption of drugs

The process of adsorption and its medical and pharmaceutical applications have been dealt with in some detail in Chapter 5. The use of adsorbents to remove noxious substances from the lumen of the gut is considered there. Adsorbents generally are nonspecific so will adsorb nutrients, drugs and enzymes when given orally. It is not uncommon for adsorbents to be administered in combination with various drugs and it becomes a matter of practical importance to determine the extent to which adsorbents will interfere with the absorption of the drug substance from the gastrointestinal tract.

Several consequences of adsorption are possible. If the drug remains adsorbed until the preparation reaches the general area of the absorption site, the concentration of the drug presented to the absorbing surfaces will be much reduced. The driving force for absorption would then be reduced, resulting in a slower rate of absorption. During the course of absorption of the drug, it is probable that the adsorbate will dissociate in an attempt to re-establish equilibrium with drug in its immediate environment, particularly if there is competition for absorption sites from other substances in the gastrointestinal tract. As a consequence, the concentration of free drug in solution would be maintained at a low level and the absorption rate would be reduced. Alternatively, the release of drug from the adsorbent might be complete before reaching the absorption site, possibly hastened by the presence of electrolytes in the gastrointestinal tract, in which case absorption rates would be virtually identical to those in the absence of adsorbent. Figure 11.14 shows the reduced amounts of promazine excreted in the urine when the promazine was administered with activated charcoal – evidence of a reduced absorption rate of this drug in this situation.

Figure 11.14   Cumulative amounts of promazine equivalents excreted in the urine following administration of various dosage forms to humans: ■ promazine in simple aqueous solution; ▼, promazine plus activated attapulgite; ●, promazine plus activated charcoal.
Reproduced from Sorby DL, *J Pharm Sci*, 1965; 54: 677.

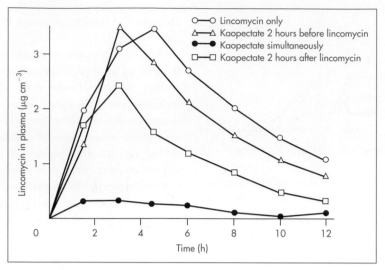

Figure 11.15 The influence of Kaopectate (kaolin and pectinic acid) on the absorption of lincomycin in humans after oral application; note the decrease in plasma levels caused by the simultaneous administration of the absorbent.
Reproduced from Wagner JG, *Can J Pharm Sci*, 1966; 1: 55.

A further example is the delayed absorption of lincomycin (**XX**) when administered with kaolin and pectinic acid (Kaopectate) (Fig. 11.15). The dramatic effect of several antacids on the adsorption of digoxin from elixirs is shown in Fig. 11.16. In view of the relatively low doses of these glycosides, these adsorption effects are likely to impair digoxin bioavailability.

If the possibility of adsorption onto formulation ingredients is not kept in mind, erroneous conclusions

Figure 11.16 Adsorption of digoxin from Lanoxin paediatric elixir at $37 \pm 0.1°C$ by: ●, Aluminium Hydroxide Gel BP (10% v/v); △, Magnesium Trisilicate Mixture BPC (10% v/v); ▲, Gelusil suspension (10% v/v); □, Lanoxin elixir diluted 1 : 10 with water.
Reproduced from Khalil SAH, *J Pharm Pharmacol*, 1974; 26: 961.

may be drawn from bioavailability studies, as was the case in the suspected *in vivo* interaction between *p*-aminosalicylic acid (PAS) and rifampicin. It was thought that PAS impaired the intestinal absorption of rifampicin, reducing its serum levels to about half those occurring when it was administered by itself (Fig. 11.17). It was later found that bentonite, a naturally occurring mineral (montmorillonite), consisting chiefly of hydrated aluminium silicate, present in the PAS granules was adsorbing the antibiotic and delaying its absorption[13] (Fig. 11.17). It can readily be seen how the initial erroneous conclusion was drawn.

Loss of activity of preservatives can arise from adsorption onto solids commonly used as medicaments. Benzoic acid, for example, can be adsorbed to the extent of 94% by sulfadimidine. Adsorption can be suppressed, however, with hydrophilic polymers. In solid dosage forms, talc, a commonly used tablet lubricant, has been reported to adsorb cyanocobalamin and consequently to interfere with intestinal absorption of this vitamin.

11.7.1 Protein and peptide adsorption

The pharmaceutical properties of peptides and proteins are discussed in Chapter 12. Adsorption can be a problem because of the amphipathic nature of many peptides, and becomes pharmaceutically important

Figure 11.17 Plasma concentrations of rifampicin (RMP) after oral administration in solution (10 mg kg^{-1}) given alone (▲), with *p*-aminosalicyclic acid (PAS) granules (●), or with Na-PAS tablets (○); mean values (*n* = 6 patients) are indicated. Reproduced from reference 13.

when they are present in low concentrations in solution. The adsorption of peptides onto glass has been ascribed to bonding between their amino groups and the silanol groups of the glass. A decapeptide derivative of LHRH, the natural luteinising hormone-releasing hormone, has two basic amino groups positively charged at low pH, providing an opportunity for binding to silanol groups.[14] Siliconisation of the glass did not inhibit adsorption completely, suggesting that ionic binding was not the only mechanism of interaction. Phosphate buffer at 0.1 mol dm^{-3} concentration and acetate ions at 0.16 mol dm^{-3} concentration (both at pH 5) were most effective in preventing adsorption.

11.7.2 Protein aggregation and interactions

As Bee and co-authors discuss,[15] 'proteins can aggregate during processing, shipping, storage and delivery to the patient. Formulation conditions are chosen to maximise protein stability over its shelf-life. However, even thermodynamically and colloidally stable proteins may aggregate after interaction with the container-closure system, container leachates, or particulate contaminants because the stability with respect to

surfaces may involve different physical processes than those that determine stability in bulk solution.' We can classify at least some of these adverse events as incompatibilities and interactions. The following are listed by Bee *et al.*:[15]

- Nucleation of the aggregation of recombinant human platelet-activating factor acetylhydrolase has been attributed to the presence of silica nanoparticles from glass containers.
- Teflon as the cause aggregation of insulin.[16]
- Silicone rubber delivery tubing decreasing the activity of interleukin-2 by 97%.[17]
- Silicone oil syringe lubricant inducing aggregation of several model proteins.[18]
- Leachates from tungsten causing protein precipitation.
- Stainless steel particles shed from a filler pump in the laboratory environment caused aggregation of a monoclonal antibody.
- Teflon containers fostering aggregation of an IgG$_2$ during freeze-thawing.

Protein aggregation in ambulatory pumps can be serious: not only does aggregation often reduce the biological activity of macromolecules, but the aggregates can cause blockage of needles. There are several mechanisms of protein aggregation, but the two most relevant to the present chapter are nucleation-controlled aggregation and surface-induced aggregation.[19] In the first, the native monomer interacts with a nucleus and adsorbs onto the nucleus, often with partial unfolding; this can lead to growth and visible precipitation. In the latter mechanism, the native monomer adsorbs onto the surface of containers or closures and partly unfolds; this can trigger growth through aggregation.

11.8 Drug interactions with plastics

In section 7.3.7 we discussed the adsorption of insulin on to glass and plastic materials used in syringes and giving sets. The plastic tubes and connections used in intravenous containers and giving sets can adsorb or absorb a number of drugs (Fig. 11.18), leading to significant losses in some cases. Drugs that show a significant loss when exposed to plastic, in particular poly(vinyl chloride) (PVC), include insulin, glyceryl trinitrate, diazepam, chlormethiazole, vitamin A acetate, isosorbide dinitrate and a miscellaneous group of drugs such as phenothiazines, hydralazine hydrochloride and thiopental sodium.

A theoretical treatment to account for the loss of glyceryl trinitrate from solution to plastic containers has been developed,[20] see Box 11.1.

Figure 11.18 The possible modes of interaction between a drug formulation and the plastic of a giving set.

Adsorption of drug to plastic

Adsorption of proteins to syringe

Partitioning of drug into plastic

Leaching of plasticiser into formulation

Box 11.1 Adsorption of glyceryl trinitrate onto plastic containers

Consider a two-stage loss of drug:

$$A \underset{k_1}{\overset{k_2}{\rightleftharpoons}} B \overset{k_3}{\longrightarrow} C$$

where

    A = glyceryl trinitrate in aqueous solution

    B = adsorbed glyceryl trinitrate

    C = glyceryl trinitrate dissolved in the matrix

Then,

$$\frac{dA}{dt} = -k_1 A + k_2 B \qquad (11.3)$$

$$\frac{dB}{dt} = k_1 A - k_2 B - k_3 B \qquad (11.4)$$

and

$$\frac{dC}{dt} = k_3 B \qquad (11.5)$$

It is found that $dB/dt \gg dC/dt$. At steady state, $dB/dt = 0$, and at $t = 0$, $A = A_0$, $B = 0$ and $C = 0$. Rate constant k_1 is a function of the amount of drug in solution, the surface area available for adsorption and the nature of the plastic, and k_3 is a function of the volume of the plastic matrix and the solubility of the glyceryl trinitrate in the plastic matrix. The ratio k_3/k_2 describes the partitioning of the drug between the plastic and the aqueous phase. So, if P is the partition coefficient,

$$\frac{k_3}{k_2} = aP \qquad (11.6)$$

a being a proportionality constant related to the mass of the plastic, the volume of the solution and other parameters. The ratio k_1/k_2 can be related to a Langmuir type of adsorption constant. The final form of the equation accurately predicts the amount (A) of glyceryl trinitrate remaining in solution:

$$A = 8.957e^{-0.028t} + 14.943e^{-0.235t} \qquad (11.7)$$

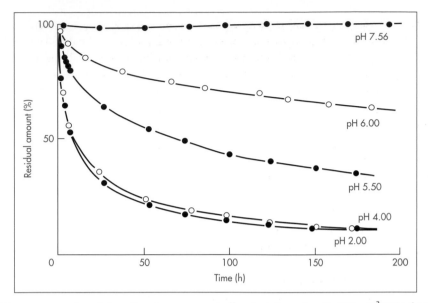

Figure 11.19 Disappearance of warfarin sodium from aqueous buffered solutions stored in 100 cm^{-3} PVC infusion bags at room temperature.
Reproduced with permission from reference 21.

Some idea of the rate and extent of disappearance of warfarin sodium from PVC infusion bags can be gained from Fig. 11.19. The marked effect of pH is seen. Losses can obviously be significant. When medazepam is present at an initial concentration of 40 µg cm^{-3} in 100 cm^3 normal saline stored in similar bags, a 76% loss of the drug occurs in 8 hours at 22°C (Table 11.8).[21]

Preservatives such as the methyl and propyl parabens present in formulations can be sorbed into rubber and plastic membranes and closures, thus leading to decreased levels of preservative and, in the extreme, loss of preservative activity.

11.9 Protein binding

This is a topic that requires a chapter to itself for full coverage. Here we have space only for a treatment of mechanisms of protein binding that might enable readers to recognise molecules likely to be protein-bound. High levels of protein binding alter the biological properties of the drug as free drug concentrations are reduced. The bound drug assumes the diffusional and other transport characteristics of the protein molecule. In cases where drug is highly protein-bound (around 90%), small changes in binding lead to drastic changes

in the levels of free drug in the body. If a drug is 95% bound, 5% is free. Reduction of binding to 90% by, for example, displacement by a second drug, doubles the level of free drug. Such changes are not evident when binding is of a low order.

Most drugs bind to a limited number of sites on the albumin molecule. Binding to plasma albumin is generally easily reversible, so that drug molecules bound to albumin will be released as the level of free drug in the blood declines. Drugs bound to albumin (or other proteins) are attached to a unit too large to be transported across membranes. They are thus prevented from reacting with receptors or from entering the sites of drug metabolism or drug elimination until they dissociate from the protein.

Plasma albumin consists of a single polypeptide chain of molecular weight $67\,000 \pm 2000$ Da. Human albumin contains between 569 and 613 amino acid residues. It is a globular molecule with a diameter of 5.6 nm (calculated assuming the molecule to be an anhydrous sphere). With an isoelectric point of 4.9, albumin has a net negative charge at pH 7.4, but it is amphoteric and capable of binding acidic and basic drugs. Subtle structural changes can occur on the binding of small molecules. Fatty acid binding produces a volume increase and a decrease in the axial ratio. This is due primarily to nonpolar interaction between the

Table 11.8 Loss of drugs from normal saline solutions in poly(vinyl chloride)(PVC) bags stored at 22 °C for 8 h[a]

Drug	Initial solute conc. ($\mu g\ cm^{-3}$)	% loss PVC (100 cm³)	% loss PVC (500 cm³)
Diazepam	40	60	31
	120	58	31
Medazepam	40	76	–
Oxazepam	40	22	12
Nitrazepam	40	15	10
Warfarin sodium[b]	20	49	–
Warfarin sodium	20	29	–
Glyceryl trinitrate	200	54	–
Thiopental sodium[c]	30	25	–
Pentobarbital sodium	30	0	0
Hydrocortisone acetate	20	0	0

[a] Reproduced from reference 21.
[b] At pH 2 and pH 4.
[c] At pH 4.0 and pH 7.2.

hydrocarbon tail of the fatty acid molecule and the binding site, and reflects the adaptability of the albumin molecule. When a hydrophobic chain penetrates into the interior of the globular albumin molecule, the helices of the protein separate, producing a small change in the tertiary structure of the protein.

What are the binding sites? Organic anions are thought to bind to a site containing the amino acid sequence Lys-Ala-Try-Ala-Val-Ala-Arg (see Chapter 12). The five nonpolar side-chains of these residues form a hydrophobic 'pool'. A cationic group is present at each end. It has been proposed that the ε-amino group of lysine is the point of attachment for anionic drugs. Albumin is, however, capable of binding molecules that are not ionised at all, such as cortisone or chloramphenicol. Acidic drugs such as phenylbutazone, indometacin and the salicylates may establish primary contact with the albumin by electrostatic interactions, but the bond can be strengthened by hydrophobic

interactions. The dual interaction would therefore limit the number of possible binding sites for anionic organic drugs. In spite of electrostatic interactions, a number of drugs bind to albumin according to their degree of lipophilicity. Evidence for the importance of the hydrophobic interaction has been obtained from studies of the binding of phenol derivatives, which depends mainly on the hydrophobic character of the substituent, the phenolic hydroxyl group playing no significant role in the binding process. Similarly, penicillin derivatives and phenothiazines bind in a manner that depends on the hydrophobic characteristics of side-chains. It has been concluded that binding to albumin is a process comparable to partitioning of drug molecules from a water phase to a nonpolar phase. The hydrophobic sites are not necessarily 'preformed'. Fatty acids and warfarin are both capable of inducing conformational changes that result in the formation of hydrophobic 'pools' in the protein.

Plasma proteins other than albumin may also be involved in binding; examples of such interactions are shown in Fig. 11.20. Blood plasma normally contains on average about 6.72 g of protein per 100 cm³, the protein comprising 4.0 g of albumin, 2.3 g of globulins and 0.24 g of fibrinogen. Although albumin is the main binding protein, dicoumarol is also bound to β- and γ-globulins, and certain steroid hormones are specifically and preferentially bound to particular globulin fractions.

An expression allowing the determination of the fraction of drug bound to a protein can be derived as shown in Box 11.2.

Box 11.2 Estimation of the degree of protein binding

Protein binding can be considered to be an adsorption process obeying the law of mass action. If D represents drug and P the protein we can write

$$D + P \rightleftharpoons (DP)\,(\text{protein} - \text{drug complex})$$

At equilibrium,

$$D_f + (P_t - D_b) = D_b \tag{11.8}$$

where D_f is the molar concentration of unbound drug, P_t is the total molar concentration of protein, and D_b is the molar concentration of bound drug (= molar concentration of complex). If one assumes one binding site per molecule, the equilibrium constant, K, is given by

$$K = \frac{k_1}{k_{-1}} = \frac{\text{rate constant for association}}{\text{rate constant for dissociation}} \quad (11.9)$$

From equation (11.8)

$$K = \frac{D_b}{D_f(P_t - D_b)} \quad (11.10)$$

It is obvious that $k_1 > k_{-1}$. The rate constant for dissociation, k_{-1}, is the rate-limiting step in the exchange of drug between free and bound forms. From equation (11.10) we obtain

$$KD_fP_t - KD_fD_b = D_b \quad (11.11)$$

That is,

$$KD_fP_t = D_b + KD_fD_b = D_b(1 + KD_f) \quad (11.12)$$

Therefore,

$$\frac{KD_fP_t}{1 + KD_f} = D_b \quad (11.13)$$

or

$$\frac{D_b}{P_t} = r = \frac{KD_f}{1 + KD_f} \quad (11.14)$$

where r is the number of moles of drug bound to total protein in the system. If there are not one, but n, binding sites per protein molecule, then

$$r = \frac{nKD_f}{1 + KD_f} \quad (11.15)$$

or

$$\frac{1}{r} = \frac{1}{n} + \frac{1}{nKD_f} \quad (11.16)$$

Protein binding results are often quoted as the fraction of drug bound, β. This fraction varies generally with the concentration of both drug and protein, as shown in equation (11.17), which relates β with n, K and concentration:

$$\beta = \frac{1}{1 + D_f/(nP_t) + 1/(nKP_t)} \quad (11.17)$$

11.9.1 Thermodynamics of protein binding

Estimation of the thermodynamic parameters of binding allows interpretation of the mechanisms of interaction. Table 11.9 gives the thermodynamic parameters of binding of a number of agents to bovine serum albumin. The negative value of ΔG implies that binding is spontaneous. ΔH is negative, signifying an exothermic process and a reduction in the strength of the association as temperature increases. ΔS is positive, most likely signifying loss of structured water on binding. A diagrammatic representation of this last process is shown in Fig. 11.21. This diagram shows the change in the ordered water in the hydrophobic cavity of the albumin and around the nonpolar portion of the drug. The loss of the structured water gives rise to the positive entropy change, which contributes to a negative free-energy change.

11.9.2 Lipophilicity and protein binding

Given the data in Table 11.9 it is not surprising to find that the extent of protein binding of many drugs is a linear function of their partition coefficient P (or $\log P$). A linear equation of the form $\log(\text{percentage bound/percentage free}) = 0.5 \log P - 0.665$ has been found to be applicable to serum binding of penicillins. Although there may be an electrostatic component to the interaction, the binding increases with the degree of lipophilicity, suggesting, as is often the case, that more than one binding interaction is in force.

 Clinical point

Binding to protein outside of the plasma may determine the characteristics of drug action or transport. Muscle protein may bind drugs such as digoxin and so act as a depot. Differences in the bioavailability of two antibiotics following intramuscular administration have been ascribed to differences in protein binding. Dicloxacillin, 95% bound to protein, is absorbed more slowly from muscle than ampicillin, which is bound only to the extent of 20%.

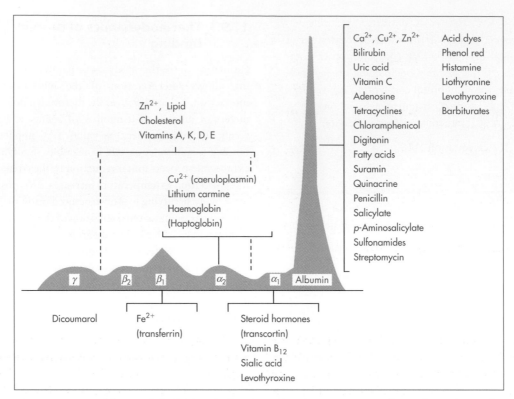

Figure 11.20 Interactions of drugs and chemicals with plasma proteins; plasma proteins are depicted according to their relative amounts.

Modified from Putnam FW, in: Neurath H, ed., *The Proteins*, 2nd edn, vol. 3, New York: Academic Press; 1965.

Figure 11.21 Electrostatic contact and hydrophobic binding of a molecular model with anionic and hydrophobic properties.

Reproduced from Hasseblatt A, *Proc Eur Soc Study Drug Toxic*, 1972; 13: 89.

Table 11.9 Thermodynamic parameters of binding of drugs to bovine serum albumin[a]

Drug	Percentage bound	ΔG	ΔH	ΔS
		(kJ mol⁻¹) at 22°C	(kJ mol⁻¹)	(J mol⁻¹ K⁻¹)
Aminopyrine (aminophenazone)	24.7	−17.7	−5.19	+42.2
Antipyrine (phenazone)	21.4	−17.1	−4.98	+41.0
4-Aminoantipyrine	22.7	−17.4	−5.27	+41.0
Phenylbutazone	84.6	−28.9	−6.1	+77.4
Oxyphenylbutazone	80.3	−27.4	−5.90	+73.2

[a] Reproduced from Ozeki S, Tejima K, *Chem Pharm Bull*, 1974; 22: 1297.

Drug binding often changes with drug concentration and with protein concentration. On increasing the drug/protein ratio, saturation of some sites can occur and there may be a decrease in binding (as indicated by total percentage). Hence the importance of determining binding at realistic albumin concentrations (about $40\,g\,dm^{-3}$). There may be more than one binding site for a drug.

In determining the pharmacological importance of protein binding, several factors have to be considered. If drug molecules not bound to plasma protein are freely distributed throughout the body, on leaving the blood they enter a volume 13 times as large as the plasma volume. Entry into the cerebrospinal fluid (CSF) depends on the concentration of free, diffusible drug in the plasma. Sulfanilamide enters CSF faster than sulfamethoxypyridazine because less is bound to serum albumin. Such binding factors may override the intrinsic lipophilicities, which in some cases may suggest a different order of penetration from that observed.

When binding occurs with high affinity and the total amount of drug in the body is low, drug will be present almost exclusively in the plasma. Drugs with lower association constants ($K \sim 10^6$ or 10^7) will be distributed more in the body water spaces. When the number of available binding sites is reduced by a second drug, it will appear as if there has been an increase in overall drug concentration.

Although drugs are predominantly bound to albumin, the amount taken up by erythrocytes must not be neglected, as can be seen in Fig. 11.22. More directly, the effect of protein binding on antibiotic action is worth considering.

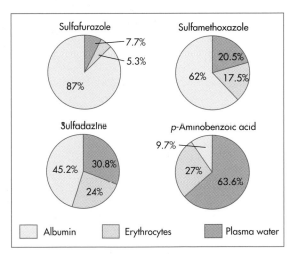

Figure 11.22 Distribution of three sulfonamides and *p*-aminobenzoic acid between albumin, plasma water and erythrocytes in humans. Log *P* values for octanol/water are: sulfafurazole 1.15; sulfamethoxazole 0.88; and sulfadiazine 0.13. Binding to albumin correlates with lipophilicity.
Reproduced from Berneis K, Boguth W, *Chemotherapy*, 1976; 22; 390.

Table 11.10 Protein binding and other characteristics of some penicillins and cephalosporins[a]

Antibiotic	Log P[b]	Serum protein binding (%)	Serum concentration ($\mu g\,cm^{-3}$) during continuous infusion (500 mg h^{-1})		Peak serum levels after 500 mg kg^{-1}	
			Total	Free	Total	Free
Dicloxacillin	3.24	96–98	25	1	15	0.3
Cloxacillin	2.49	94–96	15	0.9	–	–
Oxacillin	2.38	92–94	10	0.8	15	0.8
Nafcillin	–	89–90	9	0.9	6	0.6
Benzylpenicillin	1.72	59–65	16	5.6	4.5	1.6
Methicillin	1.06	37–60			16	10
Ampicillin	–	20–29	29	23.2	12	9
Carbenicillin	–	50	73	36.5	–	–
Ceftriaxone	–	95	–	–	–	–
Cefazolin[c]	–	89	–	–	–	–
Cefditoren	–	88	–	–	–	–
Cefalotin	0.5	65	18	6.3	7.6	2.6
Cefaloridine	–	20	24.7	19.7	18.5	14.8
Cefalexin	0.7	15	27	23	–	–
Cefradine[c]	–1.2	14	–	–	–	–

[a] Reproduced from Lien EJ *et al.*, *Drug Intell Clin Pharm*, 1974; 8: 470.

[b] log *P* values from Ryrfeldt A, *J Pharm Pharmacol*, 1971; 23: 463 and Jack DB, *Handbook of Chemical Pharmacokinetic Data*, London: Macmillan; 1992.

[c] Additional values from Singhri SM *et al.*, *Chemotherapy*, 1978; 24: 121.

 Clinical point

Penicillins and cephalosporins bind reversibly to albumin. Only the free antibiotic has antibacterial activity. Oxacillin in serum at a concentration of $100\,\mu g\,cm^{-3}$ exhibits an antibacterial effect similar to that of $10\,\mu g\,cm^{-3}$ of the drug in water. A high degree of serum protein binding may nullify the apparent advantage of higher serum levels of some agents (Table 11.10). An increase in the lipophilicity of penicillins results in decreased activity, although one normally expects that this should enhance penetration of bacterial cell walls and also absorption. The hydrophobic binding of penicillins to serum proteins reduces their potency *in vivo* by decreasing their effective concentration.

Comparisons between antibiotics are best made with activity–time plots and not serum concentration profiles, as the free levels often differ from the total antibiotic levels (see, for example, values for cloxacillin and benzylpenicillin in Table 11.10).

The second important consequence of protein binding is related to the fact that only free drug is able to cross the pores of the capillary endothelium. At equilibrium, levels of free drug on both sides of the capillary wall are equal. Albumin levels in most sites are considerably less than those in serum, so there is little bound drug in extravascular regions. There is, however, no correlation between the degree of protein binding and peak serum levels of the penicillins and cephalosporins of Table 11.10; other factors such as rates of elimination also determine the peak levels. Protein binding will affect transport into other tissues, however, as the gradient that determines movement is the gradient caused by free drug. Both ampicillin ($50\,mg\,kg^{-1}$ every 2 h) and oxacillin ($50\,mg\,kg^{-1}\,h^{-1}$) produced similar peak levels in the serum when given as repeated intravenous boluses. Levels of free drug are markedly different, however, as oxacillin is 75% bound and ampicillin is 17.5% bound in rabbit serum.

11.9.3 Penetration of specialised sites

Muscle, bone and synovial and interstitial fluid are readily accessible to intravascular antibiotics by way of aqueous pores in the capillary supply. The CSF, brain, eye, intestines and prostate gland lack such pores, and entry into these areas is by way of a lipoidal barrier. There is evidence that extensive protein binding may prevent the access of antibiotics into the eye and the inflamed meninges.

The level of free drug in serum is important in determining the amount of drug that reaches tissue spaces.[22] The total concentration of a drug in tissue fluid can be predicted from the serum concentration, the extent of serum protein binding, and the protein binding in the tissue fluid. Equation (11.18) has been shown to be highly predictive under equilibrium conditions:[22]

$$C_t = \frac{C_s f_s}{f_t} \tag{11.18}$$

where C_t is the tissue fluid drug concentration, C_s is the serum drug concentration, and f_s and f_t are the free fractions of drug in serum and tissue fluid, respectively. If protein binding in the serum and tissue fluid is identical then, provided the same proteins are present in both 'phases', the tissue fluid drug concentration will equal the serum concentration; this is true for both high and low protein-containing extravascular fluid.

 Clinical point

In the treatment of bacterial prostatitis; most currently available antibiotics do not readily pass across the prostatic epithelium. The pH of the prostatic fluid is lower than that of plasma, being around 6.6; milk has a pH of 6.8. In passage of drugs both into prostatic fluid and into milk, the degree of dissociation of the drug appears to be the most important factor determining the degree of penetration. The partition coefficient plays a secondary role.

When the prostatic fluid/plasma ratios of sulfonamides were studied it was found that the results could be predicted more closely from the ratio of undissociated/dissociated drug rather than from $\log P$ values. It is probable that this is because lipophilic drugs will be highly protein-bound and thus unable to penetrate the boundary membranes.

Summary

This chapter has dealt with the wide range of physicochemical factors that might cause changes in formulations or drug absorption processes. These have included effects of pH and solvent, interactions between cations and anions, salting-in and salting-out, ion-exchange reactions, adsorption and interactions with plastics, as well as protein binding often mediated by hydrophobic interactions. It is, as always, difficult to anticipate the exact quantitative nature of the events that follow from these effects, especially in the body, where there are many compensating and contradictory influences. However, a knowledge of the theoretical possibilities allows us to rationalise what has been observed. By analogy we should therefore be able to predict likely effects with new drugs. One has to be cautious, aware that what we anticipate theoretically may not take place *in vivo*, where a dynamic situation exists. But the physicochemical basis of interactions and incompatibilities must be appreciated if we are to rationalise interactions.

The Appendix contains tables of drug interactions that could be considered to be physicochemically driven. However, it is important that continuously updated sources are consulted such as Stockley's *Drug Interactions*.[23] For injectables the latest edition of *Handbook on Injectable Drugs*[24] is a source of authoritative and current knowledge.

Appendix Drug interactions based on physical mechanisms

The following information was taken originally from a comprehensive listing of drug interactions published in New Zealand (Ferguson R, *Drug Interactions of Clinical Significance*, Auckland: I.M.S.; 1977). **This selection is intended for illustrative purposes only and must *not* be used as a definitive source.**

A: Interactions affecting absorption of drugs

Drugs	Effect	Mechanism/Note	Recommendation
Calcium therapy + aluminium hydroxide	Chronic aluminium hydroxide antacid intake (600 cm³ weekly) can cause osteomalacia	Calcium absorption is prevented	Use alternative antacid. Especial care should be taken with people with calcium deficiency
Chlorpromazine + aluminium hydroxide, magnesium oxide, magnesium trisilicate	Reduced blood levels of chlorpromazine, with possible inhibition of therapeutic effect	Possibly due to alteration of GI pH by the antacid	Doses should be spaced by 2–3 h
Dicoumarol, warfarin + colestyramine	Anticoagulant absorption is reduced and slowed (25% lower blood levels)	Binding to colestyramine	Space doses by 2–3 h
Dicoumarol, warfarin + laxatives	Chronic laxative administration may cause loss of anticoagulant control	Two possible effects: lubricant oil action may cause decreased absorption of anticoagulant; decreased absorption of vitamin K, particularly with oils and emulsions	Periodic long-term monitoring of prothrombin times in all suspect patients
Dicoumarol + magnesium hydroxide, magnesium oxide	Opposite effects have been reported: (i) Decreased absorption and lower blood levels (up to 75%) of dicoumarol (ii) Increased absorption	Possibly adsorption on drug leading to decreased absorption. Chelation might lead to more lipophilic species increased absorption	Space doses by 2–3 h
Digitalis glycosides + docusate sodium (DOSS)	Increased absorption of digitalis to a possibly toxic level	Surface-active properties of DOSS increases wetting and perhaps solubility and absorption of poorly absorbed digitalis	Space doses by 2–3 h
Digoxin, digitoxin + colestyramine	Greatly reduced absorption of digitalis alkaloids with concurrent administration	Binding effect (anionic resin)	Space doses by about 8 h

(continued opposite)

A: Interactions affecting absorption of drugs *(continued)*

Drugs	Effect	Mechanism/Note	Recommendation
Digoxin + disodium edetate	Disodium edetate chelates calcium ions thus antagonising the action of digoxin	Chelation of digoxin in the plasma	May be necessary to monitor blood calcium levels
Digoxin + magnesium trisilicate	Absorption of digoxin reduced by up to 90%	Surface absorption effect	Space doses 2–3 h. Use alternative antacid
Lincomycin + kaolin	Reduced GI absorption of lincomycin by up to 90%	Absorption of drug to kaolin	Space doses by 2–3 h
Oxyphenonium bromide + magnesium trisilicate	Reduced blood levels of oxyphenonium with reduced effect	Oxyphenonium adsorbed on to the surface of magnesium trisilicate, reducing availability	Space doses by at least 2–3 h
p-Aminosalicyclic acid (granule formulation) + rifampicin	Reduced blood levels of rifampicin and hence impaired effect	Impaired GI absorption rifampicin due to binding to bentonite	Space doses by 8–12 h
Propantheline bromide + magnesium trisilicate	Reduced blood levels (with reduced action) of propantheline	Adsorption of propantheline to magnesium trisilicate, reducing availability for absorption	Space doses by 2–3 h
Salicylates + colestyramine	Greatly decreased absorption of salicylates	Adsorption to ion-exchange resin	Space doses by 4–5 h
Tetracycline + iron preparations	Lower blood levels of tetracycline, possibly below minimal active concentration	Chelation effect	Either space doses at least 2–3 h or alternative antibiotic therapy
Tetracycline + milk products, aluminium, bismuth, calcium and magnesium ions	GI absorption of tetracycline and blood levels of tetracycline greatly reduced	Chelation effect	Space doses by 2–3 h; possible exception minocycline
Tetracycline + sodium bicarbonate (NB: Sodium bicarbonate is present in many antacid and effervescent preparations)	Impaired absorption of tetracycline	pH increase in GI tract prevents dissolution of complete dose	Space doses by 2–3 h
Thiazide diuretics + colestyramine	Decreased absorption and effect of diuretic	Colestyramine can bind thiazide	Space doses by 2–3 h
Thyroid hormones + colestyramine	Absorption of thyroid hormone prevented	Thyroid hormones become bound to the anionic resin	Space doses by 2–3 h

B: Interactions involving protein binding

Drugs	Effect	Mechanism/Note	Recommendation
Chlorpropamide, tolbutamide + sulfonamides	Increased blood level of hypoglycaemic drug. Hypoglycaemic shock reported	Displacement from protein binding and possible metabolic inhibition, competition for excretion	Not reported with sulfadimethoxine, sulfafurazole, sulfamethoxazole. Monitor patient
Chlorpropamide, tolbutamide + salicylates	Introduction of oral salicylate therapy can result in a hypoglycaemic reaction	Displacement from protein binding, salicylates increase tissue glucose uptake	Warn patients against high dose or chronic salicylate therapy. With long-term

(continued overleaf)

B: Interactions involving protein binding *(continued)*

Drugs	Effect	Mechanism/Note	Recommendation
			salicylate therapy patients should be monitored and restabilised if necessary
Dicoumarol, warfarin + indometacin	Possible elevated blood levels of anticoagulant with risk of haemorrhage. Risk of GI bleeding	Displacement from protein	This combination best avoided
Dicoumarol, warfarin + methandienone, norethandrolone, oxymetholone	Increased hypothrombinaemia with several reported cases of haemorrhage.	Possibly due to displacement from protein	If combination is definitely indicated, patients should be carefully monitored
Dicoumarol, warfarin + p-aminosalicyclic acid	Increased anticoagulant serum levels with risk of haemorrhage	Displacement from protein	Monitor anticoagulant effect, especially with initiation or cessation of therapy
Dicoumarol, warfarin + paracetamol	With especially large doses, increase in anticoagulant effect	Possibly displacement from protein. Depression of clotting factor synthesis	Use low doses of paracetamol. Probably the safest mild analgesic to use with oral anticoagulants
Dicoumarol, warfarin + sulfadimethoxine, sulfamethoxypyridazine, sulfaphenazole	Increased anticoagulant blood levels with risk of haemorrhage	Displacement from protein by strongly bound sulfonamide	Use alternative chemotherapy. Monitor patient with initiation of cessation of therapy
Methotrexate + salicylates	Potentiation of methotrexate toxicity	Displacement of methotrexate from protein binding sites	Owing to severity of methotrexate toxicity, salicylates should not be given to patients receiving methotrexate
Methotrexate + sulfonamides	Potentiation of methotrexate with high risk of toxicity	Displacement from protein binding (sulfafurazole reduces methotrexate binding from 70% to 28%)	Owing to severity of methotrexate toxicity, sulfonamides that are protein bound should never be administered
Penicillin + probenecid	Threefold increase in serum penicillin level with increase also in spinal fluid levels but decreased brain level	Displacement from protein binding, decreased renal tubule secretion and decrease biliary excretion	Combination can be used when high serum and spinal fluid levels are required
Thyroid hormones, levothyroxine + phenytoin	Rise in thyroxine blood levels with reported tachycardia	Displacement of thyroxine by phenytoin from protein binding	Great care should be taken in administering parenteral phenytoin to people on thyroid therapy
Warfarin + aspirin	Significant increase in anticoagulant effect with possible severe GI blood loss	Displacement from protein	Combination should be avoided if possible. Use alternative analgesic such as paracetamol or pentazocine
Warfarin + clofibrate	Higher blood levels of warfarin with risk of haemorrhage	Displacement from protein	Warfarin dose may require a reduction of one-third to one half according to coagulation test
Warfarin + etacrynic acid	Increased blood level of warfarin with haemorrhage risk	Displacement from protein	Monitor patient with initiation and cessation of therapy

(continued opposite)

B: Interactions involving protein binding *(continued)*

Drugs	Effect	Mechanism/Note	Recommendation
Warfarin + mefenamic acid	Enhanced anticoagulant blood levels with risk of haemorrhage and enhanced risk of GI bleeding	Displacement from protein	Concurrent administration is best avoided. If necessary, coagulation times should be monitored
Warfarin + nalidixic acid	Possible hypothrombinaemia with associated haemorrhage risk	Displacement from protein (NB: *In vitro* evidence)	Combination administration should be used with care and patient coagulation monitored
Oral anticoagulants + naproxen	Increased anticoagulant effect and risk of GI bleeding	Naproxen has ulcerogenic potential. Displacement from protein	Best to avoid concurrent administration. Monitor patient

References

1. Allwood MC, Kearney MCJ. Compatibility and stability of additives in parenteral nutrition admixtures. *Nutrition* 1998;14:697–706.
2. Lipton JH. Incompatibility between sulfamethizole and methenamine mandelate. *N Engl J Med* 1963;268:92–3.
3. Jusko WJ *et al.* Precipitation of diazepam from intravenous preparations. *J Am Med Assoc* 1973;225: 176.
4. Langdon DE *et al.* Thrombophlebitis with diazepam used intravenously. *J Am Med Assoc* 1973;223: 184–185.
5. Marshall TR *et al.* Pharmacological incompatibility of contrast media with various drugs and agents. *Radiology* 1965;84:536–539.
6. Barbara AC *et al.* Physical incompatibility of sulfonamide compounds and polyionic solutions. *N Engl J Med* 1966;274:1316–1317.
7. Sanchez AR *et al.* Tetracycline and other tetracycline-derivatives staining of the teeth and oral cavity *Int J Dermatol* 2004;43:709–715.
8. Ambre JJ, Fischer LJ. Effect of coadministration of aluminum and magnesium hydroxides on absorption of anticoagulants in man. *Clin Pharm Ther* 1973;14:231–237.
9. Ikeda K *et al.* Inclusion complexes of β-cyclodextrin with antiinflammatory drugs fenamates in aqueous solution. *Chem Pharm Bull* 1975;23:201–208.
10. Ikeda K *et al.* Circular dichroism study on inclusion complexes of β-cyclodextrin with antiinflammatory fanamates. *J Pharm Sci* 1974;63:1168–1169.
11. Gross L, Brotman M. Hypoprothrombinemia and hemorrhage associated with colestyramine therapy. *Ann Intern Med* 1970;72:95–96.
12. uptake of radio-vitamin B_{12} by colestyramine. *Proc Soc Exp Biol Med* 1973;142:1341–1344.
13. Boman G *et al.* Mechanism of the inhibitory effect of PAS [*p*-aminosalicylic acid] granules on the absorption of rifampicin. Adsorption of rifampicin by an excipient, bentonite. *Eur J Clin Pharm* 1975;8:293–299.
14. Anik ST, Hwang J-Y. Adsorption of D-Nal(2)^{6}LHRH, a decapeptide, onto glass and other surfaces. *Int J Pharm* 1983;16:181–190.
15. Bee JS *et al.* Monoclonal antibody interactions with micro- and nanoparticles: adsorption, aggregation and accelerated stress studies. *J Pharm Sci* 2009;98: 3218–3228.
16. Sluzky V *et al.* Mechanism of insulin aggregation and stabilisation in agitated aqueous solutions. *Biotech Adv* 2007;25:318–324.
17. Tzannis ST *et al.* Adsorption of a formulated protein on a drug delivery device surface. *J Colloid Interface Sci* 1997;189:216–228.
18. Jones LS *et al.* Silicone oil induced aggregation of proteins. *J Pharm Sci* 2005;94:918–927.
19. Philo JS, Arakawa T. Mechanisms of protein aggregation. *Curr Pharm Biotechnol* 2009;10:348–351.
20. Malick AW *et al.* Loss of nitroglycerin from solutions to intravenous plastic containers: a theoretical treatment. *J Pharm Sci* 1981;70:798–801.
21. Illum L, Bundgaard H. Sorption of drugs by plastic infusion bags. *Int J Pharm* 1982;10:339–351.
22. Peterson LR, Gerding DN. Protein binding and antibiotic concentrations. *Lancet* 1978;2:376.
23. Stockley I. *Drug Interactions.* London: Pharmaceutical Press; 2010.
24. Trissel LA. *Handbook on Injectable Drugs.* Bethesda, MD: American Society of Health-System Pharmacists; 2011.

12

Peptides, proteins and other biopharmaceuticals

An increasing number of therapeutic substances are peptides or proteins, either natural or synthetic in origin or produced by recombinant DNA technology or from transgenic animals. Most peptides and proteins are not absorbed to any significant extent by the oral route and the most available formulations of protein pharmaceuticals are therefore parenteral products for injection or inhalation (Table 12.1). DNA, RNA and various oligonucleotides are being used increasingly in gene therapy. These share some of the problems of proteins as therapeutic agents, principally owing to their high molecular weight, relative fragility and ionic nature. Monoclonal antibodies have after a long gestation reached the clinic in increasing numbers.

The object of this chapter is to provide some background for the appreciation of the pharmaceutics of proteins, peptides DNA, oligonucleotides and monoclonal antibodies as therapeutic entities. From an understanding of the nature of amino acids and their physical properties comes an appreciation of the physical nature and properties of peptides, polypeptides and proteins. The solution properties of proteins in simple and complex media has to be understood, together with the factors affecting the stability of proteins in solution. Problems in the formulation and clinical use of proteins to be overcome will then become clearer.

First some definitions:

- *Peptides* have a short chain of residues with a defined amino acid sequence; therapeutic peptides include ciclosporin, octreotide and somatostatin.
- *Polypeptides* have longer amino acid chains, usually of defined sequence and length.
- *Polyamino acids* have random amino acid sequences of varying lengths generally resulting from nonspecific polymerisation of one or more amino acids. One such is available as a drug for the treatment of multiple sclerosis – glatiramer (Copaxone).

- *Proteins* are those polypeptides that occur naturally and have a definite three-dimensional structure under physiological conditions.
- *Nucleotides* are the building block of nucleic acids, consisting of a five-carbon sugar covalently bonded to a nitrogenous base (adenine, thymine, guanine, cytosine, or uracil) and a phosphate group.
- *Oligonucleotides* are short (10–25) sequences of nucleotides.
- *Plasmid DNA* is a circular piece of DNA that exists apart from the chromosome and replicates independently of it.

Other oligomeric substances such as the antisense oligonucleotides and DNA fragments are being used therapeutically and, for these as with proteins, no systematic approaches to their pharmacy have been defined. New modes of delivery of many or all of these agents will need to be developed if they are to be used to their maximal advantage. It is misleading to assume that because many are either natural substances or their close analogues they are safe. Injection of abnormal doses even of endogenous agents at sites where they do not naturally exist can often induce bizarre side-effects. Hence the need for optimised formulations, delivered in appropriate ways to the most appropriate target sites.

Development of improved formulations and delivery systems requires a good understanding of the physical pharmacy of these molecules if we are to avoid typical problems of degradation, unwanted adsorption to glassware and plastics and aggregation in delivery devices such as reservoirs or pumps.

12.1 Structure and solution properties of peptides and proteins

12.1.1 Structure of peptides and proteins

The *primary* structure of a protein is the order in which the individual amino acids are sequenced. This tells us little about the shape that the protein will assume in solution, although the primary structure determines the *secondary*, *tertiary* and even *quaternary* forms. These amino acid building blocks (Table 12.2) give the key to structure and behaviour. The standard three-letter (Glu, Arg, Trp, etc.) and one-letter (E, R, W, etc.) abbreviations for amino acids are also listed: their use makes structural descriptions more accessible.

Secondary structures include the coiled α-helix, and pleated sheets, discussed below and shown in Figs. 12.1 and 12.2. Chain folding, arising from crosslinking through hydrogen bonding, the hydrophobic effect and salt bridges, leads to a definition of tertiary structure, and association of these structural units leads to quaternary forms.

Representations in a stylised diagrammatic form of three proteins (interleukin-1β, zinc insulin dimers, and the Fc fragment of immunoglobulin) are shown in Fig. 12.3. The nature of the three-dimensional structure shows how difficult it is to define proteins in conventional ways, and how they must be considered in a new light as pharmaceutical entities. They are in many ways fragile molecules. Loss of the unique tertiary or quaternary structure, through denaturation, can occur from a variety of insults that would not affect smaller molecules.

Complex structures are formed in solution because of interactions between the structural amino acids. Unfortunately, knowing the amino acid sequence of a protein is not enough to enable us to predict its physical behaviour. Function is determined by the way the linear chains of amino acids fold in solution to give specific three-dimensional structures comprising the coils, sheets and folds (Figs. 12.1 and 12.2). Strides are being made in understanding the 'grammar' of protein folding, through the synthesis of synthetic peptides and sequences and observation of their structures. Some of the primary structures are so complex that it is not possible to predict their physicochemical properties, although modern molecular modelling techniques have made great inroads into understanding tertiary structure and behaviour.

Table 12.1 Some therapeutic proteins and peptides, their molecular weights and actions[a]

Protein/peptide	Size (kDa)	Use/action
Oxytocin	1.0	Uterine contraction
Vasopressin	1.1	Diuresis
Leuprolide acetate	1.3	Prostatic carcinoma therapy
LHRH analogues	~1.5	Prostatic carcinoma therapy
Somatostatin	3.1	Growth inhibition
Calcitonin	3.4	Ca^{2+} regulation
Glucagon	3.5	Diabetes therapy
Parathyroid hormone (1–34)	4.3	Ca^{2+} regulation
Insulin	6	Diabetes therapy
Parathyroid hormone (1–84)	9.4	Ca^{2+} regulation
Interferon gamma	16 (dimer)	Antiviral agent
TNF-α	17.5 (trimer)	Antitumour agent
Interferon α-2	19	Leukaemia, hepatitis therapy
Interferon β-1	20	Lung cancer therapy
Growth hormone	22	Growth acceleration
DNase	~32	Cystic fibrosis therapy
α_1-Antitrypsin	45	Cystic fibrosis therapy
Albumin	68	Plasma volume expander
Bovine IgG	150	Immunisation
Catalase	230	Treatment of wounds and ulcers
Cationic ferritin	400+	Anaemias

[a] Reproduced from Niven RW, *Pharmaceutical Technology*, 1993(July): 72.

12.1.2 Hydrophobicity of peptides and proteins

Amino acids have a range of physical properties, each having a greater or lesser degree of hydrophilic or hydrophobic nature. Naturally, if amino acids are spatially arranged in a molecule so that distinct hydrophobic and hydrophilic regions appear, then the polypeptide or protein will have an amphiphilic nature. Table 12.3 lists the relative hydrophobic character of a range of amino acids, where Gly is considered to have a value of zero. The amino acids range from very hydrophobic to very hydrophilic. The side-chains of selected amino acids are shown in the table where their relative hydrophobic properties are shown. Some values of $\log P$ (octanol/water) are also given, demonstrating the trend in hydrophobic parameters.

An idea of the overall hydrophobicity of a peptide or protein may be gained from the use of indices of the hydrophobicity of the individual amino acids. Secondary and tertiary structures are important in determining the actual hydrophobic nature of the polypeptide, however, and this complicates the prediction of their physicochemical properties such as solubility and adsorption.

If alternating hydrophilic and hydrophobic amino acid sequences in synthetic peptides are at the right distances in space, the molecule coils with the hydrophobic amino acids on the inside of each coil and the hydrophilic ones to the outside. There are still, however, many structural mysteries: the interior of many protein structures with myriad side-chains, and the way in which metal ions can stabilise three-dimensional structures, have been likened to a *terra incognita*.

12.1.3 Solubility of peptides and proteins

As most proteins are delivered parenterally in solution it is important to understand their properties. In physiological conditions the aqueous solubilities of proteins vary enormously from the very soluble to the virtually insoluble. In section 4.2.4 we discussed the solubility profiles of zwitterions, including tryptophan, which all have biphasic solubility–pH profiles. One would expect proteins with terminal $-NH_2$ and $-COOH$ groups to behave similarly, although the effect will be complicated by the behaviour of the multitude of the intermediate amino acids, as can be seen from the pH–solubility profile of insulin in Fig. 10.5. Figure 12.4

Table 12.2 Nomenclature and structure of the principal amino acids. The common name, the three-letter code and the single-letter code are given

Glycine (Gly) G   Alanine (Ala) A   Valine (Val) V   Serine (Ser) S   Threonine (Thr) T

Methionine (Met) M   Phenylalanine (Phe) F   Tryptophan (Trp) W   Proline (Pro) P   Glutamine (Gln) Q

Leucine (Leu) L   Isoleucine (Ile) I   Cysteine (Cys) C   Tyrosine (Try) Y   Asparagine (Asn) N

Aspartic acid (Asp) D   Glutamic acid (Glu) E   Lysine (Lys) K   Arginine (Arg) R   Histidine (His) H

shows the general solubility behaviour of a protein as a function of pH at two ionic strengths.

The solubility of globular proteins increases as the pH of the solution moves away from the isoelectric point (IP), which is the pH at which the molecule has a net zero charge and does not migrate in an electric field. Some examples of the isoelectric points of amino acids are shown in Table 12.4. At its IP a protein has no net charge and has a greater tendency to self-associate. As the net charge increases, the affinity of the protein for the aqueous environment increases and the protein molecules also exert a greater electrostatic repulsion. However, extremes of pH can cause protein unfolding, which not infrequently exposes further nonpolar groups.

Table 12.3 Relative hydrophobic character of amino acid side-chains (Gly = 0)

Side-chain	Amino acid	Hydrophobic character[a]	Log P[b]
(Most hydrophobic)			
$CH_3CH_2CH(CH_3)-$	Isoleucine	1.83	−1.72
$CH_3CH(CH_3)CH_2-$	Leucine	1.80	−1.61
$C_6H_5CH_2-$	Phenylalanine	1.69	
	Tryptophan	1.35	
$CH_3CH(CH_3)-$	Valine	1.32	−2.08
$CH_3-S-CH_2CH_2-$	Methionine	1.10	
	Proline	0.84	
$HSCH_2-$	Cysteine	0.76	
$HOC_6H_5CH_2-$	Tyrosine	0.39	
CH_3-	Alanine	0.35	−2.89
(Standard)	Glycine	0	
$CH_3CH(OH)-$	Threonine	−0.27	
$HOCH_2-$	Serine	−0.63	
	Histidine	−0.65	
$H_2NCOCH_2CH_2-$	Glutamine	0.93	
H_2NCOCH_2-	Asparagine	−0.99	
$H_2NCH_2CH_2CH_2-$	Ornithine	−1.50	
$H_3N^+-CH_2CH_2CH_2CH_2-$	Lysine	−1.54	−3.31
$HOOCCH_2-$	Aspartic acid	−2.15	−3.38
(Least hydrophobic)			

[a] **High positive values indicate very hydrophobic amino acids, and negative values indicate amino acids with hydrophilic character.** From Dressler D, Potter H, *Discovering enzymes*, New York: Scientific American; 1991.

[b] From Pliska V *et al.*, *J Chromatogr*, 1981; 216: 79.

Figure 12.1 (a) The α-helix forms because —NH and —C=O groups interact through hydrogen bonding pulling the backbone into a spiral, as shown in this diagram in a 9-amino peptide: in (A) here only the central carbon atoms are shown for clarity; in (B) the nitrogen and carbons of the backbone are shown, and in (C) the oxygen and hydrogen atoms have been added. All the —NH groups point in the same direction 'up' and the —C=O groups point 'down' to allow the formation of —C=O $\cdots$ H—N— bonds. In (D) the side-chains are added and point outwards from the α-helix. Hydrophobic interactions between some helix-promoting side-chains (the more hydrophobic chains, see Table 12.3) help to stabilise the helix. (b) An idealised α-helix, drawn as a ribbon, showing typical stabilising intrahelical interactions. Specific hydrogen-bonded interactions are said to 'cap' the ends of the chain, known specifically as the N-terminal and C-terminal ends of the helix. Free energies (ΔG) of the interactions, compared with the free energy of hydrophobic bonding involving an isobutyl side-chain ($-4.18\,\text{kJ}\,\text{mol}^{-1}$), are:

N-cap, $4.2–8.4\,\text{kJ}\,\text{mol}^{-1}$

C-cap, $\sim 2\,\text{kJ}\,\text{mol}^{-1}$

Side-chain–side-chain electrostatic interactions, $\sim 2\,\text{kJ}\,\text{mol}^{-1}$

Reproduced from Bryson JW *et al.*, *Science*, 1995; 270: 935.

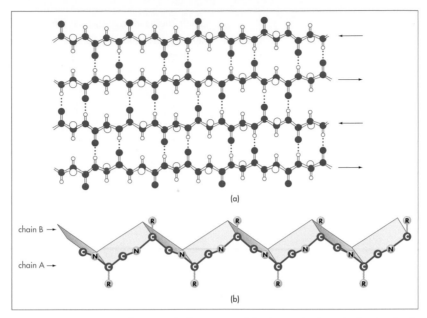

Figure 12.2 (a) A representation of β-sheet formation by four antiparallel polypeptide chains (to be visualised as being in and out of the plane on the paper). The interactions that determine β-sheet stability are more variable than those determining α-helix stability. Different amino acids have different propensities for forming β-sheets. (b) A representation of the concertina shape of a β-sheet showing two antiparallel polypeptide chains, A and B, associated by hydrogen bonding as in (a). Exposed amides at the edge of a β-sheet can hydrogen-bond to other sheets, leading to the formation of insoluble aggregates.

Figure 12.3 Ribbon diagrams of (a) interleukin 1-β, (b) zinc–insulin dimer and (c) the Fc fragment of immunoglobulin.

Reproduced from Lesk AM, *Protein Architecture*, Oxford: IRL Press; 1991.

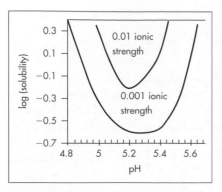

Figure 12.4 A plot of the logarithm of the aqueous stability of β-lactoglobulin versus pH at two different ionic strengths, 0.001 and 0.01 mol kg^{-1}. When the protein is charged at pH values below and above pH 5.3, solubility increases from its lowest point at the isoelectric point. Increased ionic strength shifts the isoelectric point to lower pH values, around 5.2. See also Fig. 12.6.

The relative hydrophilicities of the side-chains of the amino acids correlate well with the hydration of the side-chain; proteins are surrounded by a hydration layer, equivalent to about 0.3 g H_2O per gram of protein, which represents about two water molecules per amino acid residue. Disturbing this layer has an impact on the behaviour of the protein in solution.

The phase behaviour of protein solutions is affected by pH, ionic strength and temperature. Protein–water solutions sometimes exhibit critical solution temperatures (see Chapter 4 for a discussion of phase separation). Phase transitions are important not only in manufacture and formulation but also because they have some pathophysiological implications. Phase separation of gamma-crystallins causes opacification of the lens of the eye in certain cataracts; Figure 12.5 shows the phase diagram obtained.

In section 4.2.3 we discussed the effect of salts on the solubility of organic electrolytes. The parabolic effects of salts on protein solubility (Fig. 12.6) might, at first sight, seem unexpected. Data on haemoglobin solubility, produced many decades ago (Fig. 12.6b) show a general increase in solubility with increasing ionic strength of salts such as NaCl, KCl and $(NH_4)_2SO_4$. However, decrease in solubility occurs at higher ionic strengths – a salting-out effect. Several effects are responsible: (i) the preferential interaction of salts with bulk water, and (ii) the effect of the salts on the surface tension of water, which is related to the energy of cavity formation. In fact, the degree to which

a salt increases the surface tension of water is proportional to its tendency to salt-out proteins.

The presence of other polymers in the solution will also tend to reduce protein solubility because of the volume exclusion effect. The addition of a water-soluble polymer (such as polyoxyethylene glycol (PEG)) can lead to the formation of two distinct liquid phases, owing to changes in the energy required to accommodate the protein molecules and to the unfavourable interaction of PEG with charges on the surface of the protein.

Table 12.4 Values of pK and isoelectric point (IP) of common L-amino acids

Amino acid	pK_1 (COOH)	pK_2 (NH_3^+)	pK_3	IP
Alanine	2.34	9.69	–	6.00
Asparagine	2.02	8.80	–	5.41
Aspartic acid	1.88	3.65 (COOH)	9.60 (NH_3^+)	2.77
Cysteine	1.96	8.18	10.28 (SH)	5.07
Glutamic acid	2.19	4.25 (COOH)	9.67 (NH_3^+)	3.22
Glutamine	2.17	9.13	–	5.65
Glycine	2.34	9.60	–	5.97
Histidine	1.82	6.00 (imidazole)	9.17 (NH_3^+)	7.59
Isoleucine	2.36	9.68	–	6.02
Leucine	2.36	9.60	–	5.98
Lysine	2.18	8.95(α)	10.53 (ε-NH_3^+)	9.74
Methionine	2.28	9.21	–	5.74
Phenylalanine	1.83	9.13	–	5.48
Proline	1.99	10.96	–	6.30
Serine	2.21	9.15	–	5.68
Threonine	2.71	9.62	–	6.16
Tryptophan	2.38	9.39	–	5.89
Tyrosine	2.20	9.11	10.07 (OH)	5.66
Valine	2.32	9.62	–	5.96

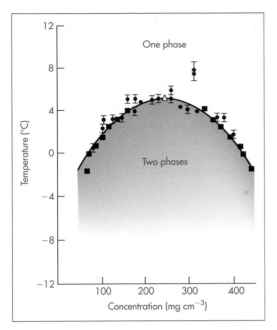

Figure 12.5   The temperature–concentration phase diagram for aqueous gamma-crystallin (mol wt $\sim$20 000) systems (pH $= 7$, $I = 0.24$ mol kg^{-1}). ●, cloud point measurements; ■ concentration measurements of separated phases; $\Delta =$ critical point.

Reproduced from Thompson JA *et al.*, *Proc Natl Acad Sci USA*, 1987; 84: 7079.

PEG molecules grafted to proteins, however, favourably change the properties of therapeutic proteins as we will discuss later.

 Key points

- Proteins have, in increasing order of complexity,
  - *Primary* structure – the order in which the individual amino acids are arranged
  - *Secondary* structures – include coiled α-helix and pleated sheets
  - *Tertiary* structure – the three-dimensional arrangement of helices and coils, and sometimes
  - *Quaternary* forms, which are the association of ternary forms (e.g. the hexameric form of insulin).

- Proteins have solubilities ranging from very soluble to virtually insoluble. The solubility of globular proteins increases as the pH of the solution moves away from the *isoelectric point* (IP), which is the pH at which the molecule has a net zero charge and a tendency to self-associate.
- Proteins are surrounded by a hydration layer, equivalent to about two water molecules per amino acid residue.
- Aqueous solutions of proteins may exhibit phase transitions. Addition of electrolytes such as NaCl, KCl and $(NH_4)_2SO_4$ decreases solubility and at high ionic strengths proteins precipitate – a *salting-out* effect. Organic solvents tend to decrease the solubility of proteins by lowering solvent dielectric constant.

12.2 The stability of proteins and peptides

In Chapter 3 we examined how the stability of drug formulations may be improved from a knowledge of the principal routes of degradation and the kinetics of breakdown. It has been implicitly assumed that the drugs under discussion were typical low-molecular-weight compounds and it is clear that for this type of drug there is a large body of knowledge relating to all aspects of their stability. The formulation of this important class of compound presents more of a challenge.

Protein pharmaceuticals can suffer both physical and chemical instability: the major pathways are summarised in Fig. 12.7. Physical instability refers to changes in the higher-order structure (secondary and above), whereas chemical instability can be thought of as any kind of modification of the protein via bond formation or cleavage, yielding a new chemical entity. For each degradation route we will look at the effect of formulation parameters such as pH and ionic strength on stability and also discuss the application of accelerated stability testing procedures. We will concentrate on the physical aspects of the problem.

Figure 12.6 (a) A generic plot of log(solubility) as a function of square root of ionic strength ($I^{1/2}$) for proteins. (b) The plot for haemoglobin at 25°C, indicating the influence of the nature of the salt. Solubility is expressed as grams per 1000 grams H_2O.

Reproduced from Green AA, *J Biol Chem*, 1932; 95: 47–66.

12.2.1 Physical instability

Physical instability is a phenomenon that is rarely encountered with small organic molecules but that arises in peptides and proteins because of the many conditions under which proteins can lose their native three-dimensional structure. Unfolding of stable forms can lead to adsorption, aggregation or further chemical reactivity. Aggregation can lead to precipitation. Loss of the unique biologically active three-dimensional structure (denaturation), can be caused by heating and, conversely, by cooling or freezing, extremes of pH, and contact with organic chemicals and denaturants. Most of these act through their influence on solubility or conformation, hence the importance of understanding protein–solvent interactions. It is generally thought that denaturation must first occur

before the other processes such as aggregation, adsorption and precipitation can proceed.

Denaturation: reversible and irreversible

Denaturation refers to a disruption of the tertiary and secondary structure of the protein molecule. The denaturation can be *reversible* or *irreversible*. When caused by an increase of temperature, the process is said to be reversible if the native structure is regained on decreasing the temperature. Irreversible denaturation implies that the unfolding process is such that the native structure cannot be regained simply by lowering the temperature. In many cases the protein may become more compact, exposing hydrophobic residues that are normally buried within its core. It is the interaction between these hydrophobic residues in the protein

Figure 12.7 Schematic of the major pathways of protein degradation, which may be physical or chemical in origin.

interior that determines the physical stability of the proteins. When they become exposed to the solvent, these residues can interact with other hydrophobic surfaces such as the container walls or the exposed residues of other denatured proteins, leading to the localised accumulation of denatured protein molecules that results in the formation of aggregates. Increase of temperature results in greater flexibility of the proteins and an increased tendency for collision, leading to aggregate formation. An increase of the ionic strength may lead to neutralisation of the surface charge on the protein molecules that is responsible for their mutual repulsion, again resulting in aggregation. Charge neutralisation and subsequent aggregation can also occur when the pH of the solution approaches the isoelectric point of the protein. In both cases, molecules in the aggregated state can undergo denaturation with time as a result of subtle changes in their conformation and the aggregation process becomes irreversible.

Two basic pathways have been observed for proteins during denaturation and folding. The simplest is a two-state model. If we refer to the native state as N and the unfolded, denatured state as D, we can write

$$N \rightleftharpoons D$$

Once critical hydrophobic residues are exposed to solvents they can interact with other surfaces (containers or the air–water interface). The process may involve the formation of intermediate conformations (I) which

may be stable and may self-associate during folding. The second general pathway for denaturation includes these stable intermediate species and may be written

$$N \rightleftharpoons I_n \rightleftharpoons \cdots \rightleftharpoons I_2 \rightleftharpoons I_1 \rightleftharpoons D$$

The equation shows the unfolding of a native protein to form an intermediate, I_n, which then unfolds to form other intermediates. If the two-state model is assumed, the concentration of denaturant required to achieve equal concentrations of N and D will give some indication of the process. If the fraction of denatured protein, f_d, is calculated under given conditions (temperature, concentration of additive, etc.) we can write

$$f_d = \frac{[D]}{[N] + [D]} = \frac{K_{ND}}{1 + K_{ND}} \quad (12.1)$$

where K_{ND} is the equilibrium constant for denaturation ($K_{ND} = [D]/[N]$), related to the free energy of denaturation $\Delta G_{ND}^{\ominus}$ by

$$K_{ND} = \exp\left(\frac{-\Delta G_{ND}^{\ominus}}{RT}\right) \quad (12.2)$$

Hence,

$$\Delta G_{ND}^{\ominus} = -2.303RT\log K_{ND} \quad (12.3)$$

When 50% of the molecules are unfolded [D] = [N] and $K_{ND} = 1$, therefore $\Delta G_{ND}^{\ominus} = 0$. The temperature at which this occurs is referred to as the melting temperature, T_m. An increase of T_m is indicative of an increase of stability; for example, T_4 lysozyme (lysozyme from bacteriophage T_4) is more stable at pH 6.5 where T_m is 65°C than at pH 2 where T_m is 42°C.

Aggregation/association

Some proteins self-associate in aqueous solution to form oligomers. Insulin, for example, exists in several associated states; the zinc hexamer of insulin is a complex of insulin and zinc that dissolves slowly into dimers and eventually monomers following its subcutaneous administration, so giving it long-acting properties. In most cases, however, it is desirable to prevent association such that only monomeric or dimeric forms are present in the formulations and a more rapid absorption is achieved. Recent studies have been directed towards engineering insulin molecules which are not prone to association,[1,2] or the prevention of association through the addition of surfactants.[3] Protein self-association is a reversible process, i.e. alteration of the solvent properties can lead to the re-formation of the monomeric native protein. There is an important distinction between this association process and the aggregation of proteins, which relates to the usually nonreversible interaction of protein molecules in their denatured state. Aggregation therefore implies that the proteins have undergone some form of denaturation prior to their interaction.

If an intermediate forms that has a solubility less than that of N or D, this can lead to aggregation and eventually to precipitation. For example, the addition of moderate amounts of denaturant to bovine growth hormone (bGH) can generate a partially unfolded intermediate of low solubility that aggregates. Similarly, γ-interferon (IFN-γ) is inactivated by acid treatment or by the addition of salt because the dimeric native state is converted into monomers, which are partially denatured. For both proteins the formation of intermediates leads to inactivation.

Surface adsorption and precipitation

The adsorption of proteins such as insulin on surfaces such as glass or plastic in giving sets is important as it can reduce the amount of agent reaching the patient. It can also lead to further denaturation, which can then cause precipitation and the physical blocking of

delivery ports in insulin pumps, for example. Insulin adsorption on the surface of the containers and the subsequent 'frosting' effect, due to the presence of a finely divided precipitate on the walls (Fig. 12.8), is accelerated by the presence of a large headspace allowing a greater interaction of the insulin with the air–water interface, which facilitates denaturation.

12.2.2 Formulation and protein stabilisation

There are several possible ways in which the physical stability of the protein can be improved through formulation. We will examine methods for minimising this and chemical degradation in the following sections.

Prevention of adsorption

Some measures can be taken to eliminate, or at least minimise, protein denaturation resulting from surface adsorption. The surface of glass is conducive to adsorption and it is preferable in principle to use more hydrophilic surfaces, although this may not be feasible in practice. Alternatively, when the use of glass cannot be avoided, components may be added to the protein solution to prevent adsorption to the glass surface. These additives can act by coating the surface of glass or by binding to the proteins. For example, serum albumin can be included in the formulation since this will compete with the therapeutic protein for the binding sites on the glass surface and so reduce its

Figure 12.8 A vial of insulin showing the frosted appearance of flocculated and adsorbed protein.

From diabetesindogs.com.

adsorption. A similar effect can be achieved by the addition of surfactants such as poloxamers and polysorbates to the protein solution. Consideration must be given, however, to the effects of the surfactants on the pharmacology of the protein and to the toxicological effects of the surfactant itself.

Minimisation of exposure to air

Significant denaturation of proteins can occur when the protein solutions are exposed at the air–solution interface. In this respect the air interface is behaving as a hydrophobic surface and the extent of denaturation is found to be dependent on the time of exposure of the protein at the interface. Agitation of protein solutions in the presence of air or application of other shear forces, such as those that occur when the solutions are filtered or pumped, may also cause denaturation. Again, the inclusion of surfactants can reduce denaturation arising from these processes. Stability testing of protein-containing formulations often involves subjecting the solutions to shaking for several hours and the subsequent assessment of the protein configuration. If the protein has retained its native state and has not aggregated, the formulation is considered to be stable against surface- or shear-induced denaturation.

Addition of cosolvents

Some excipients and buffer components added to the protein solution are able to minimise denaturation through their effects on solvation. These compounds, including polyethylene glycols and glycerol, are referred to as cosolvents. They may act either by causing the preferential hydration of the protein or alternatively by binding to the protein surface. Preferential hydration results from an exclusion of the cosolvent from the protein surface due to steric effects (as in the case of polyethylene glycols); surface tension effects (as with sugars, salts and amino acids) or some form of chemical incompatibility such as charge effects. As a result, more water molecules pack around the protein in order to exclude the additive and the protein becomes fully hydrated and stabilised in a compact form (Fig. 12.9). Alternatively, the cosolvent may stabilise the protein molecule either by binding to it nonspecifically or by binding to specific sites on its surface.

Optimisation of pH

In order to avoid stability problems arising from charge neutralisation and to ensure adequate solubility, a pH must be selected that is at least 0.5 pH units

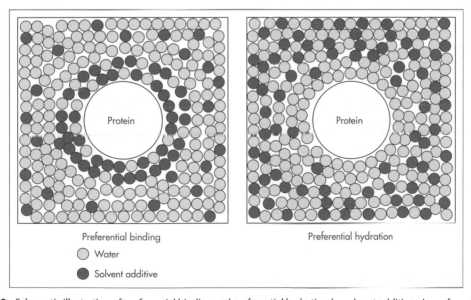

Figure 12.9 Schematic illustration of preferential binding and preferential hydration by solvent additives. In preferential binding the additive occurs in the solvation shell of the protein at a greater local concentration than in the bulk solvent, while preferential hydration results from the exclusion of the additive from the surface of the protein.

Reproduced from Timasheff SN, Arakawa T, in Creighton TE, ed., *Protein Structure: A Practical Approach*, Oxford: IRL Press; 1989: 331–345.

above or below the isoelectric point. This is often difficult to achieve, however, since a pH range of 5–7 is usually required to minimise chemical breakdown and this frequently coincides with the isoelectric point.

Characterisation of degradation

If the formulation does not prevent denaturation and aggregation of the protein, then the pharmacology, immunogenicity and toxicology of the denatured or aggregated protein must be studied to determine its safety and efficacy. Several studies must be performed to determine the extent of degradation that is acceptable for administration. If the aggregates are soluble there may be a significant effect on the pharmacokinetics and immunogenicity of the protein. On the other hand, insoluble aggregates are generally unacceptable and instructions are usually given not to administer protein solutions containing precipitates.

Key points

- *Denaturation* is the disruption of the tertiary and secondary structure of the protein molecule; it can be reversible or irreversible. When caused by an increase of temperature, the process is said to be reversible if the native structure is regained on decreasing the temperature. Irreversible denaturation implies that the unfolding process is such that the native structure cannot be regained simply by lowering the temperature. Hydrophobic residues become exposed to the solvent and can interact with other hydrophobic surfaces (container walls or the exposed residues of other denatured proteins), leading to the localised accumulation of denatured protein molecules and aggregate formation.
- *Aggregation.* Some proteins self-associate in aqueous solution to form oligomers. Although advantageous in some cases (the slow rate of dissolution of the zinc hexamer of insulin into dimers and monomers give it long-acting properties),

self-association is usually prevented, for example by addition of surfactant. This form of association is reversible, unlike the nonreversible aggregation of protein molecules in their denatured state.

- *Adsorption* of proteins on surfaces such as glass or plastic in giving sets reduces the amount of agent reaching the patient, and can lead to further denaturation and precipitation.
- Formulation procedures to improve the physical stability of the protein include:
  - Avoiding contact with glass (if possible) or adding compounds (e.g. serum albumin or surfactants) that coat the glass surface or bind to the proteins, so minimising surface adsorption.
  - Avoiding exposure at the air–solution interface, agitation of protein solutions in the presence of air, or application of other shear forces; inclusion of surfactants can reduce denaturation arising from these processes.
  - Addition of cosolvents such as polyethylene glycols and glycerol minimise denaturation by causing preferential hydration of the protein or by binding to the protein surface.
  - Buffering at a pH at least 0.5 pH units above or below the isoelectric point to avoid stability problems arising from charge neutralisation and to ensure adequate solubility.

12.2.3 Chemical instability

Chemical instability can involve one or more of a variety of chemical reactions including:

- *Deamidation*, in which the side-chain linkage in a glutamine (Gln) or asparagine (Asn) residue is hydrolysed to form a carboxylic acid.

- *Oxidation*: the side-chains of histidine (His), methionine (Met), cysteine (Cys), tryptophan (Trp) and tyrosine (Tyr) residues in proteins are potential oxidation sites.
- *Racemisation*: all amino acid residues except glycine (Gly) are chiral at the carbon atom bearing the side-chain and are subject to base-catalysed racemisation.
- *Proteolysis*, involving the cleavage of peptide (CO-NH) bonds.
- *Beta elimination*: high-temperature treatment of proteins leads to destruction of disulfide bonds as a result of β-elimination from the cystine residue.
- *Disulfide formation*: the interchange of disulfide bonds can result in an altered three-dimensional structure.

Table 12.5 lists the amino acids or sequences that are subject to chemical degradation and lists the formulation approaches used to overcome the problems.

12.3 Protein formulation and delivery

It has been said[4] that 'drug delivery represents the potential Achilles' heel of biotechnology's peptide drug industry'. The reasons for this include the range of instabilities discussed above, the inherent low membrane transport by diffusion because of molecular size and hydrophilicity, and often the need for temporal and site control of delivery.

12.3.1 Protein and peptide transport

For a series of 11 model peptides in an *in vitro* intestinal cell monolayer system, a good correlation was found between the permeability coefficient, P, and the log of the partition coefficient of the peptides between heptane and ethylene glycol (rather than octanol and water) (Fig. 12.10), results that also suggest that the principal deterrent to peptide transport is the breaking of hydrogen bonds.[5] Molecular volume (or size) will increasingly be a factor as the molecular weight of the peptide increases.

The diffusion of proteins and peptides in solution is dictated by the same considerations as those

Table 12.5 Amino acids or sequences susceptible to chemical degradation, together with formulation strategies to reduce degradation[a]

Amino acid or sequence	Mechanism of degradation	Formulation strategy
Cysteine–cysteine	Aggregation	Addition of surfactants, polyalcohols and other excipients
Glutamine, asparagine	Deamidation	pH 3–5
Tryptophan, methionine, cysteine, tyrosine, histidine	Oxidation	pH < 7
Methionine	Oxidation	Protect from oxygen
Tryptophan	Photodecomposition	Protect from light
Lysine-threonine	Copper induced cleavage	Chelating agents
Asparagine-proline, asparagine-tyrosine	Hydrolysis	pH > 7

[a] Reproduced from Parkins DA, Lashmar UT, *PSST*, 2000; 3: 129–137.

discussed in section 2.6. The rate of translational movement depends on the size of the molecule, its shape and interactions with solvent molecules. The rate of translational movement is often expressed by a frictional coefficient, f, defined in relation to the diffusion coefficient D, by equation (12.4):

$$f = \frac{k_B T}{D} \qquad (12.4)$$

where k_B is the Boltzmann constant and T is the temperature in kelvins. Many proteins are nearly spherical in solution, but if their shape deviates from sphericity this is reflected in a frictional ratio, f/f_0, above unity, where f_0 is the rate of diffusion of a molecule of the same size but of spherical shape. The frictional ratio of lysozyme is 1.24 and that of trypsin is 1.187. Globular proteins have values of f/f_0 in the range 1.05–1.38.

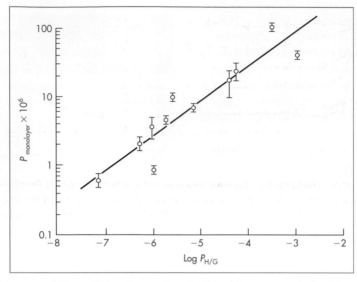

Figure 12.10 A plot of the permeability coefficient P across Caco-2 cell monolayers versus the log P (heptane/glycol) for a series of synthetic peptides to illustrate relationships between lipophilicity and transport.

Reproduced from Paterson DA *et al., Quantitative Structure–Action Relationships,* 1994; 13: 4–10.

The diffusion coefficients and translational movements of proteins are important in considering the release of proteins from hydrogel matrix devices and other delivery vehicles, and in membrane transport, as far as this can be considered to be a passive diffusion process. Changes in shape during membrane transport in a lipid environment may also have to be considered. Table 12.6 gives some values of the diffusion coefficients of a number of therapeutic peptides and proteins.

12.3.2 Lyophilised proteins

Because of their potential instability in solution, therapeutic proteins are often formulated as lyophilised powders. Even in this state several suffer from moisture-induced aggregation. Proteins such as insulin, tetanus toxoid, somatotropin and human albumin aggregate in the presence of moisture, which can lead to reduced activity, stability and diffusion.

In the presence of water vapour at 37°C, lyophilised recombinant human albumin (rHA) experiences intermolecular thiol–disulfide interchange and forms high-molecular-weight, water-insoluble aggregates.[4] The use of excipients (low- and high-molecular-weight sugars, organic acids, etc.) to prevent such effects leads

to the conclusion that the stabilising effect is correlated with the ability of the additives to preferentially absorb water. Figure 12.11 illustrates the effects on rHA solubility and the influence of sorbitol on the changes in solubility.

Table 12.6 Diffusion coefficients and molecular weights of peptides and proteins[a]

Compound	MW	$10^6 D$ (cm^2 s^1)
Oxytocin	1 007	4.30
Lys-vasopressin	1 056	4.18
Arg-vasopressin	1 084	4.27
Somatostatin	1 638	3.74
Calcitonin	3 418	2.76
Insulin	5 807	1.14
Calculated (insulin)		
Monomer	5 807	2.03
Hexamer	34 845	0.93

[a] Reproduced from Hosoya O *et al., J Pharm Pharmacol,* 2004; 56: 1501–150.

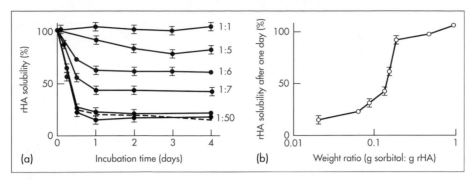

Figure 12.11   Stabilisation of rHA against aggregation afforded by co-lyophilised sorbitol. (a) The time-dependent change of solubility of rHA co-lyophilised with sorbitol at various sorbitol-to-rHA weight ratios, as indicated (the dashed line depicts the time course of rHA aggregation in the absence of sorbitol). (b) rHA solubility after a one-day incubation as a function of sorbitol-to-rHA weight ratio, taken from the data in plot (a).

Reproduced from reference 4.

12.3.3 Water adsorption

Because of the sensitivity of proteins to moisture, the ability to measure sorption of water is vital in preformulation. Water sorption isotherms from recombinant bovine somatotropin (rbST), a protein with 191 amino acids, molecular weight 22 000 Da, show water content versus the relative vapour pressure (p/p_0) for the sodium salt and the 'internal' salt of rbST (Fig. 12.12). These were fitted to modified BET isotherms which have an additional state of interacting water intermediate to the free water and the strongly bound water states.[5,6] Calculations reveal that a monolayer of water is formed from 88 moles of H_2O per mole of protein for the lyophilised sodium salt of rbST, which is equivalent to about 7.3 g per g of protein. The much higher apparent surface areas obtained using water (as opposed to nitrogen) adsorption isotherms (typically $264 \, m^2 \, g^{-1}$, compared with $1.3 \, m^2 \, g^{-1}$ with nitrogen) suggest that water penetrates the powder and that the isotherm represents adsorption and absorption. The practical implications of moisture load are seen in Fig. 12.13, which shows the rate of decomposition of rbST (albeit at 47°C) following incubation in sealed vials.

Both solubility and stability have to be addressed, as well as the mode of delivery. The wide range of biodegradable polymers used for the controlled delivery of proteins and peptides include natural substances, starch, alginates, collagen and a variety of proteins such as crosslinked albumin, a range of synthetic hydrogels, polyanhydrides, polyesters or orthoesters, poly(amino acids) and poly(caprolactones). Poly(lactide-glycolide)

(PLGA) is one of the commonest polymers used in microsphere form to deliver, *inter alia*, growth hormone-releasing factor, a somatostatin analogue, ciclosporin, and LHRH antagonists.[7,8]

12.3.4 PEGylation of peptides and proteins

Polyoxyethylene glycol (PEG) is a versatile molecule. It is used pharmaceutically in molecular weight ranges from 200 to 10 000 Da. The polyoxyethylene chain forms an integral part of many nonionic surfactants (polysorbate 80, Triton X-100). PEG is used as a vehicle

Figure 12.12   Comparison of fits obtained by the BET (dashed lines) and GAB (solid lines) models for the sorption isotherms of the sodium (■) and internal (□) salts of bovine somatropin.

Reproduced from reference 5.

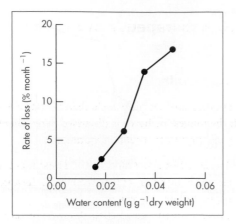

Figure 12.13 The increasing rate of decomposition of a lyophilised rbST formulation with increasing water content following incubation in sealed vials at 47°C.

Reproduced from reference 5.

for drug delivery: higher-molecular-weight fractions are used in suppository bases and lower-molecular-weight species (200–300 Da) that are liquid at room temperature are useful drug solvents. The molecule can be coupled in a range of molecular weights and hence lengths to peptides and proteins, enhancing their native properties by creating a hydrophilic 'envelope' around proteins and antibodies (Fig. 12.14). A variety of techniques is also used to modify the properties of liposomes and nanoparticles to reduce their uptake by the reticuloendoethelial system. The PEG chains act to prevent opsonisation and hence RES scavenging, thus increasing their half-life *in vivo*.

Pegylation is the term used to describe this modification of proteins, peptides or indeed nonpeptide molecules by linking one or more polyethylene glycol (PEG) chains to the molecule[9]. Polyoxyethylene glycol is non-toxic, non-immunogenic, non-antigenic and highly soluble in water. The PEG–drug conjugates also have a prolonged circulation time after IV administration; they are less susceptible to degradation by metabolic enzymes; and their immunogenicity is reduced. The hydrophilic halo is thus important, sometimes increasing the water solubility of the molecule and potentially its biological activity through modification of interactions with biological target sites. The section on colloid stability should be consulted (Chapter 6) to see how PEG molecules affect the physical stability of emulsions and particles.

Naturally the physical properties of the PEGylated molecules are altered by their acquired hydrophilic chains. Clearly their molecular radius increases: haemoglobin has a molecular weight of 64 kDa and a radius of 3.1 nm. As the molecular weight of the PEG chains increases, so too does the radius, more than doubling to 7 nm with large PEG chains of 450 ($-OCH_2CH_2-$) units. The viscosity of solutions increased by nearly 5-fold over native haemoglobin solutions. Because of the variety of possible linkages between the PEG molecules and the protein concerned, and because of the choice of PEG molecular size and indeed number of attached molecules, it is vital that the exact structural properties of these modified products are known, especially when generic versions of therapeutic proteins are available. The structure and properties of proteins and monoclonal antibodies prepared by different methods, and

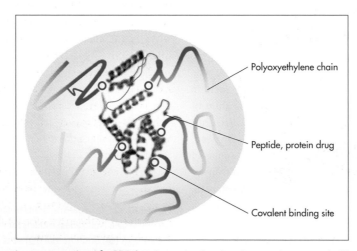

Figure 12.14 A schematic representation of a PEGylated protein, showing the protein surrounded by a PEG protective sheath.

processed in different ways with nonidentical excipients are rarely identical. Thus generic macromolecular products are termed 'bio*similars*' to make this point. Many of the issues surrounding bisomilars are dealt with in reference 10.

12.3.5 Routes of delivery

Table 12.7 lists the invasive and noninvasive routes of delivery for peptides and proteins, involving direct injection of solutions, depot systems and a variety of oral, nasal, topical and other formulations. Figure 12.15 summarises some of the issues involved in delivery of peptides and proteins by different routes. Cyclic peptides such as ciclosporin (**I**) can be absorbed orally; the bioavailability of ciclosporin is of the order of 15%. Such cyclic peptides, although molecularly large, bear a closer resemblance to conventional drugs in many ways, but absorption is quite compound-specific.

Structure I Ciclosporin in two different modes of representation.

12.4 A therapeutic protein and a peptide

12.4.1 Insulin

It is appropriate that the protein therapeutic substance with the longest pedigree is discussed here. There are three main types of insulin preparations:

- Those with a *short* duration of action that have a relatively rapid onset (soluble insulin, insulin lispro and insulin aspart)
- Those with an *intermediate* duration of action (isophane insulin and insulin zinc suspension)
- Those with a slow action, slower in onset and lasting for *long* periods (crystalline insulin zinc suspension)

Some aspects of insulin were dealt with in section 10.2.5. Table 12.8 lists some of the insulin formulations designed to produce different durations of onset and action. Insulin is generally self-administered subcutaneously with injection pens, needle-free devices or pumps.

Precipitation of insulin and other proteins

Precipitation of insulin in pumps due to the formation of amorphous particles, crystals or fibrils of insulin can lead to changes in release pattern or to blockage that prevents insulin release. 'Amorphous' or 'crystalline' precipitates can be caused by the leaching of divalent metal contaminants or lowering of pH (due to CO_2 diffusion or leaching of acidic substances), but can be prevented. More difficult to solve is the tendency of insulin to form fibrils as illustrated in Fig. 12.16.

The interactions leading to fibril formation result from the monomeric form, and from change in monomer conformation and hydrophilic attraction of the parallel β-sheet forms. Fibril formation is also encouraged by contact of the insulin solution with hydrophobic surfaces.

Propylene glycol, glycerol, nonionic and ionic surfactants and calcium ions have been used in formulations to achieve greater stability, reducing fibril formation, but the most successful strategy is the addition of calcium ions or zinc, which appear to protect the hexameric form of the insulin (see section 10.2.5).

Table 12.7 Routes of delivery for proteins and peptides[a]

Delivery routes	Formulation and device requirements	Commercial products[b]
Invasive		
Direct injection: intravenous (i.v.), subcutaneous (s.c.), intramuscular (i.m.), intracerebral vein (i.c.v.)	Liquid or reconstituted solid, (syringe)	Activase (alteplase) Nutropin (somatrotropin) RecombiVax (hepatitis B vaccine)
Depot system (s.c. or i.m.)	Biodegradable polymers, liposomes, permeable polymers (not degradable) microspheres, implants	Lupron Depot (leuprolide) Zoladex (goserelin) Decapeptyl (triptorelin)
Noninvasive		
Pulmonary	Liquid or powder formulations, nebulisers, metered dose inhalers, dry powder inhalers	Pulmozyme (dornase alfa)
Oral	Solids, emulsions, microparticulates, with or without absorption enhancers	
Nasal	Liquid, usually requires permeation enhancers	Synarel (nafarelin)
Topical	Emulsions, creams or pastes (liposomes)	
Transdermal	Electrophoretic (iontophoresis), electroporation, chemical permeation enhancers, prodrugs, ultrasonics	
Buccal, rectal, vaginal	Gels, suppositories, bioadhesives, particles	

[a] Modified from reference 7.

[b] Activase (recombinant human tissue plasminogen activator), Nutropin (recombinant human growth hormone) and Pulmozyme (recombinant human deoxyribonuclease I) are all products of Genentech; RecombiVax (recombinant hepatitis B surface antigen) is produced by Merck; Lupron Depot (leuprolide acetate – PLGA) is a product of Takeda Pharmaceuticals; Zoladex (goserelin acetate – PLGA) is produced by AstraZeneca; Decapeptyl is produced by Debiopharm; Synarel (nafarelin acetate) is produced by Roche.

Recombinant human insulin: insulin lispro and insulin aspart

Chemical modifications to an endogenous protein, however minor, can lead to significant differences in properties and activity. Species differences can also be great. Salmon calcitonin is 10 times more potent than human calcitonin, for example. Recombinant human protein analogues may be subtly different, as in the case of insulin lispro in which the sequence of proline and lysine at positions 28 and 29 in the B protein chain has been reversed (Fig. 12.17a). This sole difference leads to formation of hexamers, which more rapidly dissociate to monomers on injection, giving a faster onset of action than human insulin in which the B28 is proline and B29 is lysine (such as the recombinant product Humulin S, which is injected up to an hour before meals).

Insulin glargine (Lantus, Aventis) has two arginines added to the B30 position (Fig. 12.17b). Its isoelectric point changes from a pH of 5.4 to 6.7, making it a soluble (and thus clear) solution in the acid medium of pH 4 in which it is supplied. When it is injected subcutaneously, however, glargine precipitates at the physiological pH of 7.4, which delays its absorption and prolongs its action. Substituting glycine for asparagine at the A21 position and adding zinc stabilises the hexamer and delays absorption further.

Glargine has a similar insulin receptor affinity to that of NPH (Neutral Protamine Hagedorn, an intermediate-acting insulin that initially achieves slower action through the addition of protamine to short-acting insulin) so that once absorbed in the circulation, glargine is equipotent to NPH. The result is a relatively

Figure 12.15 A schematic diagram referring to the different routes of administration of protein and peptide drugs, namely the parenteral, nasal, oral and pulmonary routes and by pumps and patches. Of all these the oral route is the most problematic. Other potential routes, dermal, vaginal, anal and ocular are listed. AE = absorption enhancers; EI: enzyme inhibitors; EP: electroporation or iontophoresis. RT; respiratory tract.

Reproduced from Agu RU *et al.*, *Respir Res*, 2001; 2: 198–202.

constant supply of insulin with an onset of approximately 2 hours and a duration of action of approximately 24 hours.

12.4.2 Calcitonin

Calcitonin, a peptide hormone of 32 amino acids having a regulatory function in calcium and phosphorus metabolism, is used in various bone disorders such as osteoporosis. Salmon, human, pig and eel calcitonin are used therapeutically. Human calcitonin (hCT) has a tendency to associate rapidly in solution and, like insulin, form fibrils, resulting in a viscous solution.[11] The fibrils are 8 nm in diameter and often associate with one another. Heating fibrillated hCT solutions in 50% acetic acid–water converts the system back to soluble monomers. hCT has a pK of 8.7, while salmon calcitonin (SCT) has a pK of 10.4. This accounts for

the high stability of SCT at pH 7.4, as electrostatic interactions between calcitonin monomers play a role. At pH 7.4, SCT monomers will be charged and will repel each other.

12.5 DNA and oligonucleotides

12.5.1 DNA

DNA of varying molecular weights is used in gene therapy. Figure 12.18 shows the well-known primary structure of DNA and the charge-determining phosphate groups connected to the deoxyribose rings. As DNA is a large hydrophilic, polyanionic and sensitive macromolecule, its successful delivery to target cells and the nucleus within these cells is an issue. Shearing of high-molecular-weight DNA while stirring in solution

Table 12.8 Effect of insulin formulation on its pharmacokinetics after subcutaneous injection

Product[a]	Formulation	Pharmacokinetics[b]
Humulin R Novolin R	Zinc-insulin crystalline suspension (acid regular)	Rapid onset, short duration Start, 0.5 h; peak, 2.5–5 h; end, 8 h
Humulin N Novolin N	Isophane suspension protamine, zinc crystalline insulin (buffer water for injection)	Intermediate-acting, slower onset, longer duration than regular insulin
		Start, 1.5 h; peak, 4–12 h; end, up to 24 h
Humulin 70/30[c] Novolin 70/30[c]	70% isophane suspension 30% zinc crystalline	Intermediate-acting, faster onset longer duration
		Start, 0.5 h; peak, 2–12 h; end, up to 24 h
Humulin U	Extended zinc-insulin suspension – all crystalline	Slow-acting, slow onset, longer, less-intense duration than R or N forms
Humulin L Novolin L	70% zinc-insulin crystalline suspension 30% amorphous insulin (cloudy suspension)	Intermediate-acting, slower onset, longer duration Start, 2.5 h; peak, 7–15 h; end, 22 h
Humulin BR	Zinc crystalline insulin dissolved in sodium diphosphate buffer	Rapid onset, short duration; use in pumps only

[a] Humulin products (Eli Lilly & Company) contain recombinant human insulin derived from *Escherichia coli*; Novolin products (Novo Nordisk) are recombinant human insulin derived from *Saccharomyces cerevisiae*; both companies also sell other forms of recombinant human insulin and may have additional forms (formulations or new drugs) in clinical trials.

[b] The pharmacokinetics of each formulation may vary greatly among different individuals; the onset of therapeutic levels of insulin is referred to as the start of the effect, the maximum serum level of insulin is denoted the peak, and the time at which the insulin levels are below therapeutic levels is listed as the end of the therapeutic time course.

[c] Solution consists of 70% N form and 30% R form for both products.

(a)   (b)

Figure 12.16 Transmission electron micrographs of insulin fibrils formed (a) at 37°C, (b) at 80°C (×100 000).

Reproduced from Brange J, *Galenics of Insulin*, Berlin: Springer; 1987.

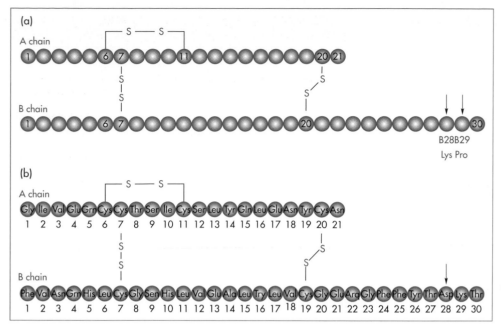

Figure 12.17 (a) Insulin lispro, a product of recombinant DNA technology, is an analogue of human insulin in which the natural sequence of proline and lysine at positions B28 and B29 (shown arrowed) of human insulin has been reversed. (b) Insulin aspart (Novo Nordisk) has an aspartame at B28 (see arrow) replacing the proline of the natural insulin. Insulin glargine has a glycine at position A21 and two arginines at B30.

can lead to breakage of the molecule. One approach to delivery is to complex the DNA with polymers or particles of opposite charge to produce, by condensation, more compact species. Many studies have been conducted to condense the DNA with cationic polymers (e.g. polylysine and chitosan), cationic liposomes and dendrimers, to produce nano-sized complexes that retain an overall positive charge and are able to transfect cells more readily than native or naked DNA. The interaction of DNA with polycationics like chitosan is akin to a coacervation process[12] (Fig. 12.19).

Through the formation of particulates (Fig. 12.20) cell-uptake characteristics and stability are improved, although transfection inside the cell depends ultimately on the successful release of DNA from the complex and its uptake into the nucleus.

12.5.2 Oligonucleotides

Antisense oligonucleotides (**II**) (used for the sequence-specific inhibition of gene expression) are polyanionic single-strand molecules comprising between 10 and 25 nucleotides. They resemble single-stranded DNA or RNA. They have molecular weights ranging from

Structure II Oligonucleotide.

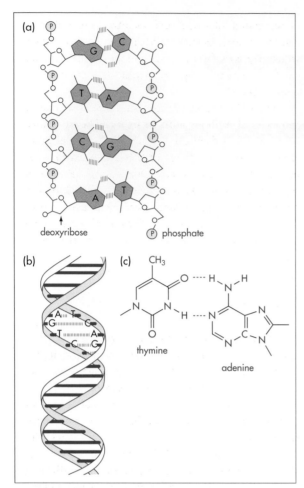

(a)

deoxyribose   ℗ phosphate

(b)   **(c)**   CH₃

thymine

adenine

Figure 12.18 (a) Diagrammatic representation of the interactions between two oligonucleotide strands. ////// represents hydrogen-bonding interactions between the base pairs G–C, T–A, C–G, A–T. P represents the phosphate groups, which confer the negative charge on the molecule. (b) Representation of the double helix again illustrating the hydrogen-bonding interaction that is key to the helical conformation. (c) The detailed primary structure showing the phosphate–deoxyribose–base point sequence for T–A.

3000 to 8000 Da and are hydrophilic, having a log P of approximately −3.5. Like DNA they clearly do not have the appropriate properties for transfer across biological membranes. They are also sensitive to nucleases and nonspecific adsorption to biological surfaces, and hence require to be formulated to achieve delivery and nuclear uptake. Chemical modification of oligonucleotides, which is outside of the scope of this book, can increase the stability and activity of the molecules.

Figure 12.19 Ternary phase diagram of complex co-acervation between pRE-luciferase plasmid DNA and chitosan at 55°C in 50 mmol dm⁻³ Na₂SO₄. Sodium sulfate solution was regarded as one component, since the concentration change in the experiment range was minimal. The region to the right of line the ABC depicts the conditions under which phase separation occurs. The concentration ranges in the small grid area yield distinct particles.

Reproduced from Mao H-Q *et al.*, *J Control Release*, 2001; 70: 399–421.

12.6 Therapeutic monoclonal antibodies

There are now a number of monoclonal antibodies (MAbs)(antibodies produced from a single clone of cells) available for use in the clinic.[13] Although they have been available since the mid-1970s, there have been problems, not least with their poor distribution and tissue penetration. They are large molecules with molecular weights of the order of 150 kDa and thus they diffuse slowly in tissues, and especially in tumours or inflamed sites. The intravenous route has been most commonly used for their delivery, so formulation has often concentrated on the development of stable solutions. Physical chemistry can explain in part their properties, such as blocking the action of target antigens, binding to antigens and their diffusion and translocation in tissues.[13] Typical MAbs include anti-HER2 monoclonal antibody, Herceptin for breast cancer, and anti-CD20 monoclonal antibody and Rituximab for malignant lymphoma. While there has been evidence suggesting that antibodies against the beta-amyloid plaques can reverse cognitive deficits in early Alzheimer disease, these promising agents do not cross the blood–brain barrier. Antibodies with a

(a)

(b)

Figure 12.20 (a) Electron micrograph of naked plasmid DNA; (b) the same sample after condensation with a cationic partial dendrimer. The size, shape, charge and stability of such complexes depend on the ionic strength of the medium, lipid composition, lipid/DNA ratio and concentration, and even on mixing procedures. Manufacturing issues include those of reproducibility, avoiding aggregation of the resulting colloidal suspension and lyophilisation, as discussed by RI. Mahato *et al.* (*Pharm Res* 1997; 14: 853–859).

Reproduced from Ramaswamy C, Florence AT, *J Drug Del Sci Technol*, 2005; 15: 307–311.

molecular size larger than 150 kDa are easily prevented from passage through the blood–brain barrier. The cerebrospinal fluid level of Rituximab in patients is reported to be only 0.1% of that of serum levels.

Many are also low-potency molecules in spite of their specificity; they have doses in the range of mg/kg IV or SC. With the SC route there is a need to reduce the volume administered, so there is the need for concentrated solutions. Such solutions pose problems: their viscosity is increased and they may be more prone to aggregation.[14] Even small amounts of silicone oil used as lubricants for syringes can lead to antibody aggregation.[15]

Figure 12.21a shows the structure of a typical monoclonal antibody with the light and heavy chains. The variable and constant regions of the model structure are also shown. In (b) a MAb is represented interacting with a target. Panel (c) shows a much-simplified representation of a MAb–drug conjugate and in (d) a conjugate showing the labile disulfide linkage, one of several that can be employed. The rate of release of the drug from the conjugate is of course a key element in its biological activity.

Summary

This chapter has not attempted to provide a complete overview of proteins and peptides and other complex therapeutics such as DNA, oligonucleotides and monoclonal antibodies. It has concentrated on giving a flavour of some of the unique physical properties that the substances discussed here have. It has tried to give some feeling for the properties of peptides and proteins and how their physical properties are dictated not only by the properties of their individual amino acids but also by the spatial arrangement of the amino acids in their polypeptide chains, and of course their interaction with water and other ingredients that might be in formulations. Hydrophobic amino acids alternating with hydrophilic, or charged amino acids can produce tertiary and quaternary structures that are quite different from those induced by the spatial separation of hydrophobic and hydrophilic amino acids. The stability of proteins and peptides is of prime pharmaceutical significance. Maintenance of chemical and physical stability is a prerequisite for clinical use. The macromolecular and generally hydrophilic character of all but the smallest peptides makes this class of compound one that is challenging in terms of delivery for therapeutic ends. Some of the issues involved in the formulation of proteins are also discussed.

Figure 12.21 (a) Representation of a typical monoclonal antibody (MAb) showing the light and heavy chains. The variable and constant regions of the model structure are also shown. (b) A MAb interacting with a target. (c) A much simplified representation of a MAb–drug conjugate, the form that many therapeutic approaches now take. (d) (not to scale) A conjugate showing the labile S–S–linkage, one of several that can be employed. The rate of release of the drug from the conjugate can be a key element in its biological activity.

References

1. Brange J *et al*. Monomeric insulins and their experimental and clinical implications. *Diabetes Care* 1990;13: 923–954.
2. Brems DN *et al*. Altering the self-association and stability of insulin by amino acid replacement. In: Cleland J, ed. *Protein Folding: In Vivo and In Vitro*. ACS Symposium Series 526. Washington, DC: American Chemical Society; 1993: 254-269.
3. Shao Z *et al*. Differential effects of anionic, cationic, nonionic, and physiologic surfactants on the dissociation, alpha-chymotryptic degradation, and enteral absorption of insulin hexamers. *Pharm Res* 1993;10: 243–51.
4. Costantino JR *et al*. Aggregation of a lyophilized pharmaceutical protein, recombinant human albumin: effect

of moisture and stabilization by excipients. *Biotechnology* 1995;13:493–496.

5. Hageman MJ *et al*. Prediction and characterization of the water sorption isotherm for bovine somatotropin. *J Agric Food Chem* 1992;40:342–347.

6. Zografi G. States of water associated with solids. *Drug Dev Ind Pharm* 1988;14:1905–1906.

7. Cleland JL, Langer R. Formulation and delivery of proteins and peptides: design and development strategies. In: Cleland JL, Langer R, eds. *Formulation and Delivery of Proteins and Peptides*. Washington DC: American Chemical Society; 1994: 1-19.

8. Ye M *et al*. Issues in long term protein delivery using biodegradable microparticles. *J Control Rel* 2010;146: 241–260.

9. Veronese FM, Pasut G. PEGylation, successful approach to drug delivery. *Drug Deliv Today* 2005;10:1451.

10. Schellekens H. Biosimilar therapeutics – what do we need to consider? *NDT Plus* 2009;2(Suppl1):i27–i36.

11. Arvinte T *et al*. The structure and mechanism of formation of human calcitonin fibrils. *J Biol Chem* 1993;268:6415–6422.

12. Mao HQ *et al*. Chitosan-DNA nanoparticles as gene carriers: synthesis, characterisation and transfection efficiency. *J Control Release* 2001;70: 399–421.

13. Breedveld FC. Therapeutic monoclonal antibodies. *Lancet* 2000;355:735–740.

14. Yadav S *et al*. Factors affecting the viscosity of high concentration solutions of different monoclonal antibodies. *J Pharm Sci* 2010;99:4812–4829.

15. Thirumangalathu R *et al*. Silicone oil- and agitation-induced aggregation of a monoclonal antibody in aqueous solution. *J Pharm Sci* 2009;98:3167–3181.

13

Physical assessment of dosage forms

It is important to have means of studying the quality and behaviour of formulations. Obviously their performance in patients is their ultimate test. However, tests in the laboratory to measure physical properties *in vitro* can give insights into the quality of the product. After all, formulations are physical constructs and various aspects of their physical chemistry can inform us about differences between batches of products, and can sometimes explain behaviour, aberrant or otherwise.

This chapter presents the basics of some *in vitro* tests that can be applied to pharmaceutical products, using the background physical chemistry discussed in earlier chapters. In particular, we will examine how we can measure the influence on drug release rates or product performance of some of the key parameters of pharmaceutical systems, such as particle size, viscosity, adhesion, swelling, flotation or formulation. It is necessary to appreciate the importance of *in vitro* testing in formulation development and in batch-to-batch control of uniformity but also in assessing product defects. *In vitro* tests might be preferred to *in vivo* measures when there is a good correlation between the two, but it should be appreciated that such correlations and physiological verisimilitude are not essential for validity in quality control, where reproducibility of a product is often in itself a goal.

It is hoped that this brief account of tests – some simple, some complex – will stimulate thought on how in practice we can assess the products we handle.

13.1 Dissolution testing of solid oral dosage forms

One of the commonest tests applied to solid oral dosage forms in particular is to measure the rate of release of the drug using a dissolution test.

Equations such as the Noyes–Whitney equation cannot readily be applied to deal with the situation of tablet and capsule dissolution because of the constantly changing surface area of the disintegrated tablet components. The presence of additives such as wetting agents, which may alter solubility as well as wettability and the tablet matrix or coating, will also determine release rates. However, the rate of solution of a solid drug substance from a granule or a tablet is dependent to a large extent on its solubility in the solvent phase and its concentration in that phase. Test conditions should provide a reasonable and realistic challenge to the dosage form in terms of degree of agitation, temperature, volume and pH of the dissolution medium. *In vitro* tests thus will provide the opportunity to make precise and reproducible release measurements to distinguish between different formulations of a drug or the effect of ageing, processing or production changes (batch-to-batch variation). The tests do not replace the need for clinical work, but they can pinpoint factors of importance in determining drug release.

Dissolution testing, whether routine or during development is necessary when:

- The drug has low aqueous solubility.
- The dissolution is poor or variable when tested by an official compendial test procedure (BP or USP).
- There is evidence that particle size may affect bioavailability.
- The physical forms of drug – polymorphs, solvates or complexes – have varying solubility and hence likely dissolution characteristics.
- Specific excipients alter dissolution or absorption.
- There is evidence that tablet or capsule coating may interfere with disintegration or dissolution.

The above list refers to solubility, dissolution rate, particle size, polymorphism, excipient interactions and film coating, some of the complexities of formulation.

In vitro dissolution test methods may be divided into two types, involving either *natural convection* or *forced convection*. Most practical methods fall into the latter category, as there is a degree of agitation *in vivo*. In natural-convection methods in which, for example, a pellet of material is suspended from a balance arm in the dissolution medium, the conditions are unnatural. In forced-convection methods, a degree of agitation is introduced. These can, in turn, be divided into those that employ non-sink conditions and those that achieve sink conditions in the dissolution medium.

Sink conditions exist when the concentration of solute in the solvent is low and does not affect the dissolution process. In the opposite case of non-sink conditions the concentration of solute is significant and slows down the dissolution process.

13.1.1 Pharmacopoeial and compendial dissolution tests

The dissolution test method now widely used and described in the British Pharmacopoeia is a variant of the rotating basket method shown in Fig. 13.1a. Figure 13.1b shows the alternative rotating paddle system. The specification of precise dimensions shown in the diagram emphasises the importance of standardisation of equipment to ensure consistency between laboratories.[1]

Tablets or capsules are placed in a basket of wire mesh, the mesh being small enough to retain broken pieces of tablet but large enough to allow entry of solvent without wetting problems. The basket may be rotated at any suitable speed, but most monographs specify 50, 100 or 1500 rpm. The effect of rotation speed on the dissolution profile of a sulfamethizole formulation is shown in Fig. 13.2, an effect that would be predicted from our understanding of particle dissolution.[2] In all the methods the appropriate pH for the dissolution medium must be chosen, not one that maximises dissolution but one that is physiologically reasonable.

With drugs of very low solubility it is sometimes necessary to consider the use of *in vitro* tests that allow sink conditions to be maintained. This generally involves the use of a lipid phase into which the drug can partition; alternatively, it may involve dialysis or physical replacement of the solvent phase. Mixed-solvent systems such as ethanol–water or surfactant systems may be used to enhance the solubility of

Speed (rpm) as specified in monograph
25–150 rpm (± 4% USP/NF; ± 5% BP)

Shaft
USP/NF: 6–10.5 mm diameter
BP: approximately 6 mm diameter
2 mm vent in drive disc

Centring (or tilt)
± 2 mm at all points

Eccentricity
USP/NF: no significant wobble
BP: no perceptible wobble

Sampling point
USP/NF: midway from top of basket
to top of fluid and no closer than
1 cm to side of flask
BP: halfway between basket and
side at middle of basket

Flask
USP/NF: cylindrical with spherical
bottom, 16–17.5 cm high, inside
diameter 10–10.5 cm, plastic or glass
BP: cylindrical, flat bottomed, glass

Basket

Basket position
USP/NF: 2.5 ± 0.2 cm
BP: 2.0 ± 0.2 cm

(a)

Paddle

Paddle position
USP/NF: 2.5 ± 0.2 cm

Stainless or glass helix may be
attached to floating dosage forms

(b)

Figure 13.1 The rotating basket and rotating paddle versions of the official method for dissolution testing of solid oral dosage forms. (a) The rotating basket – method 1, USP/NF. This method is official for USP/NF and BP. Current specifications describing the geometry and positions for each compendium are shown. (b) The rotating paddle – method 2, USP/NF.

Reproduced with permission from Hanson W, *Handbook of Dissolution Testing*, 2nd edn, Eugene, OR: Aster Publishing; 1991.

Figure 13.2 Single-tablet dissolution profiles for a sulfamethizole formulation in dilute HCl with USP XVIII method at three stirring rates.

Reproduced from reference 2.

Figure 13.3 A recommended standard design for a flow-through cell: the cell is cylindrical in shape and constructed of glass or other suitable material. A, an internal volume not exceeding 20 cm³ between barrier and filter. B, a bottom barrier of either a porous glass plate or a bed of 1 mm diameter glass beads designed to disperse flow and provide uniform distribution over the dosage chamber A. C, a suitable filter of approximately 25 mm diameter. D, fluid flow from bottom to top.

sparingly soluble drugs, but some prefer the use of flow-through systems in these cases. Both human and simulated gastric fluids have been used in dissolution tests.[3]

13.1.2 Flow-through systems

A variant on the dissolution methods discussed uses neither basket nor paddle; convection is achieved by solvent flow through a chamber such as that in Fig. 13.3. Dissolution data obtained from this type of system, where continuous monitoring of drug concentration is achieved, must be interpreted with care as the concentration–time profile will be dependent on the volume of solvent, its flow rate and the distance of the detection device from the flow cell, or rather the void volume of solvent.

Clearly there is no absolute method of dissolution testing. Whatever form of test is adopted, results are of most use on a comparative basis, where batches of a product are compared or where a branded product, say, is compared with a generic, and so on.

Factors affecting the release of drugs from other dosage forms can usefully be examined. These include suppositories, topical ointment and cream preparations, and transdermal devices. It is of course always useful to have good *in vitro–in vivo* correlations.

13.2 *In vitro–in vivo* correlations

Some factors that influence the sensitivity and degree of *in vitro–in vivo* correlations are shown in Scheme 13.1. Some relate to the dissolution method, some to the dosage form and some, of course, to *in vivo* behaviour.

13.3 Evaluation of suppositories and topical preparations

13.3.1 Suppository formulations

Suppositories are probably more difficult to study than many other dosage forms because it is not a simple matter to simulate conditions in the rectal

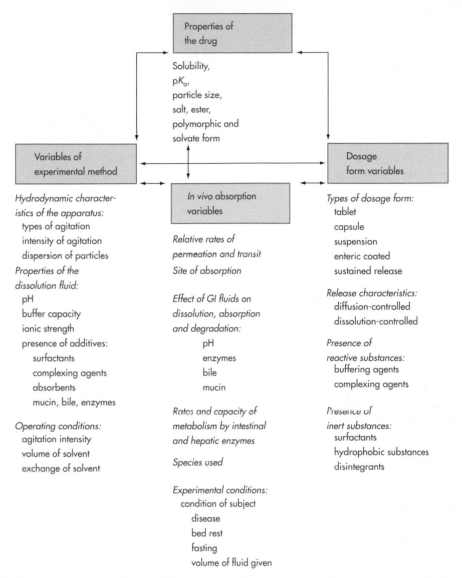

Scheme 13.1 Some interacting variables that influence the sensitivity and degree of *in vivo* correlation of *in vitro* methods for measuring drug release and dissolution.

Modified from Barr WH, *Pharmacology*, 1972; 8: 55.

cavity. In one system,[4] shown in Fig. 13.4, a suppository is placed in a pH 7.8 buffer in a dialysis bag. This bag is placed in a second dialysis bag filled with octanol, and the whole is suspended in a flow system at 37°C. The amount of drug released into the outer liquid is monitored. The results must be interpreted with care as it is possible for substances that complex with the drug to reduce transport across the dialysis membrane, something that may or may not happen in the body.

A variant on this arrangement was used[5] to obtain the data in Fig. 13.5 which shows the value of such tests, in this case illustrating the reduction in aminophylline release from a Witepsol H15 base as a function of product age.

13.3.2 *In vitro* release from topical products and transdermal systems

Ointments and transdermal systems encounter little water in use but, in the spirit of using release tests to

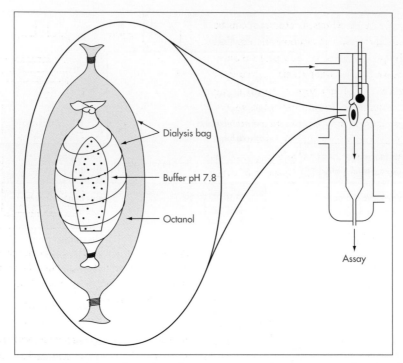

Figure 13.4 An *in vitro* system for studying drug release from suppositories. The suppository is placed in a buffer with a dialysis bag that itself resides in a dialysis bag containing octanol to simulate partitioning into tissue. The amount of drug eluted into a flowing aqueous phase is then measured.

Modified from reference 4.

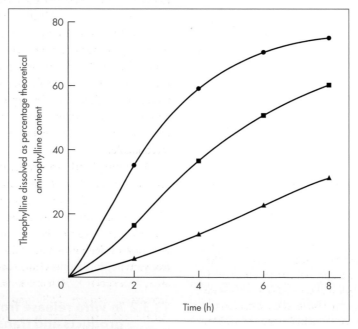

Figure 13.5 Dissolution profiles for aminophylline (theophylline and ethylenediamine mixture) suppositories stored at 35°C: ●, 2 months old; ■, 8 months old; ▲, 12 months old.

Reproduced from reference 5 with permission.

compare basically similar products, useful data can be obtained by measuring release into aqueous media. This information can be predictive of *in vivo* performance. Sometimes an attempt can be made to simulate a lipid biophase to mimic the skin. Some topical products can be tested simply in volunteers. Steroid formulations, for example, can be tested using the vasoconstrictor activity of the steroid to quantitate the results. An *in vitro* system[6] using isopropyl myristate as the 'solvent phase' or 'biophase' is shown in Fig. 13.6. The amount of drug

Figure 13.7 A system to measure the release of drug from an ointment via a synthetic membrane into a temperature-controlled and stirred receptor medium.

Reproduced from reference 7.

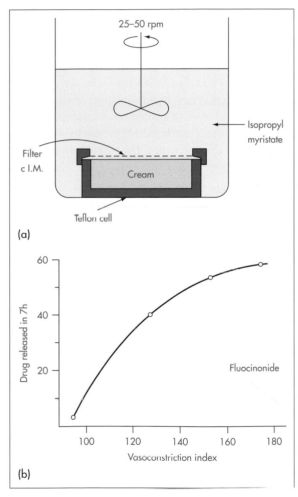

Figure 13.6 (a) An apparatus for the examination of the release of a steroid from a cream formulation: the cream is placed in a Teflon receptacle and covered with a membrane impregnated with isopropyl myristate, and the concentration of fluocinonide is monitored in the bulk isopropyl myristate layer. (b) Release *in vitro* compared with results of vasoconstrictor tests on four formulations.

Modified from reference 6.

released in 7 hours correlates with the vasoconstriction index for four formulations of fluocinonide. Vasoconstriction evidenced by skin blanching correlates with steroid potency in topical preparations.

A variant of this simple apparatus is that shown in Fig. 13.7 based on the Franz diffusion cell, which has been used to measure the release rate of tacrolimus from an ointment.[7] When a membrane has to be employed to keep the product in a compartment, as with suppositories and most semisolids, the retarding properties of the membrane and loading should be measured before the key formulation and design parameters are determined. Examples in Fig. 13.8 demonstrate how the influence of total drug loading and mean particle size may be seen, in this case with terconazole.[8]

A rotating bottle apparatus allows the study of the release of glyceryl trinitrate from Deponit transdermal patches (Fig. 13.9).[9] The influence of temperature and pH on release can be examined with this apparatus, confirming that release is essentially determined by the diffusion of drug in the adhesive layer of the product (see section 10.3) but is clearly proportional to surface area, as expected. Release increases as temperature increases; between 32°C and 37°C an increase in release rate of between 1 and $2\,\mu g\,cm^{-2}\,h^{-1}$ is detected. The BP specifies a distribution (release) test for transdermal patches based on the paddle apparatus for tablet and capsules.

Figure 13.8 An illustration of the usefulness of *in vitro* tests in drug formulation development: the effect on terconazole release rate *in vitro* of (a) drug loading and (b) particle size.

Reproduced from reference 8.

13.4 Rheological characteristics of products

The rheological behaviour of liquids and semisolids has been described in other chapters. Viscosity monitoring can be used as a quality control procedure, and some practical rheological tests are valuable, as discussed here.

The injectability of nonaqueous injections, which are often viscous and thus difficult to inject, can be assessed by a test for *syringeability*. Sesame oil has a viscosity of 56 cP (56 mPa s), but added drugs and adjuvants can increase the viscosity of such vehicles.

The desired physical properties of various topical preparations are listed in Table 13.1. The terms 'soft and unctuous' and 'hard and stiff' are difficult to quantify, but it is useful at least to consider the variety of descriptions that may be applied in a consistency profile of an external pharmaceutical product. Scheme 13.2 lists these comprehensively as primary, secondary and tertiary characteristics. The tertiary properties are probably the most elusive.

13.5 Adhesivity of dosage forms

A study of the adhesion of dosage forms to epithelial surfaces is important because of the possibility of enhancing contact between oral dosage forms and the gut wall to slow the rate of transit down the

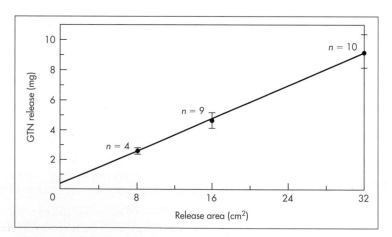

Figure 13.9 *In vitro* glyceryl trinitrate (GTN) release (24 h) into 80 cm³ isotonic NaCl versus release area of Deponit TTS.

Reproduced from reference 9 with permission.

Table 13.1 Properties of some topical preparations[a]

Class	Nature	Required physical properties
1	Ophthalmic ointments	Softest type of ointment
2	Other commonly used ointments	Soft and unctuous, but stiff enough to remain in place when applied
3	Protective ointments, e.g. zinc oxide paste	Hard and stiff; remain in place when applied to moist ulcerated areas

[a] Reproduced from Sherman P, *Rheol Acta*, 1971; 10: 121.

gastrointestinal tract. But it is also relevant in understanding the unwanted adhesion of products to the oesophagus and other epithelial surfaces. Adhesive preparations have been formulated for diverse tasks such as the topical treatment of stomatitis and the administration of insulin. The adhesive nature of

transdermal patches is important, as is the adhesion of film coats to tablet surfaces. An investigation of adhesion of erythrocytes and bacterial cells to polymer surfaces is also important for an understanding of the blood compatibility of polymers and bacterial infection mediated by catheters.

Some examples of solid–solid adhesion processes are shown diagrammatically in Fig. 13.10. Peeling tests for film coats (the separation diagrams in the figure demonstrate the geometry of such tests) are a part of pharmaceutical development and similar tests for the adhesion of transdermal particles to skin have been used. The measurement of film coat adhesion is discussed in Chapter 7.

Several methods of testing oral dosage forms for adhesivity are in use. One involves the raising of the dosage form through an excised porcine oesophagus[10] (Fig. 13.11). Another assesses the adhesion of a moistened capsule or tablet to a tissue surface using a strain gauge[11] (Fig. 13.12).

The effects of polymer concentration and composition and of additives on the adhesivity of film coating

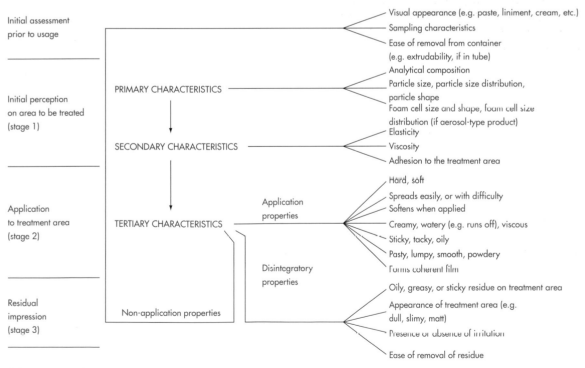

Scheme 13.2 Consistency profile for pharmaceuticals employed externally.

Reproduced from Sherman P, *Rheol Acta*, 1971; 10: 121.

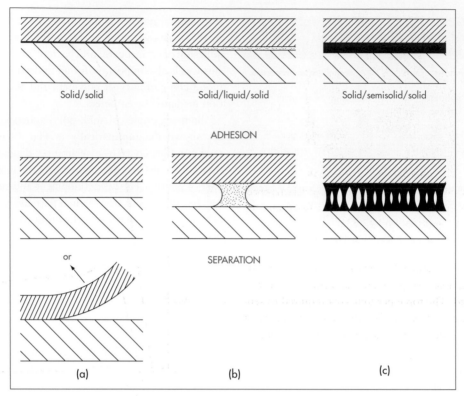

Figure 13.10 Diagrammatic representation of adhesion between solid surfaces at rest: (a) no adhesive layer; (b) a viscous liquid at the interface; and (c) a semisolid adhesive layer. On separation, the nature of the intervening film is shown: (a) no film, (b) a necking filament of liquid, (c) multiple filaments of the semisolid layer.

Figure 13.11 A system for measurement of the force required to detach a solid dosage form from an isolated porcine oesophagus.

Reproduced from reference 10.

Figure 13.12 A device to measure the force of detachment of tablets or capsules from porcine oesophageal tissue, used to determine the values given in Fig. 13.13.

materials can be studied using this apparatus, and the force, f, required to separate tablet from substrate can be measured. The force per unit area required to separate two circular plates of radius r initially in contact through a liquid layer of thickness h and viscosity η over time t is

$$f = \frac{3k'}{4t}\left[\frac{r^2\eta}{h^2}\right] \qquad (13.1)$$

where k', is a constant. This equation applies only when the surfaces are pulled apart slowly.

Clearly the viscosity of the liquid (η) is a key determinant of the force of separation. The 'tackiness' of a system is not, however, simply related to viscosity.[12] High-molecular-weight materials must be present in aqueous solutions for example to provide an elastic element to the viscous flow. Rubbery polymers that have partly liquid and partly elastic characteristics are employed as adhesives in surgical dressings and adhesive tapes. It is still unclear what factors influence the adhesivity of high-molecular-weight soluble polymers such as hydroxypropylmethylcellulose (HPMC). HPMC is a component of film coating materials. Figure 13.13 shows the detachment force required to separate tablets from a glass surface when coated with HPMC-606 from a 4% solution, shown here as a function of the thickness of the film coat.[13] The effect of the presence of high concentrations of polyoxyethylene glycol 6000 is to reduce adhesivity, presumably because the glycol solution is less tacky.

The variables likely to affect the process of adhesion of coated tablets to mucosal surfaces are shown in diagrammatic form in Fig. 13.14: film coat thickness,

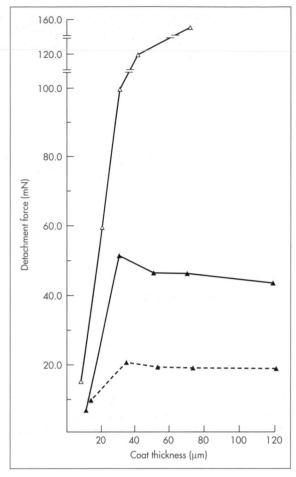

Figure 13.13 The effect of film thickness on the adhesiveness of tablets coated with HPMC-606 from a 4% solution ($\triangle$) and in the presence of 4% PEG 6000 ($-\blacktriangle-$) and 6% PEG 6000 ($\cdots \blacktriangle \cdots$), i.e. 1:1 and 1:1.5 ratios of HPMC to PEG respectively.
Reproduced from reference 13 with permission.

the nature of the film coat, its rate of solution or hydration, the rheology of the solution formed, its surface tension and its elongational characteristics. Eight stages have been identified. Stage I (before contact occurs) defines the system and the variables of film coating thickness, the nature of the coating and the nature of the tissue surface. In stage II the presence of moisture or water is postulated, and here the wetting characteristics of the film will be important. In stage III the film coat begins to dissolve and we assume that contact is made, or is about to be made with the tissue; the forces bringing the tablet and the tissue together are not controllable because contact is made by collision and is dependent to some extent on the ratio of

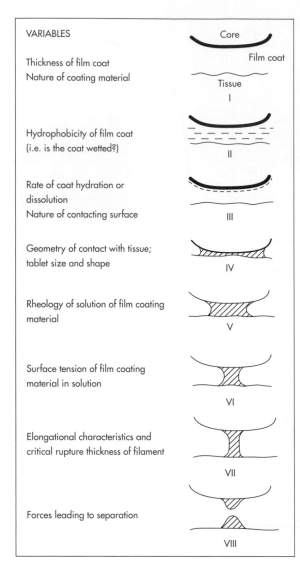

VARIABLES

Thickness of film coat
Nature of coating material

I

Hydrophobicity of film coat
(i.e. is the coat wetted?)

II

Rate of coat hydration or
dissolution
Nature of contacting surface

III

Geometry of contact with tissue;
tablet size and shape

IV

Rheology of solution of film coating
material

V

Surface tension of film coating
material in solution

VI

Elongational characteristics and
critical rupture thickness of filament

VII

Forces leading to separation

VIII

Core

Film coat

Tissue

Figure 13.14 Diagrammatic representation of the possible sequence of events in the adhesion of a tablet to a mucosal surface and its subsequent separation, with a partial listing of the many variables in the process.

Reproduced from Florence AT, Salole EG, *Formulation Factors in Adverse Reactions*, London: Wright; 1990.

tablet size to oesophageal diameter. Stage IV represents contact, when the angle of approach, together with the tablet size and shape, will determine the opportunity for adhesion. Stages V to VIII represent the detachment process initiated, for example, by swallowing food or water or dry swallowing; here the rheological and elongational characteristics of the adhesive material are important.

13.6 Gastro-retentive systems: buoyancy tests

Often in practice one seeks to find out differences between branded and generic products. There are now several gastro-retentive systems that rely for their function on their buoyancy in the stomach and hence their retention for reasonable lengths of time. So, in the words of Timmermans and Moës,[14] how well do floating systems float? It seems that the bulk density is not the most appropriate measure of flotation, but apparent density is.[15] The apparent density is a function of the porosity of the system: the greater the porosity, the lower the apparent density.

13.7 Evaluation of aerosols

Analysis of the particle size distribution of aerosol formulations during formulation, development and clinical trial or after storage is of obvious clinical relevance (see section 10.7). Aerosols are not easy to size, primarily because in use they are dynamic and inherently unstable systems, as propellants and drug solvents evaporate.

The most widely used instrument in categorising airborne particles is the cascade impactor. It attempts to mimic the obstructions and changes of direction that aerosols experience in the body, albeit in a crude way. Large particles leave the airstream and impinge on baffles or on glass microscope slides. The airstream is then accelerated at a nozzle, providing a second range of smaller sized particles on the next baffle and so on (Fig. 13.15). Progressively finer particles are collected at the successive stages of impingement owing to jet velocity and decreasing jet dimension. For more routine examination of medicinal aerosols, 'artificial throat' devices are useful. With these, comparative studies of the behaviour of aerosols can be carried out. In such devices the particles are segregated according to size. Analysis of the collecting layers at the several levels of the device allows the monitoring of changes in released particle size. In devices with an artificial mouth, this can be washed to reveal the extent of fall-out of large particles. The smallest particles of all reach the collecting solvent.

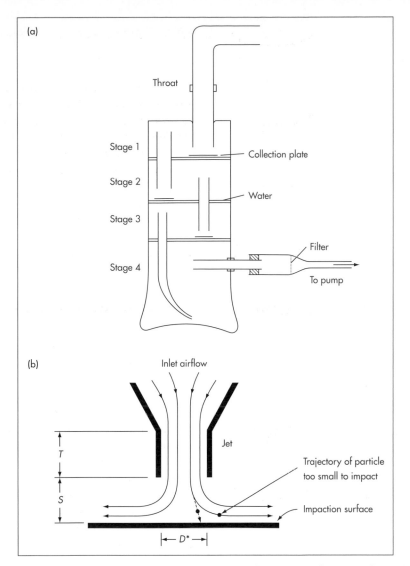

Figure 13.15 (a) The multistage liquid impinger. (b) The principal features affecting the performance of inertial impactors: air flow, the dimensions S and T, the diameter of the jet, D^*, the density, ρ, and the diameter of the particles, d. The trajectory of particles that are too small to deposit is shown.

Reproduced from Hallworth GW, in: Ganderton D, Jones T, eds, *Drug Delivery to the Respiratory Tract*, Chichester: Ellis Horwood; 1987. (a) Reproduced from G. W. Hallworth GW, *Br J Clin Pharm*, 1977; 4: 689.

Because of the need for standardisation of test equipment, the British Pharmacopoeia and other compendia have adopted detailed specifications for impinger devices. Two impinger devices have been adopted by the British Pharmacopoeia. Apparatus 'A' is shown in Fig. 13.16. All these operate by dividing the dose emitted from an inhaler into the respirable and nonrespirable fractions. The device in Fig. 13.16 employs the principle of liquid impingement

and has a solvent in both chambers to collect the aerosol. Air is drawn through the system at $60\,\text{dm}^3$ min^{-1} and the inhaler is fired several times into the device. There are several impaction surfaces at the back of the glass throat about 10 cm away from the activator (similar to human dimensions). The upper impinger has a cut off at a particle size of around 6.4 µm, with the first impact surface known as stage 1 and the last impact surface being in the

Figure 13.16 Impinger apparatus A, showing dimensions (mm) in order to ensure indenticality between equipment used in quality control.

Source: *British Pharmacopoeia*: HMSO.

Figure 13.17 An *in vitro* technique for evaluating inhaled nasal delivery systems in which particles/microspheres are deposited on a cell monolayer. Drug that is absorbed through the monolayer can be measured in the basolateral chamber.

Reproduced from Forbes B *et al.*, *STP Pharma Sci*, 2002; 12: 75–79.

lower impinger (stage 2), which is considered to be the respirable fraction.

Apparatus B (not illustrated) is made of metal and can be engineered to finer tolerances than the glass apparatus A; it is considered to be a superior apparatus for quality control testing and product release.

Typical of the result achieved with Apparatus B are those for two formulations, 1 and 5. Product 1 delivers 1 mg and Product 5 delivers 5 mg per shot. *In vitro*, the respirable fraction was found to be 25% and 20% respectively, while estimates of the percentage of the dose reaching the lung were 12.0% and 8.8% respectively. Some equipment, such as multistage impingers for aerosols, can be predictive of *in vivo* behaviour, or can at least give an assurance of consistency of effect.

An interesting test system for evaluating inhaled nasal delivery systems (Fig. 13.17) combines a physical device with cells in culture so that the interaction of microparticles with living cells can be studied directly. As new delivery systems appear, new tests will be required – as will ingenuity.

Key points

- A selection of tests can be conducted to measure the key parameters of a variety of formulations.
- Tests are not necessarily predictive of performance *in vivo*, but can be used to ensure batch-to-batch consistency.
- When good *in vitro–in vivo* correlations have been established, laboratory-based

tests can be predictive of clinical performance.

- Tests can be applied to rectal and transdermal products by adapting methods used for oral products, altering the receptor phase to mimic the medium in that the formulation will experience *in vivo*.
- Key parameters are different for different routes of delivery and different formulations: particle size is a key factor in inhalation products and in topical preparations where the drug is dispersed rather than dissolved in the vehicle.
- Adhesivity of oral dosage forms may be a factor in determining their efficacy (as in buccal treatments and delivery) or in causing adverse events (as in oesophageal injury); adhesion of transdermal patches to the skin is clearly important.
- The rheological properties of topical preparations and formulations for nasal administration are important, and a key factor is the syringeability of injectables.

Summary

No laboratory test can mimic the complexity of the biological environment and the dynamic factors involved in drug absorption in patients, but well-designed laboratory experiments can elucidate whether different formulations are comparable in terms of their key features. At best, *in vitro* tests are predictors of quality of performance in the patient; at the least they can ensure consistency of response. For example, where assays of drug content in generic products may give identical results, release studies may show differences due to drug–excipient and other interactions that may be of significance. We should always be on the look-out for novel ways of assessing dosage forms before they are used in the clinic. Sometimes simple tests can reveal much. Complex equipment is not always required.

References

1. Hanson R, V. Gray V. *Handbook of Dissolution Testing*, 3rd edn. Hokessin, DE: DissolutionTechnologies; 2004.
2. Mattock GL, McGilveray IJ. Comparison of bioavailabilities and dissolution characteristics of commercial tablet formulations of sulfamethizole. *J Pharm Sci* 1972;61:746–749.
3. Pedersen BI *et al.* A comparison of solubility of danazol in human and simulated gastro-intestinal fluids. *Pharm Res* 2000;17:891–894.
4. Ritschel WA, Banarer M. Correlation between *in vitro* release of proxyphylline from suppositories and *in vivo* data obtained from cumulative urinary excretion studies. *Arzneim Forsch* 1973;23:1031–1035.
5. Taylor JB, Simpkins DE. Aminophylline suppositories: *in vitro* dissolution and bioavailability in man. *Pharm J* 1981;227:601–603.
6. Ostrenga JA *et al.* Vehicle design for a topical steroid, fluocinolide. *J Invest Dermatol* 1971;56:392–399.
7. Yoshida H *et al. In vitro* release of Tacrolimus from Tacrolimus ointment and its speculated mechanism. *Int J Pharm* 2004;270:55–64.
8. Corbo M *et al.* Development and validation of *in vitro* release testing methods for semi-solid formulations. *Pharm Tech Int* 1993;17(9):112–118.
9. Wolff M *et al. In vitro* and *in vivo*-release of nitroglycerin from a new transdermal therapeutic system. *Pharm Res* 1985;1:23–29.
10. Marvola M *et al.* Development of a method for study of the tendency of drug products to adhere to the esophagus. *J Pharm Sci* 1982;71:975–877.
11. Al-Dujaili H *et al. In vitro* assessment of the adhesiveness of film-coated tablets. *Int J Pharm* 1986;34:67–74.
12. Marvola M *et al.* Effect of dosage form and formulation factors on the adherence of drugs to the esophagus. *J Pharm Sci* 1983;72:1034–1036.
13. Al-Dujaili H *et al.* The adhesiveness of proprietary tablets and capsules to porcine oesophageal tissue. *Int J Pharm* 1986;34:75–79.
14. Timmermans J, Moës AJ. How well do floating dosage forms float? *Int J Pharm* 1990;62:201–216.
15. Sauzet C *et al.* An innovative floating gastro-retentive dosage system: formulation and *in vitro* evaluation. *Int J Pharm* 2009;378:23–29.

Index